W0082600

Advances in Endovascular Management
of Abdominal Aortic Aneurysms

Advances in Endovascular Management
of Abdominal Aortic Aneurysms

Series Editor
DIMITRIOS K. FILIPPOU, MD, PhD
General Surgeon, Visiting Professor of Anatomy Athens, Greece

Chief Editors
THEODOSSIOS P. PERDIKIDES, MD
Director of Vascular Surgery Department, Hellenic AirForce Hospital, Athens, Greece

WOLF J. STELTER, MD
Professor of Surgery Chirurgische Klinik, Stadtische Kliniken Frankfurt a.M.-Hochst, Germany

FRANK J. VEITH, MD
Division of Vascular Surgery, The Cleveland Clinic and New York University Medical Center. Cleveland, Ohio, New York, NY

GEOFFREY H. WHITE, MD, FRACS
Department of Surgery, University of Sydney and Department of Vascular Surgery, Royal Prince Alfred Hospital, Sydney, Australia

Associate Editors
EFTHIMIOS D. AVGERINOS, MD
DIMITRIOS K. FILIPPOU, MD, PhD

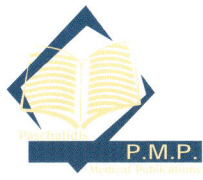

PMP (Paschalidis Medical Publications, Ltd.).
14th, Tetrapoleos str., Athens, 115 27, Greece
Tel.: 003-210-7789125, 003-210-7793012, Fax: 0030-210-7759421,
e-mail:
orders: paschalidis@medical-books.gr
© information: gp@medical-books.gr, cp@medical-books.gr

ADVANCES IN ENDOVASCULAR MANAGMENT OF ABDOMINAL AORTIC ANEURYSMS

Dedications

*To my wife Argyro and
to my children Theodora and Konstantinos*

Dimitrios K. Filippou
Series Editor

*This textbook is dedicated to the Hellenic AirForce, in grateful recognition
of the foresight displayed, as well as the generous educative material and
high-end equipment supplied, to the Vascular Surgery and Interventional
Radiology Departments, which have tremendously improved the quality of
care for patients with Aortic Aneurysms.*

*Last but far from least, I wish to express my gratitude to my family,
Christine my wife, Cecilia my daughter and Angelo my son, for their
continuous tolerance and support.*

Theodossios P. Perdikides
Chief Editor

Albertini Jan Nöel, MD
Vascular Surgery Department. Hopital Robert Debre. Reims. France
E-mail: jnalbertini@chu-reims.fr

Avgerinos D. Efthimios, MD
Resident in Vascular Surgery
Vascular Surgery Department, Athens University Medical School, Athens, Greece
E-mail: eavgerinos@prontomail.com

Baas F. AnNette, MD
Julius Center for Health Sciences and Primary Care, University Medical Center Utrecht,
The Netherlands
E-mail: A.F.Baas@umcutrecht.nl

Baxter Keith, MD, FRCSC
Department of Vascular Surgery, Royal Prince Alfred Hospital, University of Sydney, Australia

Bessias Nikos, MD
Vascular Surgeon
Vascular Surgery Department, Red Cross Hospital, Athens, Greece
E-mail: bessias@hol.gr

Blankensteijn D. Jan, MD
Department of Vascular Surgery, Radboud University Nijmegen Medical Center,
The Netherlands
E-mail: j.blankensteijn@chir.umcn.nl

Busch Kathryn DipApplSc (MedRad), DMU (Vasc), AMS
Camperdown Vascular Laboratory, Sydney, NSW, Australia

Buskens Eric, MD
Julius Center for Health Sciences and Primary Care, University Medical Center Utrecht, The Netherlands

Cairols A. Marc
Service of Vascular Surgery, Bellvitge University Hospital, L'Hospitalet de Llobregat, Barcelona, Spain
E-mail: mcairols@csub.scs.es

Can Aysel, MD
Department of Vascular Surgery, St.Franziskus Hospital Muenster, Germany
E-mail: aysel.can@sfh-muenster.de

Cao Piergiorgio, MD, FRCS
Professor of Vascular Surgery
Division of Vascular and Endovascular Surgery, University of Perugia, Ospedale S. Maria della Misericordia, Perugia, Italy
E-mail: pcao@unipg.it

Capdevilla C. MD.
Vascular Surgery Department. Hopital Robert Debre. Reims. France

Chronopoulos Anastasios, MD
Vascular Surgeon
Vascular & Endovascular Surgery Department, Henry Dunant Hospital, Athens, Greece
E-mail: anachronopoulos@hol.gr

Chuter A. Timothy, MD
Professor of Surgery
Division of Vascular Surgery, University of California San Francisco, USA
E-mail: chutert@surgery.ucsf.edu

Clement Claude, MD
Vascular Surgery Department. Hopital Robert Debre. Reims. France

Deaton H. David, MD
Chief, Endovascular Surgery, Associate Professor, Vascular Surgery, Georgetown University Hospital, Washington DC, USA
E-mail: david@deaton.md

Dias V. Nuno, MD, PhD
Endovascular Unit, Vascular Center
Malmö-Lund, Malmö University
Hospital, Malmö, Sweden
Email: nunovdias@hotmail.com

Diehm Nicolas, MD
Baptist Cardiac and Vascular Institute,
Department of Interventional Radiology,
Miami, Florida
Swiss Cardiovascular Center, Division of
Clinical and Interventional Angiology,
Inselspital, University of Bern,
Switzerland
E-mail: nicolas.diehm@insel.ch

Dowdall Joseph, MD
Department of Vascular Surgery, Cleveland
Clinic, Cleveland, Ohio, USA
E-mail: dowdallj@gmail.com

Erz Kerstin, MD
General and Vascular Surgery Dpt
Chirurgische Klinik, Stadtische Kliniken
Frankfurt a.M.-Hochst, Germany
E-mail: k.erz@gmk.de

Filippou K. Dimitrios, MD, PhD
General Surgeon
Visiting Professor of Anatomy
Athens, Greece
E-mail: d_filippou@hotmail.com

Fotis Theofanis, RN, MSc
Department of Vascular Surgery, Hellenic
AirForce Hospital, Athens, Greece
E-mail: thfotis@nurs.uoa.gr

Gargiulo J. Nicholas III, MD
Division of Vascular Surgery,
Montefiore Medical Center
New York, NY
E-mail: ngargiul@montefiore.org

Georgiadis S. George, MD
Lecturer in Vascular Surgery
Department of Vascular Surgery,
"Demokritos" University Hospital,
Alexandroupolis, Greece
E-mail: ggeorgia@med.duth.gr

**Giachetta-Ryan Denise, MPA, RN,
CNOR**
Kingsborough Community College,
Brooklyn, New York, NY
E-mail: Giaryan@aol.com

Giannopoulou Pinelopi, MDD, MSc
Director in a privet clinic
E-mail: kplagios@yahoo.com

Goodman Marcel, MD
Vascular Surgeon. Department of Vascular
Surgery, Mount and St. John of God
Hospitals, Perth, Western Australia,
Australia
E-mail: mgoo1609@bigpond.net.au

Goutzios Panayiotis, MD
Department of Interventional Radiology,
Hellenic AirForce Hospital, Athens, Greece.
E-mail: pgoutzios@yahoo.gr

Greenberg K. Roy, MD
Director, Endovascular Research,
Cleveland Clinic Health Systems
Department of Vascular Surgery, Cleveland
Clinic, Cleveland, Ohio, USA
E-mail: greenbr@ccf.org

Hackett Robert, MBChB FANZCA
VMO Anaesthetist Royal Prince Alfred
Hospital
Clinical Tutor University of Sydney and
University of New South Wales
E-mail: r_hackett74@yahoo.com.au

Halandras Pegge, MD
Assistant Professor of Surgery
Division of Vascular Surgery, Emory
University School of Medicine,
Atlanta, GA, USA
E-mail: pegge.halandras@emoryhealth-
care.org

**Harris P. John, MS, FRACS, FRCS,
FACS, DDU**
Department of Vascular Surgery,
Royal Prince Alfred Hospital,
University of Sydney,

New South Wales, Australia
E-mail: j_harris@med.usyd.edu.au

Hartley David, FRANZCR (Hon.)
Director Cook R&DWA
  Perth Australia
E-mail: dhartley@cookaust.com.au

Hinchliffe J. Robert
St George's Vascular Institute St George's
  Hospital London, U.K.
E-mail: rhinchli@sgul.ac.uk

Hopkinson R. Brian, MD
Vascular Surgery Department. Queen's
  Medical Centre. Nottingham
  United Kingdom
E-mail: Brian.Hopkinson@nottingham. ac.uk

Huilgol Ravi, MB BS FRACS
Fellow in Vascular Surgery, Royal
  Prince Alfred Hospital, University
  of Sydney, Australia
E-mail: ravi.huilgol@svhm.org.au

Ivancev Krassi, MD
Endovascular Unit, Vascular Center
  Malmö-Lund, Malmö University
  Hospital, Malmö, Sweden
E-mail: Krassi.Ivancev@med.lu.se

Javerliat Isabelle, MD
Vascular Surgery Department, Hopital
  Robert Debre, Reims, France

Kaperonis A. Elias, MD
Vascular Surgeon
Vascular Surgery Department, Athens
  University Medical School,
  Athens, Greece

Katzen T. Barry, MD
Baptist Cardiac and Vascular Institute
Department of Interventional Radiology,
  Miami, Florida, USA
E-mail: barryk@baptisthealth.net

Kiskinis Dimitrios, MD
Professor of Vascular Surgery.
1st Department of Surgery, Aristotle

University of Thessaloniki, Papageorgiou
  Hospital, Thessaloniki, Greece
E-mail: kiskinis@med.auth.gr

**Konstantinou Evangelos, RN,
  MSc, PhD**
Assistant Professor of Nurse
  Anesthesiology,
Surgical Nursing Department,
  Athens University Nursing School,
  Athens, Greece
E-mail: ekonstan30@yahoo.com

Lagios Konstantinos, MD
Interventional Radiologist. Director of
  Interventional Radiology Department,
  Hellenic AirForce Hospital,
  Athens, Greece
E-mail: kplagios@tellas.gr

Lazarides K. Miltos, MD
Professor of Vascular Surgery
Department of Vascular Surgery, Demokritos
  University Hospital, Thrace, Greece
E-mail: mlazarid@med.duth.gr

Lee W. Anthony, MD
Associate Professor of Surgery
Division of Vascular Surgery and
  Endovascular Therapy
  University of Florida
E-mail: anthony.lee@surgery.ufl.edu

Liapis D. Christos, MD, FACS, FRCS
Professor of Vascular Surgery
Vascular Surgery Department, Athens
  University Medical School, Athens,
  Greece
E-mail: liapis@med.uoa.gr

Macierewicz Jan, MD
Vascular Surgery Department. Northern
  General Hospital. Sheffield. United
  Kingdom

Malina Martin MD, PhD
Chief, Vascular Center Malmö-Lund,
  Malmö-University Hospital, Malmö,
  Sweden.
E-mail: MalinaMD@Gmail.com

Matsarides Dimitrios, MD
Interventional Radiology Department,
 Hellenic AirForce Hospital, Athens,
 Greece.
E-mail: dkmatsar@yahoo.co.uk

**May James, MD, MS, FRACS,
 FACS**
Department of Surgery, University
 of Sydney
E-mail: vascsurg@med.usyd.edu.au

**McCulloch Timothy, MBBS, BSc (Med),
 FANZCA**
Senior Staff Specialist, Royal Prince
 Alfred Hospital. Clinical Lecturer
 University of Sydney

Mehta Manish, MD
Associate Professor of Surgery,
 Albany Medical College/
 Albany Medical Center Hospital,
 Director of Endovascular
 Services, The Vascular Group, PLLC/
 The Institute for Vascular
 Health and Disease, Albany, NY
E-mail: mehtam@albanyvascular.com

Melas Nikolaos, MD
Resident in Vascular Surgery
1st Department of Surgery, Aristotle
 University of Thessaloniki,
 Papageorgiou General Hospital,
 Thessaloniki, Greece
E-mail: melasnikos2000@yahoo.gr

Milner Ross, MD
Assistant Professor of Surgery
 Division of Vascular Surgery,
 Emory University School of Medicine,
 Atlanta, GA, USA
E-mail: ross.milner@emoryhealthcare.org

Muhs E. Bart, MD, PhD
Assistant Professor of Vascular
 Surgery and Radiology Co-Director,
 Endovascular Program, Yale
 Univercity, School of Medicine,
 New Haven, CT.
E-mail: bart.muhs@yale.edu

Ohrlander Tomas, MD
Vascular Center Malmö-Lund, Malmö
 University Hospital, Malmö, Sweden
E-mail: tomas.ohrlander@gmail.com

Orend Karl - Heinz, Prof. Dr. Med.
Assistant medical director,
 Chirurgische Universitaetsklinik
 und Poliklinik fuer Thorax und
 Gefaesschirurgie, Ulm,
 Germany.
E-mail: Karl-Heinz.Orend@uniklinik-ulm.de

Parlani Gianbattista, MD
Division of Vascular and Endovascular
 Surgery, University of Perugia,
 Ospedale S. Maria della Misericordia,
 Perugia, Italy

Parodi C Juan, MD
University of Miami
E-mail: JParodi@med.miami.edu

Perdikides P. Theodossios, MD
Vascular Surgeon.
Director of Vascular Surgery
 Department, Hellenic AirForce Hospital,
 Athens, Greece
E-mail: perd@otenet.gr

Prinssen Monique, MD
Division of Vascular Surgery,
 Department of Surgery, University
 Medical Center Utrecht, The Netherlands

Qingsheng Lu, MD
Department of Vascular Surgery,
 Cleveland Clinic, Cleveland,
 Ohio, USA

Quaranta Federico, MD
Istituto Universitario di Scienze Motorie,
 Roma, Italy

Reid B Donald MD, FRCS
Consultant Vascular & Endovascular
 Surgeon, Vascular & Endovascular
 Institute, Wishaw Hospital,
 Scotland, UK
E-mail: dreid@doctors.org.uk

Romano Lydia, MD

Division of Vascular and Endovascular
   Surgery, University of Perugia,
   Ospedale S. Maria della Misericordia,
   Perugia, Italy

Ruppert Volker, MD

Department of Vascular Surgery,
   Staedtische Kliniken Ingolstadt, Germany
E-mail: volker.ruppert@klinikum-
   ingolstadt.de

Saratzis Athanasios, MD

First Department of Surgery, Aristotle
   University of Thessaloniki, Papageorgiou
   General Hospital, Thessaloniki, Greece
E-mail: a_saratzis@hotmail.com

Saratzis Nikolaos, MD

Assistant Professor of Vascular Surgery
1st Department of Surgery, Aristotle
   University of Thessaloniki,
   Papageorgiou General Hospital,
   Thessaloniki, Greece
E-mail: saratzis@germanosnet.gr

Schlösser J.V. Felix, MD

Section of Vascular Surgery, Yale
   University School of Medicine, New
   Haven, CT, USA and the Department of
   Vascular Surgery, Erasmus Medical
   Center, Rotterdam, and University
   Medical Center Utrecht, The Netherlands

Semmens B. James, MD

Professor of Population Health Research
   School of Public Health, Curtin
   University of Technology, Bentley,
   Western Australia, Australia
E-mail:James.Semmens@curtin.edu.au

Shina Evangelia

Interventional Radiology Department,
   Hellenic AirForce Hospital, Athens Greece

Sonneson Björn, MD, PhD

Vascular Center Malmo-Lund, Malmo
   Univercity Hospital,
   Malmo, Sweden
E-mail: b.sonesson@gmail.com

Soong V. Chee, MD

Vascular Surgery Department. City
   Hospital. Belfast. United Kingdom

Stelter J. Wolf, MD, PhD

Professor of Surgery
Chirurgische Klinik, Stadtische Kliniken
   Frankfurt a.M.-Hochst, Germany
E-mail: stelter@surgery-franfurt.de

Subramanian Murali FRCS

Vascular & Endovascular Institute,
   Wishaw Hospital,
   Scotland, UK

Tessarek Joerg, MD

Department of Vascular Surgery,
   St. Franziskus Hospital Muenster,
   Germany
E-mail: joerg.tessarek@sfh-muenster.de

Torsello Giovanni, MD, PhD

Department of Vascular Surgery,
   St. Franziskus Hospital Muenster,
   Germany
E-mail: giovanni.torsello@sfh-muenster.de

Tsoukas I. Athanassios, MD

Baptist Cardiac and Vascular Institute,
   Department of Vascular Surgery,
   Miami, Florida, USA
E-mail: tsoukas@pol.net

Tzilalis D. Vasilios, MD, PhD

Department of Vascular Surgery,
   401 General Military Hospital,
   Athens, Greece
E-mail: vtzil@yahoo.gr

Umscheid Thomas, MD

Department of Vascular Surgery,
   St.Franziskus Hospital Muenster,
   Germany
E-mail: thomas.umscheid@sfh-muenster.de

Veith J. Frank, MD

Division of Vascular Surgery, The Cleveland
   Clinic and New York University Medical
   Center. Cleveland, Ohio, New York, NY
E-mail: FJVMD@msn.com

Verhagen J.M. Hence, MD, PhD
Department of Vascular Surgery,
   Erasmus University Medical Center,
   Rotterdam, and University
   Medical Center Utrecht,
   The Netherlands
E-mail: h.verhagen@erasmusmc.nl

Verzini Fabio, MD
Division of Vascular and Endovascular
   Surgery, University of Perugia,
   Ospedale S. Maria della Misericordia,
   Perugia, Italy
E-mail: fverzini@unipg.it

White H. Geoffrey, FRACS
Department of Surgery, University
   of Sydney and Department
   of Vascular Surgery, Royal
   Prince Alfred Hospital,
   Sydney, Australia
E-mail: ghwhite@mail.usyd.edu.au

Yezerski D. Sol, MBBS FANZCA
Director, Vascular Anaesthesia,
   Royal Prince Alfred Hospital,
   Sydney, NSW Australia
E-mail: yezerski@bigpond.net.au

Zarmpis Nikolaos, MD, PhD
Clinic of Thoracic and Vascular Surgery,
   University Ulm, Ulm, Germany
E-mail: nikolaosiz@gmail.com

Yu Weiyun MB, BS
Department of Vascular Surgery, Royal
   Prince Alfred Hospital, University of
   Sydney, Australia

Ziegler Peter, MD, PhD
Consultant Surgeon and Vascular Surgeon
Chirurgische Klinik, Stadtische Kliniken
   Frankfurt a.M.-Hochst,
   Germany
E-mail: Peter.Ziegler@skfh.de

It is for me a pleasure to write a prologue for the book entitled:

"Advances in Endovascular Management of Abdominal Aortic Aneurysms"
by Theodossios Perdikides, Wolf Stelter, Frank Veith and Geoffrey White

What was a fantasy more than three decades ago came into reality as one of the most revolutionary procedures seen in vascular surgery. Endografts did not come as a continuation of stents, endografts were conceived when stents were not yet in use. The idea of lining the aorta was created in 1976 and it took decades to enter the clinical arena. Nobody could initially understand how a hostile environment like the aorta could stand having a foreign body composed of wires and fabric inside the lumen without producing damage to the wall, breaking off or migrating. The initial times were not easy but today we count with level 1 evidence that endografts placed in patients harboring aneurysms with suitable anatomy for EVAR are better than surgery, advantages continue after at least four years in terms of aneurysm related deaths.

Many physicians contributed to allow the method to achieve a high level of perfection. Today we are all proud of the development and eager to continue to improve the method. Many of the pioneers and leaders in the field are writing chapters in this book. Readers will find in this book the last updates of this still evolving field

For many of us reality is still hard to believe and when we see patients effectively treated under local anesthesia using a percutaneous approach and going home in 12 hrs with his or her aneurysm excluded we cannot prevent a smile to come to our lips.

Branched or fenestrated endografts, endosutures, local or systemic administration of drugs or cell seeding are part of the future for this technology that will bring it to unimaginable levels.

Physicians are helping patients better and preventing unnecessary suffering.

Juan C. Parodi MD,
University of Miami

Since 1991, when Dr Parodi introduced endovascular aneurysm repair, this treatment modality has undergone an explosive evolution. Vascular surgeons and interventionalists fueled by the minimally invasive concept and the increasing public demand for such procedures have embraced modern endovascular technology and brought it to a current state of widespread acceptance. Today endovascular abdominal aortic aneurysm repair (EVAR) has reached its maturity. Experience and knowledge on EVAR technology and device behavior have expanded and an even broader range of patients with more complicated anatomies are targeted.

This book presents in its state of the art chapters the compiled knowledge of pioneers and experts in the field of endovascular aortic aneurysm repair. Preoperative planning, perioperative considerations, optimal endograft fixation, management of challenging anatomy and EVAR complications, emergencies, clinical trials and contemporary training perspectives are all discussed in a comprehensive manner together with the direction of currently evolving advances. Such a volume can serve as an excellent resource not only for residents but also for practicing vascular surgeons and interventional specialists who wish to expand their skills to *advanced techniques for endovascular aneurysm repair* such as fenestrated or branched endografting.

We would like to thank all the contributors to this book for their excellent efforts in the preparation of the chapters. It has been our privilege to put all these chapters together in this volume which provides a comprehensive overview of the field of endovascular abdominal aortic aneurysm repair as of 2008.

The Editors

Dear friends, we have the pleasure to present you the second book of the series under the general title "Advances" focused on important and interesting subjects in the field of surgery. The first edition entitled Advances in Obstructive Jaundice Diagnosis and Treatment is already available via Elsevier in almost every part of the world. The first book referred the currents concepts and advances in a field familiar to general surgeons, hepatologists, radiologists and gastroenterologists.

The present book presents in detail a subject that is familiar mainly to interventional radiologists and vascular surgeons. Interventional vascular radiology with minimally invasive approaches is considered a revolution in the treatment of various vascular diseases and entities. The most impressive application of these minimally invasive approaches is on the treatment of the abdominal aortic aneurysms. In the past these operations were difficult to perform and presented significant morbidity and even mortality. All these things changed significantly after the development of various techniques for the Endovascular Management of Abdominal Aortic Aneurysms. The present books analyses on detail the advances in the filed of Endovascular Management of Abdominal Aortic Aneurysms.

We have the pleasure and the honor to have as Editors in Chief of the present edition well known experts in the endovascular surgery who were among the pioneers who invented and developed this therapeutic alternative. I would like as Series Editor to thank first of all Dr. Theodossios Perdikides, who had the responsibility to collaborate with excellent scientists from all over the world and outlined the contents in order to represent the real advances in endovascular aortic aneurysms treatment. The contribution of the experts Dr. Frank Veith from USA, Dr. Wolf Stelter from Germany, and Geoffrey White from Australia was essential and we would also like to thank them from heart. The Editors as well as all the other authors worked hard on this edition preparing a really modern, informed and detailed book that should read from anybody that is interested on this subject.

I would also like to thank the Publishers fro their help and their stuff for the excellent work. Our purpose is to present to medical community a complete and useful modality and reference guide in the field of the Endovascular Management of Abdominal Aortic Aneurysms. I think that you will find our work interesting and educational.

Finally I would like to remind to announce that the following editions of the series entitled: Advances in Hydatid Disease Diagnosis and Treatment and Advances in Obesity (Part 1), will be available within the next months.

Athens, October 15th 2008
Dimitrios K. Filippou, MD, PhD
Series Editor

Contents

Contents

Section 2: Contemporary application of double tube graft techniques
Thomas Umscheid, Joerg Tessarek, Volker Ruppert, Wolf Stelter, Giovanni Torsello

Preoperative assessment and postoperative follow-up of EVAR using TeraRecon, M2S, and 3Surgery

Anthony W. Lee, Hence J.M. Verhagen

INTRODUCTION

Accurate preoperative assessment of the aortoiliac system is critical to the early and late success of endovascular aortic repair (EVAR). The proper selection of devices and the actual execution of the procedure are dependent on this stage of the overall treatment plan. It can be said that 90% of the "battle" is won or lost before stepping into the operating theater using plans and devices based on proper preoperative imaging.

While cross-sectional volumetric data may be acquired using either CT (computed tomography) or MR (magnetic resonance) imaging, the gold standard modality remains CT angiography (CTA).[1,2] Today, there is almost no role for conventional angiography in the preoperative assessment for EVAR.[3] CTA is performed using a timed-bolus intravenous contrast enhanced technique and is extremely accurate and fast, especially with currently available 32- and 64-slice multirow detectors. Oral contrast should not be used. The scan should typically be performed at a maximum of 2 mm slice thickness to enable sufficient z-axis resolution during the image recon-

struction. A consequence of this type of imaging technique is that the resultant datasets are enormous and becomes almost impractical to view and adequately extract all the available information using conventional printed film, so that they are ideally viewed electronically using a dedicated DICOM (Digital Imaging and Communications in Medicine) software.

Three-dimensional (3D) reconstructions of these datasets enable a variety of morphologic assessment tools that are not possible using conventional axial imaging.[4] There are several commercially available systems that can process DICOM datasets and produce different types of 3D renderings. Some are specific to the actual image acquisition hardware (i.e. the actual CT scanner) and come standard with the equipment and others are stand-alone systems that have been validated for medical diagnostic application and can be purchased for individual use. Three such systems, the TeraRecon Aquarius Workstation (San Mateo, California), the M2S Medical Metrx System (West Lebanon, New Hampshire), and 3Surgery Vascular Imaging Workstation (3mensio Medical Imaging, Biltoven, The Netherlands) will be discussed in this chapter.[5] Although all have similar basic features, for more advanced post-processing, there are substantial differences which are reflected in the cost of the respective systems.

PREOPERATIVE ASSESSMENT

Preoperative assessment for EVAR involves dimensional and morphologic analysis. Dimensional analysis consists of diameter measurements of the infrarenal aortic neck and the iliac arteries and the lengths from the lowermost renal artery to the aortic bifurcation and to the origins of the right and left hypogastric arteries. These measurements will determine the device sizes which will be used for the repair. Morphologic analysis consists of qualitative and semi-quantitative assessments of angulation, tortuosity, calcifications, and intraluminal thrombus that will influence the conduct of the procedure in terms of which side to introduce the endograft main body, its orientation, the proximal and distal landing zones, and the potential problems which may lie ahead. These assessments are as critical, if not more so, than the actual selection of the device and can significantly impact the short-term seal and long-term durability of the repair.

For most experienced endovascular aortic therapists, these assessments do not occur in a serial manner but using tools such as the TeraRecon Workstation, the M2S or the 3Surgery Vascular Imaging Workstation, the elements of the dimensional and morphologic assessments occur in a parallel and recursive manner. More specifically, while one is in the process measuring diameters and lengths for a particular segment of the treatment zone, the tortuosity of iliac arteries may influence the distal extent of the iliac limb which in turn may require a shorter or longer device to be used. Conversely, an angulated and conical neck may require

the main body to be implanted lower or higher than anticipated and, therefore, change the reference diameter and the device selection.

AQUARIUS, M2S AND 3SURGERY WORKSTATIONS

The TeraRecon Aquarius Workstation is a stand alone system that runs on a Windows PC platform with proprietary hardware for dedicated 3D image processing. This combination allows real-time manipulation of the data and rapid rendering of images from one format to another. The system can import DICOM datasets from virtually any source and has a large storage capacity that can archive over 1000 individual datasets. The entire system costs approximately US$40,000-$60,000 depending on the desired software features.

The M2S is a centralized postprocessing service where the user submits a DICOM dataset electronically, and for a fixed fee per study (approximately US$ 300/ study), a 3D rendering of the aortoiliac vasculature is created with some ability for user manipulation of the image and quantitative analysis of the anatomy.

The 3surgery VI workstation is a stand alone workstation. The workstation can be configured on a laptop or on a standard deskstop computer. This is possible because of the technology that is being used for the 3D processing; GPU (Graphics Processing Unit) technology which in its turn is derived from the gaming industry. This technology allows rapid 3D rendering on standard PC's. Even on a laptop based workstation the system can import DICOM data from every modality. The imported data are stored in a database which can contain up to 1000 datasets. The costs of a 3surgery VI workstation are approximately $25,000, that depends whether it is a laptop or a desktop computer based workstation (Figures 1, 2, 3).

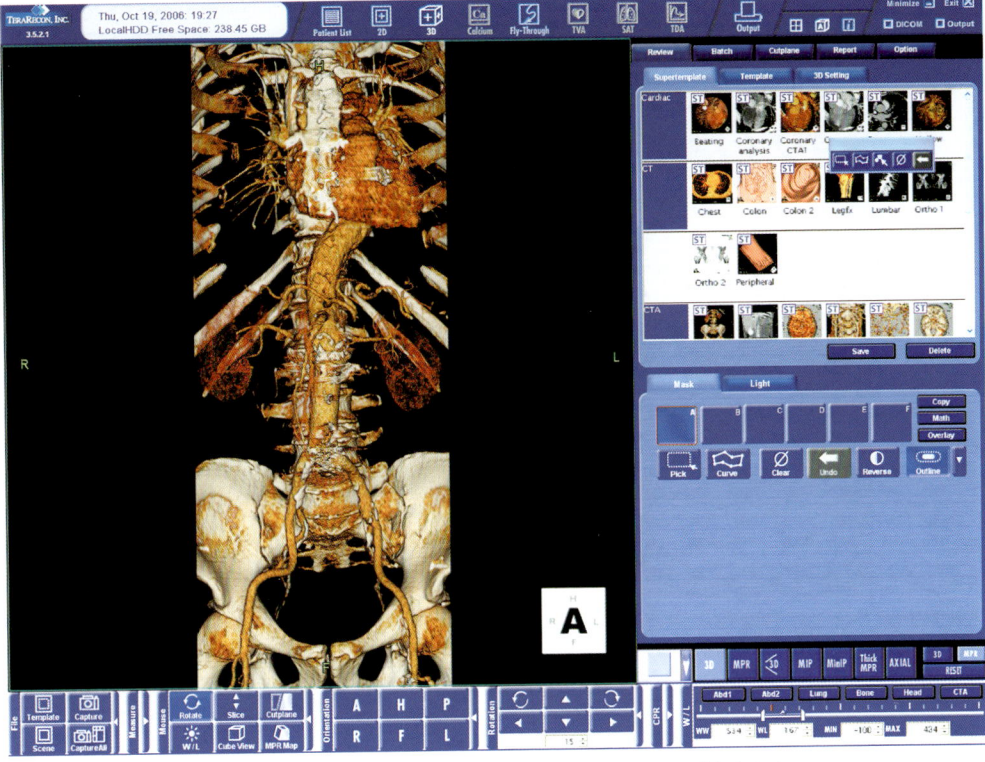

FIGURE 1: Initial user-interface of the TeraRecon Aquarius Workstation.

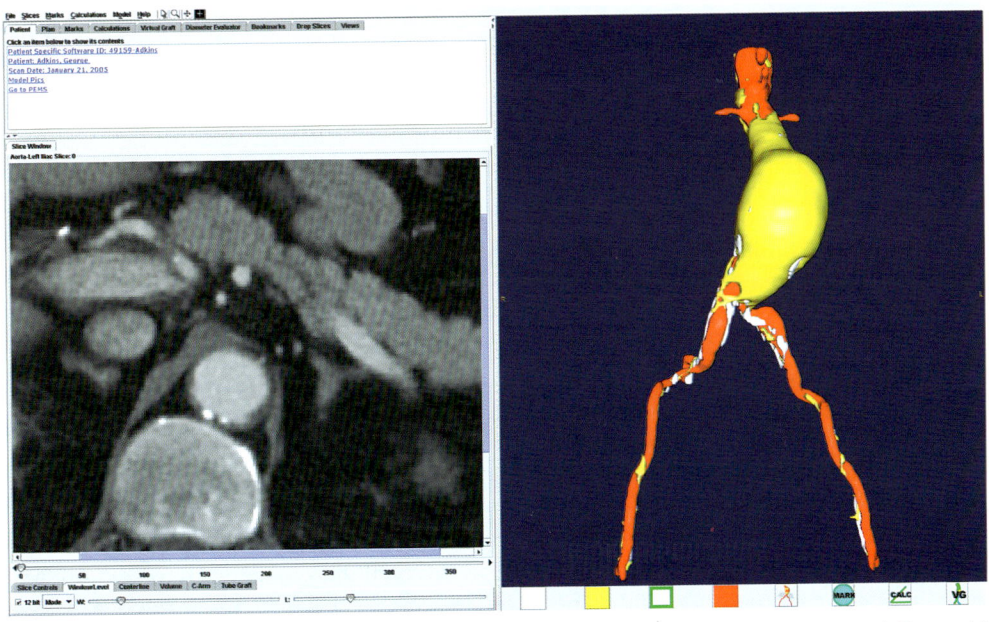

FIGURE 2: Initial user-interface of the M2S. Notice that the soft tissues and bone have been removed. The model is color-coded to show the flow lumen (*red*), thrombus (*yellow*), and calcifications (*white*).

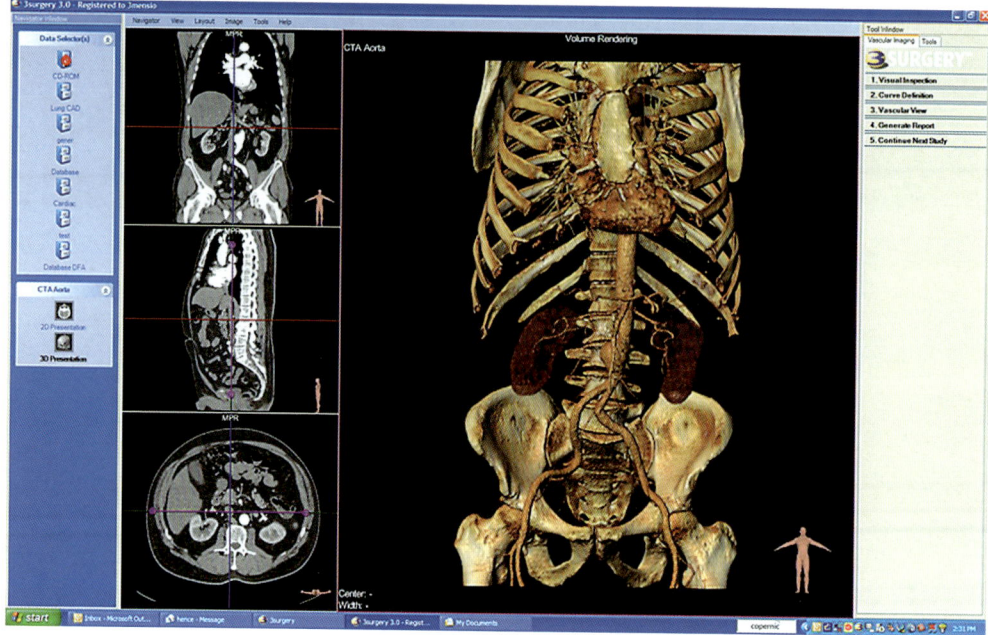

FIGURE 3: Initial user-interface of the 3surgery™ Vascular Imaging Workstation.

Preoperative assessment starts with segmentation of the anatomy of interest. Segmentation involves removing the soft and hard tissues around the arteries such that the user can visualize the aortoiliac anatomy unimpeded. The ability for the image to be properly segmented automatically with minimum operator intervention is dependent on the timing of the contrast bolus and selective opacification of the arterial system without significant venous contamination. In the TeraRecon system, the operator selects out a segment of the arterial vasculature that is to be segmented and using that as a nidus, the surrounding arterial tree is automatically "grown" automatically based on a threshold Hounsfield value (Figure 4). In the M2S system, the aortic vasculature is manually segmented out by a trained technician to generate the model (Figure 2). In the 3Surgery system, preoperative assessment starts with segmentation of the vessel concerned by removing the bones surround-

ing it. This will provide a visual inspection of the calcification of the vessel through MIP visualization. Furthermore, in 3D rendering, the segmented bones can be shown in 'Dimmed Background' mode, to create a significant contrast between the aorta and surrounding bones.

In all three systems, this color-surface shaded model can be spun in 3D space to qualitatively assess for tortuosity and angulations.

Due to the way each system generates this surface-shaded model, their respective anatomic representations are slightly different. For TeraRecon and 3Surgery, because the segmentation is largely automated, only those voxels that are highly attenuated, such as a contrast-filled lumen or calcifications are visualized. Those intravascular elements, such as thrombus, with low soft-tissue attenuation are not visualized. In order to see these features in the model, the low attenuation elements must be manually circumscribed by the

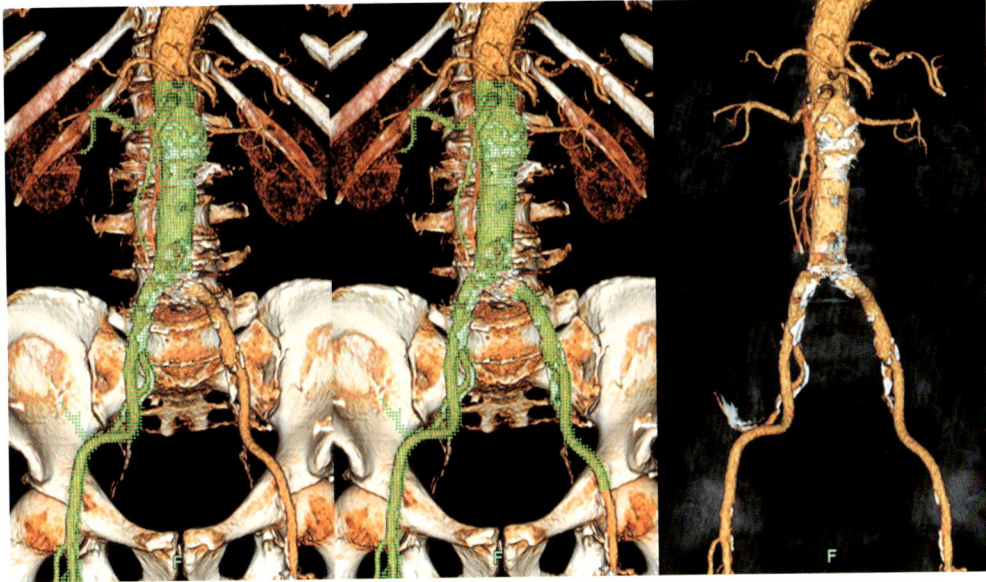

FIGURE 4: In TeraRecon, a point in the arterial vasculature is selected by the user and the surrounding arterial vasculature is progressively grown (*green*) until the entire region of interest is segmented out.

operator and "added" to the model as a separate mask. This is one of the advantages of the M2S system, where the three primary components, blood, thrombus, and calcifications, are all represented and color-coded for easy identification. Further, because these components are separately modeled internally, each component can be removed or made translucent within the overall model itself (Figure 5). In the TeraRecon and 3Surgery systems, the extravascular structures may be opacified to variable degrees ("landmarking") to allow the user to visualize the spatial rela-

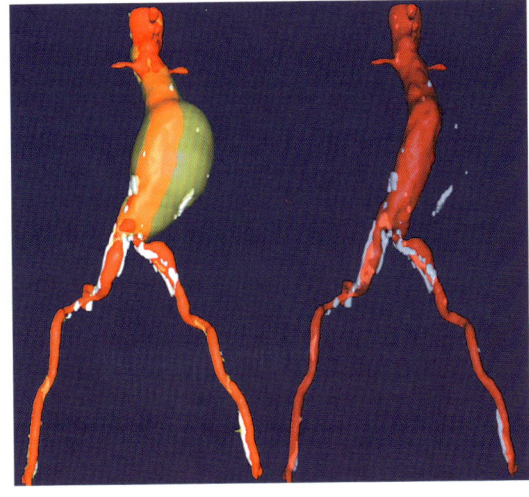

FIGURE 5: In M2S, the intravascular elements may be selectively made translucent or completely removed. The left image shows the thrombus partially transparent and the right image shows the thrombus completely removed with the flow lumen and the calcifications partially transparent.

tionships between one area of the aorta and the surrounding bone or soft tissue. This is useful during the EVAR procedure when key anatomic structures, such as the renal arteries, can be localized relative to their position along the bony spine (Figure 6, 7).

The next step in the preoperative assessment is to generate a centerline within the flow lumen. For endovascular abdominal aortic aneurysm repair, two centerlines are generated that extend to each iliac artery (Figure 8). One must keep in mind that this centerline does not necessarily represent the true lie of the endograft. Indeed, the problem of path length determination is a complex computational problem that is device dependent. In practice the centerline measurement is slightly longer than the actual graft path length due to the fact that in tortuous anatomies the endograft has a tendency to appose the inner curve. This must be taken into account during selection of device lengths. It is better to err slightly on a shorter device than longer as it is safer to extend a

limb than suffer inadvertent coverage of important branch vessels.

Based on this centerline, orthogonal multiplanar reformations (MPR) are created. These images give a truer representation of the aortic cross-section than axial images which can distort the luminal contour due its tangential cuts across an angulated aorta (Figure 9). When working with axial images, the short axis of the aorta is the closest approximation of the aortic diameter. Using orthogonal MPR a closer approximation of the aortic diameter can be obtained. Contrary to conventional belief, however, the aortic neck is not truly circular. There is an intrinsic eccentricity to the aortic lumen such that if one is implanting a circular device, the cross-sectional shape of the aorta should be modeled as an imperfect ellipse, and the average of the long and short axes of the lumen taken as the "reference diameter". Another confounding factor in diameter measurement is that the CT scan is acquiring the images at variable points in the cardiac cycle. Even with cardiac gat-

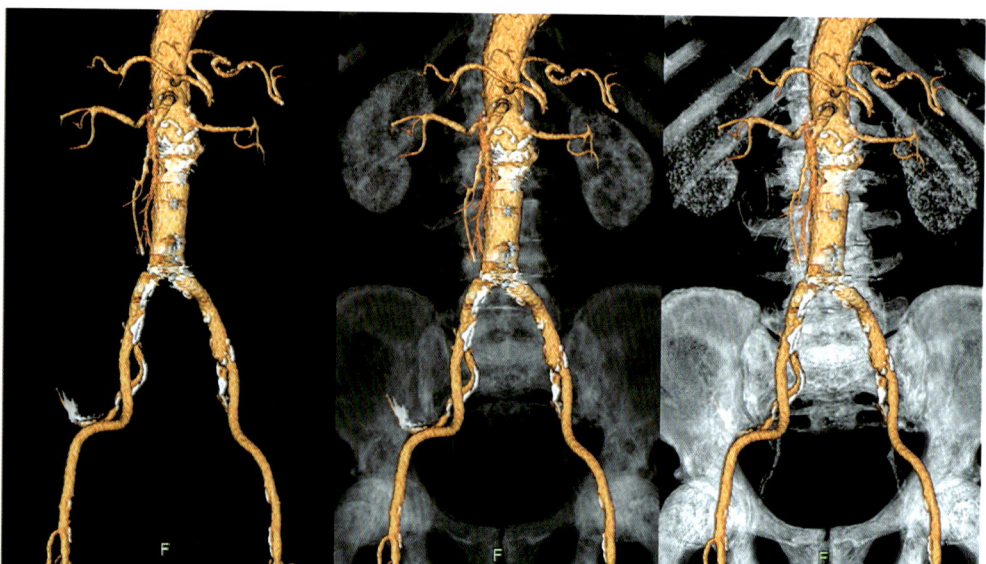

FIGURE 6: Landmarking in the TeraRecon workstation. Going from left to right, the bone and soft tissues are progressively opacified. The renal arteries are located at the level of the bottom half of the first lumbar vertebral body.

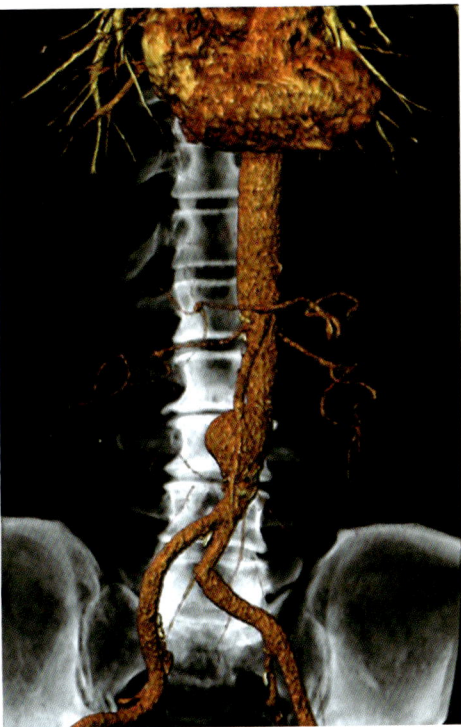

FIGURE 7: Landmarking in the 3Surgery Medical Imaging Workstation. The renal arteries are located between the first and second lumbar vertebral body.

ing, due to the variations in the transmission of the aortic pulse and its reflected waves, there can be 10-15% variability in the degree of aortic distension. Although for an individual patient the extent of this variability is unpredictable due to the loss of compliance that occurs with age, this occurs to a smaller extent in the abdominal aorta as compared to the thoracic aorta due to the decreased elastin content. Some devices require inner wall (intima)-to-inner wall (intima) measurement and others outer wall (adventitia)-to-outer wall (adventitia). In the former instance, the inner wall is the actual inner wall of the aorta-it does not mean the luminal wall of the aorta, which can be lined with thrombus.

Putting all of these concepts together, the anatomy can now be quantitatively as-sessed in preparation for endovascular repair. The steps are as follows:

1) The lowermost renal artery that will be preserved is identified. This represents the proximal extent of the aortic neck. While the clinical sequelae of covering accessory renal arteries are minimal, on occasion a large accessory renal artery may need to be preserved. Next, the top of the aneurysm is identified. This is the bottom of the proximal neck. In certain cases of a conical neck, the end of the neck and the beginning of the aneurysm may be poorly defined. In these and other cases where one is faced with a long but irregular anatomic neck, the 15-20 mm segment that will serve as the landing zone is the functional neck for endovascular repair. After identification of the aortic neck (or the landing zone), at least 2-3 diameter measurements are made. These measurements characterize the morphology of the neck, i.e. funnel, conical, barrel, or parallel in shape. From these set of measurements, a single reference diameter should be determined which will be used to select the appropriate endograft size.

2) The aortic bifurcation is identified and the centerline distance from the lowermost renal artery to the aortic bifurcation is measured. Within this segment, the maximum diameter of the AAA and the aortic bifurcation are measured. On occasion, especially in women, the aortic bifurcation is extremely narrowed due to calcific occlusive disease. In most instances, using "kissing" angioplasty techniques either before or after (preferred) endograft placement, the aortic bifurcation may be dilated to decrease the risk of limb thrombosis from extrinsic compression. However, there is a small risk of aortic rupture that can complicate the repair. In general, the long axis measurement of the aortic diameter should be at least 60% of the sum of the diameters of the two limbs of a bifurcated device.

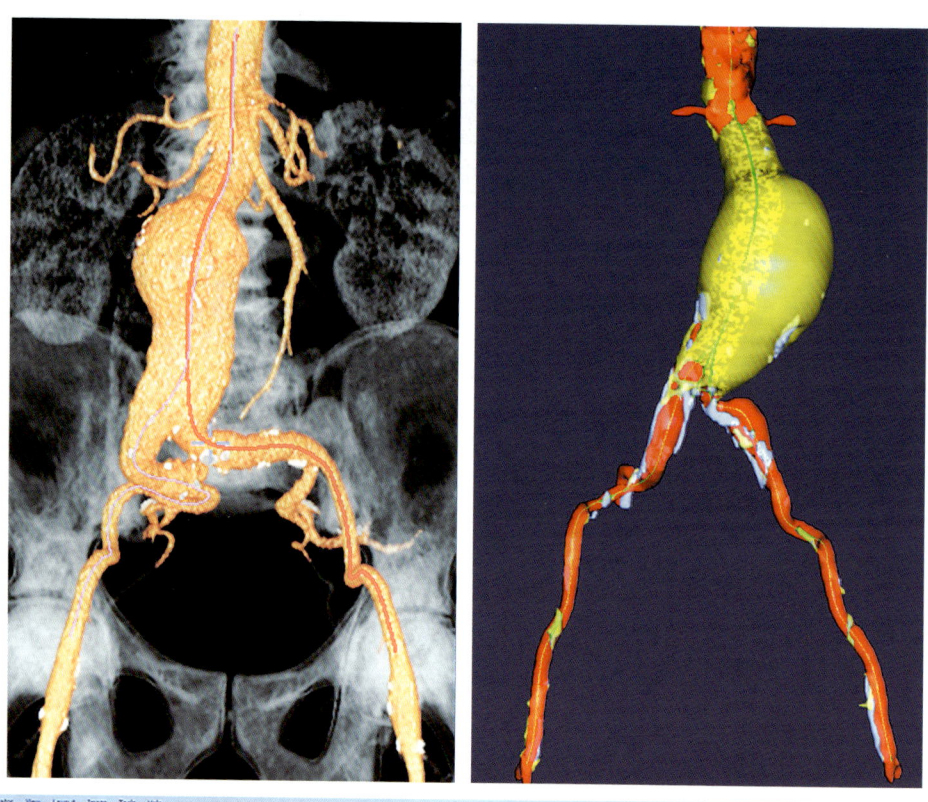

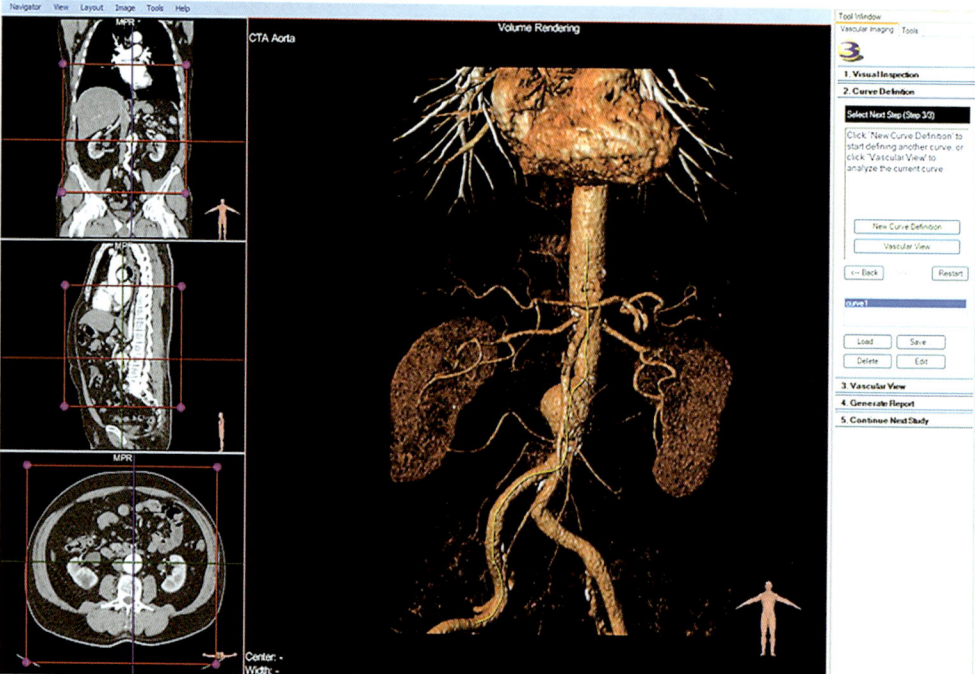

FIGURE 8: Centerlines for length and orthogonal MPR. Left image is from TeraRecon (*right-pink, left-orange*), the left image is from M2S (*green*), and the bottom picture is from 3Surgery.

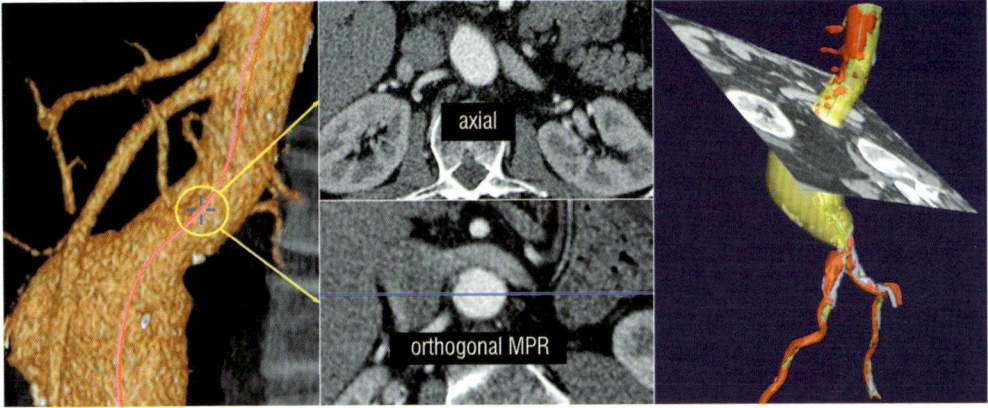

FIGURE 9: Orthogonal MPR. In plain axial images, the aorta is cut at a tangential angle (*top middle panel*). When the data is reformatted perpendicular to the centerline, the elliptical appearance of the aortic lumen is corrected (*bottom middle panel*). The right panel illustrates this concept using the M2S system, the bottom panel shows 3Surgery.

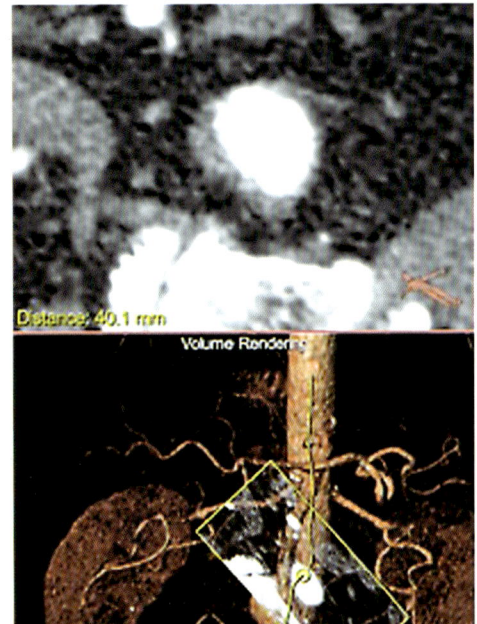

3) The distance along the centerline from the lowermost renal artery to the right and left hypogastric arteries are measured. The diameters of the right and left common iliac arteries are measured at a minimum of 2-3 points along the length of each iliac artery. Again, a reference diameter is determined to select the proper endograft limb. Typically, 15-20 mm is discounted from the actual centerline path for the reasons cited above.

4) The diameters of the access vessels are next measured. The access vessels refer to the common femoral and external iliac arteries. Unlike the outer wall measurements of the aortoiliac vasculature in the previous steps, to determine adequacy of vessel size for safe delivery of endovascular devices, the inner diameter of the access vessels are measured. The conversion from millimeters to French is 1 mm = 3.14 French.

5) After all the dimensional measurements are obtained, the side through which the main body device will be introduced is determined. The overriding factor is the size and quality of the access vessels. In terms of quality, tortuosity, calcification, and severity of occlusive disease are all important in determining the better of the two sides. However, all things being

equal, secondary considerations include the aortoiliac angle, which can impact ease of catheterization of the contralateral gate, and the lateral deviation of the proximal neck for ortho-symmetric deployment of the main body (Figure 10).

After the endografts are chosen based on the above measurements, the M2S system allows preoperative assessment of the device selections using a feature called a "Virtual Graft". A virtual bifurcated endograft with the dimensions of the main body and iliac limbs specified by the operator is fitted into the surface shaded 3D model. Proper endograft oversizing and apposition can be visually confirmed by the relationships of the color-coded endograft to the blood flow lumen. This still does not solve the graft path length problem since the virtual endograft is modeled around the centerline path.

POSTOPERATIVE ASSESSMENT

The postoperative assessment after EVAR consists of evaluation of aneurysm size, detection and characterization of endoleaks, migration, and conformational changes.[6,7] Regarding AAA size, whatever method is used to measure the sac diameter should be used consistently throughout the course of follow-up. The baseline diameter which will be used to monitor subsequent aneurysm size should be based on the first postoperative CT scan and not the preoperative scan. The presence of an endograft within the aorta can subtly change the axial orientation of the aortoiliac system. Therefore, if one uses plain axial images to follow sac diameters, this method should be used in all subsequent follow up imaging, and conversely if one uses 3D reconstructions with orthogonal MPR based on the centerline of the right iliac limb, this should be used in all future measurements for that particular patient.

Endoleaks can be reliably diagnosed using a triple-phase contrast CT angiogram. The three-phases include a non-contrast, timed-bolus, and delayed series of images. The non-contrast images allow discrimination of high-attenuation artifacts in the aneurysm sac, such as calcifications, from endoleaks. The delayed series can detect slow endoleaks from branch vessels that may be missed during the contrast phase. Three-dimensional analysis can aid in the localization of the source of the endoleak which has obvious prognostic and therapeutic implications. Using MPR reconstructions, continuity of the contrast pool in the sac can be traced to its source (Figure 11). Unlike dynamic imaging modalities such as a duplex ultrasound, the inflow and outflow vessels are not easily determined.

Endograft migration is an important failure mode of endovascular aneurysm repair. This is particularly true for those devices without active fixation. Although very gross migrations may be detectable on plain x-ray, due to parallax effects more subtle migrations may not be reliably detected. Three-dimensional reconstruction is the most sensitive method of detecting migrations and planning for remedial secondary procedures (Figure 12). The distance from the lowermost renal artery or the original implantation site to the top of the main body and to the endograft bifurcation can be measured, and thus determine the need for any intervention. Typically, almost any migration associated with a Type IA endoleak should be repaired, whereas even clinically silent migrations of 10 mm should strongly be considered for elective revision. The distance from the renal artery to the flow-divider of the endograft will determine what kind of revision (proximal cuff or aortouni-iliac conversion with femoral-femoral bypass) and any adjunctive procedures (main body retraction) will be required. Frequently proximal or distal migrations or limb separations are

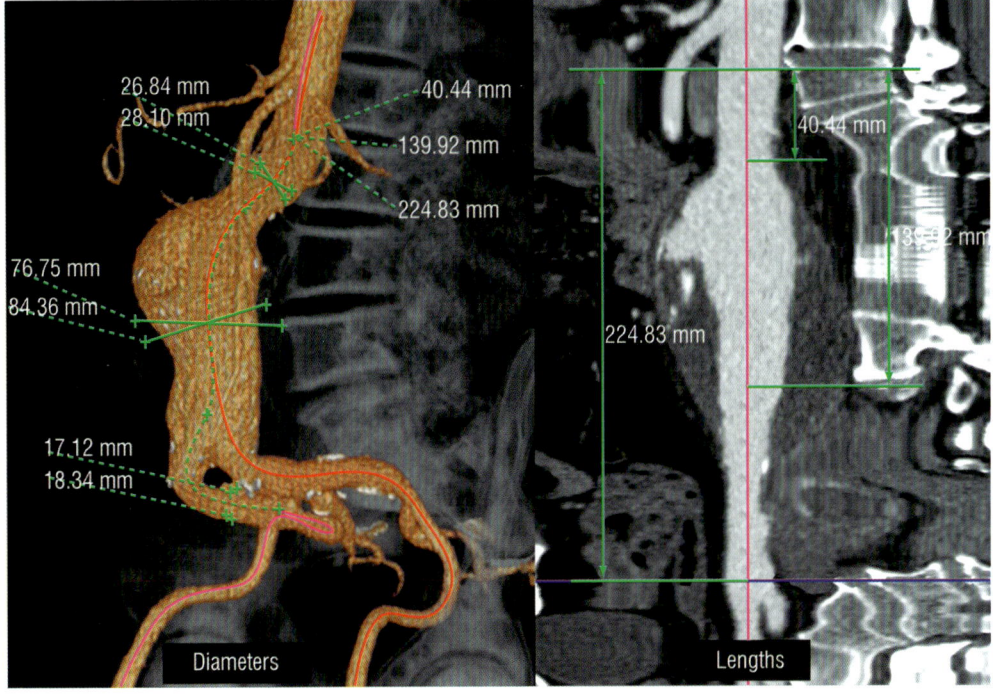

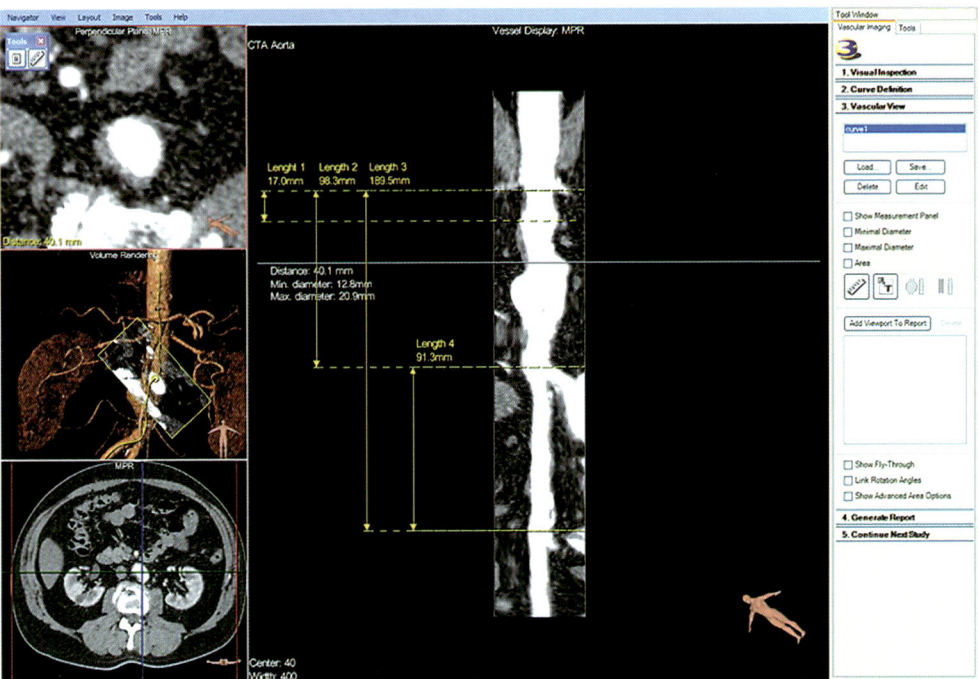

FIGURE 10: This figure illustrates the complete set of dimensional measurements typically obtained during preoperative assessment for EVAR using the TeraRecon (*top*) or 3Surgery (*bottom*) system. The right panel is an example of a stretch CPR (*curved planar reformation*) that facilitates measurements of centerline lengths between two points.

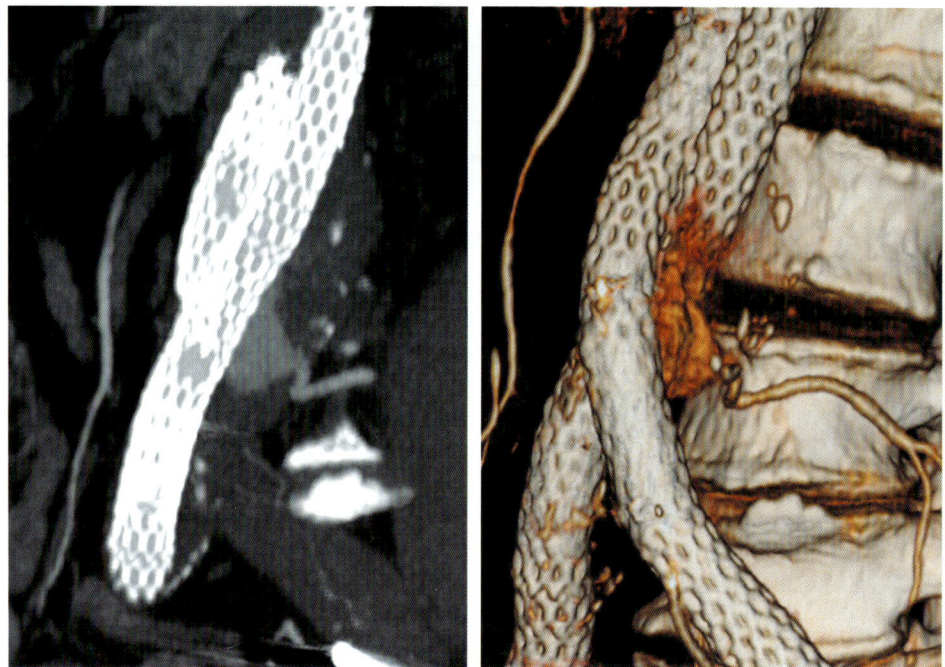

FIGURE 11: The figure shows a Type II endoleak that is in continuity with a lumbar artery as demonstrated using a thin-cut MIP (maximal intensity projection) (*left*) and a color surface shaded model (*right*).

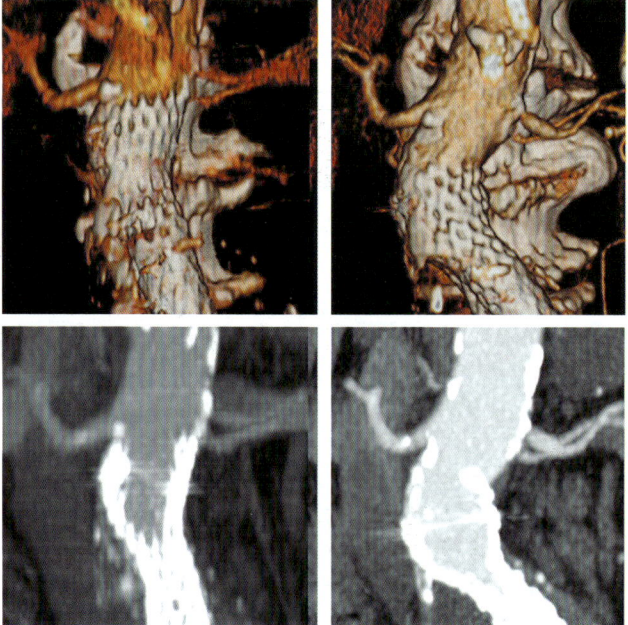

FIGURE 12: The left side of this figure shows the immediate postoperative CTA after EVAR reconstructed using Ter-aRecon workstation (*top, surface shaded model, bottom, MPR*). The right panels show corresponding images of a 2 cm migration of the proximal attachment 3 years later.

associated with conformational changes of the endograft either due to chronic hemodynamic forces endured by the endograft or AAA sac changes involved with either enlargement or shrinkage (Figure 13).

Stent integrity was typically assessed using multi-view plain abdominal x-rays whose technique was optimized for visualization of metallic elements. With 3D-maximum intensity projection (MIP) reconstruction, the metallic stents of the endografts can be imaged with greater clarity (Figure 14). The double density of the metal stents allows clear visualization of overlap at the junction of two endografts. Conformational changes that may result in late limb separation can be easily identified and prophylactically treated. Furthermore, one is not limited by 2 or 4 projections as is the case for plain films, but similar to the surface shaded model, the MIP

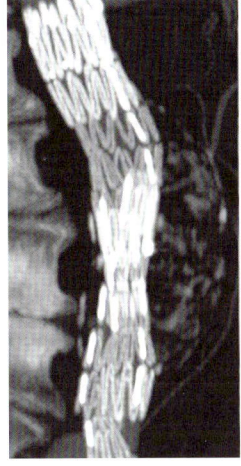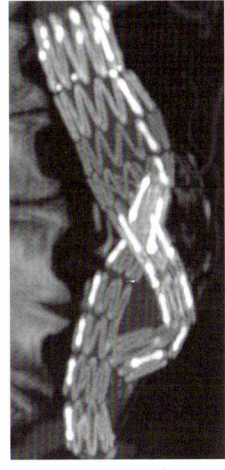

FIGURE 13: Two years after a successful EVAR, the aneurysm has decreased by 12 mm in size. On follow up this caused a conformational change of the endograft that resulted in the retraction of the right limb from the common iliac artery attachment site with a large Type IB endoleak.

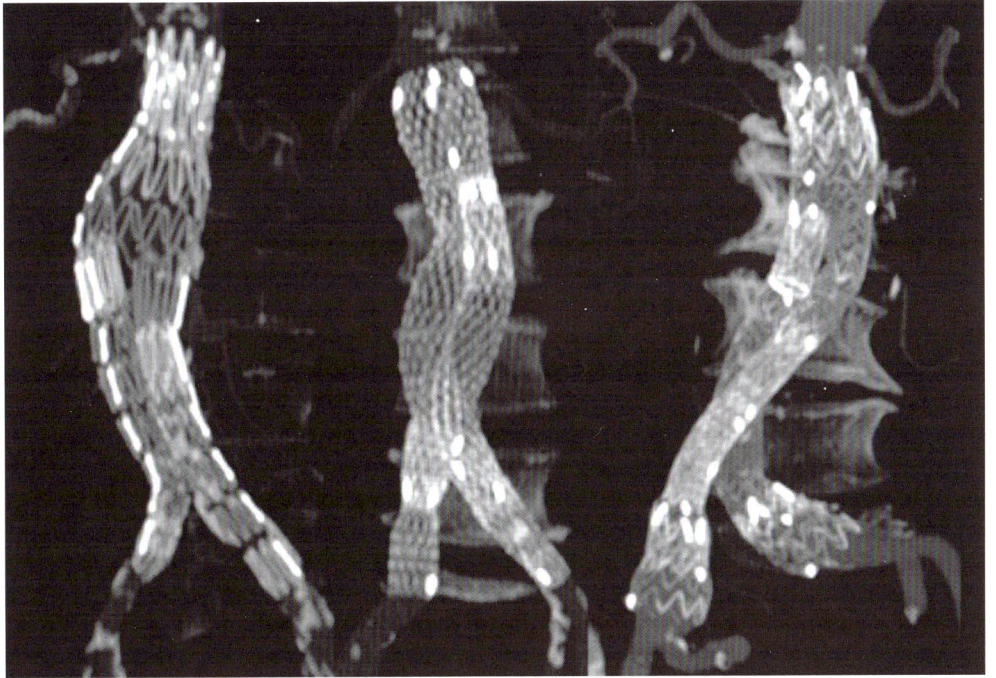

FIGURE 14: MIP images of three different abdominal endografts that are commercially available in the US. Note how the individual stent struts are clearly visible and the areas of junctional overlap can be identified by the double-density of the metal.

model can be rotated and magnified in an infinite number of projections such that even subtle defects can be detected, and can be generated from a non-contrast CT scan as the stents are radiopaque. MIP imaging has obviated the need for conventional x-rays in the postoperative assessment of EVAR patients.

CONCLUSION

In conclusion, volumetric data from cross-sectional imaging modalities such as CT angiograms can be rendered into a variety of 3D reconstruction formats. The concepts are broadly applicable across different software and hardware platforms, but there may be considerable variability in the representation of the anatomic structures. These tools have allowed accurate preoperative assessment of the aortoiliac system such that endovascular aortic repairs can be performed more safely and efficiently. Equally important, they have played an important role in the postoperative surveillance of these repairs, which may be the most critical component of the overall success of this therapy.

REFERENCES

1. Lutz AM, Willmann JK, Pfammatter T, Lachat M, Wildermuth S, Marincek B, Weishaupt D: Evaluation of aortoiliac aneurysm before endovascular repair: comparison of contrast-enhanced magnetic resonance angiography with multidetector row computed tomographic angiography with an automated analysis software tool. J Vasc Surg 2003, 37:619-27.
2. Flamm SD: Cross-sectional imaging studies: what can we learn and what do we need to know? Semin Vasc Surg 2007, 20:108-14. Review.
3. Wyers MC, Fillinger MF, Schermerhorn ML, Powell RJ, Rzucidlo EM, Walsh DB, Zwolak RM, Cronenwett JL: Endovascular repair of abdominal aortic aneurysm without preoperative arteriography. J Vasc Surg 2003, 38:730-8.
4. Parker MV, O'Donnell SD, Chang AS, Johnson CA, Gillespie DL, Goff JM, Rasmussen TE, Rich NM: What imaging studies are necessary for abdominal aortic endograft sizing? A prospective blinded study using conventional computed tomography, aortography, and three-dimensional computed tomography. J Vasc Surg 2005, 41:199-205.
5. Lee WA: Endovascular abdominal aortic aneurysm sizing and case planning using the TeraRecon Aquarius workstation. Vasc Endovascular Surg 2007, 41:61-7.
6. Teutelink A, Muhs BE, Vincken KL, Bartels LW, Cornelissen SA, van Herwaarden JA, Prokop M, Moll FL, Verhagen HJ: Use of dynamic computed tomography to evaluate pre- and postoperative aortic changes in AAA patients undergoing endovascular aneurysm repair. J Endovasc Ther 2007, 14:44-9.
7. Bromley PJ, Kaufman JA: Abdominal aortic aneurysms before and after endograft implantation: evaluation by computed tomography. Tech Vasc Interv Radiol 2001, 4:15-26.

Intravascular ultrasound in endovascular repair of abdominal aortic aneurysm

Murali Subramanian, Donald B. Reid

INTRODUCTION

Since ultrasound was introduced into clinical medicine, there has been an explosion in its various diagnostic applications, and miniaturization of ultrasound probes has been a further advance which has allowed access to previously unseen territories.[1,2] Catheter based vascular procedures were introduced as early as 1963 by Fogarty to extract arterial thrombi and emboli.[3] This was followed by transluminal dilatation for the treatment of atherosclerotic obstruction in 1964.[4] In the 1970's the predecessors of the current intravascular ultrasound (IVUS) catheters were developed, which were capable of cross-sectional imaging. Modern IVUS catheters are of two configurations: rotating mirror catheters and multiple phased array transducers. The former consists of an acoustic mirror assembly incorporated into the catheter tip: this rotates through a cable which is driven by a motor drive. The signal travels from the rotating mirror, producing a cross-sectional image. Phased array IVUS contains an integrated circuit in the tip of the catheter which sweeps around the catheter electronically, the advantage being that there are no moving parts and the catheter can configure with the guide wire coaxially.[5]

PRINCIPLES OF INTRAVASCULAR ULTRASOUND

Current IVUS catheters use frequencies in the range of 10-40 MHz. Low frequency catheters are required to visualize the larger diameter aortic circumference, especially in aneurysms. The catheter tip (Figure 1) is positioned parallel to the vessel wall so that the ultrasound beam is at 90 degrees to the luminal surface. Eccentric position-

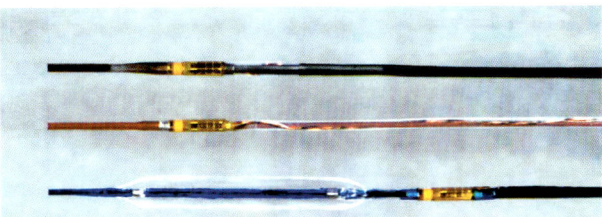

FIGURE 1: Phased array IVUS probes.

ing of the catheter causes an artefact of wall thickness and shape. The greyscale images are transmitted to the IVUS unit (Figure 2) where the measurements of luminal diameters and cross-sectional areas can be calculated. A three-dimensional longitudinal greyscale image can be produced by the IVUS unit by stacking cross-sectional images which provide an image similar to an angiogram. The differences between normal vessel wall, plaque, thrombus, or dissection flap are appreciated with the longitudinal imaging as well as providing the luminal profile. Colour flow IVUS helps appreciate the luminal blood flow without using the Doppler effect (Figure 3). IVUS captures up to 30 frames per second to generate the image.[6, 7]

While considering the role of IVUS in endovascular aneurysm repair it is worthwhile remembering the criteria for successful patient selection (Table 1).[8,9]

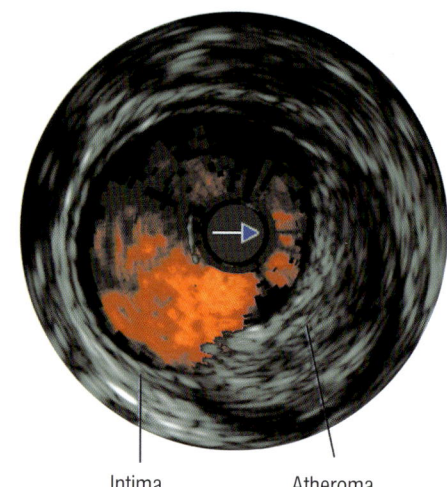

Intima   Atheroma

FIGURE 3: Colour flow IVUS, showing the blood flow in red and an eccentric atheromatous plaque.

While all these criteria are relative contraindications, there is no doubt that in our practice, we have found IVUS to be very useful in selecting cases for EVAR where we would not have anticipated endoluminal repair being feasible, and also in excluding some other cases. Unlike CT scanning, it is often the same interventionalist who performs the IVUS and then the endovascular repair - which is advantageous.

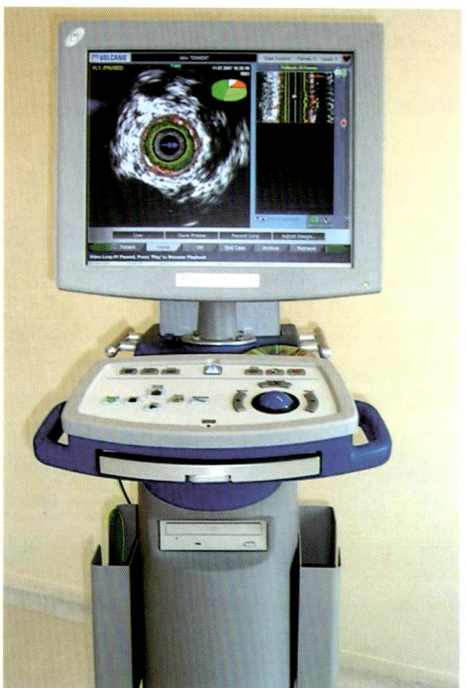

FIGURE 2: IVUS machine (S5, Volcano Corporation, Rancho Cordova, CA, USA).

TABLE 1	RELATIVE EXCLUSION CRITERIA FOR EVAR[9]

1 Extensive mural thrombus at the neck

2 Aortic neck diameter >32 mm, neck length <15 mm, aortic neck angulations >60 degrees

3 Severe iliac tortuosity

4 Access artery <7 mm

5 Aortic bifurcation diameter <12 mm

6 Bilateral common iliac aneurysms requiring coverage of both hypogastric arteries

7 Essential accessory renal artery

Currently there are several modalities of assessment of AAA: conventional angiography, magnetic resonance angiography (MRA) and computerised tomography angiography (CTA). IVUS is generally used in conjunction with one or more of these investigations.

Conventional angiography needs biplanar assessment in cases of tortuosity and irregularity, and images only the vessel lumen. This may be insufficient to delineate the complete anatomy and it is also known to underestimate the size of the lesion.[5] CT scanning is the preoperative gold standard investigation prior to endoluminal stenting. Lutz et al compared CT scanning and MRA in the evaluation of AAA preoperative planning. It was observed that they were similar in all respects apart from the fact that MRA was unable to detect calcification, (and may even miss the diagnosis of aortic aneurysm).[10]

IVUS is generally used following CT angiography to accurately assess the luminal neck diameters and then to obtain a guide to the length of the aneurysm neck and the distance from the caudal renal artery to the hypogastric artery. It can also provide information about the mesenteric branches of the aorta. Once the stent graft is deployed IVUS is used again to check the accuracy of placement of the stent and any endoleaks.[11,12]

TABLE 2	INFORMATION GAINED THROUGH IVUS[11]
Lumen diameters of necks, aorta and iliacs
Wall thickness
Lesion length, shape and volume
Lesion type: fibrous or calcified
Presence of dissection flap and extent
Presence and amount of thrombus

IVUS TECHNIQUE

In our institution, all patients scheduled for repair of AAA routinely undergo IVUS evaluation to assess the suitability of treatment for stent grafting. As long as there is satisfactory renal function, an aortogram is performed to provide road mapping. The IVUS catheter is introduced percutaneously over a 0.35 inch guide wire. A manual pullback is commenced. This entails very slow withdrawal of the catheter. Information is gathered from cross-sectional imaging and the longitudinal reconstruction (Figure 4 and 5). The important assessments with regard to suitability for stenting are accurate diameters of the proximal neck and distal landing zones, the presence of accessory renal arteries

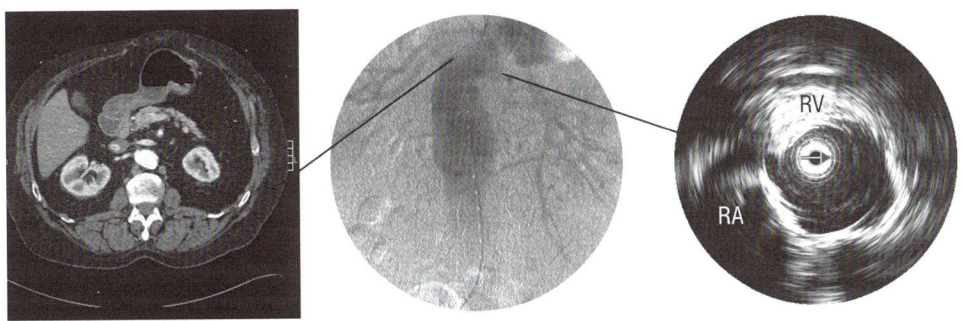

FIGURE 4: CTA, aortography and IVUS showing the level of the renal arteries.

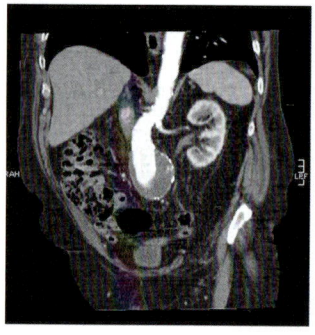 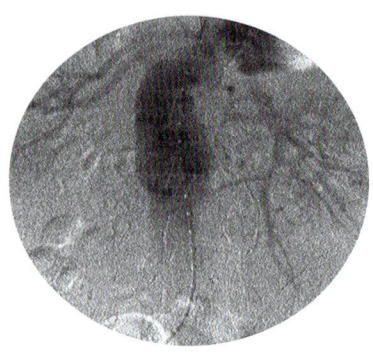  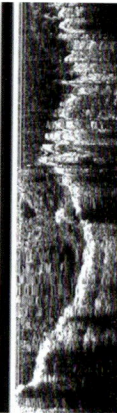

FIGURE 5: CTA, aortography and 3D longitudinal greyscale IVUS of an AAA before endoluminal repair.

and the diameters of the iliac arteries for access as well as deployment. The importance of accurate assessment cannot be overemphasised. Upon deployment of the stent, IVUS is performed again to assess the completeness and accuracy of stent deployment.

DISCUSSION

Some centres have investigated the use of IVUS in comparison to other imaging modalities. Verbin et al compared the utility of CT and IVUS in the evaluation of aortic necks in a canine model and artificially constructed AAAs. It was noted that IVUS was able to show proximal and distal landing zones with greater detail as well as the presence of intraluminal thrombus. IVUS was found to be superior during planning, during and after deployment.[13]

Nolthenius et al compared the differences in measurements between helical CT and IVUS prior to stent grafting in 54 patients. There was a 26% discrepancy in the diameter of the neck and 39% discrepancy in length measurements between CT and IVUS.[14] Garrett et al, in their series of 78 patients undergoing IVUS during AAA stenting, noted a 28% discrepancy in the

aortic neck diameter and/or length of aneurysm as compared to the pre-operative CT (there were no type I endoleaks reported in their series).[15,16]

Van essen et al compared the use of angiography, CT and IVUS in 15 patients. Four proximal necks which were absent on angiography were shown on CT and IVUS. Furthermore, angiography failed to identify three of five distal necks. The neck measurements were 3.5% smaller on IVUS as compared to CT.[17]

Plaque morphology was assessed in another series of 140 patients.[18] 15% had no atherosclerotic plaque; 59.3% had grade 2 plaque; 21.4% had grade 3 plaque and 4.3% had grade 4 plaque. It has been shown that increased plaque burden causes an increased risk of major complications. Presence of thrombus in the neck was associated with type I endoleak, graft migration and embolic complications.[18]

Routine use of IVUS can reduce contrast load in patients with renal insufficiency. Von Segesser et al used an average of 190 mls of contrast in 80 patients who underwent aortic stent grafting. Forty nine patients had their procedures performed purely with IVUS. They had to use angiography twice, due to failure of IVUS probes. There were no differences with regard to conversion, hospital stay and mortality but significant differences were noted in early endoleaks: IVUS (6.1%) vs angiography (25.8%).[19] Marty et al observed that their fluoroscopy time was reduced to 19 minutes in their series of 88 patients who underwent endovascular repair of AAA using systmatic IVUS guidance.[20] We have used IVUS instead of angiography in an acutely ruptured AAA to perform EVAR, in order to avoid the high pressure of intra aortic injection of contrast, as well as to protect an impaired renal function.

IVUS has limitations. The apparent high cost of IVUS is a prohibitive factor in many centres. Appreciation of the limitations of IVUS measurements in tortuous vessels is essential for accurate assessment: the IVUS catheter ideally should be placed in the centre of the lumen in order to avoid artefacts.[12,21]

SUMMARY

IVUS is an invaluable tool for a vascular interventionalist in all aspects of endoluminal assessment and repair, and particularly in endovascular repair of AAA. It is used as an adjunct to other assessment modalities and can play a major role in the assessment of suitability for EVAR. It provides accurate measurements for selection of stent size and then checks the accuracy of endograft deployment.

REFERENCES

1. Donald I. How and why medical sonar developed. Ann R Coll Surg Eng 1974;54:132-140.
2. Reid DB, Douglas M, Dietrich EB. The clinical value of three-dimensional intravascular ultrasound imaging. J Endovasc Surg 1995;2:356-364.
3. Forgarty TJ, Cranley jj, Krause RJ. A method of extraction of arterial emboli and thrombi. Surg Gynae Obstet 1963;116:241-244.
4. Dotter CT, Judkins MP. Transluminal treatment of atherosclerotic obstruction: Description of a new technique and preliminary report of its application. Circulation 1964;30:659-670.
5. Nishanian G, Kopchok GE, Donayre CE et al. Impact of IVUS on endovascular interventions. Sem Vasc Surg 1999;12:285-99.
6. Irshad K, Reid DB, Miller PH et al. Early clinical experience with colour three dimentional intravascular ultrasound in peripheral interventions. J Endovasc Ther 2001;8:329-338.
7. Lee JT and White RA. Basics of intra vascular ultrasound: An essential tool for the endovascular surgeon. Sem Vasc Surg 2004;17:110-18.
8. Parodi JC, Plamaz JC, Barone HD Transfemoral intraluminal graft implantation for abdominal aortic aneurysms Ann vasc Surg 1991;5:491-499.
9. Carpenter JP, Baum RA, Barker CF et al. Imapact of exclusion on patient selection for endovascular abdominal aortic aneurysm repair. J Vasc Surg 2001;34:1050-4.
10. Lutz AM, Willman JK, Pfammatter T et al. Evaluation of aortoiliac aneurysm before and endovascular repair: Camparison of contrast enhanced magnetic resonance angiography with multidetector row computed tomogrphic angiography with automated analysis software tool.
11. Scoccianti M, Verbin C, Kopchok GE et al. Intravascular ultrasound guidance for peripheral vascular interventions. J Endovasc Surg 1994;1:71-80.
12. Song TK, Donayre CE, Kopchok GE et al. Intravascular ultrasound use in the treatment of thoracoabdominal dissections, aneurysms and transections. Sem Vasc Surg 2006;19:145-9.
13. Verbin C, Scoccianti M, Kopchok G et al. Comparison of the utility of CT scans and intravascular ultrasound in endovascular aortic grafting. Ann Vasc Surg 1995;9:434-440.
14. Nolthenius RPT, van den Berg JC, Moll FL. The value of intraoperative intravascular ultrasound for determining stent graft size with the modular system. Ann Vasc Surg 2000;14:311-17.
15. Garrett HE, Abdullah AH, Hodgkiss TD et al. Intravascular ultrasound aids the performance of endovascular repair of abdominal aortic aneurysm. J Vasc Surg 2003;37:615-8.
16. Zanchetta M, Rigatelli G, Pedon L et al. IVUS guidance of thoracic and complex abdominal aortic

aneurysm stent-graft repairs using an intracardiac echocardiography probe: Preliminary report. J Endovasc Ther 2003;10:218-26.

17. Van Essen JA, Gussenhoven EJ, van der Lugt A et al. Accurate assessment of abdominal aortic aneurysm with intravascular ultrasound scanning: Validation with computed tomographic angiography. 8.

18. Gitlitz DB, Ramaswami G, Kaplan D et al. Endovascular stent-grafting in the presence of aortic neck filling defects: early clinical experience. J Vasc Surg 2001;33:340-44.

19. Von Segesser LK, Marty B, Ruchat P et al. Routine use of intravascular ultrasound for endovascular aneurysm repair: Angiography is not necessary. Eur J Vasc Endovasc Surg 2002;23:537-42.

20. Marty B, Tozzi P, Ruchat P et al. Systematic and exclusive use of intravascular ultrasound for endovascular aneurysm repair- The Lausanne experience. Interactive cardiovascular and thoracic surgery 2005;4:275-9.

21. The SHK, Gussenhoven EJ, Zhong Y et al. Effect of balloon angioplasty on femoral artery evaluated with intravascular ultrasound imaging. Circulation 1992;86:483-93.

Dynamic imaging of the aorta for endovascular aortic aneurysm grafting

Felix J.V. Schlösser, Hence J.M. Verhagen, Bart E. Muhs

ABSTRACT

Purpose: New imaging techniques with ultrasound, computer tomography and magnetic resonance imaging have been introduced. The potential of dynamic imaging, which involves a time sequence of images, in the diagnosis, pre-operative work-up and follow-up of patients undergoing endovascular aortic aneurysm repair, is becoming more evident during recent years.

Methods: Available articles about the potentials of these new techniques in clinical applications and research are reviewed with special regard to endovascular aortic aneurysm repair.

Results: Dynamic imaging with ultrasound, computer tomography and magnetic resonance imaging has offered more insight into aortic wall motions, both before and after aortic aneurysm repair. These wall motions are considerable and have implications for stent-graft design. Many articles reported on benefits of dynamic imaging in the detection and characterization of endoleaks after endovascular aortic aneurysm repair. Some authors showed that more oversizing of endografts might be recommended in some patients with extensive aortic wall movements to reduce the post-operative risks of type I endoleak and graft migration.

Conclusions: Computer tomography, ultrasound and magnetic resonance imaging can be successfully used to characterize aortic wall movements. With further improvements of these technologies, their clinical applicability and importance in the clinical setting is likely to increase. Future studies about dynamic imaging with more extensive study of clinical outcome and larger patient cohorts, might improve our knowledge and result in improved future stent-graft design and patient prognosis.

INTRODUCTION

Angiography is since decennia regarded as the "gold standard" for diagnostic imaging of aortic diseases, but angiography is an invasive procedure and is associated with a low, but significant risk of morbidity and mortality.[1] Besides, an hospital admission is often required in patients undergoing angiography. Some newer techniques have been introduced and have increased our knowledge during the last period and are likely to do so in future: Ultrasound, Magnetic Resonance Imaging (MRI) and Computed Tomography (CT). With further improvements of these techniques, the position of angiography as the "gold standard" is becoming more and more into question.

Since the advent of endovascular aneurysm repair (EVAR) in 1991, improved diagnostic techniques were required for the pre-operative work-up and follow-up examinations after surgery.[2-5] Precise imaging of aortic measurements, most importantly aneurysm diameter and proximal length of the aneurysm neck, are essential for a good prognosis after endovascular aortic aneurysm repair. Further improvements in stent-graft design and more insight in the pathological mechanisms of complications after endovascular aortic aneurysm repair could possibly increase the number of patients in whom endovascular aortic aneurysm repair is suitable and might reduce the risk of endoleaks and other complications. Dynamic imaging is a three dimensional imaging method with the acquisition of time, and dynamic imaging with ultrasound, CT or MRI can possibly be valuable to provide more insight in the aforementioned topics.

The available evidence about the potentials of these new techniques in clinical applications and research will be discussed in this article with special regard to endovascular aortic aneurysm repair.

ULTRASOUND SCANNING

Ultrasonography is an ultrasound-based, inexpensive, noninvasive technique to visualize the size, structure, and pathologies of soft tissue body structures. Duplex ultrasound or Doppler can be used to visualize the structure and hemodynamics within a vessel. Disadvantages include the fact that accuracy of diagnostic testing with ultrasound is highly operator-dependent and that ultrasound has limited bone penetration. Methods to reduce the high operator-dependability have been described. Lanne et al. described that ultrasound reliability in diagnostics of abdominal aortic aneurysms can be improved by implementing an echo-tracking system using electronics markers on the aortic walls.[6,7] Ultrasound has been described as an accurate modality to assess sizes of abdominal aortic aneurysms,[8,9] with an inter- and intraobserver coefficient of variation that has been described to be in the range of 2 to 3%.

Ultrasound scanning can also have clinical implications after aortic aneurysm surgery. Pulsatile wall motion of aortic aneurysms can be assessed noninvasively with ultrasound scanning. Malina[10] reported that the pulsatile wall motion of abdominal aortic aneurysms (AAA) differed significantly before and after endovascular repair. Besides, they found that the pulsatile wall motion of aneurysms in patients with endoleaks was 50% higher compared to aneurysms in patients without endoleaks (p-value <.01). Bargellini[11] also described the potential of ultrasound in detecting endoleaks. Type II lumbar endoleaks had different hemodynamic features that could be identified by contrast-enhanced ultrasound scanning. This might subsequently be associated with aneurysm expansion rates, risk of rupture and need for re-intervention.

COMPUTED TOMOGRAPHY

Since its introduction in 1973, Computer Tomography has been settled as an important medical imaging technique in addition to X-rays and ultrasound scanning.[12] Computed tomography is currently the most frequently used imaging modality for the pre-operative evaluation of the aneurysm and aorta in patients planned for endovascular aortic aneurysm repair.[13,14] Important disadvantages of Computed Tomography is the necessity of radiation exposure and administration of contrast. When ECG-gating is used, the radiation exposure from CTA will even be higher.[15] This is especially important in patients with aortic aneurysms, during watchful waiting or follow-up after endovascular aortic aneurysm repair, because of the likelihood of many follow-up examinations. Another disadvantage is that CT is not suitable for patients who are critically ill and cannot be transported to the Computed Tomography room.

The newest multi-slice CT systems, up to 256 slices, are described to render images with excellent qualities of vascular images.[16,17,18] Dynamic cine-CT is a sequence of axial images, with both a spatial and temporal resolution. Several authors have reported useful applications of dynamic computed tomographic angiography. Dynamic CT has valuable applications in the pre-operative work-up and follow-up of patients undergoing aortic aneurysm surgery. A Dutch study described the value of dynamic CT imaging for identifying patients with large pulsatility of the aorta in whom the standard regime of 10% to 15% oversizing may be insufficient to prevent stent-graft migration or intermittent type I endoleaks. In a prior study they described that the largest change in diameter in patients with abdominal aortic aneurysms was at the level of the suprarenal part of the aneurysm neck and a considerable longitudinal movement occurs in the aorta during the cardiac cycle.[19] Altered renal artery movement after endovascular abdominal aortic aneurysm repair has also been detected with the use of ECG-gated dynamic CTA.[20] Dynamic cine-CT angiography of the thoracic aorta revealed a maximal diameter change of 10% of the thoracic aorta during the cardiac cycle.[21] Rydberg[22] reported that dynamic CTA is a useful tech-

nique in the detection, classification and localization of endoleaks. The endoleaks of five patients out of 104 patients could not be classified accurately with non-dynamic CTA. With dynamic CTA, these five endoleaks and inflow and outflow branches could be localized accurately.

Dynamic CTA can also offer valuable information for future endograft design. Van Prehn[23] showed with the use of dynamic cine-CTA a significant movement of the ascending thoracic aorta in all three spatial dimensions. The forces which the thoracic graft has to withstand during the continuingly repeating cardiac cycle, should be regarded carefully to improve the design of future stent-grafts. With future improvements of techniques, Computed Tomography is likely to expand its clinical applications in patients with aortic aneurysms, planned for surgery or after aneurysm repair.

MAGNETIC RESONANCE IMAGING

Magnetic Resonance Imaging is another technology that can be used for visualizing aortic aneurysms. It is noninvasive, offers high resolution imaging, requires no radiation exposure and contrast administration is often not required. Disadvantages include that this modality is time consuming and some patients are not suitable, for example critically ill patients.[24] If a gadolinium-based contrast is used to enhance vascular imaging, it is regarded as less nephrotoxic than iodinated contrast media used for CT or angiography.[25] Dynamic cine MR uses ECG-gated imaging to provide a sequence of axial images. Dynamic cine MRI has considerably changed during recent years with important improvements in data acquisition and imaging qualities.[26]

Several authors have reported potential applications of dynamic contrast-enhanced MRI in patients undergoing aortic endografting or after the procedure. Dynamic contrast-enhanced MRI has a great sensitivity in the pre-operative work-up of patients undergoing endovascular thoracic aortic aneurysm repair by detecting the artery of Adamkiewicz, a structure that is important in the blood supply of the anterior spinal artery. Interruption of this blood supply, for example due to endografting, can induce spinal cord ischemia. Hyodoh et al.[27] reported that this artery was detected in 42 out of 50 patients with dynamic contrast-enhanced MR angiography (84%) and this had clinically implications, because the surgical approach could be adjusted to provide maximal protection of this artery. Subsequently, all these patients had no spinal cord ischemia and no neurologic complications after surgery.

Several authors have investigated aortic wall motions before and after endovascular AAA repair. Van Herwaarden[28] described that aortic diameter sizes proximal to and at the level of the aneurysm neck change during the cardiac cycle. The diameter changed asymmetrically and up to 8.9% pre-operatively and 11.5% post-operatively. They hypothesized that 10 to 15% oversizing of an endograft may be insufficient for some patients undergoing AAA repair. A study by Faries et al.[29] stated that endovascular AAA repair resulted in decreased aortic wall motion during the cardiac cycle and patients who had a type I endoleak had higher aortic wall pulsatility than patients without type I endoleak. They could not detect a significant difference in aortic wall movement in patients with and without a type II endoleak. Vos and collegues[30] have also performed a study to evaluate stent-graft and aneurysm wall motions during the cardiac cycle using dynamic cine-MRI. They detected increased longitudinal translation of both the aneurysm and stent-graft after endovascular AAA repair, which is possibly caused by downward pulling forces at

the proximal fixation site of the stent-graft. An increased angulation of the stent-graft during cardiac systole was also observed, which can be important for improved future stent-graft design. Van Herwaarden and colleagues[31] have shown that dynamic MRI is a technique that offers more possibilities than only measuring of the aortic aneurysm sizes. They described the feasibility of dynamic MRI in characterization of aortic stiffness and elastic modulus during the cardiac cycle. Both aortic stiffness and elastic modulus were highest at the level of the aneurysm sac and endovascular AAA repair appeared to be associated with further increase of these variables. The aortic stiffness of the aneurysm neck increased with 94% after endovascular AAA repair and the elastic modulus with 60%. This may have implications for future endograft design. Endoleaks did not appear to have an effect on these indexes of aortic wall compliance.

Van der Laan[32] has described that dynamic contrast-enhanced MR angiography has an additional value in the classification of endoleaks. In 6 out of 23 patients with an endoleak, dynamic contrast-enhanced MRI made classification of these endoleaks possible, while the regular, non-dynamic MRI did not allow this classification. All type I and type III endoleaks could be classified with dynamic contrast-enhanced MR angiography. MRI techniques are still continuing to improve. High-resolution contrast-enhanced MR angiography with cardiac gating can produce images with a high quality and this will lead to improvements in the accuracy of diagnosis in these patients.[33] Markl et al.[34] reported recently a feasible powerful magnetic resonance technique, "prospectively ECG-gated cine three-dimensional MR velocity mapping with improved navigator gating, real-time adaptive k-space ordering and dynamic adjustments of the navigator acceptance criteria", that is a possible solution for artifacts related to breathing motion. The resulting images had an excellent quality, especially with regard to the visualization of the aorta. Future studies using dynamic MRI might improve our knowledge of determinants of aneurysm growth, rupture risk, effects of stent-grafts and pathologic mechanisms of complications after endovascular AAA repair, subsequently resulting in improved stent-graft design and patient prognosis.

CONCLUSIONS

The potential of dynamic imaging of the visualization of aneurysm wall motion during the cardiac cycle and aneurysm wall compliance has been shown. These new techniques, including ultrasound, magnetic resonance imaging and CT, are becoming more importantly in diagnosis, pre-operative work-up and follow-up of patients with aortic aneurysms undergoing endovascular surgery.

Each of the different techniques has its own benefits and disadvantages and several clinical applications have been demonstrated. Changes in aneurysms before and after endovascular aortic aneurysm repair were shown. Computed tomography and magnetic resonance imaging could be successfully used to characterize aortic wall movements. Several studies described the potential of dynamic imaging as an adjunct diagnostic modality for the detection and characterization of endoleaks.

With further improvements of these technologies, their clinical applicability and importance in the clinical setting is likely to increase. Future studies about dynamic imaging with more extensive study of clinical outcome and larger patient cohorts, might improve our knowledge of determinants of aneurysm growth, rupture risk, effects of stent-grafts and pathologic mechanisms of complications after endo-

vascular AAA repair, subsequently resulting in improved stent-graft design and patient prognosis.

REFERENCES

1. Young N, Chi KK, Ajaka J, McKay L, O'Neill D, Wong KP. Complications with outpatient angiography and interventional procedures. Cardiovasc.Intervent.Radiol. 2002;25:123-6.
2. Parodi JC, Palmaz JC, Barone HD. Transfemoral intraluminal graft implantation for abdominal aortic aneurysms. Ann.Vasc.Surg. 1991;5:491-9.
3. Rubin GD, Shiau MD, Leung AN, et al. Aorta and iliac arteries: single versus multiple detector-row helical CT angiography. Radiology. 2000;215:670-6.
4. Prince MR, Narasimham DL, Stanley JC, et al. Breath-hold gadolinium-enhanced MR angiography of the abdominal aorta and its major branches. Radiology. 1995;197:785-92.
5. Durham JR, Hackworth CA, Tober JC, et al. Magnetic resonance angiography in the preoperative evaluation of abdominal aortic aneurysms. Am.J.Surg. 1993;166:173-8.
6. Sonesson B, Hansen F, Stale H, et al. Compliance and diameter in the human abdominal aorta-the influence of age and sex. Eur.J.Vasc.Surg. 1993;7:690-7.
7. Lanne T, Sandgren T, Mangell P, et al. Improved reliability of ultrasonic surveillance of abdominal aortic aneurysms. Eur.J.Vasc.Endovasc.Surg. 1997;13:149-53.
8. Goldberg BB, Lehman JS. Aortosonography: ultrasound measurement of the abdominal and thoracic aorta. Arch.Surg. 1970;100:652-5.
9. Wheeler WE, Beachley MC, Ranniger K. Angiography and ultrasonography. A comparative study of abdominal aortic aneurysms. Am.J.Roentgenol. 1976;126:95-100.
10. Malina M, Lanne T, Ivancev K, et al. Reduced pulsatile wall motion of abdominal aortic aneurysms after endovascular repair. J.Vasc.Surg. 1998;27:624-31.
11. Bargellini I, Napoli V, Petruzzi P, Cioni R, Vignali C, Sardella SG, Ferrari M, Bartolozzi C. Type II lumbar endoleaks: hemodynamic differentiation by contrast-enhanced ultrasound scanning and influence

on aneurysm enlargement after endovascular aneurysm repair. J.Vasc.Surg. 2005;41:10-8.

12. Hounsfield GN. Computerized transverse axial scanning (tomography). 1. Description of system. Br.J.Radiol. 1973;46:1016-22.

13. Broeders IA, Blankensteijn JD, Olree M, et al. Preoperative sizing of grafts for transfemoral endovascular aneurysm management: a prospective comparative study of spiral CT angiography, arteriography, and conventional CT imaging. J.Endovasc.Surg. 1997;4:252-61.

14. Parker MV, O'Donnell SD, Chang AS, et al. What imaging studies are necessary for abdominal aortic endograft sizing? A prospective blinded study using conventional computed tomography, aortography, and three-dimensional computed tomography. J.Vasc.Surg. 2005;41:199-205.

15. Schertler T, Glucker T, Wildermuth S, Jungius KP, Marincek B, Boehm T. Comparison of retrospectively ECG-gated and nongated MDCT of the chest in an emergency setting regarding workflow, image quality, and diagnostic certainty. Emerg.Radiol. 2005;12:19-29.

16. Kalender WA, Seissler W, Klotz E, et al. Spiral volumetric CT with single-breath-hold technique, continuous transport, and continuous scanner rotation. Radiology. 1990;176:181-3.

17. Klingenbeck-Regn K, Schaller S, Flohr T, et al. Subsecond multi-slice computed tomography: basics and applications. Eur.J.Radiol. 1999;31:110-24.

18. Mizuno N, Funabashi N, Imada M, Tsunoo T, Endo M, Komuro I. Utility of 256-slice cone beam tomography for real four-dimensional volumetric analysis without electrocardiogram gated acquisition. Int.J.Cardiol. 2007;120:262-7.

19. Teutelink A, Rutten A, Muhs BE, et al. Pilot study of dynamic cine CT angiography for the evaluation of abdominal aortic aneurysms: implications for endograft treatment. J.Endovasc.Ther. 2006;13:139-44.

20. Muhs BE, Teutelink A, Prokop M, et al. Endovascular aneurysm repair alters renal artery movement: a preliminary evaluation using dynamic CTA. J.Endovasc.Ther. 2006;13:476-80.

21. Muhs BE, Vincken KL, van Prehn J, et al. Dynamic cine-CT angiography for the evaluation of the thoracic aorta; insight in dynamic changes with implications for thoracic endograft treatment. Eur.J.Vasc.Endovasc.Surg. 2006;32:532-6.

22. Rydberg J, Lalka S, Johnson M, Cikrit D, Dalsing M, Sawchuk A, Shafique S. Characterization of endoleaks by dynamic computed tomographic angiography. Am.J.Surg. 2004;188:538-43.

23. Van Prehn J, Vincken KL, Muhs BE, Barwegen GK, Bartels LW, Prokop M, Moll FL, Verhagen HJ. Toward endografting of the ascending aorta: insight into dynamics using dynamic cine-CTA. J.Endovasc.Ther. 2007;14:551-60.

24. Khalil A, Tarik T, Porembka DT. Aortic pathology: aortic trauma, debris, dissection, and aneurysm. Crit.Care Med. 2007;35:S392-400.

25. Rieger J, Sitter T, Toepfer M, Linsenmaier U, Pfeifer KJ, Schiffl H. Gadolinium as an alternative contrast agent for diagnostic and interventional angiographic procedures in patients with impaired renal function. Nephrol.Dial.Transplant. 2002;17:824-8.

26. Ho VB, Foo TK. Impact of "cine MR imaging: potential for the evaluation of cardiovascular function." Am.J.Roentgenol. 2006;187:605-8.

27. Hyodoh H, Kawaharada N, Akiba H, Tamakawa M, Hyodoh K, Fukada J, Morishita K, Hareyama M. Usefulness of preoperative detection of artery of Adamkiewicz with dynamic contrast-enhanced MR angiography. Radiology. 2005;236:1004-9.

28. van Herwaarden JA, Bartels LW, Muhs BE, et al. Dynamic magnetic resonance angiography of the aneurysm neck: conformational changes during the cardiac cycle with possible consequences for endograft sizing and future design. J.Vasc.Surg. 2006;44:22-8.

29. Faries PL, Agarwal G, Lookstein R, et al. Use of cine magnetic resonance angiography in quantifying aneurysm pulsatility associated with endoleak. J.Vasc.Surg. 2003;38:652-6.

30. Vos AW, Wisselink W, Marcus JT, et al. Aortic aneurysm pulsatile wall motion imaged by cine MRI: a tool to evaluate efficacy of endovascular aneurysm repair? Eur.J.Vasc.Endovasc.Surg. 2002;23:158-61.

31. van Herwaarden JA, Muhs BE, Vincken KL, et al. Aortic compliance following EVAR and the influence of different endografts: determination using dynamic MRA. J.Endovasc.Ther. 2006;13:406-14.

32. Van der Laan MJ, Bakker CJ, Blankensteijn JD, Bartels LW. Dynamic CE-MRA for endoleak clas-

sification after endovascular aneurysm repair. Eur.J.Vasc.Endovasc.Surg. 2006;31:130-5.

33. Groves EM, Bireley W, Dill K, Carroll TJ, Carr JC. Quantitative analysis of ECG-gated high-resolution contrast-enhanced MR angiography of the thoracic aorta. Am.J.Roentgenol. 2007;188:522-8.

34. Markl M, Harloff A, Bley TA, Zaitsev M, Jung B, Weigang E, Langer M, Hennig J, Frydrychowicz A. Time-resolved 3D MR velocity mapping at 3T: improved navigator-gated assessment of vascular anatomy and blood flow. J.Magn.Reson.Imaging. 2007;25:824-31.

Anaesthesia considerations in endovascular aneurysm repair

Robert Hackett, Timothy McCulloch, Sol Yezerski

INTRODUCTION

Endovascular aneurysm repair (EVAR) is an increasingly popular alternative to conventional open abdominal aortic aneurysm (AAA) repair. It is rapidly replacing the need for open surgery and all the morbidity associated with this procedure. The less invasive nature of EVAR has allowed for modification of anaesthetic technique, and has enabled less invasive modes of anaesthesia to be utilized.

Since commercially produced grafts started trials in 1994,[1] the technology for EVAR has spread worldwide, and has been continually improved and refined. Improvements have included the development of slimmer catheters, stents which self expand allowing more rapid delivery and deployment, and stents of tailored design to meet the needs of the patient. The ability of proceduralists to perform this less invasive surgery has also improved, leading amongst other things to shorter surgical times. EVAR has allowed AAA repair in patients considered unfit for open repair or general anaesthesia, and has provided a valuable alternative in the management of emergency AAA repair. Anaesthetic practice, in turn, has been adapted in response to the changing requirements of endovascular surgery.

Whilst EVAR represents a revolution in the operative management of aneurysms, anaesthetists need to be aware of the potential advantages and disadvantages of the endovascular techniques. Numerous trials including the recent multicentre randomized controlled EVAR1[2] and DREAM trials[3] have clearly demonstrated the short-term benefits of EVAR. Surgically, EVAR is a less invasive procedure with potential rewards in terms of short term mortality,[2,3] reduced morbidity, reduced physiological stress including cardiac, pulmonary, and renal impairment, reduced blood loss with decreased need for intraoperative blood transfusion, reduced requirement for ICU admissions, earlier ambulation, and an earlier return to normal activities. Disadvantages of EVAR over open repair include cost,[2] the need for experienced staff and dedicated equipment, the risk of endoleak development, and the need for long-term postoperative surveillance.

ANAESTHETIC MANAGEMENT

The anaesthetic management of patients having EVAR must attain several goals, and several considerations unique to endovascular surgery need to be taken in to account:

- The principal goal of perioperative management during any surgical procedure is to conserve organ function and optimise patient comfort.
- Compared to open aortic surgery, endovascular surgery is relatively non-invasive. The absence of laparotomy and aortic cross clamping dramatically reduces the physiological stress of the procedure. However, disruption of the aorta or the iliac vessels can occur suddenly. The anaesthetist needs to be vigilant, prepared for the possibility of sudden massive blood loss, and prepared for rapid conversion to laparotomy with aortic cross clamping.
- The patient needs to remain still for the duration of the procedure, which is usually just over 2 hours but may be prolonged. Immobility is particularly important during stent deployment and intermittent cooperation with a breath hold may be required to optimise digital subtraction angiography.
- Management must aim to minimize postoperative impairment of renal function. Several mechanisms may cause renal insult including contrast-induced nephropathy, hypovolaemia, dehydration from fasting and bowel preparation, renal artery occlusion, and thromboemboli.

Preoperative assessment

The preoperative assessment for patients having EVAR needs to be thorough, as patients with vascular disease often have several co-morbidities. Within our institution, patients presenting for elective EVAR are seen in a dedicated Vascular Pre-Anaesthetic Assessment Clinic.

Vascular disease is often the end product of generalized disease and is frequently present in many arteries leading to multiple end organ insufficiency. The risk factors for having an AAA include advanced age, smoking >40 years, hypertension a low serum HDL cholesterol, a high plasma fibrinogen, and a low platelet count.[4] Patients with an abdominal aortic aneurysm have been shown to have the following rates of co-morbidities:[3,5]

- coronary artery disease (50-70%)
- previous myocardial infarction (40-60%)
- hypertension (25-70%)
- silent myocardial ischaemia (20-60%)
- hyperlipidemia (50%)
- chronic lung pathology (25-50%)
- carotid artery disease (15%)
- chronic renal failure (5-15%)
- diabetes mellitus (8-12%)

Patients in the DREAM trial were aged 70 ±7 years and 90% male.[3] Their preoperative medical therapy reflected the high rates of co-morbidities; 48% of patients were taking beta blockers, 40% statins, 40% antiplatelet drugs, 31% angiotensin converting enzyme (ACE) inhibitors, 18% calcium channel blockers, and 13% anticoagulants. Outside of randomised trials, one group of patients has an even higher rate of severe co-morbidities; these are the patients with an aortic aneurysm who are considered unfit for an open procedure, or even unfit for general anaesthesia, and are offered EVAR.

Given the above information, it can be assumed that a typical patient with an aortic aneurysm has an almost 100% chance of having some degree of heart disease; regardless of whether significant disease was detected on preoperative assessment. The American Heart Association (AHA) guidelines on preoperative cardiac investigations are based on the patient's risk factors, the patient's ability to exercise, and the risk associated with the surgical procedure.[6,7] Aortic surgery is classified as a high risk procedure and most patients presenting for AAA repair would, according to these guidelines, require non-invasive cardiac investigation such as stress-ECG, echocardiography (with or without exercise or pharmacologically-induced stress), and/or cardiac scintigraphy. However, the perioperative mortality with EVAR is significantly lower than with traditional AAA repair[2,3] and we classify EVAR as an intermediate risk procedure. Hence, we only refer patients for further cardiac evaluation if they are at high risk based on clinical predictors: e.g. unstable coronary syndromes, uncompensated cardiac failure, known or suspected severe valvular abnormalities, arrhythmias, or inability to perform moderate exercise such as climbing two flights of stairs.

There is evidence that patients who have had successful coronary artery bypass surgery within the previous 5 years are at no greater risk of a perioperative cardiac event than patients who have no evidence of significant coronary disease.[8] Percutaneous coronary revascularisation may not confer the same protection.[9] Patients who have recently had coronary stenting and are taking platelet inhibiting medications present a particular challenge. Depending on the type of stent, the risk of ceasing antiplatelet medications preoperatively can be associated with a very high risk of thromboembolic phenomena. In most cases, the surgeons in our institution do not cease drugs such as clopidogrel prior to EVAR. If cessation of these drugs is considered, close liaison is required between the patient's cardiologist, the proceduralist, and the anaesthetist.

In our institution preoperative testing prior to EVAR includes electrolytes, blood sugar, creatinine, liver function tests, full blood count, coagulation screen, blood grouping and screening for antibodies to red cell antigens. All patients have a preoperative electrocardiograph and patients with respiratory disease have spirometry. Further investigations are guided by the clinical situation, including cardiac investigations as discussed above.

Premedication may include some form of anxiolysis. The patients' usual cardiovascular medications are continued on the morning of the procedure including, in our practice, ACE inhibitors. Intravenous fluid can be administered to overcome the potential dehydration caused by bowel preparation and fasting. However, this cannot usually be commenced prior to arrival in the operating theatre as currently most patients arrive in hospital on the day of surgery. N-acetylcysteine is administered preoperatively in those considered to have an increased risk of nephrotoxicity from intravenous contrast.

Procedure location

Within our institution EVAR is always performed in a dedicated vascular theatre. Repeated angiograms need to be carried out throughout the procedure to check the position of the stent, and in some hospitals suitable quality angiograms may only be obtainable in the radiology department. Also, as technology improves and surgical experience increases there is a tendency to prepare less for the unlikely event of sudden conversion to open surgery. Thus in some institutions the procedure is performed in the radiology suite.

The use of the radiology suite for the provision of anaesthesia for EVAR poses several risks. The fluoroscopic equipment is often bulky, taking up much space within the room. The layout of radiology suites is rarely designed with the needs of the anaesthetist in mind as it is often cramped and may be located in a remote site. Thus the use of the radiology suite should be reserved for those cases where the operators are experienced, the procedure is deemed to be straightforward, and there is ready access to an operating theatre should it be required.

If EVAR is performed in the radiology suite it is necessary to ensure that a suitable environment is created for safe anaesthesia. Requirements include adequate equipment, drugs, and personnel similar to those normally available in a theatre suite. Also, there needs to be a well-rehearsed and workable plan for the institution of resuscitative measures and transfer to theatre if required. Everyone in the radiology suite needs to be ready to deal with the rare event of acute aortic rupture as the time from diagnosis to treatment is critical. As well as aortic rupture, situations that require transfer to operating theatre may include retroperitoneal cut down to the iliac arteries, and open repair related to a difficulty with EVAR.

Equipment

Prior to commencing EVAR several pieces of anaesthetic equipment should be considered and prepared in advance. It is important to be well prepared for rare adversities, especially during the learning curves of new practitioners.

There needs to be sufficient large bore intravenous access, availability of rapid fluid infusion systems with fluid warmers, and ready availability of blood products. Intraoperative cell salvage is not routinely required for elective EVAR as the average blood loss is only 250 to 550 mL.[10,11]

Hypothermia is known to have detrimental effects on coagulation as well as cardiovascular, respiratory, metabolic, central nervous, and neuromuscular systems. It is also a contributing factor to impairing wound healing and prolonging recovery room stay. One study reported that maintaining normothermia was associated with a reduced risk of ischaemic ECG changes in the immediate postoperative period.[12] We utilise a forced-air warming blanket in all patients undergoing EVAR. However, blood flow through the femoral arteries is interrupted during the procedure so active warming should not be applied to the lower limbs. Heel rests and other padding should be used to prevent pressure effects on ischaemic tissue and nerve entrapment where soft tissues or nerves are at risk.

It is important that all staff involved in the procedure take adequate precautions to minimize exposure to radiation. This includes the use of lead aprons, thyroid collars, and radiation goggles.

Monitoring

We use invasive blood pressure monitoring with a radial arterial line in all patients undergoing EVAR. This allows complications such as hypotension from massive blood loss or acute myocardial ischaemia to be detected earlier. Invasive monitoring also facilitates sampling of arterial blood for blood gas analysis and other tests including serial haematocrit measurement.

A 5-lead ECG monitor mode with ST segment analysis is useful for detection of ischaemic events. The routine use of a central venous catheter or pulmonary artery catheter during elective EVAR is not necessary as fluid shifts are usually minimal. We reserve central venous pressure monitoring for patients with severe cardiac disease and patients undergoing emergency surgery for aortic rupture or dissection.

A urinary catheter is helpful for monitoring intraoperative renal function, guiding fluid therapy, and avoiding discomfort due to over-distension of the bladder during prolonged procedures or when regional anaesthesia is employed.

As patients having EVAR often have multiple co-morbidities, they may fall into a group of patients with an increased risk of awareness under relaxant general anaesthesia.[13] The bispectral index (BIS), or similar hyphenated monitors of hypnotic depth, can be used with the aim of decreasing the risk of awareness. If a general anaesthetic is administered to elderly patients with cardiovascular disease, we find BIS monitoring useful to guide a reduction in the doses of anaesthetic agents and thus reduce the requirements for pharmacological support of the blood pressure.

Intraoperative management

The median duration of surgery for EVAR is around 2 hours however the procedure may be prolonged, for example during the early learning curve for proceduralists, if there is difficulty with access via the iliac arteries, or if complex procedures are undertaken such as placement of fenestrated supra-renal stents. The surgical stimulus during EVAR is mainly caused by surgical incision of the groin and insertion of the sheath through the arteriotomy. Nociceptive stimulation may also be caused by ischaemia of the limb distally and, possibly, by mechanical traction of the stent on the aortic wall. There is usually only moderate postoperative pain which is localized in the groin.

To aid fluoroscopic imaging and stent positioning it is important that the patient remains still. Breath holding for a period of around 15 to 20 seconds is useful for optimising digital subtraction angiography. This is easily achieved during general anaesthesia but if the procedure is performed with regional or local anaesthesia, the patient needs to be sufficiently cooperative to remain still. Movement from gut peristalsis also causes artefacts on digital subtraction angiograms and this can be prevented by administering intravenous hyoscine. However adequate images can usually be obtained despite normal gut peristalsis and the benefit of hyoscine must be weighed against the potential detrimental effects of tachycardia.

Historically, in early EVAR anaesthesia at our hospital, induced hypotension was often employed during stent deployment to prevent distal migration of the stent by the propulsive forces of systolic pressure, and to minimize hypertension which may occur proximal to the stent. Several methods of induced hypotension have been used in the past including increasing anaesthetic depth, short acting beta blockers such as esmolol, infusions of vasodi-

lating agents such as glyceryl trinitrate or sodium nitroprusside, and intravenous adenosine. With currently used self-expanding stents haemodynamic changes during stent deployment are rarely observed and the stent position can be adjusted without the need for systemic hypotension.

Blood loss during EVAR is usually minimal but it may be insidious and can amount to a substantial amount over time. The insertion and manipulation of access sheaths and stents through the arteriotomy can cause a steady ooze of blood, and bleeding may be brisk at times. Average estimated blood loss during the procedure is 250 to 550 mL, with the lower volumes being quoted in more recent trials.[10,11] A retrospective review by Baker et al of 100 patients from 1992 to 1996 showed that there was a fourfold increase in the incidence of death in the group of patients who had a haemoglobin level documented at <80 g/L in the intra or postoperative period.[14] The DREAM trial had a median blood loss of 250 mL, an interquartile range of 100 to 500 mL, and only 6% received an intraoperative blood transfusion.[11] Intravenous fluid requirements during EVAR are approximately 2000 to 2500 mL.[15]

Renal failure remains a risk related to EVAR. The anaesthetist can utilize several practices to minimize the risk of postoperative renal impairment. These include preoperative intravenous fluids (this has become more difficult with most patients presenting for their procedure on the day of surgery), avoiding hypovolaemia, monitoring urine output aiming to maintain a high flow of dilute urine, and minimizing the volume of radio-opaque dye used. In the DREAM trial the mean volume of intravenous contrast used was 167 mL, with an interquartile range of 120 to 200 mL.[3]

Perioperative oral N-acetylcysteine (NAC) is frequently prescribed to patients with renal impairment undergoing EVAR. A small trial in patients with normal creatinine undergoing EVAR reported significant sub-clinical renal impairment postoperatively with no difference between patients given NAC and those given placebo.[16] The evidence for a protective effect from NAC in patients at risk of contrast-induced nephropathy is equivocal.[17] However, as this therapy is inexpensive and has minimal side effects, it may be reasonable to administer it to higher-risk patients. Within our institution we administer 600 mg NAC twice daily to all patients with a preoperative creatinine greater than or equal to 130 mmol/L. This commences on the day prior to surgery, and continues if their creatinine level remains above 130 mmol/L, until they have had their postoperative CT scan on day 3.

Despite extensive study, mannitol has not been proven to prevent acute renal failure attributed to radiocontrast dye,[18] and has been shown to impair renal function more than saline does.[19] In their review of 100 patients Baker et al found that a rise in serum creatinine of greater than 100 mol/L occurred more commonly in those given mannitol than those who did not receive it (16% versus 4%).[14] Although the mechanism for a possible harmful effect from mannitol is not known, one possibility is that the diuresis causes dehydration and subsequent impairment of renal perfusion.

The extent and duration of impaired tissue perfusion is drastically reduced with EVAR compared to open surgery. However if EVAR is prolonged then the reduced perfusion of the lower limbs may produce a reperfusion response. This manifests as transient hypotension which is usually readily controlled with sympathomimetic agents. If the effect persists then the surgeon could be asked to temporarily re-occlude the femoral artery and gradually release it until the patients haemodynamic status is more effectively managed. Rarely, a complex procedure may be very prolonged, in which case leg ischaemia could cause permanent tissue damage.

Heparinization is usually requested prior to clamping of the femoral artery. This involves a bolus intravenous dose of 0.5-0.75 mg/kg (50-75 units/kg), which may be repeated if the procedure is prolonged. Deep venous thromboprophylaxis with low molecular weight heparin (LMWH) is usually commenced 6 to 8 hours after surgery. Evidence suggests that LMWH may also have a beneficial effect on the endoluminal prosthesis site.[20]

Prophylactic antibiotic therapy for vascular procedures focuses on the likely pathogens which include *Staphylococcus aureas*, *Staphylococcus epidermis*, Gram negative *bacilli* and *Enterococcus*. Usually a single intravenous dose of a third generation cephalosporin e.g. Ceftriaxone given within 1 hour prior to surgical incision is sufficient.

Postoperative management

Postoperatively most patients who have had successful EVAR may be managed in a general ward after sufficient time in recovery. The appropriate environment in which to nurse these patients may alter if they have significant co-morbidities or if the procedure is complicated. Postoperative analgesic requirements are usually minimal and regional analgesia is usually unnecessary. Pain originates from the arteriotomy sites and is often controlled with simple analgesics such as paracetamol, along with parenteral opioids if required. The patient is usually mobilized on the first postoperative day.

ANAESTHETIC TECHNIQUE

A variety of anaesthetic techniques have been utilized for EVAR including general anaesthesia, several different regional anaesthesia modalities (epidural, combined spinal epidural, and spinal anaesthesia), and local anaesthesia. During the early development of EVAR general anaesthesia was primarily used, providing ideal operating conditions with a still patient, and providing airway security in case of the need for urgent conversion to laparotomy. Early after EVAR was introduced local and regional anaesthesia were also shown to be viable anaesthetic alternatives. The perceived benefits of regional or local anaesthesia have allowed EVAR to be performed on those patients considered unfit for general anaesthesia.

General anaesthesia

When EVAR was first introduced patients were anaesthetized with a general anaesthetic technique.[21] As other modalities of anaesthesia were introduced early reports showed that most surgeons preferred their patients to have a general anaesthetic as they were more comfortable operating on a motionless patient.

Advantages
- General anaesthesia can be performed rapidly, providing control over airway and breathing, and allowing high concentrations of oxygen to be delivered.
- General anaesthesia provides an immobile patient which can be vital during stent deployment. Also it allows rapid conversion to more extensive surgery e.g. if open surgery needed. However in the EUROSTAR registry early conversion was rare amounting to 0.5% for those in whom a loco regional anaesthetic technique was used.[22]
- Hypotension may be easily induced if required by increasing inspired volatile or intravenous anaesthetic agent prior to stent deployment.

Disadvantages
- The use of induction agents such as propofol or thiopentone causes vasodilatation and decreased cardiac contractility which may compromise blood pressure.
- The volatile anaesthetic agents also cause some vasodilatation leading to hypotension.

- The hypertensive response with intubation could increase the risk of cardiac morbidity or aneurysmal rupture.
- Positive pressure ventilation can reduce cardiac output.

General anaesthesia may be the preferred option where the proceduralist is inexperienced, if the aneurysmal anatomy appears difficult, or where the risk of conversion to open repair is high.

Regional anaesthesia

Numerous trials have documented the feasibility of regional anaesthesia for EVAR.[21,22,23]

Advantages
- Regional anaesthesia preserves respiratory function.
- Regional anaesthesia has been shown to have a number of advantages over general anaesthesia for patients undergoing vascular surgery, including dampened hormonal stress response, and better peripheral circulation. Whether these advantages exist in patients having EVAR is debatable.[23,24,25] There are claims that regional anaesthesia may obtund the immune response following surgical procedures, modifying the inflammatory response syndrome seen after EVAR.[26]
- In hypertensive patients the sympathectomy produced by regional block may decrease the risk of aneurysmal rupture. Also controlled hypotension if requested prior to stent placement can be achieved by extending an epidural block.
- Regional anaesthesia may be extended to cover dissection of the iliac arteries if required.

Disadvantages
- Insertion of regional anaesthesia takes more time than that required for induction of general anaesthesia.
- It may be difficult for the patient to lie

still for the sometimes unpredictable duration of the procedure.

- Regional analgesia is rarely required postoperatively for EVAR.
- The sympathectomy caused by regional blockade produces several concerns. Regional anaesthesia is contraindicated for emergency aneurysm surgery with haemodynamic instability. Also if general anaesthesia is required abruptly after regional blockade, for example for aneurysmal rupture, the sympathetic blockade could create a cycle of hypotension without physiological compensation.
- Vasculopathic patients are often taking anticoagulant medications, and considering the need for the intraoperative administration of intravenous heparin, there may be an increased risk of neuraxial haematoma. The motor and sensory deficits caused by regional techniques may also mask the presentation of a neuraxial haematoma.

Anticoagulation and neuraxial anaesthesia

Attention should be paid to existing guidelines regarding administration of anticoagulants and the timing of regional blockade and catheter removal as neuraxial haematoma can lead to catastrophic and irreversible paralysis.[27,28] At least 3 societies have published official guidelines for thromboembolism prophylaxis and regional anaesthesia. These include the American Society of Regional Anesthesia and Pain Medicine,[29] the German Society of Anesthesiology and Intensive Care Medicine,[30] and the Spanish Consensus Forum.[31] However, whilst clear guidelines exist there needs to be a good understanding of the complexity of this issue. 40% of patients in the DREAM trial were taking antiplatelet therapy, whilst 10-15% were taking anticoagulants.[11] Often there will be interplay between a number of medications, including herbal therapies, and the patients underlying coagulation

status. It is important to perform a careful preoperative assessment of the patient regarding bleeding or bruising tendency, and other factors which could contribute to bleeding. Ultimately the benefits and risks of performing neuraxial anaesthesia should be considered on an individual basis, particularly as alternative anaesthetic and analgesic techniques exist for EVAR.

Regional anaesthesia may be particularly useful in those patients with respiratory compromise or those deemed unfit for general anaesthesia. Whilst several different modes of regional anaesthesia have been used, it may be wise to avoid a single shot spinal technique when there are concerns that the duration of the procedure may exceed that of the block.

Local anaesthesia

Local anaesthetic techniques in conjunction with sedation have been successfully used for EVAR. It has proved particularly useful in the initial anaesthetic management of a ruptured AAA having EVAR. The incidence of procedures performed with local anaesthesia varies considerably between institutions and between different countries. EVAR has been less commonly performed under local anaesthesia in the United States, possibly related to a publication by De Virgilio et al which did not find a positive effect of local anaesthesia with regard to cardiopulmonary morbidity and mortality.[22,32]

To date the largest published series of EVAR with local anaesthesia was by Verhoeven et al who have described the details of their technique.[33] They reported that local anaesthesia was well tolerated. In the study of 239 patients having EVAR, the strategy was to use local anaesthesia for all the procedures. Absolute exclusion criteria for local anaesthesia were the need for an additional retroperitoneal approach to the aorta or iliac arteries, the need for associated abdominal procedures (e.g. umbilical hernia repair), and patients choice. Relative exclusion criteria were patient anxiety, groin re-explorations, and a body mass index >30 kg/m^2. Using these criteria 170 of the 239 patients were treated with local anaesthesia. Verhoeven et al noted that in order to achieve good results with a local anaesthetic technique for EVAR the patients require detailed information and preparation, careful dissection with slow insertion of the main delivery sheath, the early restoration of blood flow to the lower extremities, and a short operating time of less than 2 hours.

Advantages

- Local anaesthesia is relatively simple to perform and provides better maintenance of haemodynamic stability which is particularly useful for emergency EVAR.
- Local anaesthesia provides better preservation of respiratory function than with either general or neuraxial anaesthesia.
- Overstretching of the arterial system by the delivery sheath may induce discomfort which may alert the physician to the risk of injury or rupture.

Disadvantages

- It may be uncomfortable for the patient to lie motionless during EVAR.
- Abdominal pain may occur during instrumentation of the aorta, and pain may arise related to lower limb ischaemia.
- More extensive surgery is not possible with local anaesthesia.

Comparison of anaesthetic techniques

Numerous studies have allowed comparisons to be drawn between the different anaesthetic approaches, however there is no level one evidence indicating whether the choice of anaesthetic technique affects patient outcomes. There are no prospective randomized controlled trials com-

paring the different anaesthetic modalities for EVAR. As always the type of anaesthetic used should be that considered safest for the patient taking in to account their clinical state, the potential for surgical difficulty, and the skills of the anaesthetist. In the DREAM trial 52% of patients having EVAR had a general anaesthetic, 5% had a combination of general and regional anaesthesia, 40% had a regional anaesthetic alone, and just over 5% had the procedure performed under local anaesthesia.[11] Of the three authors of this chapter, one uses epidural anaesthesia almost exclusively and one uses general anaesthesia almost exclusively.

A retrospective review of postoperative events after EVAR in 5,557 patients from the EUROSTAR Registry reported an association between anaesthetic technique and patient outcomes.[22] Duration of operation, frequency of ICU admissions, duration of hospital stay, and frequency of complications were all lowest in patients given a local anaesthetic. Outcomes were worst in patients given a general anaesthetic and the patients given a regional anaesthetic were intermediate between the other two groups. The results of this non-randomised trial must be interpreted carefully. The majority of patients operated under local anaesthesia were from a single centre. Also, selection bias probably influenced the results; for example patients in the local anaesthesia group had less complex aneurysms requiring fewer additional procedures.

With regards to open abdominal surgery, several trials have examined the potential advantages of combined epidural and general anaesthesia over general anaesthesia alone. The most influential include a cumulative meta-analysis of randomized controlled trials by Ballantyne in 1998,[34] the Veterans Affairs Study 2001,[35] and the MASTER study 2002.[36] The Veterans Affairs Study showed no overall difference between the two groups. However, a retrospectively defined subgroup who had open AAA surgery were noted to have lower mortality and major morbidity in the epidural group. The MASTER study also found that mortality was the same in both groups, but that there was less pain in the epidural group over the first 72 hours.[36] The initial report of the MASTER trial indicated less respiratory failure in the epidural group, however in a subsequent analysis it was reported that the difference was not clinically significant.[37] It is unlikely that the purported advantages of epidurals over general anaesthesia noted in the above trials hold true in the case of EVAR because of its significantly less invasive nature when compared to laparotomy and the lack of significant postoperative pain after EVAR.

Emergency endovascular repair of acute abdominal aortic aneurysm

The use of endovascular techniques for the repair of acute AAAs was first described in 1994.[38] Recently this technique has become routine practice in Europe and is being increasingly performed in the US. Most experience suggests a potential for improved perioperative patient survival with endovascular repair than after open repair.[22,38,39] EVAR is less invasive and less traumatic, the duration of the procedure is shorter, there is less blood loss - sudden decompression of intra-abdominal pressure associated with opening the abdomen being avoided, there is greater intraoperative cardiopulmonary stability, and a faster recovery.[40] The mean ICU stay is shorter,[41] whilst the overall hospital stay is variable. Also unlike the cost analysis of elective AAA repair, there may be a significant reduction in hospital costs with endovascular repair compared to open repair of acute AAA. Visser et al, after 1 year follow up, have shown that the cost for endovascular repair was Euro 23,588 versus Euro 36,488 for open repair.[42] Also the use of EVAR for the management of an acute AAA allows the use or regional and local anaesthesia.

Anaesthesia for emergency EVAR differs from that of elective EVAR in several ways. The urgency of the procedure does not allow for a thorough assessment of the patients co-morbidities and there needs to be urgent preparation for massive blood loss. Control of blood pressure becomes even more critical with ruptured aortic aneurysms to minimize blood loss and optimize organ perfusion. Several recent studies have indicated that aggressive volume resuscitation may be detrimental in the presence of an uncontrolled vascular injury.[43,44] The increased blood pressure may lead to dislodgement of clot, free rupture of the aneurysm and increased bleeding. Also the haemodilution from intravenous fluid administration may increase coagulopathies. In a study by Ohki and Veith fluid resuscitation was limited to patients in whom the systolic blood pressure fell to less than 50 mmHg.[45]

General, regional, and local anaesthetic techniques have all been used for emergency EVAR, however in those with haemodynamic instability regional anaesthesia is contraindicated. Within our institution roughly 80% of those emergency AAA repairs that make it to the operating theatre are amenable to EVAR. These are all managed initially with local anaesthetic in the presence of an anaesthetist with full haemodynamic monitoring. Once control of the leak is established and the patients condition is stable we convert to a general anaesthetic.

SUMMARY

Endovascular aneurysm repair represents an advance in the surgical care of abdominal aortic aneurysms. The technique is becoming increasingly common as grafts continue to progress, proceduralists skills improve, and through being established as a safe and effective way of managing aortic aneurysms.

Anaesthetists need to have a good understanding of the surgical complexities of the procedure, and need to be well prepared for dealing with rare catastrophes. They need to be aware of the potential advantages of EVAR, (including reduced morbidity and mortality, reduced physiological stresses, shorter duration times, and more rapid postoperative recovery) and its disadvantages (including the need for more technical equipment, likely increased cost, and the need for long term follow up). EVAR provides the possibility of surgical correction in those patients considered as an excessive risk for open repair or general anaesthesia.

Many vasculopathic patients presenting for EVAR are so medically compromised that they pose major anaesthetic challenges. They necessitate a thorough preoperative assessment and comprehensive perioperative management.

General, regional, and local anaesthetics have all proved to be acceptable techniques for EVAR. Each technique has particular advantages and disadvantages. Those studies which have compared the benefits of each are likely to have been affected by patient selection. Ultimately a prospective multicentre randomized controlled trial may clarify which anaesthetic technique is most beneficial. We feel that it is important to be able to utilize each technique. This allows for the best anaesthetic technique to be used taking in to account the patients co-morbidities, the skills of the proceduralist, the skills of the anaesthetist, and the type of surgery being performed.

REFERENCES

1. Moore, Wesley S: Repair of abdominal aortic aneurysm by transfemoral endovascular graft placement. Ann Surg 1994 Sep, 220(3):331-9.

2. Greenhalgh RM: Comparison of endovascular aneurysm repair with open repair in patients with abdominal aortic aneurysm (EVAR trial 1), 30-day operative mortality results: randomized controlled trial. Lancet 2004, 364:843-48.

3. Blankensteijn JD, de Jong SE, Prinssen M, van der Ham AC, Buth J, van Sterkenburg SM, Verhagen HJM, Buskens E, Grobbee DE: Two year outcomes after conventional or endovascular repair of abdominal aortic aneurysms. N Engl J Med 2005, 352:2398-405.

4. Singh K, Bonaa KH, Jacobsen BK, Bjork L, Solberg S: Prevalence of and risk factors for abdominal aortic aneurysms in a population based study: The Tromso Study. Am J Epidemiol 2001 Aug, 154(3):236-44.

5. Clark NJ, Stanley TH: Anesthesia for vascular surgery. Miller RD Anesthesia, 4th edition. New York: Churchill Livingstone; 1994:1851-1895.

6. ACC/AHA Task Force on Practice Guidelines: ACC/AHA guidelines for perioperative cardiovascular evaluation for noncardiac surgery. Circulation 1996, 93:1280-1317.

7. Committee to Update the 1996 Guidelines on Perioperative Cardiovascular Evaluation for Noncardiac Surgery: ACC/AHA Guideline Update for Perioperative Cardiovascular Evaluation for Noncardiac Surgery-Executive Summary: A Report of the American College of Cardiology/American Heart Association Task Force on Practice Guidelines. Circulation 2002 March, 105(10):1257-1267.

8. Hertzer NR: Basic data concerning associated coronary disease in peripheral vascular patients. Annals of Vascular Surgery 1987 Dec, 1(5):616-20.

9. Howard-Alpe GM, de Bono J, Hudsmith L, Orr WP, Foex P, Sear JW: Coronary artery stents and non-cardiac surgery. British Journal of Anaesthesia 2007, 98(5):560-74.

10. May J, White GH, Yu W, Ly CN, Waugh R, Stephen MS, Arulchelvam M, Harris JP: Concurrent comparison of endoluminal versus open repair in the treatment of abdominal aortic aneurysms: analysis of 303 patients by life table method. Journal of Vascular Surgery 1998, 27:213-221.

11. Prinssen M, Verhoeven ELG, MD, Buth J, Cuypers PWM, Sambeek MRHM, Balm R, Erik B,

Grobbee DE, Blankensteitn JD for the Dutch Randomized Endovascular Aneurysm Management (DREAM) Trial Group: A Randomized Trial Comparing Conventional and endovascular Repair of Abdominal Aortic Aneurysms. NEJM 2004 Oct, 351:1607-1618.

12. Frank SM, Fleisher LA, Breslow MJ, Higgins MS, Olson KF, Kelly S, Beattie C: Perioperative maintenance of normothermia reduces the incidence of morbid cardiac events: a randomized clinical trial. Journal of the American Medical Association 1997, 277:1127-1134.

13. Myles PS, Leslie K, McNeil J, Forbes A, Chan MTV, and for the B-Aware trial group: Bispectral index monitoring to prevent awareness during anaesthesia: the B-Aware randomised controlled trial. Lancet 2004 May 29, 363(9423):1757-1763.

14. Baker AB, Lloyd G, Fraser TA, Bookallil MJ, Yezerski SD: Retrospective review of 100 cases of endoluminal aortic stent-graft surgery from an anaesthetic perspective. Anaesthesia and Intensive Care 1997, 25:378-384.

15. Henretta JP, Hodgson KJ, Mattos MA, Karch LA, Hurlbert SN, Sternbach Y, Ramsey DE, Sumner DS: Feasibility of endovascular repair of abdominal aortic aneurysms with local anesthesia with intravenous sedation. Journal of Vascular Surgery 1999 May, 29(5):793-8.

16. Moore NN, Lapsley M, Norden AG, Firth JD, Gaunt ME, Varty K, Boyle JR: Does N-Acetylcysteine Prevent Contrast-Induced Nephropathy During Endovascular AAA repair? A Randomized Controlled Pilot Study. Journal of Endovascular Therapy: Official Journal of the International Society of Endovascular Specialists 2006 Oct,13(5):660-666.

17. Bagshaw SM, McAlister FA, Manns BJ, Ghali WA: Acetylcysteine in the prevention of contrast-induced nephropathy: a case study of the pitfalls in the evolution of evidence. Archives of Internal Medicine 2006 Jan 23, 166(2):161-6.

18. Carmichael P, Carmichael AR: Acute renal failure in the surgical setting. Aust NZ J Surg 2003, 73:144-153.

19. Solomon R, Werner C, Mann D, D'Elia J, Silva P: Effects of saline, mannitol and furosemide on acute decreases in renal function induced by radiocontrast agents. New England Journal of Medicine 1994, 331:1416-1420.

20. Ross A: HART-II (a randomized comparison of low-molecular-weight heparin and unfractionated heparin adjunctive to t-PA thrombolysis and aspirin). Clinical Cardiology 2000, 23:384.

21. Aadahl P, Lundbom J, Hatlinhus S, Myhre HO: Regional anaesthesia for endovascular treatment of abdominal aortic aneurysms. Journal of Endovascular Surgery, 4(1):56-61.

22. Ruppert V, Leurs LJ, Steckmeier B, Buth J, Umscheid T: Influence of anesthesia type on outcome after endovascular aortic aneurysm repair. An analysis based on EUROSTAR data. J Vasc Surg 2006, 44:16-21.

23. Cao P, Zannetti S, Parlani G, Verzini F, Caporali S, Spaccatini A, Barzi F: Epidural anesthesia reduces length of hospitalization after endoluminal abdominal aortic aneurysm repair. Journal of Vascular Surgery 1999 Oct, 30(4):651-7.

24. Yeager MP, Glass DD, Neff RK, Brinck-Johnsen T: Epidural anesthesia and analgesia in high risk surgical patients. Anesthesiology 1987, 66:729-736.

25. Modig J: Regional anaesthesia and blood loss. Acta Anaestesiologica Scand 1988, 32(89):44-48.

26. Kehlet H: Epidural analgesia and the endocrine-metabolic response to surgery: update and perspectives. Acta Anesthesiol Scand 1984, 28:125-127.

27. Tryba M: Ruckmarksnahe regionalanasthesie und niedermoekulare heparine: Pro. Anasth Intensivmed Notfallmed Schmertzer 1993, 28:179-181.

28. Vandermeulen EP, Van Aken H, Vermylen J: Anticoagulants and spinal-epidural anesthesia: A closed claims analysis. Anesthesiology 1999, 90:1062-1069.

29. Horlocker TT, Wedel DJ, Benzon H, Brown DL, Kayser Enneking F, Heit JA, Mulroy MF, Rosenquist RW, Rowlingson J, Tryba M, et al: Regional anesthesia in the anticoagulated patient: Defining the risks (The Second ASRA Consensus Conference on Neuraxial Anesthesia and Anticoagulation). Regional Anesthesia & Pain Medicine 2003, 28(3):172-197.

30. Gogarten W, Van Aken H, Wulf H, Klose R, Vandermeulen E, Harenberg J: Regional anesthesia and thromboembolism prophylaxis/anticoagulation. Anaesthesiol Intensivmed 1997, 12:623-628.

31. Llau JV, de Andres J, Gomar C, Gomez A, Hidalgo F, Sahagun J, Torres LM: Drugs that alter hae-

mostasis and regional anaesthetic techniques: Safety guidelines. Consensus conference. Rev Esp Anestesiol Reanim 2001, 48:270-278.

32. De Virgilio C, Romero L, Donayre C, Meek K, Lewis RJ, Lippmann M, Rodriguez C, White R: Endovascular abdominal aortic aneurysm repair with general versus local anesthesia: a comparison of cardiopulmonary morbidity and mortality rates. Journal of Vascular Surgery 2002 Nov, 36(5):988-91.

33. Verhoeven EL, Cina CS, Tielliu IF, Zeebregts CJ, Prins TR, Eindhoven GB, Span MM, Kapma MR, van den Dungen JJ: Local anesthesia for endovascular abdominal aortic aneurysm repair. Journal of Vascular Surgery 2005 Sep, 42(3):402-9.

34. Ballantyne JC, Carr DB, deFerranti S, Suarez T, Lau J, Chalmers TC, Angelillo IF, Mosteller F: The comparative effects of postoperative analgesic therapies on pulmonary outcome: cumulative meta-analyses of randomized, controlled trials. Anesthesia & Analgesia 1998 Mar, 86(3):598-612.

35. Park WJ, Thompson JS, Lee KK, and the Department of Veterans Affairs Cooperative Study #345 Study Group: Effect of epidural anesthesia and analgesia on perioperative outcome: a randomized, controlled veterans Affairs cooperative study. Ann Surg 2001, 234:560-9.

36. Rigg JR, Jamrozik K, Myles PS, Silbert BS, Peyton PJ, Parsons RW, Collins KS, MASTER Anaesthesia Trial Study Group: Epidural anaesthesia and analgesia and outcome of major surgery: a randomised trial. Lancet 2002 Apr 13, 359(9314):1276-82.

37. Peyton PJ, Myles PS, Silbert BS, Rigg JA, Jamrozik K, Parsons R: Perioperative epidural analgesia and outcome after major abdominal surgery in high-risk patients. Anesthesia & Analgesia 2003 Feb, 96(2):548-554.

38. Yusuf SW, Whitaker SC, Chuter TA, Wenham PW, Hopkinson BR: Emergency endovascular repair of leaking aortic aneurysm. Lancet 1994 Dec 10, 344(8937):1645.

39. Lee WA. Huber TS. Hirneise CM. Berceli SA. Seeger JM: Eligibility rates of ruptured and symptomatic AAA for endovascular repair. Journal of Endovascular Therapy: Official Journal of the International Society of Endovascular Specialists 2002 Aug, 9(4):436-42.

40. Scharrer-Pamler R, Kotsis T, Kapfer X, Gorich J, Sunder-Plassmann L: Endovascular stent-graft repair of ruptured aortic aneurysms. Journal of Endovascular Therapy: Official Journal of the International Society of Endovascular Specialists 2003 Jun, 10(3):447-52.

41. van Sambeek MR, van Dijk LC, Hendriks JM, van Grotel M, Kuiper JW, Pattynama PM, van Urk H: Endovascular versus conventional open repair of acute abdominal aortic aneurysm: feasibility and preliminary results. Journal of Endovascular Therapy: Official Journal of the International Society of Endovascular Specialists 2002 Aug, 9(4):443-8.

42. Visser JJ, van Sambeek MR, Hunink MG, Redekop WK, van Dijk LC, Hendriks JM, Bosch JL: Acute abdominal aortic aneurysms: cost analysis of endovascular repair and open surgery in hemodynamically stable patients with 1-year follow-up. Radiology 2006 Sep, 240(3):681-9.

43. Stern SA, Dronen SC, Birrer P, Wang X: Effect of blood pressure on hemorrhage volume and survival in a near-fatal hemorrhage model incorporating a vascular injury. Ann Emerg Med 1993, 22 (2):155-163.

44. Bickell WH, Bruttig SP, Millnamow GA, O'Benar J, Wade CE: The detrimental effects of intravenous crystalloid after aortotomy in swine. Surgery 1991, 110: 529-536.

45. Ohki T, Veith FJ: Endovascular grafts and other image-guided catheter-based adjuncts to improve the treatment of ruptured aortoiliac aneurysms. Annals of Surgery 2000 Oct, 232(4):466-79.

Contrast induced nephropathy during EVAR: Managing patients with increased creatinine levels

Manish Mehta, Frank J. Veith

INTRODUCTION

Endovascular aneurysm repair (EVAR) with intra-arterial contrast agents has become an established method for treating aortoiliac aneurysms. EVAR requires intra-arterial administration of radiographic contrast agents that are cleared from the body by glomerular filtration without any appreciable renal tubular reabsorption. Although numerous risk factors for the development of intra-arterial contrast agent induced nephropathy have been suggested, only the presence of pre-existing renal insufficiency has been directly correlated with the development of complications renal failure. Furthermore, in patients with normal renal function contrast agent related nephropathy is secondary to acute tubular necrosis which is usually self limiting, and therefore this chapter will focus on patients with chronic renal insufficiency (CRI) and elevated creatinine levels undergoing EVAR.

CRI increases the risks of contrast-induced nephrotoxicity.[1] High osmolar contrast agents, nephrotoxic drugs, diabetes mellitus, and dehydration further increase the risks of worsening renal failure.[2,3] Renal insufficiency is a well-recognized complication after open AAA repair; the inci-

dence of worsening renal function in patients undergoing open surgical AAA repair with normal preoperative renal function is approximately 5%, and increases two-to-threefold in patients with pre-existing renal insufficiency.[4,5] Since EVAR requires the use of contrast agents during the procedure as well as during life-long surveillance with computed tomography (CT) scans, CRI is also considered to be a relative contraindication and might further increase the risks for EVAR. We reviewed a five year experience with EVAR to determine how best to manage patients undergoing EVAR with elevated pre-existing CRI.

MATERIALS AND METHODS

Over a five year period, all patients with abdominal aortic aneurysms (AAAs) larger than 5.0 cm in diameter, with and without iliac involvement, that were eligible for EVAR were offered treatment with a variety of industry and surgeon-made endografts including Vanguard (Boston Scientific, Natick, MA), Talent (Medtronic, Sunrise, FL), Ancure (Guidant-EVT, Menlo Park, CA), AneuRx (Medtronic, Sunrise, FL), Excluder (WL Gore, Flagstaff, AZ), and Zenith (Cook, Bloomington, IN), and Montefiore Endovascular Grafting System (MEGS). Our techniques for EVAR have been described elsewhere.[6] Briefly, the endografts were fixed proximally just below the renal arteries, and distal fixation sites were either the common iliac, external iliac, or femoral arteries. When AIAs extended up to the iliac bifurcation, Gianturco coils (Cook, Bloomington, IN) were used to exclude flow to the hypogastric arteries, either preoperatively or intraoperatively. Routine precautions in patients with pre-existing CRI included the following: 1) preoperative intravenous hydration with 2 liters of normal saline, 2) discontinuation of all nephrotoxic drugs, 3) intraoperative us of Mannitol (0.5 gm/kg, IV), and 4) use of nonionic, low-osmolar intra-arterial contrast agent (Omnipaque-350). Furthermore, to limit the cumulative nephrotoxic effects of intravascular contrast agents, pre- and peri-operative imaging including CT scans, arteriograms, and EVAR were routinely staged at least 2 weeks apart. Although low-osmolar intra-arterial contrast agent (Omnipaque-350) was also routinely used in all patients, the use of Mannitol and preoperative intravenous hydration was not standard protocol in patients with normal preoperative serum creatinine values (Group I).

The charts, operative reports, and laboratory data were reviewed. In the initial postoperative period, serum creatinine (Cr., mg/dl) levels were measured on postoperative day 1 and 2. Patients with worsening renal function, illustrated by an increase in serum Cr. level, were followed with daily serum Cr. measurements until the acute tubular necrosis (ATN) resolved or improved. In such patients, serum Cr. levels were also measured on their postoperative office visit at 1-2 weeks. Cr.-clearance indicated measure of glomerular filtration rate (GFR) and was calculated using the Cockroft formula: [GFR = {(140-age) x Weight (kg)}/{0.81 x Serum Cr. (micromol/liter)}]. The patients were retrospectively assigned to 3 groups based on their pre-operative serum Cr. levels; Group I (n = 108) had Cr. <1.5 (normal range), Group II (n=65) had Cr. 1.5-2.0, and Group III (n = 27) had Cr. 2.1-3.5 without a history of hemodialysis (Table 1). The exclusion criteria included patients with pre-existing CRI on hemodialysis, and those requiring renal angioplasty and stent for symptomatic high grade renal artery stenosis. Analysis included Fischer's Exact test, and univariate/ multivariate analysis using binary logistic regression. All tests were two tailed and tested at the alpha = 0.05 level.

TABLE 1
DEMOGRAPHICS AND PREOPERATIVE RISK FACTORS FOR PATIENTS UNDERGOING EVAR

	Group I	Group II	Group III
Preop. Cr (mg/dl)	<1.5	1.5 - 2.0	2.1 - 3.5
Number of Patients	108	65	27
Male	91 (84%)	54 (83%)	21 (78%)
Female	17 (16%)	11 (17%)	6 (22%)
Diabetes Mellitus	27 (25%)	23 (35%)	13 (48%)
Hypertension	42 (39%)	30 (46%)	14 (52%)
Coronary Artery Disease	55 (51%)	32 (49%)	16 (59%)

RESULTS

Over the 5-year period, 200 patients underwent EVAR with the use of intra-arterial contrast agents. Of these, 108 patients had normal renal function (Group I) and 92 had pre-existing chronic renal insufficiency with a baseline Cr. ranging from 1.5-2.0 mg/dl (Group II: n = 65) and from 2.1-3.5 mg/dl (Group III: n = 27). The average age was 72.2 years, and comorbidities included coronary artery disease (Group I: 51%, Group II: 49%, Group III: 59%), hypertension (Group I: 39%, Group II: 46%, Group III: 52%), and diabetes mellitus (Group I: 25%, Group II: 35%, Group III: 48%) (Table 1). The mean aortic and iliac aneurysm diameters were 6.2 cm and 4.2 cm, respectively. Intraoperative hemodynamic instability, defined as systolic blood pressure <80 mmHg or >40% drop below normal for more than 10 minutes, and the amount of non-ionic low-osmolar contrast used during EVAR are listed in Table 2. On postoperative follow-up at 1 to 2 weeks, serum Cr. levels were routinely checked, and none of the patients with normal serum Cr. at hospital discharge presented with a delayed rise in their serum Cr. values.

The rate of postoperative complications between the 3 study groups was not significantly different (p = NS). Perioperative serum Cr. for individual patient and the mean Cr. -clearance for each group is depicted in Figures 1 and 2. In Group I, a transient increase in serum Cr. (>30% over baseline and >1.4 mg/dl) was noted in 3 patients (2.7%), 2 patients (1.9%) required temporary hemodialysis, and 1 patient (0.9%) died with renal failure. In Group II, a transient increase in serum Cr. was noted in 2 patients (3.1%), 2 patients (3.1%) required temporary hemodialysis, and 1 patient (1.5%) died with renal failure. In Group III, a transient increase in serum Cr. was noted in 2 patients (7.4%), 1 patient (3.7%) required temporary hemodialysis, and 1 patient (3.7%) died with renal failure (Table 3). The overall 30-day mortality secondary to causes other than renal failure was 3.7% (Group I), 4.5% (Group II), and 3.7% (Group III). Univariate analysis failed to indicate coronary artery disease, hypertension, and diabetes mellitus as significant risk factors for worsening renal insufficiency or death. Univariate and multi-variate analysis indicated 2 independent risk factors that had a significant negative impact on worsening CRI: 1) presence of perioperative hypotension, and 2) the use of larger contrast volumes. Furthermore, only the presence of pre-existing CRI increased the risk of dialysis (P <0.05), and perioperative hypotension increased the risk of death (P <0.03) (Table 4).

TABLE 2

INTRAOPERATIVE RISK FACTORS FOR PATIENTS UNDERGOING EVAR. INTRA-ARTERIAL CONTRAST AGENT (MEAN VOLUME): OMNIPAQUE-350

	Group I	Group II	Group III
Preop. Cr (mg/dl)	<1.5	1.5 - 2.0	2.1 - 3.5
Number of Patients	108	65	27
Amount of Intra-Arterial Contrast	210 cc	160 cc	130 cc
Intraoperative Hemodynamic Instability	3	1	1

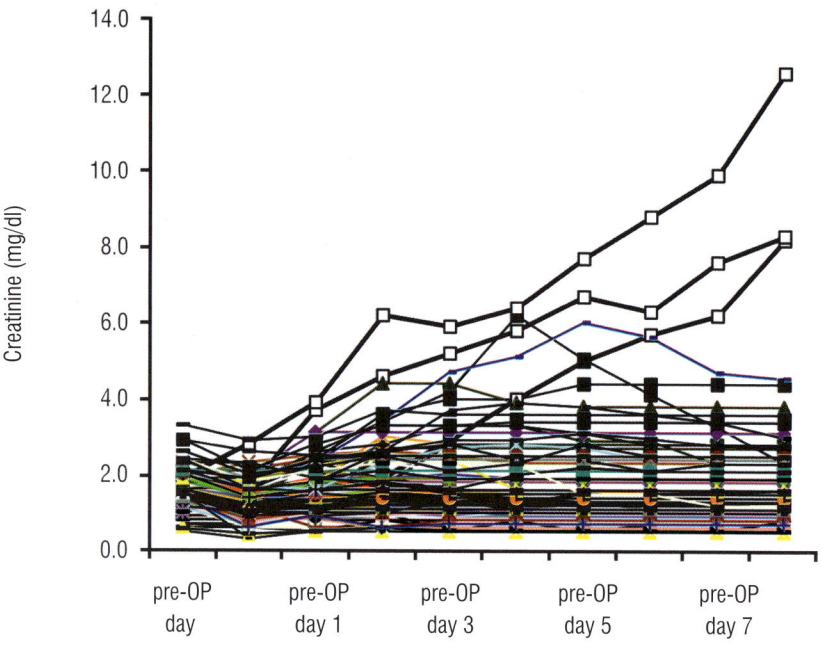

FIGURE 1: Serum creatinine levels for individual patients in the perioperative period.

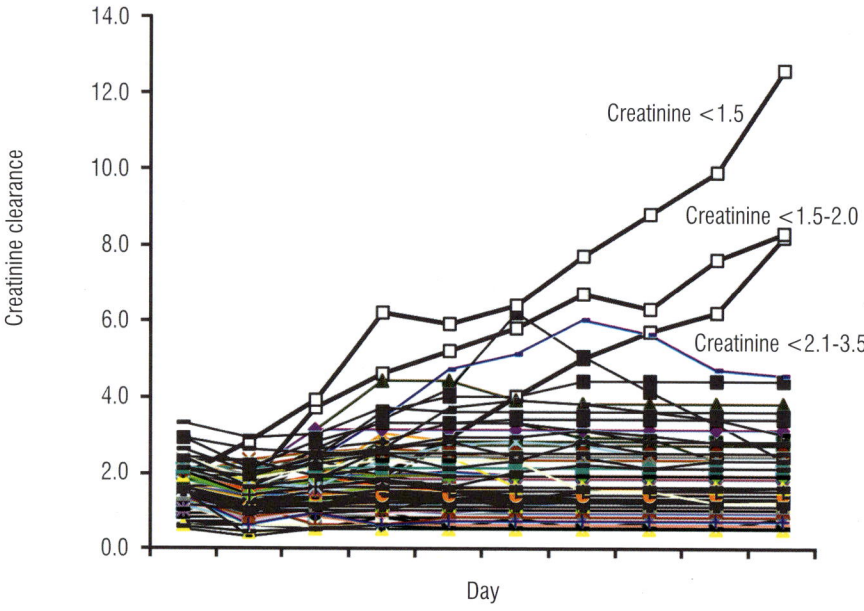

FIGURE 2: Mean Cr-Clearance in the perioperative period. Group I: Creatinine <1.5, Group II: Creatinine 1.5 - 2.0, Group III: Creatinine 2.1 - 3.5

TABLE 3

RENAL COMPLICATIONS AND MORTALITY FOLLOWING EVAR. * TRANSIENT INCREASE >30% OVER BASELINE AND >1.4 MG/DL, BG: BETWEEN GROUPS. IN A MULTIVARIATE ANALYSIS COMPARING THE 3 GROUPS, THE POWER IS LESS THAN 12%, AND THE TYPE 2 ERROR IS GREATER THAN 0.88

	Group I	Group II	Group III	P-value
Preop. Cr (mg/dl)	<1.5	1.5 - 2.0	2.1 - 3.5	BG
Number of Patients	108	65	27	
Postop. Cr Increase*	3 (2.7%)	2 (3.1%)	2 (7.4%)	NS
Temporary Postop. Dialysis	2 (1.9%)	2 (3.1%)	1 (3.7%)	NS
Death & Renal Failure	1 (0.9%)	1 (1.5%)	1 (3.7%)	NS
Death without Renal Failure	4 (3.7%)	3 (4.5%)	1 (3.7%)	NS

DISCUSSION

Chronic renal insufficiency increases the frequency of contrast induced nephrotoxicity. High-osmolar contrast agents, dehydration, nephrotoxic drugs, and diabetes mellitus further increase the risk of worsening renal failure.[7-9] Renal insufficiency is a well-recognized complication following open AAA repair, albeit its incidence following EVAR remains poorly documented.

The incidence of worsening renal function in patients undergoing open surgical AAA repair with normal preoperative renal function is 5.4%, and it increases 2 to 3-fold in patients with pre-existing CRI.[10,11] In a recent report, the mortality with associated renal failure in patients undergoing EVAR with and without pre-existing CRI was 47% and 3%, respectively.[12] Contrary to that report, the findings of the present study show that with perioperative precautions

TABLE 4

UNIVARIATE ANALYSIS: BINARY LOGISTIC REGRESSION. THE EFFECTS OF PREEXISTING COMORBIDITIES (CAD: CORONARY ARTERY DISEASE, HTN: HYPERTIONSION, DM: DIABETES MELLITUS, CRI: CHRONIC RENAL INSUFFICIENCY), PERIOPERATIVE HYPOTENSION, AND CONTRAST VOLUMES (50 CC INCREMENTS) ON WORSENING RENAL FUNCTION AND DEATH

	Increased Serum Cr		Dialysis		30-day Mortality	
	P-value	Odds Ratio	P-value	Odds Ratio	P-value	Odds Ratio
CAD	0.5	1.5	0.4	2.1	0.6	0.8
HTN	0.6	0.8	0.5	1.9	0.6	1.4
DM	0.6	1.4	0.4	1.9	0.5	0.5
CRI	0.4	1.6	0.02	5.0	0.2	2.1
Hypotension	0.001	9.1	0.1	2.1	0.03	4.8
Contrast Volume	0.001	1.6	0.8	1.0	0.4	0.9

including adequate intravenous hydration, use of low-osmolar contrast agents, avoidance of nephrotoxic drugs, and the use of Mannitol to promote diuresis, the risks of worsening renal failure is low and not significantly increased in patients with pre-existing CRI, when compared to those with normal renal function.

Endovascular aneurysm repair requires the administration of intra-arterial contrast agents that have the potential to produce hemodynamic changes in the kidney within 24-48 hours. The contrast agents induce renal vasoconstriction and interfere with water and sodium absorption by the renal tubules leading to an increase in renal vascular resistance and a decrease in the glomerular filtration rate, respectively.[13] The subsequent renal failure manifests itself as an increase in serum Cr. and a decrease in Cr.-clearance. CRI prolongs the elimination half-life of the contrast agents leading to increased renal exposure and nephrotoxicity. Patients with CRI, particularly in association with diabetic nephropathy and dehydration, are increasingly susceptible to the deleterious effects of intra-arterial contrast agents. Low-osmolar non-ionic contrast agents result in diminished reductions in renal blood flow and are associated with reduced adverse effects, when compared to high-osmolar ionic contrast agents.[9,14] The association between contrast volume and nephrotoxicity remains controversial. While some investigators have reported a significant correlation, others have found no relationship.[8,9] During our earlier experience with EVAR much larger volumes of contrast agents were used. However, over the past 2 years we have developed a number of methods to decrease contrast load in all patients, these include: 1) use of an automated volume controllable power injector to deliver intra-arterial contrast (Acist, Eden Praire, MN), 2) performing arteriography only with minimal contrast volumes after the device is in place, near the level of the renal arter-

ies, and 3) not performing contrast imaging within two weeks of the procedure.

We have adopted several strategies to reduce the amount of contrast used during EVAR. Bony lumbar vertebral landmarks are used to approximate the level of renal arteries (usually lumbar vertebrae 1-2) and position the main-body of the modular stentgraft. Automated power injectors are used to infuse low volumes of contrast agents (5-10 cc) delivered at high flow-rates (5 cc contrast @ 25 - 30 ml/sec) to mark the positions of the renal arteries. AIAs length and diameter measurements can be based on preoperative computed tomography (CT) and arteriograms. When preoperative imaging for EVAR evaluation includes only CT or magnetic resonance angiography, which is often the case in patients with pre-existing CRI, adequate intraoperative arteriograms can be obtained using as little as 15 cc of contrast agent and optimizing digital subtraction techniques. Following deployment of the main-body and cannulation of the contralateral limb, once again <10 cc of contrast can be used to mark the position of the contralateral hypogastric artery. Finally, a completion arteriogram to evaluate the adequacy of proximal and distal fixation, and the presence of endoleaks, generally requires 20-25 cc of contrast. Although with limited contrast utilization, visualization of Type II endoleaks might be inadequate, these require no further treatment during the EVAR and in patients with pre-existing CRI excessive use of contrast should be avoided.

In our experience, using less than 20 cc of contrast to evaluate endoleaks, particularly Type II and Type IV generates suboptimal images, and requires repeat arteriogram. If adequate intraoperative digital subtraction imaging is available, non-nephrotoxic Gadolinium based contrast agents can generate adequate images. In cases when low contrast volumes fail to produce adequate opacification, dilute low-osmolar non-ionic contrast agents (50:50 mixtures) can be used to further enhance the digital subtraction imaging. Although Gadolinium based contrast agents have been used over the past decade to enhance imaging in patients with CRI, recently, the administration of Gadolinium based contrast agents has been associated with a severe, potentially fatal, adverse reaction, termed nephrogenic systemic fibrosis (NSF), in patients with moderate-to-severe renal insufficiency.[25] A combination of factors, including altered renal function with elevated Cr., inflammatory burden, and exposure to Gadolinium based contrast agents may all play a role in development of NSF, and alternative contrast agents should be considered in patients with these risk factors.

In a prospective, placebo controlled, randomized trial involving patients with CRI who were at risk for contrast induced renal damage, Acetylcysteine (Mucomyst) has been shown to be beneficial in preventing renal damage.[15] Acetylcysteine is an antioxidant that at doses of 600 mg twice daily (PO), on the day before and on the day of administering intravascular contrast, was shown to prevent worsening of renal function in patients with pre-existing CRI. Fenoldopam, a derivative of Dopamine, has also been shown to be effective in preventing contrast media induced nephrotoxicity.[16] Over the past several months we have routinely used Acetylcysteine for patients with pre-existing CRI undergoing EVAR. However, during the time-period of this study, neither Acetylcysteine nor Fenoldopam were used.

To minimize the adverse effects of CRI in our patients, we routinely staged the pre- and peri-operative CT scans, arteriograms, and EVAR, discontinued all possible nephrotoxic drugs, hydrated preoperatively with normal saline, infused intravenous Mannitol (0.5 gm/kg) intraoperatively, and used limited volumes of a low-osmolar contrast agent (Omnipaque-350).

Patients with extensive AIAs extending up to the iliac bifurcation or involving the internal iliac arteries underwent flow interruption of unilateral or bilateral internal iliac arteries via coil embolization. Internal iliac artery coil embolization in patients with pre-existing CRI was always staged 1 - 2 weeks prior to the EVAR.[17] Our results indicate that differences in the incidence of postoperative increase in serum Cr., decrease in Cr.-clearance, need for temporary dialysis, and death with renal failure were surprisingly not statistically significant among patients with and without pre-existing CRI. This makes arguments to the use of CO_2 based contrast for arteriography and intravascular ultrasound to facilitate EVAR, although these are alternative agents that can also be used in select cases.[18,19]

Overall in our patients, the mean Cr.-clearance remained unchanged. Due to adequate pre- and intraoperative hydration, the Cr.-clearance initially improved within the first postoperative day, and subsequently returned to baseline over the next 2 - 3 days, implicating preservation of renal function in patients with and without pre-existing CRI (Figure II). A transient increase in the serum Cr. developed in 3 patients (2.7%) in Group I, 2 patients (3.1%) in Group II, and 2 patients (7.4%) in Group III. All of these patients were treated with conservative supportive measures, and none required dialysis. Two patients (1.9%) in Group I, 2 patients (3.1%) in Group II, and 1 patient (3.7%) in Group III required temporary dialysis. There were no isolated identifiable differences in patients with transient Cr. increase when compared to those requiring temporary dialysis. None of these patients had suprarenal bare-stent fixation, inadvertent renal artery stentgrafts coverage, developed remarkable intraoperative hemodynamic instability, or received excessive intra-arterial contrast load.

In each of the 3 groups, 1 death occurred secondary to renal failure as part of multisystem organ failure (Table 3). In all 3 patients, the intraoperative course was remarkable for either the use of excessive amounts of intra-arterial contrast agent, longer operative times, or hemodynamic instability, or coverage of the renal artery orifices with bare stents/endografts. Unrecognized microembolization secondary to catheter and wire manipulation during EVAR could have also contributed to renal and multisystem organ failure in these patients. Transrenal fixation of the uncovered portion of the proximal stentgrafts and iatrogenic injuries to the renal arteries such as dissection or stentgraft coverage are other possible causes of renal insufficiency.[20,21] Preexisting comorbidities including coronary artery disease, hypertension, and diabetes mellitus did not have an adverse effect on worsening renal function or death. The presence of perioperative hypotension was associated with an increase in serum Cr. and death (P <0.05), and the use of larger contrast volumes was associated with patients developing an increase in postoperative serum Cr. (P <0.001). Patients with perioperative hypotension had a 9-fold increased risk of developing worsening renal function, and 5-fold increased risk of death (odds ratio of 9 and 5, respectively).

Our findings of limited morbidity and mortality from use of intra-arterial contrast during EVAR are supported by several other reports documenting a low incidence of renal insufficiency following EVAR (17, 18). Chuter and colleagues reported their experience of 116 high-risk patients undergoing EVAR: twenty six patients with pre-existing CRI received mean intra-arterial contrast volume of 155 ml during EVAR, and only 1 patient developed a transient increase in serum Cr. Postoperatively.[24]

In patients with CRI, EVAR with use of intra-arterial radiographic contrast agents is believed to impair renal function, and is considered a relative contraindication to the procedure. The results of our investigation indicate that the risks of worsening renal insufficiency, dialysis, and death are only slightly and not significantly greater in patients with CRI when compared to those with normal renal function. With appropriate precautions of avoiding perioperative hypotension and limiting the volume of nonionic contrast agents, CRI need not be a contraindication for EVAR with intra-arterial contrast agents. Furthermore, alternative agents such as CO_2 and IVUS might also help limit the patient exposure to non-ionic contrast agents and limit worsening renal insufficiency and the need for dialysis.

REFERENCES

1. Parfery PA, Griffiths SM, Barrett BJ, et al: Contrast material-induced renal failure in patients with diabetes mellitus and renal insufficiency, or both: A prospective controlled study. N Engl J Med, 1988; 321:143-149.
2. Barrett BJ, Carlisle EJ. Meta-analysis of the relative nephrotoxicity of high-and low-osmolarity iodinated contrast media. Radiology 1993;188:171-178.
3. Barrett BJ. Contrast nephrotoxicity. J Am Soc Nephrol 1994;5:125-137.
4. Johnston WK. Multicenter prospective study of non-ruptured abdominal aortic aneurysms. J Vasc Surg 1989;437-447.
5 Joseph MG, McCollum PT, Lusby RJ. Abnormal preoperative creatinine levels and renal failure following abdominal aortic aneurysm repair. Aust N A J Surg 1989;59:539-541.
6 Ohki T, Veith FJ, Sanchez LA, et al. Varying strategies and devices for endovascular repair of abdominal aortic aneurysms. Semin Vasc Surg 1997; 10(4): 242-56.
7. Barrett BJ. Contrast nephrotoxicity. J Am Soc Nephrol 1994; 5: 125-37.
8. Barfrey PS, Griffiths SM, Barrett BJ, et al. Contrast material induced renal failure in patients with diabetes mellitus, renal insufficiency, or both: a prospective controlled study. N Engl J Med 1989; 320:143-9.

9. Barrett BJ, Carlisle EJ. Meta-analysis of the relative nephrotoxicity of high- and low-osmolality iodinated contrast media. Radiology 1993; 188: 171-8.

10. Johnston WK. Multicenter prospective study of nonruptured abdominal aortic aneurysms. Part II. Variables predicting morbidity and mortality. J Vasc Surg 1989; 9: 437-47.

11. Joseph MG, McCollum PT, Lusby RJ. Abnormal preoperative creatinine levels and renal failure following abdominal aortic aneurysm repair. Aust N Z J Surg 1989, Jul; 59(7): 539-41.

12. Walker SR, Yusuf SW, Wenham PW, Hopkinson BR. Renal complications following endovascular repair of abdominal aortic aneurysms. J Endovasc Surg 1998; 5: 318-22.

13. El-Sayed AA, Haylor JL, El Nahas AM, Salzano S, Marcos SK. Hemodynamic effects of water-soluble contrast media on the isolated perfused rat kidney. Br J Radiol 1992; 64: 435-9.

14. Katholi RE, Taylor GJ, Woods WT, et al. Nephrotoxicity of nonionic low-osmolality versus ionic high-osmolality contrast media: a prospective double blind randomized comparison in human beings. Radiology 1993; 186: 183-7.

15. Topel M, Giet MVD, Schwarzfeld C, Laufer U, Liermann D, Zidek W. Prevention of radiographic contrast agent induced reductions in renal function by Acetylcysteine. N Engl J Med 2000; 343: 180-4.

16. Bakris GL, Lass NA, Glock D. Renal hemodynamics in contrast media induced renal dysfunction: a role for dopamine-1 receptors. Kidney International 1999; Vol.(56): 206-210.

17. Mehta M, Veith FJ, Ohki T, Cynamon J, Goldstein K, Suggs WD, et.al. Unitaleral and bilateral hypogastric artery interruption during aortoiliac aneurysm repair in 154 patients: a relatively innocuous procedure. J Vasc Surg. 2001 Feb;33(2 Suppl):S27-32.

18. Parodi JC, Ferreira LM. Gadolinium-based contrast: an alternative contrast agent for endovascular interventions. Ann Vasc Surg 2000, Sept; 14(5): 480-3.

19. Vogt KC, Brunkwall J, Malina M, Ivancev K, Lindblad B, Risberg B, et al. The use of intravascular ultrasound as control procedure for the deployment of endovascular stentgrafts. Eur J Vasc Endovasc Surg 1997, June; 13(6): 592-6.

20. Lobato AC, Quick RC, Vaughn PL, Rogriguez-Lopez J, Douglas M, Diethrich EB. Transrenal fixation of aortic endografts: intermediate followup of a single center experience. J Endovasc Therapy 2000 Aug; 7(4): 273-78.

21. Bove PG, Long GW, Zelenock GB, et al. Transrenal fixation of aortic stentgrafts for treatment of infrarenal aortic aneurismal disease. JVS 2000 Oct; 32(4): 697-703.

22. Thompson MM, Sayers RD, Nasim A, et al. aortomonoiliac endovascular grafting: difficult solutions to difficult aneurysms. J Endovasc Surg 1997; 4: 174-81.

23. White RA, Donayre CE, Walot I, et al. Preliminary clinical ourcome and imaging criterion for endovascular prosthesis development in high-risk patients who have aortoiliac and traumatic and arterial lesions. J Vasc Surg 1996; 24: 556-69.

24. Chuter TAM, Reilly LM, Faruqi RM, Kerlan RB, Sawhney R, Canto CJ. Endovascular aneurysm repair in high-risk patients. J Vasc Surg 2000; 31: 122-33.

25. Sadowski EA, Bennett LK, Chan MR, et al. Nephrogenic systemic fitrosis: risk factors and incidence estimation. Radiology, 2007 Sept;244(3):930-31.

Chapter 6

53

6. FATE OF THE AAA SAC AFTER EVAR. ARE SIZE CHANGES ENDOGRAFT-DEPENDANT?

Fate of the AAA sac after EVAR. Are size changes endograft-dependant?

Christos D. Liapis, Elias A. Kaperonis

INTRODUCTION

The primary goal of abdominal aortic aneurysm (AAA) treatment is to exclude the aneurysm sac from the arterial circulation, protect it from the stressful influence of the arterial pressure and therefore prevent rupture, which in most cases is lethal. With the conventional approach, the sac is evacuated, wrapped protectively around the graft and definitely excluded from arterial flow. The endovascular revolution has brought a whole new approach to the management of AAAs. Flow is directed through the stent graft, the sac is excluded, but remains unchanged in size and full of its contents. Therefore the fate of the aneurysm sac after endovascular repair (EVAR), is quite crucial to the long-term success of the procedure. Aneurysm sac shrinkage is being viewed as a favorable outcome measure following EVAR, and is being considered an indication of successful sac depressurization. On the other hand, sac enlargement is strongly suggestive of the existence of arterial flow inside the aneurysm sac, that could lead to rupture, given the known association of sac size with the risk of rupture.

Sac size changes have been associated with several predictive variables.[1] Nevertheless, the presence of an endoleak is required in most cases, in order to sustain pulsatile flow inside the sac and is generally considered the Achille's heel of endovascular management. A brief classification of the different endoleak types is provided in Table 1. Some endoleaks seem to

TABLE 1 CLASSIFICATION OF ENDOLEAKS

I: Attachment site leaks
  A. Proximal attachment
  B. Distal attachment
  C. Iliac occluder

II: Branch leaks (no flow through the attachment site)
  A. Simple flow or to-and-fro (one patent branch)
  B. Complex flow or flow through (two or more patent branches)

III: Graft defect
  A. Leak at the junction
  B. Fabric hole
    Minor <2 mm (eg, suture hole)
    Major ≤2 mm

IV: Fabric porosity (<30 d after the procedure)

V: Endotension (↑ sac size with no identifiable leak)

be associated with an unfavorable prognosis (type I and III), while others have a more benign course (type II). It is the operator or the device or both, that are usually responsible for an unsuccessful exclusion of an aneurysm. Preprocedure maximum aneurysm major diameter and the presence of thrombus or plaque in the neck have also been found to be significant predictors of aneurysm sac size change. One other factor that has been reported to influence the size of the sac post EVAR is the type of the endovascular device.[2]

DEVICE SPECIFIC CAUSES

Sixteen years have passed, since the introduction of Parodi's original home made endograft. Over the years at least sixteen different devices have been used in the treatment of AAAs.[3] Only five devices have thus far been approved by the Food and Drug Administration (FDA) in the United States for use in patients with AAA and another two are in the clinical trial phase: The Gore Excluder®, the Cook Zenith®, the Medtronic Talent® (phase II clinical trials), the Guidant Ancure® (the only unibody tubular device, now off-market since 2003), the Medtronic AneuRx®, the Edwards Lifepath® (the only balloon expandable endograft, phase II clinical trials) and

the Endologix Powerlink® (the only unibody bifurcated device). Their individual characteristics are depicted in Table 2.

The initially developed devices were unibody, but by now modular devices have dominated the market. Most of the devices use a metal skeleton of self-expanding stents throughout the graft that is made from nitinol, elgiloy or stainless steel. Nitinol, a nickel titanium alloy, is versatile but fragile. It is very advantageous in manufacture and use, because of its superelasticity and thermal memory. In blood, on the surface of nitinol a layer of titanium oxide is formed, which leads to fractures and separation when stent deformation exceeds strict limits. Recent improvements in nitinol based stent-grafts include electropolishing and the avoidance of welds. Nevertheless, stent fractures are a common finding on explanted nitinol based devices. Both Talent and AneuRx are reported to have high rates of stent fracture. The connecting bar of the long limb of the main body of the Talent endograft, has been found fractured once too often. Changing connecting bar alignment from lateral to medial (Figure 1), probably by minimizing blood flow forces exerted on the bar, remedied the problem.

The Lifepath stent-graft uses elgiloy (cobalt, chromium, nickel) in its metal frame and the Powerlink uses a cobalt

TABLE 2

THE STRUCTURAL CHARACTERISTICS OF THE MOST WIDELY USED STENT-GRAFTS TO DATE

Devices	Sturcture	Skeleton	Fabric	Fixation
Ancure	Unibody	Stainless steel	Woven polyester	Infrarenal
AneuRx	Modular	Nitinol	Woven polyester	Infrarenal
Excluder	Modular	Nitinol	ePTFE	Infrarenal
Lifepath	Modular	Elgiloy	Woven polyester	Infrarenal
Powerlink	Unibody	Elgiloy	ePTFE	Infra;suprarenal
Talent	Modular	Nitinol	Woven polyester	Suprarenal
Zenith	Modular	Stainless steel	Woven polyester	Suprarenal

55

6. FATE OF THE AAA SAC AFTER EVAR. ARE SIZE CHANGES ENDOGRAFT-DEPENDANT?

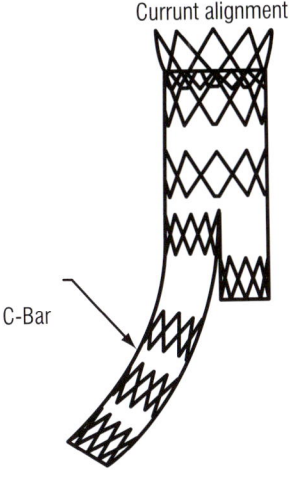

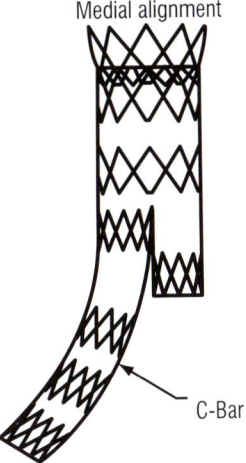

FIGURE 1: Frequent fractures of the C-Bar of the long limb of the main body of the talent device has forced medtronic to move the bar to the medial side.

chromium alloy. Both of these materials exhibit exceptional strength and resistance to high temperature and corrosion. Self-expanding stainless steel-based stent-grafts have also been seen to fracture after long term implantation. One problem has been corrosion of solder at junctions in the wireform. Another is a stent-graft configuration or stent design that produces locations of increased stress and strain. For example, the large stent just above the bifurcation of the Zenith endograft has often been found fractured in long-term implants.

The fabric used in all these devices is the same with minor modifications that has been used over the years in open procedures. Only the Excluder and the Powerlink use PTFE fabric while the rest of them use woven polyester (Dacron).[4] PTFE has demonstrated a higher degree of porosity and some believe this affects the rate of type IV endoleaks. Where the fabric comes in contact with the hard stiff metal stents, in a constantly pounding prosthesis, the risk of fabric weakening or even a tear, is present. One way around this problem is to suture the two components together at multiple points. But even then, suture penetration can disrupt spacing in the weave and create small holes. AneuRx stent-grafts for example, have an average of 1.3 holes larger than 0.2 mm per.[5] This, could explain why in AAAs treated with the AneuRx device, the aneurysm sac shrinks at a lower rate, than in those treated with other devices.[6]

Migration is probably the most important complication of endovascular treatment, since it leads, if untreated, almost certainly to type I endoleak and possibly to rupture. Factors that help to maintain stent position are friction, hook or barb penetration, suprarenal attachment, columnar strength and arterial ingrowth. Self-expanding stents with hooks or barbs, provide better fixation than those that rely on the radial force of the proximal stent. Baloon-expandable stents do not seem to depend so much on these metallic protrusions.[7] The clinical importance of the use of barbs and hooks in the proximal stent of the graft is illustrated by the difference in migration rates between the AneuRx and the Ancure devices, both of which have infrarenal fixation.

Component separation is another disastrous complication that leads to type III endoleak and plagues all modular devices. Many of the forces that cause proximal stent migration, are also exerted on the junction of different components of a modular system. All of the existing stent-grafts depend on several factors in order to stabilize the overlapping zone. Friction, strong stents and long overlap reduce the risk of separation. The relative lengths of the trunk and limbs of the grafts also play a role. Short limbs have a restricted range of movement and this lowers their chances of dislocation. None of the current devices has any mechanisms for active fixation of inter-component junctions.

Since there were no validated design parameters, or realistic models for preclinical testing, most advances in endograft design have resulted from clinical experience. All the devices with no exception, from their introduction, to the clinical trial phase, to FDA approval, and after that, have had minor or major pitfalls, which led to limited to extensive modifications or redesigning of the metal or the fabric part or the suture that keeps them together, or even withdrawal of the device. The absolute failure of EVAR is aneurysm rupture. The first step towards rupture is sac enlargement. Endoleaks, migration, component separation or fabric failure could all lead to sac enlargement. In the context of endotension, enlargement could exist without any apparent cause. Stent fractures, suture breaks, fabric holes and sac shrinkage in endografts with long limbs may all result in EVAR failure.

Successful exclusion, depressurization and sac shrinkage, incomplete exclusion and sac expansion, continued aneurysmal degeneration of adjacent segments and the internal radial force exerted by the proximal fixation stent can all induce significant changes in the sizes of the aneurismal sac and the proximal and distal necks.

OPERATOR SPECIFIC CAUSES

Not all EVAR failures can be attributed to the device. The operator should be aware that not all abdominal aortic anatomies are amenable to endovascular treatment, that the rationale "one device fits all" can lead to disastrous results, that adequate oversizing both proximally and distally is required in order to ensure satisfactory fixation and wall apposition and that sufficient overlap of the modular components of the graft can prevent kinking and component separation.

The anatomical configuration of every individual aneurysm should be studied meticulously and detailed measurements should be recorded, in order to answer three questions: first if the patient is eligible for endovascular treatment at all, second which is the appropriate device to fit the characteristics of the aneurysm and last but not least what the dimensions of the specific device should be.

There are no absolute contraindications for EVAR. Nevertheless, a short or conical or severely angulated (>120°) proximal neck, the presence of thrombus or plaque in the proximal landing zone, a critical inferior mesenteric artery, and significant occlusive disease or tortuosity of the iliac and femoral vessels, are all considered relative contraindications.[7] Anyone who violates one ore more of these conditions, risks the life of his patient and the success of his intervention.

Once the patient is eligible for endoluminal treatment, the next important step is the choice of the device. When the length of the proximal neck is marginal, an endograft with suprarenal fixation proves useful and when small access arteries are encountered (especially in females), the use

57

6. FATE OF THE AAA SAC AFTER EVAR. ARE SIZE CHANGES ENDOGRAFT-DEPENDANT?

of a low-profile device is advised. A sound knowledge of the features, the advantages and shortcomings of every device in the market, significantly helps us choose the most suitable stent-graft and greatly enhances our chances of effective and durable exclusion of the aneurismal sac.

Over sizing the proximal stent's diameter relatively to the proximal neck of the aneurysm has greatly reduced migration rates. It is now well known that, when choosing the diameter of our endograft, we should oversize by 20% or more, rather than the 5-10% originally advocated. On the other hand, excessive oversizing by 30% or more is associated with a 14-fold increase in device migration at 12 months and a 16-fold increased risk of AAA expansion at 24 months.[8] Distal movement of the proximal stent by 5mm or more is considered clinically significant. Late migration is probably related to progressive disease of the aneurysm neck and can only be prevented if the graft is hooked suprarenally.

The choice of unnecessarily long limbs and insufficient component overlap could produce kinking and exert significant forces on the overlapping zone, that could potentially lead to type III endoleak. One manufacturer (Cook Zenith®) recommends, that the iliac leg graft overlaps at least one full iliac leg stent (maximum one and a half) inside the contralateral limb of the main body (Figure 2), while another (Gore Excluder®), proposes an overlap of at least 3 cm. Generally, when overlapping, we should always keep in mind that a seal at the junction, is fundamental for the integrity of the endograft and that a distal type I endoleak is usually far less important and far easier to treat than a type III leak.

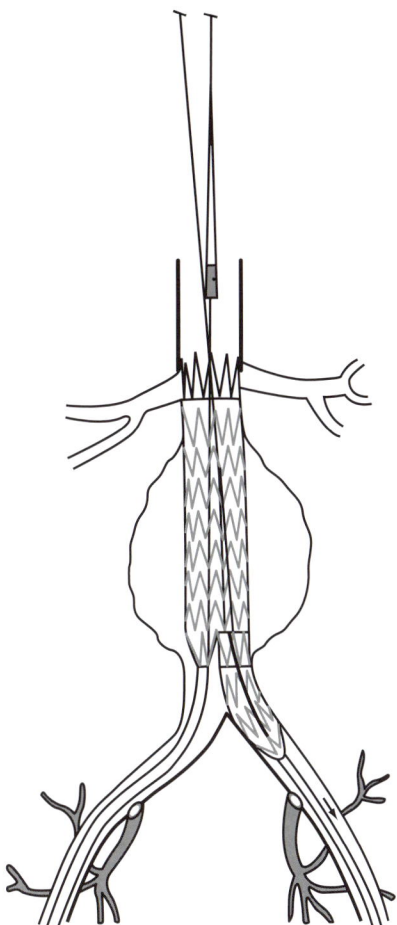

FIGURE 2: At least one stent overlap between the main body and the contralateral limb is recommended by Cook for the Zenith endograft.

SURVEILLANCE

Surveillance of the integrity and position of endovascular grafts is a lifetime neces-sity for all patients because of the clear and present danger of migration, kinking, material failure and endoleaks. Our main concern is the potential risk of aneurysm rupture.All these complications are extremely important, but their clinical significance is essentially determined by the fate and the course of the size of the aneurysm sac. Therefore the main imaging and clinical endpoint in endograft follow-up, that could be an indication for reintervention, is sac expansion. Indeed, a rein-tervention rate of 10% per year has been reported, for treatment of problems identified on follow-up.[9]

Central to surveillance, is the establishment of a baseline reference against which any change can be detected. Most centers use a combination of four-view abdominal radiographs, duplex ultrasonography, and computed tomographic angiography (CTA). According to the recommended surveillance routine, follow-up is done at 1, 6, 12 months and annually thereafter. If an endoleak is detected, the frequency of the scans increases to every 6 months until resolution of the endoleak. MRI can also be used for graft surveillance. A recent development in endograft follow-up is the monitoring of sac pressure within treated aneurysms through an implanted sensor device. The association of matrix metalloproteinases and AAA pathophysiology, could lead in the future to a simple biochemical test, that could predict which AAAs treated with EVAR are at inherent risk for aneurysm sac growth.

The plain radiograph is a universal tool for monitoring any metallic prosthesis and can demonstrate certain changes in an endograft more easily than can be seen on CT. While the other modalities used in surveillance, can replace one another, the radiograph is practically irreplaceable. Wire fractures, anchor stent separation, kinking, limb dislocation and migration can be detected by careful examination of the stent-graft's structure and position relatively to anatomical landmarks (lumbar vertebral bodies etc.) and by comparing the follow-up exam to the baseline radiograph. Computed tomographic angiography has been the benchmark of follow up imaging of endoluminally treated aneurysms, because it generates high quality axial images suitable for measuring changes in sac dimensions. With the use of contrast medium, CT scans can also confirm device patency and identify endoleaks. CT has been found superior to duplex ultrasound for endoleak detection.[10] Nevertheless, only a small percentage (20%) of the endoleaks missed by duplex ultrasound required treatment.[11]

Ultrasonography provides an effective means for identification of endoleaks and can measure changes in the size of the residual aneurysm sac. The increasing use of ultrasonography contrast agents can further enhance the sensitivity of this technique. However, a skilled technologist is required in order to identify and classify an endoleak. In this regard, the main limitation of this technique is that it is user-dependent and can require an extended examination period to complete an accurate endoleak study. Some groups recommend the use of MRI and MRA (magnetic resonance angiography), as more sensitive tools for endoleak identification. One advantage of this modality is that gadolinium contrast is safe for patients with an elevated creatinine. However, stainless steel leads to severe artifact, which makes the study difficult to interpret and patients with certain aortic endografts cannot be accurately evaluated by MRI technology. Moreover, the cost of this modality is the highest of all competing surveillance imaging techniques.

There is a tendency in many centers to minimize surveillance. Some advocate CT scan elimination in favor of duplex ultrasound, because they consider that the risk of radiation exposure and contrast administration is not balanced by appropriate patient benefit, if all endoleaks are not routinely treated. Others, prefer an unenhanced CT scan that can detect changes in aneurysm size and plain films that can assess for device fatigue or migration. If the sac size is stable or shrinking, then the imaging study is complete, but if sac size increases, then contrast can be administered to identify an endoleak. This change in surveillance protocol is becoming common practice in many European centers.

59

6. FATE OF THE AAA SAC AFTER EVAR. ARE SIZE CHANGES ENDOGRAFT-DEPENDANT?

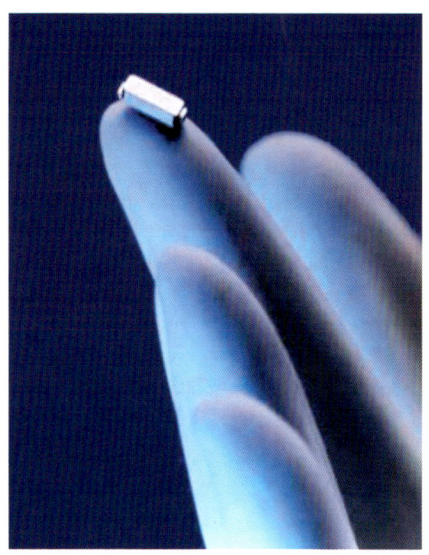

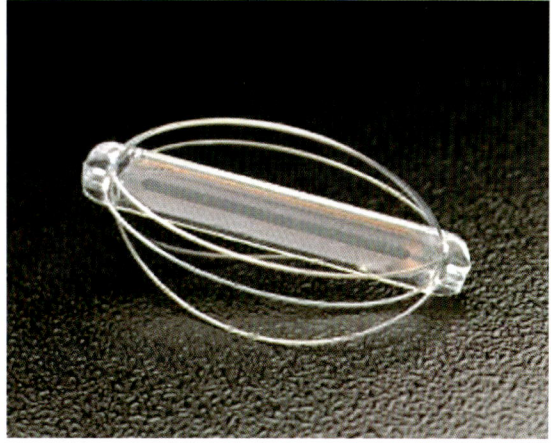

FIGURE 3: Two different pressure sensors that can be implanted on the outside surface of stent-grafts have been developed in Israel (Remon) and USA (Cardiomems).

The increased demand for perfection of endograft surveillance has led to the investigation of new technologies. The most promising technique identified thus far is remote pressure sensing. Remote pressure sensors allow for measurement of the systolic and diastolic pressures within the residual aneurysm sac at any given point in time. Two different sensors have been developed (Figure 3), none of which was cleared from FDA for chronic surveillance of endografts.[12] There are still unresolved issues, making diffusion of this innovative technology outside specific trials, impossible for the time being. First, the capacity of remote pressure sensing to replace the current standard of care for long-term patient surveillance has not yet been confirmed. A clinical trial to assess the safety and efficacy of the EndoSure Wireless AAA Pressure Sensor in comparison to CTA for long-term follow-up is underway. Second, the cost-effectiveness of this new technology has not been defined. The current cost of an EndoSure Wireless AAA Pressure Sensor is equivalent to that of an aortic extension cuff. Finally, it remains to be determined whether this technology will lead to earlier identification of endoleaks with a concomitant reduction in aneurysm-related complications, such as rupture. With the new technology, radiation and contrast media administration are avoided. Surveillance with pressure sensors is cheaper and the exam can be performed anytime at home. If the method proves also equivalent to CT in endograft follow-up, the tiny sensor will probably replace it (Figure 4).

DIFFERENT DEVICES AND SAC SIZE

Different endografts have indeed behaved differently, as regards the fate of the aneurysm sac size. Several theories have been proposed as mechanisms for explaining differential sac shrinkage rates. Type of graft material, presence or absence of structural support, stent construct, modularity, main body length, and inherent anatomy are all examples of potentially influential factors.

Beginning with the Talent device, in a recent multicenter study of 165 patients with a long follow-up, sac shrinkage (>5 mm) occurred in 64.2% of the patients

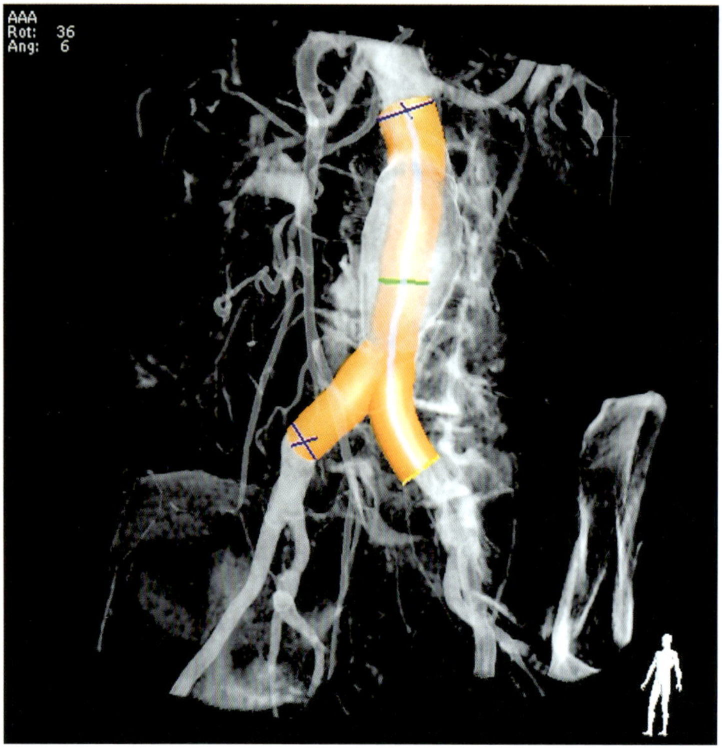

FIGURE 4: Virtual stenting of AAA.

while enlargement in only 8.5%. Only endoleaks were significantly correlated with sac enlargement. Freedom from secondary intervention was 77.4% at 7 years.[13] While only 12.1% were treated for endoleak, migration or rupture, an alarming 6.1% were treated for endograft thrombosis. Adverse aortic anatomy did not influence sac size, risk for a secondary procedure, or the clinical success rate. In a small group treated with the same device, the authors had an endoleak rate (early and late included) of 36.7%. Surprisingly, more than half of early endoleaks were type I. Endoleaks were not associated with morbidity or mortality and they were not predictive of sac expansion.[14] Dynamic magnetic resonance angiography has been used in a very original work, in order to determine elastic modulus and aortic stiffness as indexes of wall compliance during the cardiac cycle, pre- and postoperatively in patients treated with different devices.[15] After implantation, the measurements at the aneurysm neck in patients treated with the Excluder endograft, were 94% and 60% higher, respectively, compared to those in patients treated with the Talent device (p <0.05). This difference may be attributable to the different proximal fixation system between the two grafts.

In the Ancure experience with the phase II and III clinical trials, the sac shrinkage rate increased from 51.3% at 12 months to 68.5% at 24 months, while for the same time period, sac enlargement rate decreased from 2.1% to 1.1%. The endoleak rate also decreased between the first and the second year of follow-up, but it could not predict sac size changes.[16] The same group, have compared the results of the non-supported Ancure with those of the fully supported Excluder endograft. Endoleak rate at 1 month was significantly higher in the Ancure group (25% vs. 18%). Nevertheless, initial endoleak status did not affect sac shrinkage rates at 12 and 24 months. On the contrary, patients treated with the Ancure device, had significantly greater sac shrinkage at 2 years.[17] There was no significant difference in endoleak rates or sac regression at 1 year, between aneurysms excluded with the Ancure or the Talent endograft.[18]

In a significant US multicenter trial, the Zenith endograft exhibited a remarkably low endoleak rate at two years follow-up (5.4%), and an impressive sac shrinkage (>5 mm) rate of 66% at the first year and 75% at the end of the second one. Migration (>5 mm) was detected in four (2%) patients through 12 months; none was greater than 10 mm or associated with adverse events through 24 months 19. Oversizing is very important when we plan an endovascular procedure and it is usually around or a little over 20%. When we oversize by >30% with the Zenith device, this was associated with a higher type II endoleak rate (11% vs. 4.7%) and an increased migration risk at 24 months (14% vs. 0.9%). Sac enlargement was much higher in the excessive oversizing group (9.5% vs. 0.6%), while sac shrinkage was significantly reduced (48% vs. 77%). Aortic neck diameter also increased significantly by 6 months follow-up but after that it remained stable.[8] Although with the Zenith endograft, endoleak and migration rates are remarkably low and sac shrinkage rates impressively high, the device has faced over the years some limited integrity issues (barb separation with no clinical sequelae, 2% incidence and suprarenal stent detachment, 6 cases worldwide). A design alteration with a double suture attachment seems to have solved the problem.[20] A few months ago we have had the first report of strut failure of the Zenith device. It was about three patients that have had clinically insignificant wire fractures in the inferior

body of the graft but above the bifurcation.[21] Migration both of 5 and 10 mm with the Zenith device is significantly lower than with the AneuRx at 4 years follow-up. Aortic neck length was shorter in migrators, but still greater than the acceptable limit of 15 mm.[22]

The experience with the Excluder endograft has shown low sac shrinkage rates at 4 years (36.8%) although the endoleak rates were fairly normal or even low.[23] In the annual clinical update of the manufacturing company for the Excluder AAA bifurcated endoprosthesis, that appeared in the site on February 2006, the main shortcoming of the endograft is highlighted: in the Gore Excluder Pivotal Trial data, there is 36% sac enlargement (>5 mm) (53% without endoleak attributed to device permeability) but no rupture. Since then three ruptures in the absence of endoleak have been reported.[24] In the same trial, in the subgroup of patients with sac expansion, 39% of patients had endoleaks. Volume was a more sensitive indicator of aneurysm sac growth than diameter (79% vs. 41%, p<0.001). The difference in the detection of sac enlargement, between the two methods was more pronounced in the first year (56% vs. 8%). Enlargement was detected by volume criteria 18m earlier and at a smaller diameter.[25] All this data led to the development of the new low porosity Excluder device almost two years ago. A comparative study between the old the new Excluder and the Zenith endograft (known for its high sac shrinkage rate), showed that the new device has significantly lower endoleak rate, higher sac regression rate and 1 year mean diameter reduction than the old one and is equivalent to the Zenith device in all three parameters.[26]

In a significant explant analysis of AneuRx stent grafts, structural findings (fractures, holes and suture breaks) were documented in most of the explanted devices although the mean implant duration was only 22 months. However, they were not associated with endoleaks, sac enlargement, device failure and late conversion. It should be noted that it was the manufacturer's Special Team that performed the explanted grafts' analysis and device improvements (increasing flexibility and decreasing porosity) were made during and after the study.[27] In a large sample of patients treated with the AneuRx endograft, with a mean follow-up of 3 years, sac enlargement was observed in 12%, and sac shrinkage in 36%. AAA expansion with or without endoleaks was the main reason for secondary endotreatment or conversion. While sac enlargement was associated with increased age and the presence of endoleaks, it was not associated with increased risk of rupture or decrease in survival.[28]

The French Powerlink Multicenter Trial have found low endoleak, migration and conversion rates. Three-year mean sac diameter significantly decreased, 55.2% of the aneurysm sacs shrinked, while in 43.1% of the patients, sac diameter remained stable.[29] Experience with the same device in the US multicenter trial has been rather favorable. Although the early endoleak rate was 22.3% (mainly type II), the 4-year endoleak-free survival rate was 73%, there has been no material failure recorded and sac regression was noted in 83% of patients.[30] Finally with the Lifepath stent graft, after overcoming a major pitfall with the first generation device, fractures of the critical anchoring wireforms were significantly reduced in the second generation grafts. Mean aneurysm diameter and volume significantly decreased at 6, 12 and 24 months. Diameter reduction was seen in 58% and volume reduction in 84% of patients by the first year.[31]

The association of several variables with sac size change was investigated, in a significant study of 351 patients treated with the Zenith endograft and followed for 2 years. The presence of an endoleak, preprocedure maximum aneurysm diameter and thrombus/plaque within the proximal neck preprocedurally, were significantly related to aneurysm sac size change at 6, 12 and 24 months.[1] Endoleaks and thrombus/plaque within the proximal neck preprocedurally were associated with sac growth or less shrinkage, while larger preprocedure maximum aneurysm diameters were more likely to experience more shrinkage. The impact of endograft type on the fate of the aneurysm sac size has drawn a lot of attention lately. There are several comparative studies where more than one device was used.

The use of the Zenith device was associated with a significantly higher sac shrinkage rate (73.1%) compared to the use of the AneuRx endograft (43.1%) at 12 months. Mean reduction of sac diameter was more than double in the Zenith group compared with the AneuRx group.[32] In a large comparative study that included 703 patients and where five devices were used, no device-specific differences were detected in risk of aneurysm related death, the risk of conversion, migration and the necessity of a secondary procedure. Endoleaks and sac size were significantly different between different groups. The Excluder had the highest any endoleak and type II endoleak rate and the lowest sac shrinkage rate. The Zenith and the Talent the highest 1 year sac shrinkage rate and the Zenith used outside the multicenter clinical trials the highest sac expansion rate.[33]

In another significant study four devices were used (Ancure, AneuRx, Excluder, Talent) and the following observations were made: a) absolute decrease in size and percentage of patients with significant diameter reduction were higher for the Ancure and Talent devices, b) no detection of statistical differences in sac enlargement between the stent grafts and c) endograft type was an independent predictor of sac regression both at 1 and 2 years.[2] In another comparison between the Ancure, the Excluder and the Zenith endografts, we had similar results. The Excluder group had the lowest and the Zenith the highest rate of sac size decrease. The Ancure group had the highest and the Zenith the lowest endoleak rate. Endoleaks had a moderating effect on the rate of sac diameter decrease and initially larger sacs tended to have greater reduction regardless of graft type and the presence of endoleak.[34] All these data of course are referring to the old Excluder device and not the new low porosity one. The new low porosity graft seems to have resolved this problem and to have become almost equal to the Zenith in this regard.

The importance of the type of endograft used, for endoleaks and neck dilatation has also been investigated. Neck dilation did not differ significantly among graft types. Migration was more frequent for the AneuRx and the Lifepath systems and dilation was associated with migration and late proximal endoleaks for the Ancure, the AneuRx and the Excluder endografts. There were no differences in preoperative aneurysm sac sizes or rates of sac collapse between patients with and without dilatation for any graft type.[35] The Talent and Lifepath had an apparent lower initial rate of type II endoleaks, but this was only significant for the Talent at 6 months compared with Excluder, Zenith, and Ancure, and at 1 year compared with Excluder and Zenith. No graft had a long-term statistically significant difference in the rate of type II endoleak formation. The various grafts had a nearly identical pattern for the rate of spontaneous resolution but this was highest for Talent.[36]

SAC SIZE, VOLUME AND PRESSURE

Volume measurements tend to represent aneurysm expansion more accurately than maximum transverse diameter.[25] If there is not even a small aneurysm sac volume reduction in the first six months, then this indicates the need for closer surveillance. Volumetric change has a higher predictive accuracy for an endoleak than diameter change.[37] Sac pressure measurements are the last development in endograft surveillance. Pressure in the space between the device and the aneurysm wall, is measured either directly with an intravascular catheter, or by an ultrasound activated remote pressure transducer, fixed to the outside of the stent-graft and exposed to the arterial flow. In an effort to correlate pressure values measured with an endoluminal catheter, with aneurysm sac diameter measurements, the mean pressure index (MPI = the percentage of mean intra-sac pressure relative to the simultaneous mean intra-aortic or systemic pressure) was calculated during the follow-up of patients treated with AAA endografts. Median MPI was 19% in shrinking, 30% in stable and 59% in expanding aneurysms. Pulse pressure was also significantly higher in expanding compared with shrinking AAAs.[38]

In another study, MPI was measured with a permanently implanted remote pressure sensor and results were similar.[39] EVAR resulted in significant reduction of sac pressure in most patients. Patients with aneurysm shrinkage after EVAR had significantly lower MPI. However, the absence of shrinkage is not indicative of persistent sac pressurization. In an experimental aneurysm model, the differential distribution of strain/pressure (S/P) on the aneurysm wall was recorded.[40] Endoluminal exclusion of an aneurysm led to uniform S/P reduction in the aneurysm sac. Type I endoleak but not type II was associated with significantly higher S/P in an area of the sac adjacent to the proximal neck. The presence of thrombus had no effect on S/P distribution in the aneurysm sac. Sac pressure measurements via an indwelling catheter during EVAR and open

63

6. FATE OF THE AAA SAC AFTER EVAR. ARE SIZE CHANGES ENDOGRAFT-DEPENDANT?

repair, have shown that aneurysm sac reperfusion through patent side branches alone, although moderately increases sac pressure, does not result in persistent pressurization.[41]

Pressure sensors are being developed over the last few years, but still face problems of reliability and measurement accuracy. We have recently learned that pulsatile sensor motion can influence pressure measurements.[42] More compliant grafts are more susceptible to this phenomenon. Despite false high pressure measurements, stent-graft attached sensors seem appropriate to follow pressure trends in the aneurysm sac. In the most recently published APEX trial, the efficacy and safety of the permanently implanted Endosure wireless pressure sensor, has been studied.[43] Measurements with both the device and an angiographic catheter have shown little difference. Before deployment of the contralateral limb (type I endoleak equivalent), sensor measurements agreed closely with angiographic catheter measurements. At the completion of the procedure the two methods agreed in the detection of type I and III endoleaks in 92.1% of the measurements. While the device has been proven a useful tool during and after the procedure, the issue of its chronic use in postoperative surveillance remains unsettled.

PRECLINICAL TESTING - DEVICE IMPROVEMENT

Medical technology is rapidly moving forward. Physicians and engineers move closer in an effort to understand how prosthetic (metal, synthetic, composite etc.) devices fit anatomically, behave physiologically and interact with adjacent structures of living tissues, in the era of minimally invasive surgery. Traditionally, new products were developed by prototyping and evaluation. However, this proc-

ess is very time consuming and often fails to reveal potential problems. Finite Element Analysis (FEA), can greatly reduce testing and time to market, by allowing the designer to computer test his product in advance of any prototypes and expose and solve any design flaws before even the first product is produced.[44]

In FEA, the computer, by using specific finite element modeling software, provides a simulation of the mechanical behavior of medical devices and components. In simple words, the virtual prosthesis (practically a computer design and not a real prosthesis) is broken down into very small pieces or elements. The model calculates the forces applied on every single element by the arterial wall and the blood flow, and is trying to predict their effect (displacement, breakage or other) on this tiny element. Then the behavior of all elements are summed up, in order to have an image of the device's behavior in vivo. Material fatigue is also tested. Provided certain mathematical requirements are satisfied, the finer the mesh, (i.e. the smaller the element size) the closer the virtual behavior of the graft will be to the real-life behavior.

Computational analysis of biomechanical contributors to possible endovascular graft failure, has shown that even in the absence of endoleaks, elevated sac pressure can still be caused by fluid-structure interactions between the device, stagnant blood and the aneurysm wall.[45] AAA neck angle, iliac bifurcation angle, neck aorta-to-iliac diameter ratio, stent-graft size, aorto-uni-iliac device and hypertension play important roles in generating forces potentially leading to migration.

Computational fluid dynamics (CFD) is a branch of fluid engineering, that is investigating, among other things, the forces that arise when blood flows through an endoluminal graft. For computational convenience, the flow is assumed to be steady (non-pulsatile) and turbulent. Peak

65

6. FATE OF THE AAA SAC AFTER EVAR. ARE SIZE CHANGES ENDOGRAFT-DEPENDANT?

flow rates are used in order to approximate as much as possible the accurate value for the peak forces on the graft. The goal is to calculate the "downward" drag force that the blood flow exerts on the proximal fixation site and the specific value that is required in order to displace the proximal stent. This value seems to be higher for an endograft with a larger diameter. Increased cardiac output, increases the drag on a bifurcated graft. Attachment design at the proximal end and patient selection must take into account a safety margin to accommodate for a peak value for the forces acting on an endograft.[46]

The infinite capabilities of computer systems have also been used in order to design stent-grafts for AAAs.[47] A 3-dimensional morphological model of the aorta and its main branches has been reconstructed from contrast-enhanced helical CT slice images of abdominal aortic aneurysms. By determining the central lumen axis, accurate measurements were made. A computer graphics software is used to design the stent-graft. Then it is virtually inserted into the 3-D reconstruction of the aortic aneurysm and its anatomic compatibility is observed in detail (Figure 4).

We have had many major improvements in stent-graft design over the years. Unibody design has been largely replaced by modular design. The new design has increased versatility and makes the graft suitable for many different aortic anatomies. The initial support at the ends of the graft has stepped back in favor of metal support throughout the whole length of the device, in order to increase columnar strength and decrease migration rates. While the first generation endografts had a metallic endoskeleton, in the newer devices the metal part is outside the graft. This way, the metal is removed from circulation, the fabric is no longer directly subjected to the stress and the friction developed between the stent and the arterial wall and the direct contact of the wall with

the metal strengthens fixation. There have also been minor modifications in widely used endografts. One example is the redesigning of the Talent device. Many fractures of the connector bar of the ipsilateral limb have been observed and after detailed explant analysis they have been attributed to material fatigue possibly due to the tighter angles of the lateral side. Consequently the manufacturer moved the bar to the medial side and the problem was cured. The Excluder has faced the complication of increased aneurysm sac size after the procedure, probably due to type IV endoleak and remedied it by minimizing the porosity of the fabric.

New devices with fenestrations and side branches have been developed in order to avoid occluding aortic branches or establish a communication between the endograft and a patent artery arising from the aneurysm sac, or seal a common iliac aneurysm without occluding the internal ilac artery. This way, the range of indications of endovascular treatment of AAAs is broadened. Although implants that are fenestrated or branched are technically demanding, a few centers in the world have achieved success using endoluminal devices to treat juxtarenal, thracoabdominal and arch aneurysms. Moreover, by stent bridging the gap between the main body, or limb, fenestration or branch and the branch of the aneurysm wall or the internal iliac artery, we could minimize the rate of endloleaks (especially type IB and II) and contribute to aneurysm shrinkage. Insertion of these devices requires from the operator 3-dimensional thinking, planning, orientation and deployment, far different from that of the classic bifurcated device.

CONCLUSIONS

Endoluminal repair slowly but steadily becomes an extremely important technique in the treatment of AAAs. Endoleaks, migration and material failure, can all lead to sac enlargement and increased risk of rupture. Even sac shrinkage, long considered the Ithaca of the endovacsular adventure, can be detrimental, depending on the individual anatomy and the characteristics of the endograft. The course of aneurysm sac size determines the need for secondary intervention or even conversion. Several factors appear to influence sac behavior. The type of endograft seems to be one of them.

A number of theories have been cited as mechanisms for different sac behavior when using different endografts. Different types of metal, fabric and suture and different ways of interaction between them, could influence the fate of aneurysm sac. In order to improve their performance, all devices have been evolved, modified, redesigned and some of them even withdrawn over the years. All the improved second and third generation endografts have ameliorated device behavior, minimized structural and design problems and significantly improved complication rates. Variable sac behavior will soon probably be a thing of the past.

REFERENCES

1. Fairman RM, Nolte L, Snyder SA, Chuter TA, Greenberg RK, for the Zenith Investigators. Factors predictive of early or late aneurysm sac size change following endovascular repair. J Vasc Surg 2006;43:649-56.
2. Bertges DJ, Chow K, Wyers MC, Landsittel D, Frydrych AV, Stavropoulos W, et al. Abdominal aortic aneurysm size regression after endovascular repair is endograft dependent. J Vasc Surg 2003;37:716-23.
3. Rutherford RB, Krupski WC. Current status of open versus endovascular stent-graft repair of abdominal aortic aneurysm. J Vasc Surg 2004;39:1129-39.
4 Katzen BT, Dake MD, MacLean AA, Wang DS. Endovascular repair of abdominal and thoracic aortic aneurysms. Circulation 2005;112:1663-75.
5. Zarins CK, for the AneuRx Clinical Investigators. The US AneuRx Clinical Trial: 6-year clinical update 2002. J Vasc Surg 2003;37:904-8.
6 Resch T, Malina M, Lindblad B, Malina J, Brunkwall J, Ivancev K. The impact of stent design on proximal stent-graft fixation in the abdominal aorta: an experimental study. Eur J Vasc Endovasc Surg 2000;20:190-95.
7. Ohki T, Veith F. Patient selection for endovascular repair of abdominal aortic aneurysms: changing the threshold for intervention. Semin Vasc Surg 1999;12:226-34.
8. Sternbergh WC 3rd, Money SR, Greenberg RK, Chuter TA; Zenith Investigators. Influence of endograft oversizing on device migration, endoleak, aneurysm shrinkage and aortic neck dilation: results from the Zenith Multicenter Trial. J Vasc Surg 2004;39:20-6.
9. Ouriel K. Endovascular repair of abdominal aortic aneurysms: The Cleveland Clinic experience with five different devices. Semin Vasc Surg 2003;16:88-94.
10. Raman KG, Missing-Carroll N, Richardson T, Muluk SC, Makaroun MS. Color-flow duplex ultrasound scan versus computed tomographic scan in the surveillance of endovascular aneurysm repair. J Vasc Surg 2003;38:645-51.
11. AbuRahma AF. Fate of endoleaks detected by CT angiography and missed by color duplex ultrasound in endovascular grafts for abdominal aortic aneurysms. J Endovasc Ther 2006;13(4):490-5.
12. Milner R, Kasirayan K, Chaikof EL. Future of endograft surveillance. Semin Vasc Surg 2006; 19:75-82.
13. Torsello G, Osada N, Florek HJ, Horsch S, Kortmann H, Luska G, et al. Long-term outcome after Talent endograft implantation for aneurysms of the abdominal aorta: a multicenter retrospective study. J Vasc Surg 2006;43:277-84.
14. Seriki DM, Ashleigh RJ, Butterfield JS, England A, McCollum CM, Akhtar N, et al. Midterm follow-up of a single-center experience of endovascular repair of abdominal aortic aneurysms with use of the Talent stent-graft. J Vasc Interv Radiol 2006; 17(6):973-7.
15. van Herwaarden JA, Muhs BE, Vincken KL, van Prehn J, Teutelink A, Bartels LW, et al. Aortic compliance following EVAR and the influence of

67

6. FATE OF THE AAA SAC AFTER EVAR. ARE SIZE CHANGES ENDOGRAFT-DEPENDANT?

different endografts: determination using dynamic MRA. J Endovasc Ther 2006;13(3):406-14.

16. Makaroun MS. The Ancure endografting system: an update. J Vasc Surg 2001;33(Supp 2):S129-34.

17. Rhee RY, Garvey L, Missing-Carroll N, Makaroun MS. Does endograft support alter the rate of aneurysm sac shrinkage after endovascular repair. J Endovasc Ther 2003;10(3):411-7.

18. Farner MC, Carpenter JP, Baum RA, Fairman RM. Early changes in abdominal aortic aneurysm diameter after endovascular repair. J Vasc Interv Radiol 2003;14(2):205-10.

19. Greenberg RK, Chuter TA, Sternbergh WC 3rd, Fearnot NE, for the Zenith Investigators. Zenith AAA endovascular graft: intermediate-term results of the US multicenter trial. J Vasc Surg 2004; 39:1209-18.

20. Kaviani A, Greenberg RK. The Zenith AAA endovascular graft. Expert Rev Med Devices 2004;1(2):175-80.

21. Rumball-Smith A, Wright IA, Buckenham TM. Strut failure in the body of the Zenith abdominal endoprosthesis. Eur J Vasc Endovasc Surg 2006; 32(2):136-9.

22. Tonnessen BH, Sternbergh WC 3rd, Money SR. Mid- and long-term device migration after endovascular abdominal aortic aneurysm repair: a comparison of AneuRx and Zenith endografts. J Vasc Surg 2005;42(3):392-400.

23. Melissano G, Bertoglio L, Esposito G, Civilini E, Setacci F, Chiesa R. Midterm clinical success and behavior of the aneurysm sac after endovascular AAA repair with the Excluder graft. J Vasc Surg 2005;42(6):1052-7.

24. Gore Excluder AAA bifurcated endoprosthesis annual clinical update. W. L. Gore & Associates Inc; Feb 2006.

25. Fillinger M; Excluder Bifurcated Endoprosthesis Clinical Investigators. Three-dimensional analysis of enlarging aneurysms after endovascular abdominal aortic aneurysm repair in the Gore Excluder Pivotal clinical trial. J Vasc Surg 2006;43(5):888-95.

26. Haider SE, Najjar SF, Cho JS, Rhee RY, Eskandari MK, Matsumura JS, et al. Sac behavior after aneurysm treatment with the Gore Excluder low-permeability aortic endoprosthesis: 12-month comparison to the original Excluder device. J Vasc Surg 2006;44(4):694-700.

27. Zarins CK, Arko FR, Crabtree T, Bloch DA, Ouriel K, Allen RC, et al. Explant analysis of AneuRx stent grafts: Relationship between structural findings and clinical outcome. J Vasc Surg 2004; 40:1-11.

28. Zarins CK, Bloch DA, Crabtree T, Matsumoto AH, White RA, Fogarty TJ. Aneurysm enlargement following endovascular aneurysm repair: AneuRx clinical trial. J Vasc Surg 2004;39(1):109-17.

29. Albertini JN, Lahlou Z, Magnan PE, Branchereau A; French Powerlink Multicenter Trial Investigators. Endovascular repair of abdominal aortic aneurysms with a unibody stent-graft: 3-year results of the French Powerlink Multicenter Trial. J Endovasc Ther 2005;12:629-37.

30. Carpenter JP. The Powerlink bifurcated system for endovascular aortic aneurysm repair: four-year results of the US multicenter trial. J Cardiovasc Surg 2006;47(3):239-43.

31. Carpenter JP, Anderson WN, Brewster DC, Kwolek C, Makaroun M, Martin J, et al. Multicenter pivotal trial results of the Lifepath System for endovascular aortic aneurysm repair. J Vasc Surg 2004;39(1):34-43.

32. Sternbergh WC 3rd, Conners MS 3rd, Tonnessen BH, Carter G, Money SR. Aortic aneurysm sac shrinkage after endovascular repair is device-dependent: a comparison of Zenith and AneuRx endografts. Ann Vasc Surg 2003;17(1):49-53.

33. Ouriel K, Clair DG, Greenberg RK, Lyden SP, O'Hara PJ, Sarac TP et al. Endovascular repair of abdominal aortic aneurysms: Device-specific outcome. J Vasc Surg 2003;37(5):991-8.

34. Greenberg RK, Deaton D, Sullivan T, Walker E, Lyden SP, Srivastava SD, et al. Variable sac behavior after endovascular repair of abdominal aortic aneurysm: Analysis of core laboratory data. J Vasc Surg 2004;39(1):95-101.

35. Dillavou ED, Muluk S, Makaroun MS. Is neck dilatation after endovascular aneurysm repair graft dependent? Results of 4 US phase II trials. Vasc Endovasc Surg 2005;39(1):47-54.

36. Sheehan MK, Ouriel K, Greenberg RK, McCann R, Murphy M, Fillinger M, et al. Are type II endoleaks after endovascular aneurysm repair endograft dependent? J Vasc Surg 2006;43(4):657-61.

37. Bargellini I, Cioni R, Petruzzi P, Pratali A, Napoli V, Vignali C, et al. Endovascular repair of abdomi-

nal aortic aneurysms: analysis of aneurysm volumetric changes at mid-term follow-up. Cardiovasc Intervent Radiol 2005;28(4):426-33.

38. Dias NV, Ivancev K, Malina M, Resch T, Lindblad B, Sonesson B. Intra-aneurysm sac pressure measurements after endovascular aneurysm repair: differences between shrinking, unchanged and expanding aneurysms with and without endoleak. J Vasc Surg 2004;39(6):1229-35.

39. Ellozy SH, Carroccio A, Lookstein RA, Jacobs TS, Addis MD, Teodorescu VJ, et al. Abdominal aortic aneurysm sac shrinkage after endovascular aneurysm repair: correlation with chronic sac pressure measurement. J Vasc Surg 2006;43(1):2-7.

40. Xenos ES, Stevens SL, Freeman MB, Pacanowski JP, Cassada DC, Goldman MH. Distribution of sac pressure in an experimental aneurysm model after endovascular repair: the effect of endoleak types I and II. J Endovasc Ther 2003;10:516-23.

41. Vallabhaneni SR, Gilling-Smith GL, How TV, Brennan JA, Gould DA, McWilliams RG, et al. Aortic side branch perfusion alone does not account for high intra-sac pressure after endovascular repair (EVAR) in the absence of graft-related endoleak. Eur J Vasc Endovasc Surg 2003;25(4):354-9.

42. Hinnen JW, Koning OH, Vlaanderen E, van Bockel JH, Hamming JF. Aneurysm sac pressure monitoring: effect of pulsatile motion of the pressure sensor on the interpretation of measurements. J Endovasc Ther 2006;13:145-51.

43. Ohki T, Ouriel K, Silveira PG, Katzen B, White R, Criado F, et al. Initial results of wireless pressure sensing for endovascular aneurysm repair: The APEX Trial-Acute Pressure Measurement to Confirm Aneurysm Sac Exclusion. J Vasc Surg 2007;45(2):236-42.

44. Haridas B, Haynes C. Predictive analysis at the forefront of medical product development. Med Dev Diag Ind 1999;10:112-9.

45. Li Z, Kleinstreuer C, Farber M. Computational analysis of biomechanical contributors to possible endovascular graft failure. Biomech Model Mechanobiol 2005;4(4):221-34.

46. Liffman K, Lawrence-Brown MMD, Bui A, Semmens JB, Rudman M, Hartley DE, et al. Analytic modeling and numerical simulations of forces in an endoluminal graft. J Endovasc Ther 2001;8:358-71.

47. Imai Y, Urayama S, Uyama C, Inoue K, Ueno K, Kuribayashi S, et al. A system for computer-assisted design of stent-grafts for aortic aneurysms using 3-D morphological models. Cardiovasc Intervent Radiol 2001;24:277-9.

Advanced procedure planning: Anatomic and device considerations

Geoffrey H. White, Ravi Huilgol

INTRODUCTION

Pre-procedural planning is one of the most important aspects needed to achieve success with endovascular graft techniques for repair of abdominal aortic aneurysms (AAA). The major anatomic regions of interest in the planning process are the aortic neck and the iliac arteries. Problem features in the neck include angulation, irregular shape, short length and poor aortic wall quality. Difficult necks are a significant cause of procedure failure modes such as device migration, endoleak and late aneurysm rupture. Iliac anatomy can also be a significant influence, with angulated calcified arteries being a risk factor for failed access, iliac rupture and device thrombosis.

Anatomic measurements and procedural planning

The process of procedural planning for endovascular AAA graft operations starts with a careful assessment of the imaging studies. The essentials of the aorto-iliac and branch anatomy should be measured by electronic digital image calibration (or alternatively by caliper calibration from hard-copy images), and then recorded on a dedicated planning sheet. These as-pects include the basic dimensional details of the aortic neck (neck diameter, length, shape) as well as other characteristics such as angulation in the antero-posterior or lateral planes, wall irregularity and thrombus. In addition, note is made of the shape and diameter of the flow lumen through the sac, and the characteristics of the access arteries (iliac tortuosity, calcification and atheroma). It is important to ascertain the number of renal arteries and their relationship to the aortic neck, as well as the position of the lowest renal artery with respect to bony landmarks such as the first or second lumbar vertebrae, and any significant amount of thrombus or atheroma involving the aortic wall close to the renal orifices, or within the aortic neck. This information is then used to plan the device dimensions and the order of the procedure, including a consideration of likely difficulties or complications during the operation, and a back-up plan as to their management. Planning should also include the provision of reserve or extension grafts which can be used to deal with endoleaks or inadequate coverage; this is particularly applicable in patients with a difficult aortic neck or calcified, atherosclerotic iliac arteries. Variations in the generally recommended anatomical requirements for successful implantation of an endovascular AAA graft are provided in the instructions for use of individual graft designs.

Measurements of the diameter of the aortic neck and the iliac arteries are, in general, best obtained from the CT scan images, whereas length measurements are more accurate when obtained from 3D reconstructions or from calibrated angiography (Figure 1). When determining vessel diameters, it is important to recognize that some of the device companies recommend sizing with respect to the internal or luminal measurement of the aortic neck or iliac diameter, whereas others recommend measuring the external, adventitial diameter. Vessel diameter measurements usually assume a circular or cylindrical shape, so it is useful to verify that the true shape is not ovoid or irregular by reference to the 3D images. The angles of deployed devices should be anticipated, and consideration given as to whether this could be improved by use of different access side or technique, or by using different device components. Extra graft extensions of vari-ous sizes, balloons, access catheters and guidewires should be available. In cases where there may be access difficulties, an alternative technique of access should be pre-planned (for example, iliac conduit graft via retro-peritoneal approach) and the patient prepared and informed.

WHAT CONSTITUTES ADEQUATE IMAGING FOR ENDOGRAFT PROCEDURE PLANING?

With regards to planning AAA endograft procedures, most centers now rely primarily on a combination of the axial and re-formatted images obtained from state-of-the-art multi-slice CT scanners, with particular emphasis on 3-Dimensional reconstructions (3-D) of the aortic anatomic features. The arrival of rapid reformatting programs and specialized workstations such as those marketed by TeraRecon and 3-Mensio (see chapter 1) make this technology more accessible to the operating surgeon. Some centers also apply Magnetic

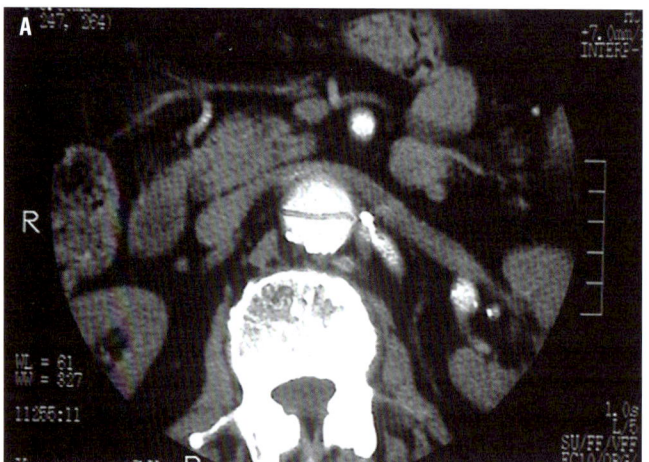 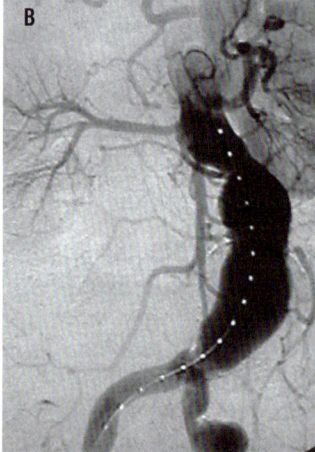

FIGURE 1: Pre-Operative Planning and Aortic Measurement. **A.** CT film images may be used for calculations of aortic neck diameter and iliac diameters. **B.** Angiography is used sparingly, but may be may be useful for accurate calculations of aortic and iliac lengths, as well as for demonstration of angulations and aortic neck morphology.

Resonance Imaging (MRI) for both pre-operative imaging and for progressive follow-up imaging studies. The role of angiography varies at different sites.

There are some situations where adjunctive angiography can still be invaluable in procedure planning. These particularly relate to advanced planning techniques for difficult anatomy as shown on CT imaging, particularly if clear and accurate 3D reformatted images are not readily available. An example is the short or severely angulated aortic neck, particularly when angulation is in the antero-posterior plane. Angiography may also be valuable in the work-up for fenestrated and branched graft designs.

How much device oversizing?

Most endovascular device companies recommend use of a graft that is oversized by approximately 10-15% compared to the diameters of the attachment zones in the aortic neck and the iliac arteries. These recommendations have largely been empirical, based on the fact that a self-expanding graft needs to deploy to a size large enough to attain both attachment and seal within these sites. There has also been an argument that allowance should be made for late spontaneous dilatation of the aortic neck,[1] although there is a contrary view that deployment of an endograft high within the aortic neck has the effect of preventing neck dilatation.[2] The true amount of oversizing that results depends on the method used for calculating the vessel diameters, for which there is no standardized technique. Usually the aortic neck diameter is calculated with respect to the external (adventitial) surface, so that the true diameter of the lumen may be considerably less and the graft diameter may therefore be oversized substantially more with respect to the lumen.

With severe oversizing, some endograft designs appear to then cause dilatation of the neck due to their inherent radial expan-sile force. Excessive oversizing (20% or more) has been shown to be associated with increased graft migration rates with at least 2 self-expanding device designs.[3,4] In one study, oversizing by more than 20% with the AneuRx graft resulted in late aortic neck dilation and high rates of device migration.[3] With the Zenith graft, oversizing of 30% in a multicenter phase II trial resulted in a 14-fold increase in migration rates, as well as increased rate of AAA sac enlargement, and early dilatation of the aortic neck at the 6-month follow-up interval, which then stabilized out to 24 months.[4] Although these changes may be device-dependant, avoidance of excessive oversizing is recommended. The characteristics of the neck itself are also important factors: a short neck or aortic neck angulation greater than 40° have significant adverse effects on the outcome.[5,6]

THE PLANNING PROCESS FOR INTRA-PROCEDURAL IMAGING

Working out the best angles for the image intensifier is an essential, and often neglected, aspect of successful and precise AAA endograft implantation. Angulations of the aortic neck in either the lateral or anteroposterior planes may mean that standard views cause considerable fore-shortening, thereby reducing considerably the apparent length of the neck (Figure 2). This can result in imprecise placement of the device. Similarly, oblique angles of the renal arteries and the iliac vessels may best be seen with oblique image intensifier views or with alterations in the cranio-caudal angulation of the x-ray beam.

General strategies for endovascular AAA repair procedures

Some of the guiding principles for endovascular repair of AAA are:

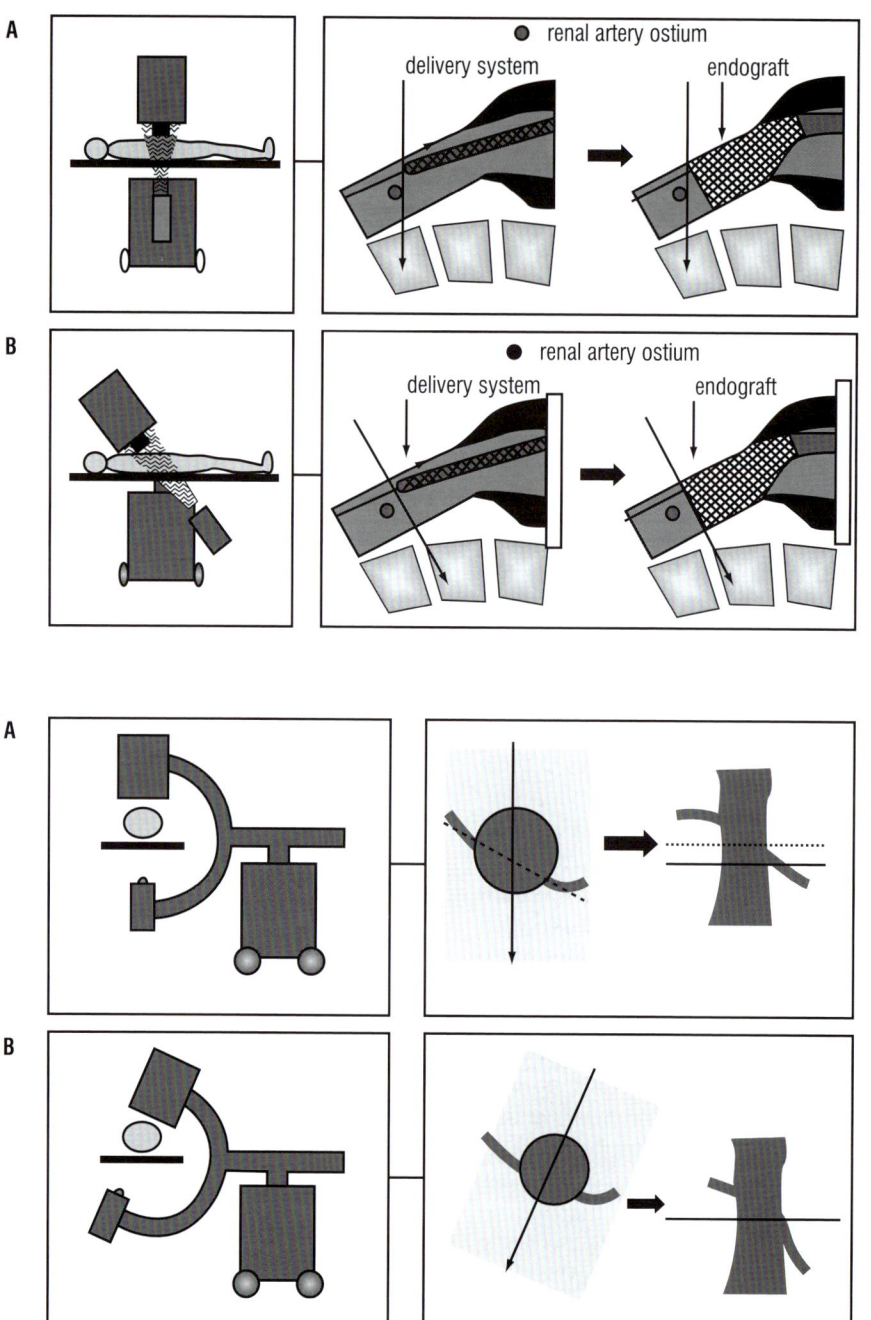

FIGURE 2: Planning correct angulation of the image intensifier during the implant procedure. **A.** Ideal cranio-caudal orientation of the fluoroscope head can be calculated from pre-operative imaging studies, allowing accurate positioning of the endovascular graft with respect to the origin of the renal arteries. **B.** Oblique image intensifier angulation (left anterior oblique or right anterior oblique angulation) can be a valuable adjunct when the aortic neck or iliac arteries are tortuous, or for increased accuracy in demonstration of the origin of renal, visceral and internal iliac arteries.

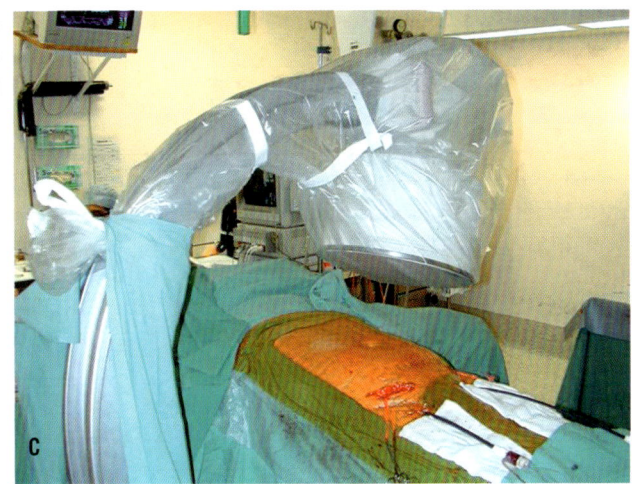

FIGURE 2: C. Intra-procedural left oblique angulation of the II head to accurately show the origin of the right internal iliac artery.

(i) Procedures should be done in a suite which is well-equipped for precise vascular imaging as well as for surgical exposure of the vessels. For the most difficult cases, it is advantageous to be prepared for emergency surgical conversion to open repair of the aorta or the iliac arteries. Anatomic grade of difficulty for the individual patient should also influence choice of procedure venue; when there are significant anatomic problems then the potential need for open surgical adjuncts or even conversion is increased.

(ii) Assisting team members should be assigned specific roles for various aspects of the procedure, particularly with respect to device preparation, care and positioning of the access and delivery sheaths, and maintenance of guidewire position throughout the procedure. It is advantageous to have one team member assigned to making sure throughout the whole procedure that the sheaths are not extruded by the force of blood flow, and that the primary guidewires are never inadvertently removed during the procedure. Sheaths are particularly vulnerable to dislodgement during passage of balloons or extension graft devices.

(iii) In most cases, the aim should be to internally line the whole length of the infrarenal aorta and the common iliac arteries, so that device coverage is from just below the renal artery orifices to just above the origin of the internal iliac arteries.

(iv) Device choice depends on anatomic features, early and especially long-term device results, operator experience and other factors. Favorable device features include active fixation components, as well as device flexibility and malleability to cater for angulated or irregular vessel shapes (especially when modified by adjunctive balloon dilatation), a wide range of device component diameters, durable materials and non-kinkable access sheaths. We prefer multi-piece modular devices which allow considerable customizing for the individual patient, and can be selected from the shelf at the time of procedure rather than requiring weeks of preparation. Bifurcated devices are always preferred over aorto-monoiliac devices, unless there is a specific overriding indication for single-sided iliac limb.

(v) Choice of the primary access side depends on factors such as diameters of the femoral and iliac vessels, vessel tortuosity, angles of entry of the common iliac arteries into the aorta, and lengths of the respective common iliac arteries. For example, if the common iliac artery is short on one side, this should usually be chosen as the contra-lateral limb side to allow more flexibility in device choice (length and diameter).

(vi) Primary operative concerns are the attachment and fixation of the proximal graft body segment within the aortic neck, good overlap and fixation of modular component pieces, and seal around the aortic and iliac grafts.

(vii) After deployment of self-expand-ing components, careful adjunctive bal-looning should be done to ensure ade-quate expansion of the supporting wire-forms or stents, particularly in the attach-ment zones and at overlap zones.

(viii) Cannulation of the contralateral stump of the bifurcated primary trunk seg-ment of modular devices can be quite a demanding technical exercise. It is useful to have available a variety of shaped angi-ographic catheters, and also to be capa-ble of backup cannulation from above us-ing guidewire and snare techniques (see below).

(ix) Confirming that the contralateral stump has been definitely accessed is im-portant to avoid placement of iliac extension grafts outside the overlap zone of the stump. This can be done by a number of techniques, including rotation of the shaped cannulation catheters within the interior of the trunk graft, inflation of a balloon within the trunk stump, injection of contrast, or di-rected passage of guidewires.

(x) If there is a suspicion of iliac or fem-oral limb compression or kink, iliac arterial pressures should be measured by con-necting pressure transducer lines to the access sheaths. If pressures are compro-mised, adjunctive ballooning may be re-peated or further bare stent support used.

(xi) Endoleaks of type I or type III clas-sification should always be corrected at the initial operation by extension or over-lap devices, wherever feasible.

(xii) Guidewire access should be main-tained for a short interval after the access sheaths have been removed, in case a rupture or tear of the iliac artery is ex-posed by sheath removal. This permits rapid re-access for inflation of a balloon, temporary plugging of any bleeding site by sheath reinsertion, or placement of secondary limb extensions which can be deployed to repair the torn vessel wall.

(xiii) Closure of the groin incisions should include careful cauterization of any regions where lymphatic vessels may have been transected or damaged, to help minimize the incidence of post-oper-ative wound seroma or lymphocoele.

Access techniques

Access to the femoral arteries is usually achieved by an open surgical approach ("femoral cut-down"), but may also be gained by percutaneous approach. In se-lected cases, a tunneled approach is made to the femoral or external iliac arter-ies to allow a relatively straight-line entry to the artery when the femoral vessels are unduly deep because of fat, bulk or de-formity (Figure 3).

● Femoral cutdown approach
An oblique transverse incision is preferred by many and may have a lower incidence of post-operative seroma or lymphocoele than a vertical incision.[7,8] The incision will usually be limited to 3-4 cm in length, since exposure of only the common femo-ral artery is required. Most access sheaths are now designed with a smooth taper so that the sheath can be inserted directly over the guidewire into the artery resulting in a gradual dilatation of the arteriotomy; use of a formal surgical arteriotomy is lim-ited to selected vessels that are severely calcified or stenotic.

● Percutaneous approach
Improvements in the profile of sheath sys-tems potentially allow for percutaneous

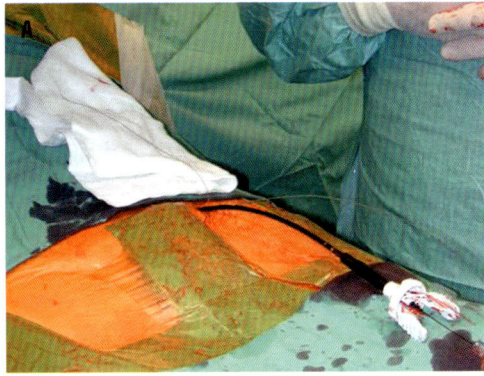
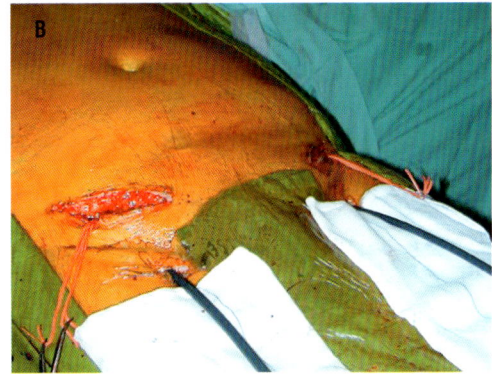
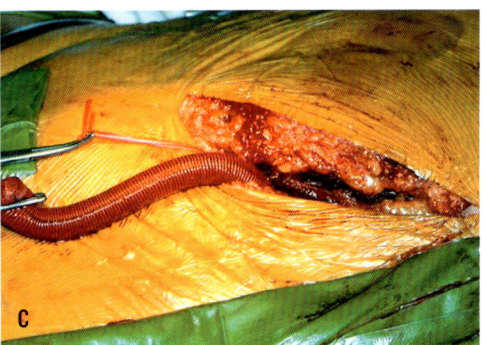

FIGURE 3: Access Techniques. **A.** Percutaneous access to the common femoral arteries. The "pre-close" technique: The sutures of the Perclose closure device are placed prior to insertion of the device. **B.** Tunneled access to the femoral artery is a useful technique in obese patients. Cutdown approach is made to the artery before oblique tunneled approach for sheath insertion. This provides a favorable angle of device introduction. **C.** Iliac conduit access technique. A polyester graft is anastomosed to the external or common iliac artery after retroperitoneal exposure, and used for sheath and device access.

access, but the widespread application of this technique is limited by a lack of approved efficient devices required to achieve effective closure of the large hole formed in the arterial wall (Figure 3a). The Perclose system (Abbott Vascular, Menlo Park, CA) is used most commonly, applying a particular method of deploying percutaneous needles and sutures prior to the passage of the endograft deployment sheath.[9-12] (These devices are not specifically approved for such an application in the USA).

• *Tunneled femoral access*
When the femoral artery is very deep, the device deployment sheath may be compromised by angulation and kinking over the ridge formed by the tissues overlying the vessel –in this situation it is often advantageous to form a narrow subcutaneous tunnel angled gradually down to the vessel from a small skin incision 5-10 cm further down the thigh (Figure 3b).

• *Alternative access*
Other access routes include use of a conduit graft anastomosed to the common or external iliac artery[13] (Figure 3c), laparoscopic-guided approach via the iliac artery, and access from neck or arm arteries.

Cannulation of the contralateral stump

When a modular device is used, there are three basic techniques available for cannulation of the contralateral stump:

• *Cannulation from below (retrograde cannulation)*
In the majority of cases, access to the contralateral stump can be achieved ex-

peditiously by guidewire and catheter technique retrogradely from the contralateral femoral access site (Figure 4). All modular devices feature a radio-opaque marking system to indicate the position of this stump and facilitate the cannulation process. Once the guidewire passes into the correct channel, exchange is made for a super-stiff wire, which is then used for passage of the delivery sheath. Various special maneuvers may be used to verify that the wire is truly within the lumen of the contralateral stump, including rotation of a pre-shaped catheter tip[14] injection of contrast, or inflation of a balloon within the stump (see Figure 4c).

• Crossover cannulation (antegrade cannulation)

An alternative technique is to pass a guidewire via an angulated guiding catheter over the graft bifurcation and down into the contralateral stump. This wire may then be further directed down the iliac artery, or may be retrieved by a snare catheter passed from the contralateral femoral site.

• Brachial artery approach

An approach from the left brachial artery may also be used if the two previous methods fail. A guide wire is passed from the left brachial artery and directed down the descending thoracic aorta by a guiding catheter to reach the aneurysm sac and then the iliac artery via the contralateral stump. The brachial approach may also be a useful adjunct in cases of extreme tortuosity in the iliac arteries. After retrieval of the brachial guide wire by snare device in the aneurysm sac, tension can be applied from the brachial and femoral ends.[15] This results in considerable straightening of the iliac arteries, allowing passage of the sheaths.

PLANNING CONSIDERATIONS FOR ILIAC ARTERY PROBLEMS Access techniques for unfavorable iliac arteries

Categories of difficult anatomy in the iliac segment include tortuosity, acute angula-

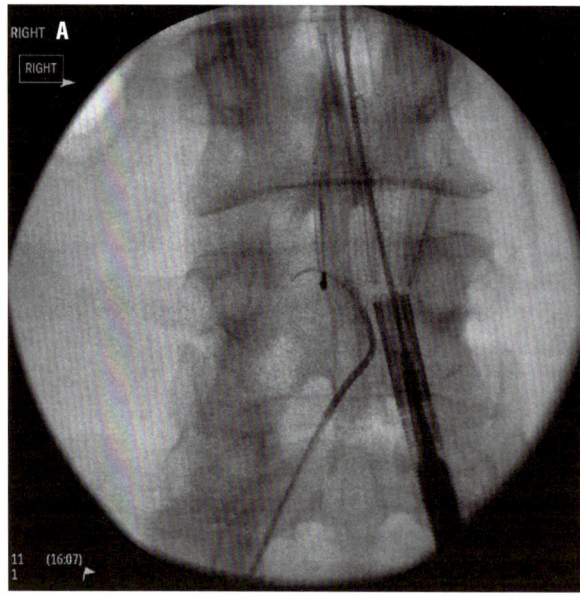

FIGURE 4: Cannulation of the contralateral stump of a modular bifurcated device. **A.** Typical technique using angulated catheter for guidewire positioning.

FIGURE 4: **B.** Following guidewire access, a number of approaches can be used to verify that the contralateral stump of the trunk device component has been successfully accessed. In this case, a calibrated pigtail angiographic catheter has been placed over the guidewire.

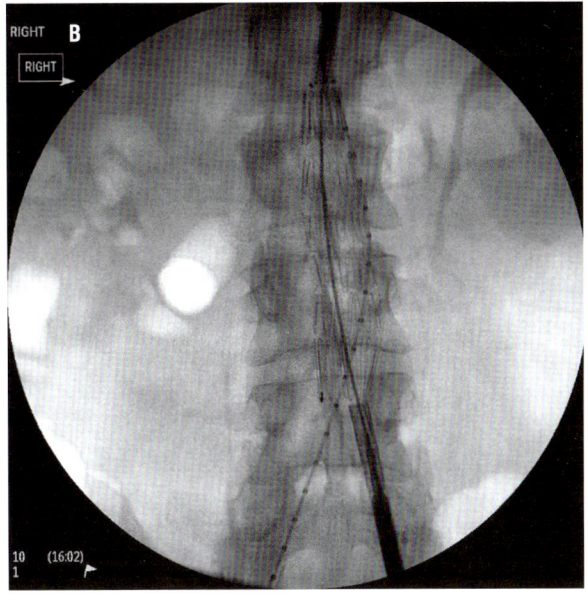

tions, narrow atherosclerotic lesions and calcified vessel wall (Figure 5). Iliac aneurysms present their own problems in management. Unfavorable iliac anatomy may present obstacles to access and successful deployment of aortic devices, as well as problems in obtaining aneurysm exclusion and secure fixation. Early or late migration of iliac limb devices may occur, whereas angulation of the limbs can lead to device occlusion.

With regards to access, adjunctive techniques include use of super-stiff guidewires of various grades (Figure 6), hydrophilic delivery catheters, arterial dilatation by angioplasty balloons or tapered sheaths, and iliac conduit grafts. External manipulation of the iliac vessels through the abdominal wall may sometimes be a helpful adjunct.[16,17]

Improved fixation and seal in ectatic or

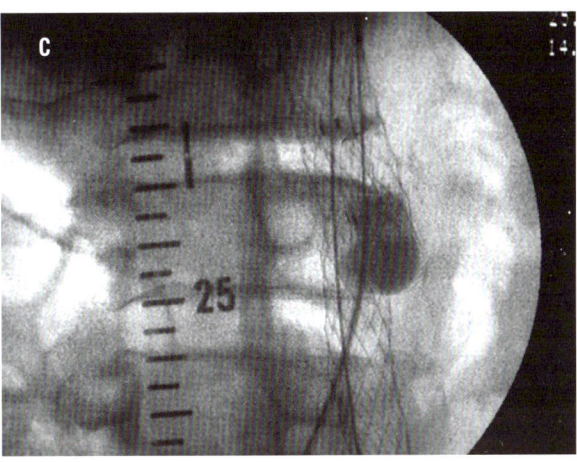

FIGURE 4: **C.** The "mushroom balloon" sign. A balloon inflated at the opening of the contralateral stump assumes this shape due to constriction of the proximal aspect within the limb stump.

aneurysmal iliac arteries usually requires the use of large diameter extension limbs, often with flared distal ends ("bell-bottom" technique). For such cases, it is helpful to have a variety of grafts in a range of diameters and lengths to allow in-situ customizing to the anatomy of the individual patient (Figure 7).

Strategies for difficult iliac artery access

Problematic iliac arteries are usually calcified, tortuous and stenosed. These features are more frequent in elderly patients, especially small-framed women, or those with chronic renal disease. Angulations may be made more favorable by use of super-stiff guidewires, such as the Lundequist wire (W L Cook) or similar (see Figure 6). The guidewire may be made less liable to distortion by the use of a through-and-through approach from brachial artery to the femoral site.[15]

There are a number of strategies available for gaining access in a patient with difficult iliac artery anatomy (Table 1). These include use of special guidewires, adjunctive balloon dilatation of focal stenotic lesions in the iliac artery, or graduated dilatation using progressively larger trocars or sheaths. In some cases, it is necessary to obtain access via a conduit graft sewn onto the external or common

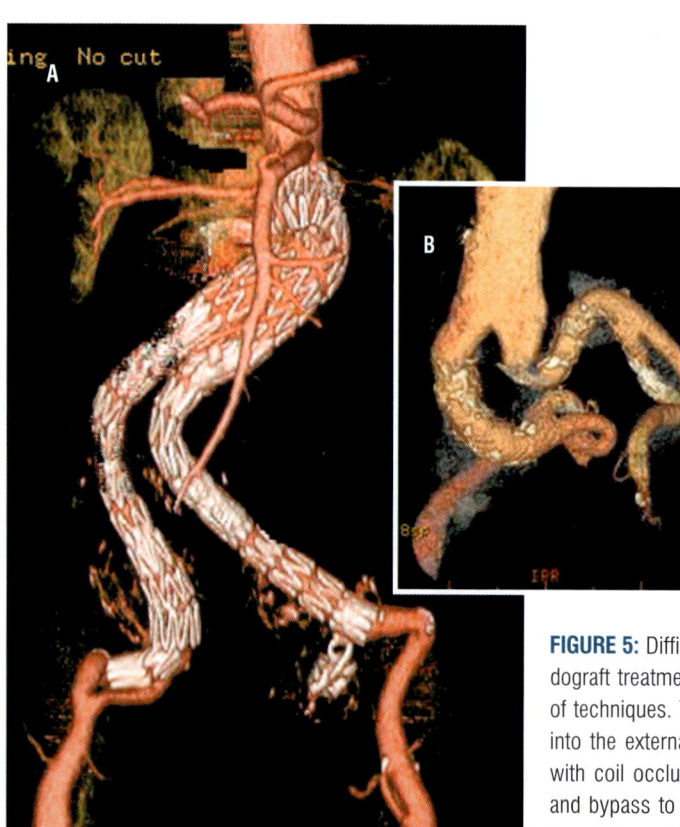

FIGURE 5: Difficult iliac arteries. **A.** Successful endograft treatment of difficult anatomy by a variety of techniques. The iliac limbs have been extended into the external iliac artery bilaterally, combined with coil occlusion of the left internal iliac artery and bypass to the right internal iliac from the external iliac artery. **B.** Unfavorable iliac anatomy. Factors which increase the difficulties of access include angulation, stenosis and calcification.

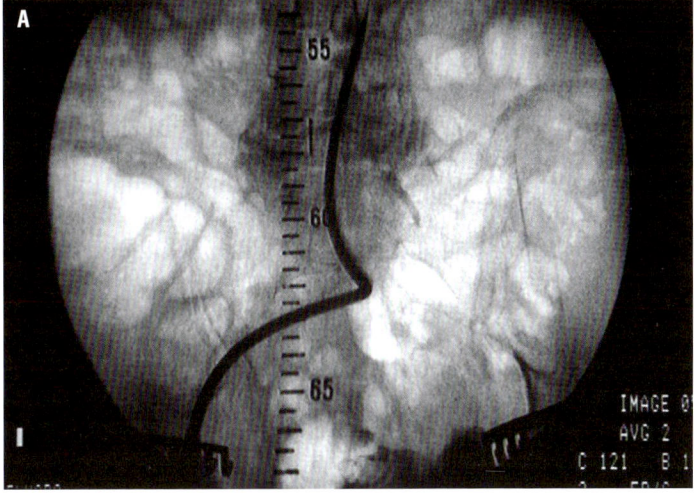

FIGURE 6: Straightening the iliac artery achieved by stiff guidewires. **A.** A tortuous iliac system has been straightened somewhat by use of an Amplatz "super-stiff" wire.

iliac artery after retroperitoneal exposure. A variation of this technique is to place an iliac-to-femoral bypass graft by open surgical method, followed by endovascular graft delivery through the bypass graft. Laparoscopic means for iliac artery access have also been trialed. Rarely, access is gained via an aortic graft or via the carotid artery.[18]

Management of the ruptured iliac artery

Excessive force or the large diameter of the access sheaths may result in iliac artery rupture in such cases. Typically this will occur at the site of narrowed external iliac segments or in regions of severe fixed angulation.

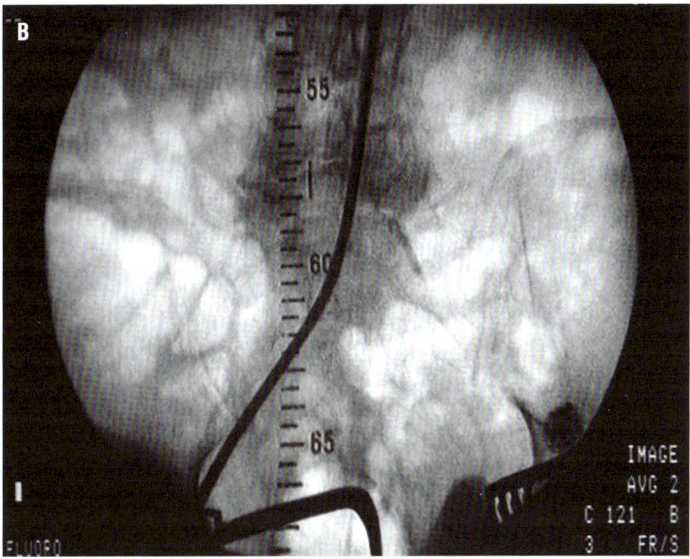

FIGURE 6: B. Further straightening was achieved in this case with an even more rigid Lunderquist wire.

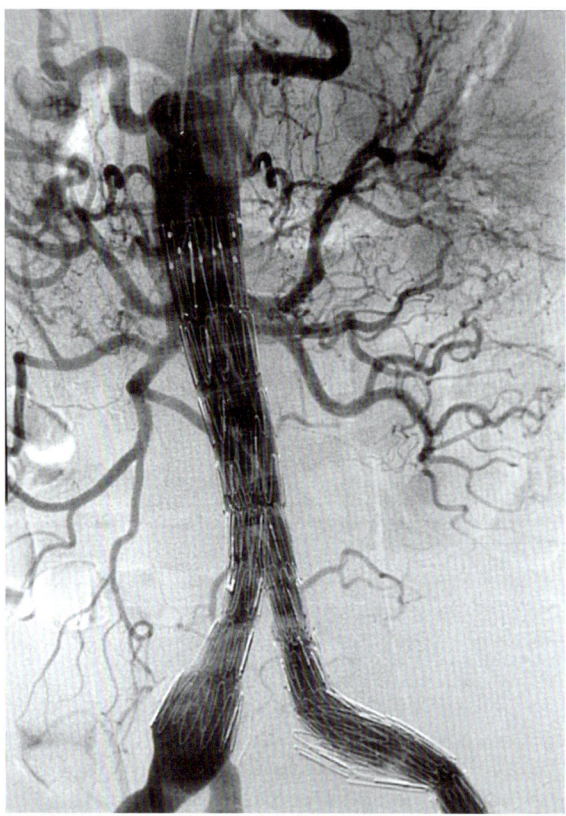

FIGURE 7: Use of "bell-bottom" shaped iliac limbs for dilated or aneurysmal iliac arteries. On the right side, a 2.2 cm diameter iliac aneurysm has been lined with a 24 mm diameter bell-bottom iliac extension limb. On the left side, a larger iliac aneurysm has been treated by extension of the iliac limb down to the external iliac artery, in conjunction with a reversed bell-bottom or 'converter' graft adjunct to block backflow from the internal iliac artery.

The first step in management of such problems is to plug the bleeding site by re-insertion of the sheath. An alternative technique is to inflate a balloon at the site. These maneuvers both require a general policy of maintaining guidewire access at all times, and careful monitoring of hemodynamic parameters at any time when difficult anatomy is encountered, especially if the sheath or artery is felt to give way during passage.

Once control of the hemorrhage is established, a decision must be made as to whether the best next move is aimed towards continuing endovascular repair techniques, or surgical retroperitoneal exposure of the iliac rupture site, with a view to direct closure or adjunctive bypass. Endovascular repair of the damaged arterial segment will often be feasible, by rapid deployment of an iliac limb graft across the perforation site, or several overlapped extension limbs. When surgical exposure is chosen, usually a bypass of the damaged vessel will be preferred, and this can be then used as the access site to continue the aortic graft deployment process.

Prevention of iliac artery rupture

The key to preventing iliac artery rupture lies in patient selection. When pre-operative imaging shows narrow and tortuous iliac arteries, the options include avoiding endovascular techniques, adjunctive use of an iliac conduit graft, trial passage of graduated dilators, or prior dilatation and graft lining.

TABLE 1

ALTERNATIVE ACCESS STRATEGIES IN THE PATIENT WITH DIFFICULT ILIAC ANATOMY

I. Transfemoral access
– use of super-stiff guidewires
– use of femoral-brachial through-and-through guidewire
– adjunctive balloon dilatation of external iliac or common iliac lesions, prior to passage of the access sheath
– iliac dilatation using graduated access trocars or sheaths
– preliminary stent-graft lining and reinforcement of the iliac arteries by iliac extension grafts

II. Iliac access
– conduit graft via retro-peritoneal exposure
– direct iliac puncture after retro-peritoneal exposure
– iliac-femoral bypass, then access via the prosthetic graft
– iliac exposure via laparoscopic access

III. Aortic access
– via distal aorta or aortic replacement graft (prior surgery)

IV. Carotid or upper limb access
– rarely used

Management of the iliac component of aorto-iliac aneurysms

Iliac artery aneurysms are commonly present in association with AAA. There are a number of options for combined treatment. These include treatment of the iliac segment by "bell-bottom" iliac extension limbs (Figure 7, 8), occlusion of the origin of the internal iliac branch as an adjunct to extension of the iliac limb graft through to the external iliac artery (Figure 7), and iliac branch graft devices.

Management of poor distal landing zones and common iliac artery aneurysms: Use of the iliac bifurcation device

The presence of a common iliac artery aneurysm (CIAA) in conjunction with an AAA is a common problem which complicates 15-30% of endovascular abdominal aortic

aneurysm repairs (EVAR).[19-21] Possible endovascular solutions include:
1. Using a flared iliac limb for small CIAAs. Flared or bell-bottom iliac limbs are available up to 24 mm diameter.
2. Internal iliac artery coiling and placement of an extension endograft into the external iliac artery.
3. Endograft extension into the external iliac artery combined with an open surgical retroperitoneal revascularization of the internal iliac artery (see Figure 5a).
4. Using a bifurcated iliac endograft (or "iliac branched device") with preservation of the IIA (see also chapter 12).

Occlusion of the IIA results in buttock claudication in 12-45% of patients. Maintenance of IIA patency may be required for sexual potency and visceral and spinal cord perfusion in some patients.[20-24] The need to preserve the IIA when performing EVAR must be assessed on a case by case basis. In the presence of bilateral CI-

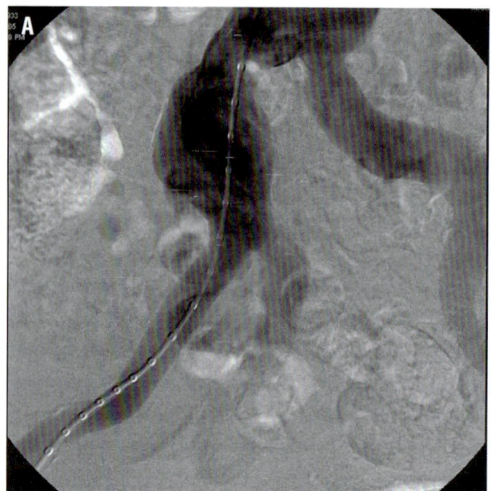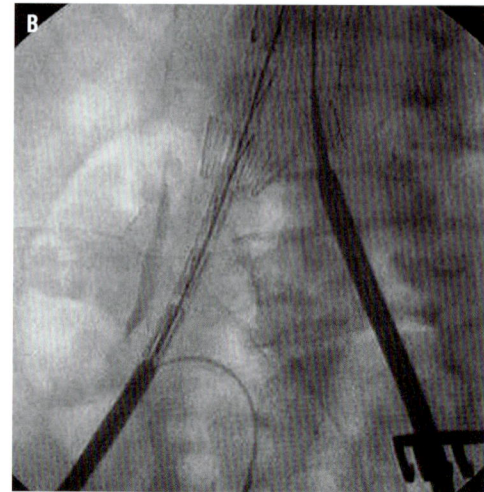

FIGURE 8: Advanced treatment of iliac aneurysm by a "double bell-bottom" graft technique. **A.** Angiogram showing an aneurysm of the right common iliac artery in association with an AAA. **B.** After implantation of an endograft into the AAA, a first bell-bottom extension has been implanted so that its widest aspect occludes the dilated orifice of the common iliac artery. Note the guidewire placed into the internal iliac artery to allow precise placement of the second overlapped iliac bell-bottom extension graft which is about to be implanted immediately proximal to this branch.

AAs it is advisable to preserve at least one internal iliac artery.[25]

The iliac bifurcation device (IBD), (Cook, Brisbane, Australia) is a branched endovascular graft which, when linked to an EVAR device achieves exclusion of an AAA and CIAA with preservation of the internal iliac artery (Figure 9). This combination of devices results in generous stent-graft overlap in an area of relative anatomic fixation and thus intuitively has a good chance of long term durability.

The IBD has a pre-mounted catheter and a wire passing from the control handle through the distal end of the internal iliac limb out through the proximal end of the device. When snared from the contralateral side this wire is used to guide a sheath into the internal iliac limb, which is then used for deployment of a stent graft into a suitable sealing zone in the internal iliac artery (Figure 9). Standard EVAR deployment follows with the main body introduced from the contralateral side. A bridg-

ing stent is placed between the main body of the EVAR device and the IBD.

Preoperative planning considerations, which are unique to the use of the IBD, include accurate assessment of:

1. CIA length. If the CIA is too short for the length of the CIA component of the IBD, cannulation of the proximal end of the device from the contralateral CIA will be difficult and brachial access may be required.
2. Distal CIA diameter. If the CIAA narrows to a normal CIA diameter at the iliac bifurcation, the internal iliac limb of the IBD will not have the required space to open up.
3. Internal iliac artery landing zone. There must be adequate landing zone in the internal iliac artery or one of its branches for a seal to be achieved with a stent graft. Also, some internal iliacs will have a diameter exceeding that covered by currently available stent grafts and this may contraindicate the use of the IBD.

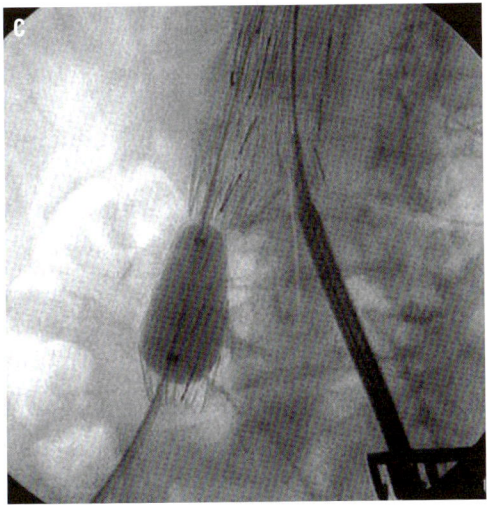
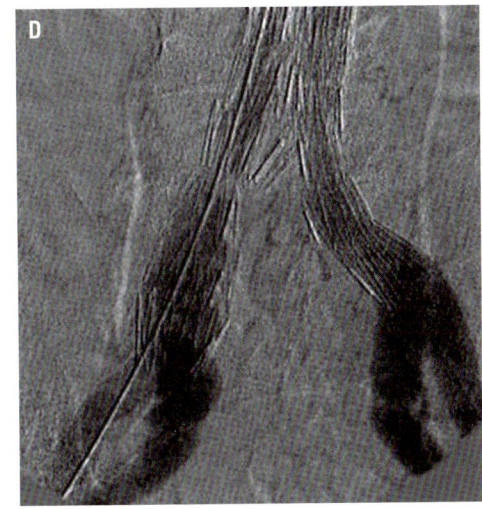

FIGURE 8: C. Following deployment of the second extension graft, its bell-bottom distal aspect is fully opened by balloon expansion technique to occlude the distal aspect of the aneurysm of the right common iliac artery. **D.** Post-deployment angiogram showing successful exclusion of the right common iliac artery aneurysm, with preservation of flow into the internal iliac artery.

The IBD can also extend a previous EVAR where CIA fixation has been lost due to aneurysmal dilation of the CIA. AAA with bilateral CIAAs may also be treated with the IBD, this requires deployment of the EVAR main body prior to deployment of bilateral IBDs with cannulation of each internal iliac limb using a brachial access sheath (Table 2).

Special Planning Considerations for the Aortic Neck Zone

Suprarenal or infrarenal attachment?

Some endovascular graft devices feature a bare-stent segment which projects superiorly from the top of the graft, above the level of graft fabric, with struts of these stents extending to the level of the suprarenal aorta. Such devices may also include projecting hooks designed to im-

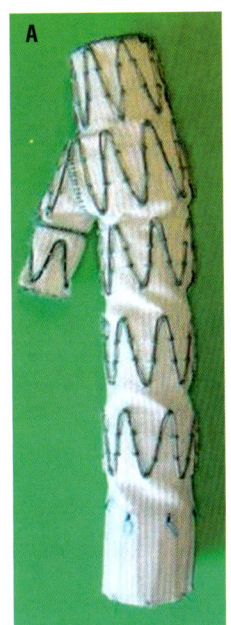
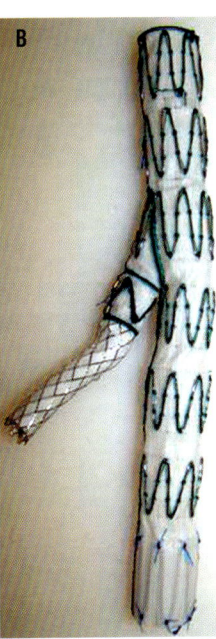

FIGURE 9: Treatment of iliac aneurysm associated with AAA using an iliac branch device. **A.** Iliac branch device (Cook Zenith, William A. Cook, Queensland, Australia). **B.** Iliac branch device, with adjunctive balloon-expandable extension limb for the internal iliac branch.

TABLE 2

COMPARISON OF SINGLE-PIECE AND MODULAR BIFURCATED ENDOVASCULAR GRAFTS

Single-piece	Modular (multi-piece)
Complex graft construction and delivery system	Simple graft components and delivery system
Graft dimensions determined at time of manufacture	Customised graft component selection may be available at time of procedure
Requires preliminary insertion of iliac crossover catheter	Requires guidewire access to the contra-lateral graft stump to place iliac limb
Single piece construction may reduce potential for fabric leak or graft failure	Potential for leakage, disconnection or stenosis at graft overlap zone
Difficult to deliver fully stented –may require addition stents implanted into graft limbs	Can be delivered as a fully supported stent-graft

prove attachment and long term fixation of the device. The main advantage of suprarenal attachment is that it may protect against early or late migration of the device by improving the resistance to displacement by flowing blood and other forces. The compromise of such devices is that the stent struts may cross the orifice of the renal arteries causing significant detrimental affects on renal function, including renal failure and an increased risk of renal infarcts due to emboli or compromised flow.[26] Despite these concerns, some centers use suprarenal attachment devices routinely, whereas other centers are selective, using infrarenal devices for routine anatomy and reserving suprarenal attachment only for selected cases with a difficult neck (short, or angulated, or containing mural thrombus). Intermediate-term results (of up to 5-10 years) have not shown any large incidence of late renal effects.

THE ANGULATED AORTIC NECK

Angulation of the aortic neck may compromise the fixation, attachment and sealing functions of the endovascular graft device, both in the early phase and also in long term follow-up. Angulation of the neck is often associated with curvature of the AAA itself as well as tortuosity of the iliac arteries, increasing the incidence of access problems and vascular complications.

How much neck angulation is acceptable for endograft implantation?

Conventional wisdom is that neck angulation of greater than 45-60 degrees constitutes a contra-indication for use of AAA endografts. Again, these criteria are somewhat arbitrary, and the true limits have not really been adequately tested and will depend on device design factors such as graft flexibility and attachment methods. Another important factor is the length of neck over which angulation occurs, with regular and gradual angulation being more favorable than an acute region of aortic kink. Of current devices, the Zenith Flex graft (Cook) and the Aorfix device appear best suited to tortuous neck anatomy, but further trials are needed to better define the ability of these devices to adapt to severe angulation and to provide durable results.

THE SHORT AORTIC NECK

Conventional graft or fenestrated device?

A neck length of 15 mm is generally considered to be the minimum requirement for reliably achieving adequate infrarenal graft fixation.[27] Preferably the neck should be cylindrical but graft oversizing may compensate for conical reverse tapered necks[4] (Figure 10). These criteria are mostly based on empirical data provided for early trials of aortic endografts, and there are a number of techniques available for use of conventional devices in less favorable neck anatomy. Precise placement of the proximal aspect of the graft immediately below the renal artery orifice (within 1-3 mm) can enhance attachment and fixation in shorter or angled necks to some extent this is also dependant on device design, so broad selection criteria are not universally appropriate. Special adjunctive techniques may include preserving patency of the renal artery by stenting, and enhancement of neck fixation by first placing an oversized proximal tube graft within the most dilated segment.[28]

For aneurysm necks that do not fit the accepted criteria, or for those that are otherwise unfavorable, the problem of proximal fixation may alternatively be solved by use of scalloped or fenestrated endografting. Fenestrated techniques may be used to treat primary juxtarenal and visceral segment aneurysms, proximal type I endoleaks after previous endoluminal repair and para-anastomotic aneurysms after previous open aneurysm repair.[27,30-32]

The most widely used technique for fenestrated EVAR requires manufacture of a custom Zenith graft (William A Cook, Brisbane, Australia) with scallops and fenestrations cut into the fabric in the appropriate positions as determined by pre-operative imaging (see also chapters 11 and 16.[29-31]

Planning a fenestrated endograft requires measurements obtained from high resolution CT angiography with 3D reconstruction.[29,31,34] Whilst many different visceral artery configurations may be accommodated, construction of the fenes-

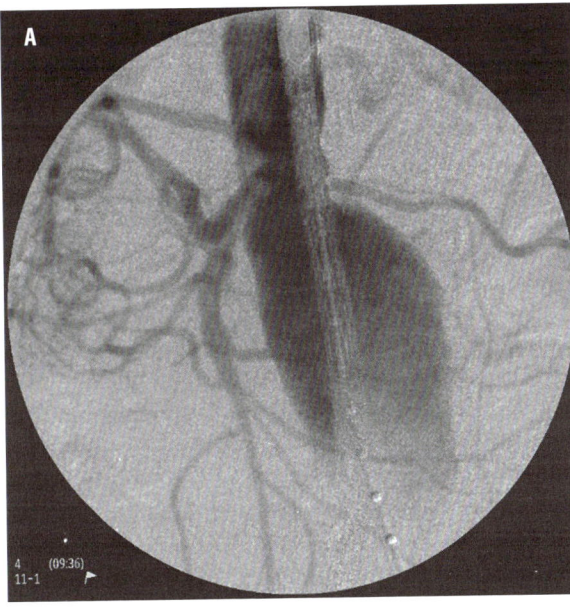

FIGURE 10: Successful endograft treatment of AAA with unfavorable neck anatomy, using standard off-the-shelf technology. **A.** Intra-operative angiogram during deployment of an endovascular graft into the very short, reversed taper neck of an AAA in a patient with significant risk factors for open surgery.

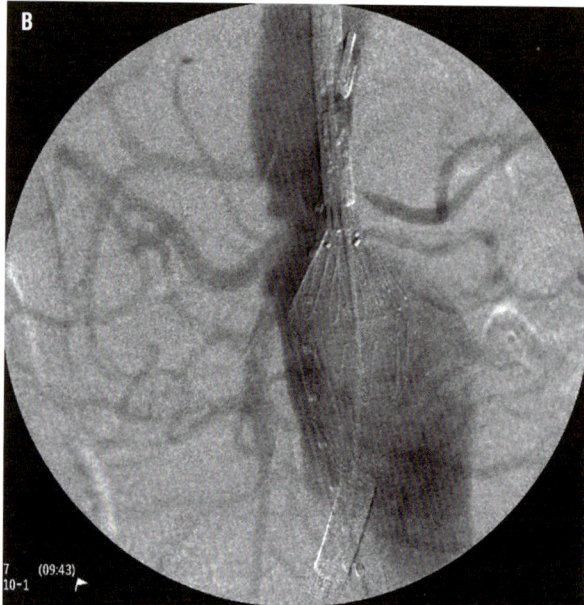

FIGURE 10: B. In such cases, precision placement of the device immediately below the renal arteries is important, together with selection of an oversized graft which will fit the larger diameter of the distal neck or proximal aneurysm segment.

trated graft may be complicated by the presence of multiple renal arteries or visceral arteries in close proximity to each other. Aneurysm neck angulation, calcifi- cation and thrombus also complicate fenestrated EVAR.[32-34]

Catheter angiography is not a prerequisite for graft planning, however, the in-

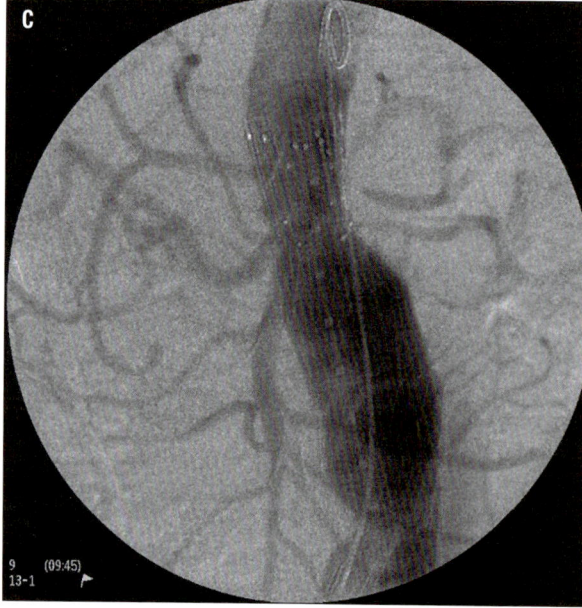

FIGURE 10: C. Angiogram after graft deployment and ballooning, showing successful exclusion of the AAA. Cases such as this demonstrate that fenestrated or branched graft configurations are not always required for successful endovascular repair in unfavorable neck anatomy.

formation obtained in regard to iliac diameters, calcification and tortuosity and the orientation of visceral arteries in relation to the aneurysm neck is valuable.[29,31]

Other considerations prior to performing fenestrated EVAR include the increased operative times, contrast volumes and screening times and the effects of these factors on the patient. The need for high resolution imaging and the prolonged screening times which make dose monitoring mandatory mean that fenestrated EVAR is best performed in an angiography suite. Consideration should be given to the use of pulsed fluoroscopy to reduce radiation exposure.[31] Familiarity with standard EVAR as well as advanced endovascular skills including visceral stenting competency is required to achieve success with the fenestrated EVAR technique.

The lower pole renal artery

Accessory renal arteries (ARAs) occur with 15-30% percent of kidneys, approximately half of these will be inferior to the main renal artery.[35] ARAs arising inferior to the main renal artery shorten the length of neck available for proximal graft fixation. In patients with normal renal function, ARA coverage may be considered to achieve adequate proximal fixation.[35-37] Alternatively, a graft fenestration or scallop may be created to maintain ARA patency.

The volume of renal parenchyma supplied by an ARA may be estimated by CT angiography or catheter angiography. For ARAs supplying less than one third of renal parenchyma, coverage results in small renal infarctions in twenty percent of cases and no discernable effect in the remainder.[35,37] The glomerular filtration rate has been found not to change after ARA coverage and hypertension is a rare complication.[35-37] For larger ARAs graft fenestration is more appropriate. Type II endoleak arising from a covered ARA is a rare occurrence whether it arises from the neck or from the aneurysm sac.[35-37]

Mural thrombus or atheroma within the neck

The presence of mural thrombus or degenerative atheroma within the aortic neck zone used to be considered a contraindication (or relative contraindication) for aortic endograft implantation. Experience has shown that these cases can be treated relatively safely (Figure 11), al-

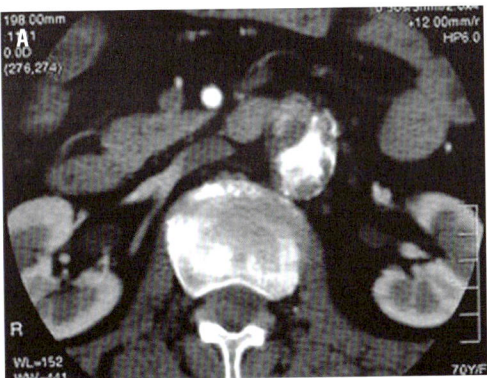 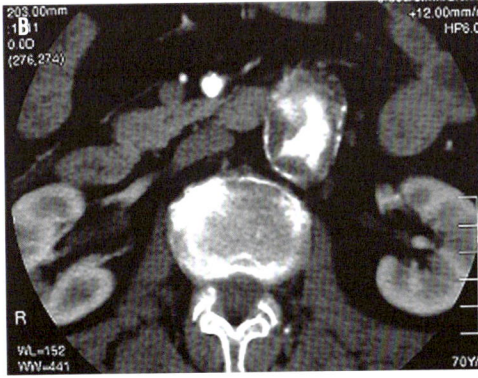

FIGURE 11: Successful endograft treatment of AAA with unfavorable neck morphology. **A. B.** CT scans through the aortic neck show irregular shape and severe atheroma or thrombus within the aortic wall. This is regarded as a relative contra-indication to endograft use in many centers.

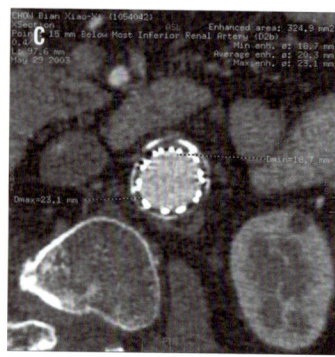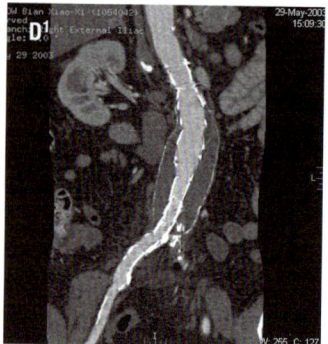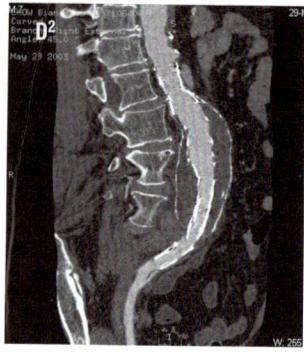

FIGURE 11: C. Post-operative CT scans through the same region of aortic neck show successful seal, with apparent remolding of the unfavorable wall features by the self-expanding device. **D.** Post-operative CT reconstruction through the plane of the iliac artery show impressive remodeling of the aortic wall and very successful outcome of endograft repair of AAA. No embolization occurred to mesenteric or distal arteries.

though there may be an increase risk of embolization to the renal arteries or to the leg vessels. In most cases, the atheroma is compressed outwardly, so that the post-implant appearance may be almost normal in the neck region. Devices with suprarenal attachment may be safer for such indications. It is generally recommended to either avoid balloon dilatation in this area, or to apply balloon dilatation judiciously.

CONCLUSIONS

Measurement, sizing and patient selection for aortic endograft procedures is sometimes complex. New modalities for imaging are being applied to gain improved anatomic data to aid in procedure planning. Device design for both aortic and iliac aneurysms will likely evolve and improve progressively, with specific designs being applied for different indications. The planning process remains one of the most important aspects in obtaining successful exclusion and repair of aneurysms by the endovascular approach.

REFERENCES

1. Cao P, Verzini F, Parlani G, Rango PD, Parente B, Giordino G, Mosca S, Maselli A. Predictive factors and clinical consequences of proximal aortic neck dilatation in 230 patients undergoing abdominal aorta aneurysm repair with self-expandable stent-grafts. J Vasc Surg 2003; 37:86-90.

2. May J, White GH, Ly CN, Jones MA, Harris JP. Endoluminal repair of asdominal aortic aneurysm prevents enlargement of the proximal neck: a 9-year life-table and 5-year longitudinal study. J Vasc Surg 2003;37:86-90

3. Connors MS, Sternbergh WC, Carter G, Tonnessen BH, Yoselevitz M, Money SR. Endograft migration one to four years after endovascular abdominal aortic repair with the AneuRx device: a cautionary note. J Vasc Surg 2002; 36:476-84

4. Sternbergh WC, Money SR, Greenberg RK, Chuter TA, Zenith Investigators. Influence of endograft oversizing on device migration, endoleak, aneurysm shrinkage, and aortic neck dilation: results from the Zenith Multicenter Trial. J Vasc Surg 2004; 39:20-26

5. Sternbergh WC, Carter G, York JW, Yoselovitz M, Money SR. Aortic neck angulation predicts adverse outcome with endovascular abdominal aortic aneurysm repair. J Vasc Surg 2002; 35:482-486.

6. Chaikof EL, Fillinger MF, Matsumura JS, Ruther-

ford RB, White GH, Blankensteijn JD, Bernard VM, Harris PL, Kent KC, May J, Veith FJ, Zarins CK. Identifying and grading factors that modify the outcome of endovascular aortic aneurysm repair. J Vasc Surg 2002 ;35:1061-6.

7. Chuter TA, Reilly LM, Stoney RJ, Messina LM: Femoral artery exposure for endovascular aneurysm repair through oblique incisions J Endovasc Surg 6:125; 1998.

8. Caiati JM, Kaplan D, Gitlitz D, Hollier L, Marin ML: The value of the oblique groin incision for femoral artery access during endovascular procedures. Ann Vasc Surg 14:248-53; 2000.

9. Rachel ES, Bergamini TM, Kinney EV, Jung MT, Kaebnick HW, Mitchell RA. Percutaneous endovascular abdominal aortic aneurysm repair. Ann Vasc Surg 2002; 16:43-9.

10. Howell M, Doughtery K, Strickman N, Krajcer Z. Percutaneous repair of abdominal aortic aneurysms using the AneuRx stent graft and the percutaneous vascular surgery device. Catheter Cardiovasc Interv 2002; 55:281-7.

11. Traul DK, Clair DG, Gray B, O'Hara PJ, Ouriel K. Percutaneous endovascular repair of infrarenal abdominal aortic aneurysms: a feasibility study. J Vasc Surg 2000; 32: 770-6.

12. Torsello GB, Kasprzak B, Klenk E, Tessarek J, Osada N, Torsello GF. Endovascular suture versus cutdown for endovascular aneurysm repair: a prospective randomised study. J Vasc Surg 2003; 38: 78-82.

13. Abu-Ghaida AM, Clair DG, Greenberg RK, Srivastava S, O'Hara PJ, Ouriel K. Broadening the applicability of endovascular aneurysm repair: the use of iliac conduits. J Vasc Surg 2002; 36: 111-7.

14. Dawson DL, Terramani TT, Loberman Z, Lumsden AB, Lin PH. Simple technique to ensure coaxial guidewire positioning for placement of iliac limb of modular aortic endograft. J Intervent Cardiol 2003; 16: 223-6.

15. Criado FJ, Wilson EP, Abul-Khoudoud O, Barker C, Carpenter J, Fairman R. Brachial artery catheterisation to facilitate endovascular grafting of abdominal aortic aneurysm: safety and rationale. J Vasc Surg 2000; 32: 1137-41.

16. Sternbergh WC, Money SR, Yoselovitz M. External transabdominal manipulation of vessels: a useful adjunct with endovascular abdominal

aortic aneurysm repair. J Vasc Surg 2001;33:886-7.

17. Ivancev K, Chuter TAM. Adjunctive manoeuvres for endovascular exclusion of abdominal aortic aneurysm. In: Endovascular Surgery For Aortic Aneurysms. Hopkinson B, Yusuf W, Whitaker S, Veith F (eds) Saunders, London, 1997 (pp 57-71)

18. Estes JM, Halin N, Kwoun M, Burch J,England M, Mackey WC. The carotid artery as alternative access for endoluminal aortic aneurysm repair. J Vasc Surg 2001 ;33:650-3

19. Armon MP, Wenham PW, Whitaker SC, Gregson RH, Hopkinson BR. Common iliac artery aneurysm in patients with abdominal aortic aneurysms. Eur J Vasc Endovasc Surg 1998;15(3):255-257.

20. Serracino-Inglott F, Bray AE, Myers P. Endovascular abdominal aortic aneurysm repair in patients with common iliac artery aneurysms - Initial experience with the Zenith bifurcated iliac side branch device. J Vasc Surg 2007;46(2):211-217.

21. Ziegler P, Avgerinos ED, Umscheid T, Perdikides T, Erz K, Stelter WJ. Branched iliac bifurcation: 6 years experience with endovascular preservation of internal iliac artery flow. J Vasc Surg 2007;46(2):204-210.

22. Malina M, Dirven M, Sonesson B, Resch T, Dias N, Ivancev K. Feasibility of a branched stent-graft in common iliac artery aneurysms. J Endovasc Ther 2006;13:496-500.

23. Greenberg RK, West K, Pfaff K, Foster J, Skender D, Haulon S, et al. Beyond the aortic bifurcation: Branched endovascular grafts for thoracoabdominal and aortoiliac aneurysms. J Vasc Surg 2006;43:879-886.

24. Haulon S, Greenberg RK, Pfaff K, Francis C, Koussa M, West K. Branched grafting for aortoiliac aneurysms. Eur J Vasc Endovasc Surg 2007;33(5): 567-574.

25. Lin P, Bush R, Chaikof E, Chen C, Conklin B, Terramani T et al. A prospective evaluation of hypogastric artery embolisation in endovascular aortoiliac aneurysm repair. J Vasc Surg 2002;36(3):500-506.

26. Bockler D, Krauss M, Mannsmann U, Halawa M, Lange R, Probst T, Raithel D. Incidence of renal infarctions after endovascular AAA repair: Relationship to infrarenal versus suprarenal fixation. J Endovasc Ther 2003; 10:1054-60.

27. Stanley BM, Semmens JB, Lawrence-Brown M, Goodman MA, Hartley DE. Fenestration in endovascular grafts for aortic aneurysm repair: New horizons for preserving blood flow in branch vessels. J Endovasc Ther 8:16-24, 2001.

28. Minion DJ, Yancey A, Patterson DE, Saha S,Endean ED. The endowedge and kilt techniques to achieve additional juxtarenal seal during deployment of the Gore Excluder endoprosthesis. Ann Vasc Surg 2006; 20:472-7.

29. Anderson JL, Berce M, Hartley DE. Endoluminal aortic grafting with renal and superior mesenteric artery incorporation by graft fenestration.. J Endovasc her 8:3-15, 2001.

30. Verhoeven ELG, Muhs BE, Zeebregts CJAM, Tielliu IJF, Prins TR, Bos WTGJ, Oranen BI, Moll RL, Van den Dungen JJAM. Fenestrated and branched stent-grafting after previous surgery provides a good alternative to open redo surgery. Eur J Vasc Endovasc Surg 33(1):84-90, 2007.

31. Verhoeven ELG, Prins TR, Tielliu IJF, Bos WTGJ, Van den Dungen JJAM, Zeebregts CJAM, Hulsebos RG, van Andringa de Kempenaer MG, Oudkerk M, van Schilfgaarde R. Treatment of shortnecked infrarenal aortic aneurysms with fenestrated stent-grafts: Short-term results. Eur J Vasc Endovasc Surg 27(5):377-83, 2004.

32. Greenberg RK, Haulon S, O'Neill S, Lyden S, Ouriel K. Primary endovascular repair of juxtarenal aneursyms with fenestrated endovascular grafting. Eur J Vasc Endovasc Surg 27(5):484-91, 2004.

33. Greenberg RK, Haulon S, Lyden SP, Srivastava SD, Turc A, Eagle MJ. Endovascular management of juxtarenal aneurysms with fenestrated endovascular grafting. J Vasc Surg 39(2):279-281, 2004

34. O'Neill S, Greenberg RK, Haddad F, Resch T, Sereika J, Katz E. A prospective analysis of fenestrated endovascular grafting: Intermediate-term outcomes. Eur J Vasc Endovasc Surg 32(2):115-123, 2006.

35. Karmacharya J. Parmer SS. Antezana JN. Fairman RM. Woo EY. Velazquez OC. Golden MA. Carpenter JP. Outcomes of accessory renal artery occlusion during endovascular aneurysm repair. J Vasc Surg 43(1):8-13, 2006

36. Kim B. Donayre CE. Hansen CJ. Aziz I. Walot I. Lippmann M. Kopchok GE. White RA. Endovascular abdominal aortic aneurysm repair using the AneuRx stent graft: impact of excluding accessory renal arteries. Ann Vasc Surg 18(1):32-7, 2004

37. Aquino RV. Rhee RY. Muluk SC. Tzeng EY. Carrol NM. Makaroun MS. Exclusion of accessory renal arteries during endovascular repair of abdominal aortic aneurysms. J Vasc Surg 34(5):878-84, 2001.

Considerations regarding the best management of young fit patients with abdominal aortic aneurysms

Nicolas Diehm, Athanassios I. Tsoukas, Barry T. Katzen

INTRODUCTION

Endovascular abdominal aortic aneurysm (AAA) repair (EVAR) was introduced in the early nineties[1] and initially regarded as an alternative to conservative treatment in patients unfit for open surgery.[2] As endograft technology developed, EVAR has been increasingly used in patients judged fit for open AAA repair (OAR) and was shown to be associated with certain advantages in the perioperative period in a wide spectrum of patients.[3,4] However, in contrast to OAR,[5] serious concerns regarding the long-term durability of EVAR have been raised.[6,7] Based on experiences with reduced durability of EVAR using first-generation devices, many physicians refrained from using EVAR in young low-risk patients.[8]

As use of contemporary endograft devices was recently shown to be a safe, effective, and durable method to prevent AAA rupture and aneurysm-related death,[9,10] expansion of indications for EVAR to young and fit patients is subject of ongoing discussion.

EVAR was shown to offer several advantages such as faster recovery time, less blood loss, shorter hospital stay and less sexual dysfunction related to the min-imal-invasiveness of the procedure.[3,4,11] Furthermore, physicians face a growing number of patients presenting with the desire for a less-invasive procedure shortened recovery time and quicker return to normal activity despite the potential impact on the durability of treatment.[12]

TRIAL DATA

While recent studies and personal series focused on the role of EVAR in elderly patients with substantial comorbidites thus rendering them at high risk for OAR,[3,4,9,13] data on clinical outcomes of younger patients undergoing EVAR is currently scarce.

To date, three landmark randomized prospective trials comparing OAR and EVAR in a wide spectrum of patients are available.[3,4,13] Mean patient age was 69.5 years in the DREAM study, whereas it was 74.0 and 76.8 in the EVAR-1 and -2 trials.

The mean patient age in the presently available large multi-centre series on EVAR is 72.8 years [14] and higher.[15,16] Furthermore, these series contained a substantial proportion of high-risk patients and do not specify results in young low-risk subgroups.

Within a large single-center series, OAR was shown to be associated with a 30-day mortality of 1.2% 5 in patients with various risk factor backgrounds having a mean age of 70.5 years. In that series, increased patient age was identified as an independent predictor of 30-day mortality.

Retrospective comparison of outcomes among various series is difficult, since the wide application of EVAR might have impacted recent results of OAR.[8]

MIAMI EXPERIENCE WITH EVAR IN YOUNG FIT PATIENTS

Between 4/1994 and 7/2005, 652 patients underwent elective EVAR at our institution. Among them were 25 patients (2 females, mean age 62.3 ± 3.3 years) classified as low-risk patients (overall risk scores 0 and 1 according to the Society of Vascular Surgery 17) below the age of 65 years. Based on patient gender and comorbidities, 25 patients undergoing OAR were selected as matched-pair controls for this series.

Open surgical AAA repair

OAR was performed under general and/or regional anesthesia by standard infrarenal implantation of Dacron prosthesis. Following mostly retroperitoneal approach and cross-clamping of the aorta (suprarenal clamping n = 1, 4%), a tube (n = 9, 36%) or bifurcated (n = 16, 64%) graft was inserted.

EVAR

EVAR was carried out by a dedicated interdisciplinary team consisting of interventional radiologists, vascular surgeons and anesthesiologists as described previously 1,18. Patients undergoing EVAR had a mean infrarenal aortic neck length of 30.0 ± 2.1mm and an infrarenal neck diameter of 22.4 ± 3.3 mm reflecting favourable anatomy for aortic endografting.[19]

30-day results

Rates of procedural death and aortic rupture did not differ significantly between the OAR and EVAR groups (Table 1). Blood transfusion was necessary in one patient (4%) after EVAR and in 4 (16%) patients undergoing OAR, but differences did not reach statistical significance.

Mean intensive care unit (ICU) time and mean length of stay (LOS) were significantly higher after OAR: ICU time was 0.2 ± 0.4 after EVAR and 5 ± 2.1 after OAR (p <0.0001), whereas LOS was 2.32 ± 0.95 and 5 ± 2.1 (p <0.0001).

Total complication rate was 20% after EVAR and 52% after OAR (p = 0.0378), but complications were confined to mild and moderate complications, whereas no severe complications occurred in both patient groups. OAR was associated with transient and spontaneously resolving renal failure in 2 (8%) patients, whereas it was not encountered in patients undergoing EVAR, but differences did not reach statistical significance. Furthermore, during the first 30 days, no patient died in either group and no AAA rupture was observed.

Long-term follow-up

Mean follow-up open after open surgical AAA repair was 5.9 ±1.8 years, whereas it was 7.1 ±3.2 years after EVAR (p = 0.1020). Two patients died during follow-up after EVAR, both deaths being related to cancer, whereas 5 patients died after open surgery with all causes of deaths being unrelated to AAA (stroke, n = 1; type A thoracic aortic dissection, n = 1; COPD, n = 1; cancer, n = 2). Cumulative long-term patient survival rates did not differ between EVAR and OS patients (p = 0.144 by log-rank).

Ruptures did not occur in follow-up

TABLE 1

30-DAY OUTCOMES COMPARING PATIENTS UNDERGOING ENDOVASCULAR AND OPEN SURGICAL ABDOMINAL AORTIC ANEURYSM REPAIR

30-day outcomes	EVAR n = 25	Open repair n = 25	P*
Procedural conversion	0 (0%)	N/A	N/A
Procedural death	0 (0%)	0 (0%)	N/A
Procedural rupture	0 (0%)	0 (0%)	N/A
Need for transfusion	1 (4%)	4 (16%)	0.3487*
Mean ICU time [days]	0.2 ± 0.4	1.1 ± 0.4	<0.0001†
Mean length of stay [days]	2.3 ± 1.0	5.0 ± 2.1	<0.0001†
30-day death	0 (0%)	0 (0%)	N/A
AAA-related 30-day death	0 (0%)	0 (0%)	N/A
Complications	5 (20%)	13 (52%)	0.0378*
Mild	4 (16%)	10 (40%)	0.1137*
Moderate	1 (4%)	3 (12%)	0.6092*
Severe	0 (0%)	0 (%)	N/A
Renal failure	0 (0%)	2 (8%)	0.4898*
30-day rupture	0 (0%)	0 (0%)	N/A

ICU = intensive care unit, † from two-tailed Student t-test, * from two-tailed Fisher test.

during OAR and EVAR. No conversions were necessary in patients who had undergone EVAR. In patients undergoing open surgery, two redo procedures related to OAR were performed: embolic occlusion of the abdominal aorta occurred 4.2 years after OAR in one patient necessitating surgical renal arterial embolectomy and aortobifemoral bypass procedure. Hernia repair related to the incision for previous OAR was performed in one patient after 0.7 years.

In patients undergoing EVAR, four endovascular redo procedures related to this procedure were performed (AAA sac thrombin injection due to endoleak type II, n = 1; coiling of AAA sac and IMA due to endoleak type II, n = 1; proximal extension due to endoleak type I, n = 1; PTA and thrombolysis due to graft limb occlusion, n = 1).

Cumulative rates of freedom from secondary procedures was not significantly different among both patient groups (p = 0.418 by log-rank). We are in the process of completing a long term evaluation of the functional status of patients from both groups, the results of which will be the published later.

DISCUSSION

With increased application of routine ultrasound screening for patients at increased risk for AAA, physicians will face a growing number of young and fit AAA patients presenting with the desire for a less-invasive procedure, shortened recovery time and quicker return to normal activity despite the potential impact on the durability of treatment.[12]

Given excellent peri-operative as well as long-term results of OAR,[5] the question of whether young healthy patients should undergo EVAR, is currently subject of debate.

Average life-expectancy of a 65 year old person today is more than 18 years in the United States.[20] Initial experiences with EVAR showed that durability of EVAR is limited using first-generation devices.[6,7] Based on these experiences, EVAR had been regarded an alternative to open surgery or conservative treatment in high-risk patients and many physicians refrained from using EVAR in low-risk young patients.[8]

At present, in the absence of dedicated answers to the question "What is the best management of young fit AAA patients?" from the three available large-scale randomized trials,[3,4,13] decision making is limited in this increasingly encountered subgroup of patients. It has been shown that EVAR and OAR result in similar quality of life adjusted life expectancy for most patients who are candidates for surgical AAA repair.[12] In that study, decision analysis suggested that OAR may be preferred for younger patients with low operative risk and EVAR may be preferred for older patients with higher operative risk. However, given the similarity in overall patient outcomes in that series, the authors concluded that patient preference should be weighed heavily in decision making. This dilemma is well depicted by Hertzer[21] who quotes the Nationwide Inpatient Sample: "Open AAA repair has less than 2% mortality rate for patients 65 or younger. This low operative risk may not justify exposure to whatever incidence of late complications the current generations of endografts may prove to have during the relatively long survival times that can be anticipated for these patients".

Our limited Institutional observational experience in young fit patients indicates that EVAR is associated with a lower rate of mild and moderate perioperative complications, shorter ICU time and length of stay as compared to OAR. These findings are well in accordance with outcomes observed in older patients at higher risk.[3,4,13]

In the present series, no significant differences in hard endpoints such as patient survival, aortic rupture and freedom from repeated intervention were found during long-term follow-up comparing EVAR to a group of age- and risk-matched patients undergoing OAR.

Data from studies assessing the outcomes of patients in whom new-generation devices had been used, suggest that EVAR is a safe, effective, and durable method to prevent AAA rupture and aneurysm-related death.[9,10] EVAR can be considered a moving target with today's complications being associated with yesterday's graft material and know-how. Since the first concerns regarding impaired long-term durability due to material fatigue, graft migration and endoleaks of EVAR emerged, endograft material and endovascular techniques have been substantially refined.

In addition to technical improvements of EVAR, the systemic implications of aneurysmal disease have recently increasingly been acknowledged. In particular, AAA patients were shown to be at significant risk for cardiovascular complications and AAA is now considered a CHD risk equivalent.[22] According to experiences from EUROSTAR, the perioperative use of statins is recommended in patients undergoing EVAR.[23] However, treatment of cardiovascular risk is currently suboptimal and could be improved, with an expected reduction in cardiovascular short- and long-term morbidity and mortality in patients undergoing OAR and EVAR alike.[24]

Our series of EVAR in young fit patients contains a large number of aortas with "favourable" anatomy and that is not accidental. It reflects our philosophy of patient selection and institutional decision making. Every patient has been evaluated by the endovascular team including both interventionalists and vascular surgeons, and our recommendations have been the result of Interdisciplinary consensus. Our guidelines evolved overtime from the daily construct-ive debate of specialists of different back-grounds. Currently we would recommend EVAR in young fit patients with favourable anatomies only (aortic neck length of ≥ 2 cm, lack of thrombus and extensive calcifi-cation). Aortic neck angulations, if encoun-tered, should be less than 45 degrees. Pa-tients should understand the risk of endole-ak, migration and potential need for sec-ondary procedures. They would have to be deemed reliable and available to enter a lifetime schedule of monitoring. Intra-oper-atively we seek to maximize coverage from the renal to the hypogastric arteries. Our In-stitutional bias favours preservation of the hypogastric vessels when possible.

The patient and medical team have to weigh the risk of transfusion, recovery time, incision related disability and sexual dysfunction against the risk of secondary procedures as well as the unknown dura-bility of EVAR over 15-20 years.

We keep in mind that as our "young fit" patients age, EVAR technology will evolve. Prosthetic graft technology took 50 years to be where it is today. We speculate that we have just seen the beginning of endo-vascular technology but we recognize that speculation about tomorrow should not be used for patient decision making today. In a cost conscious environment, the ex-pense of the device and imaging projected over the lifetime of these patients becomes another important factor.

Further large-scale studies which are mandatory to compare the impact of EVAR and OAR on hard endpoints and as well as on quality of life measures in young fit patients undergoing AAA repair may be rendered irrelevant by the evolu-tion of technology which is unfolding fast-er than it can be tested. We feel that our dedicated multidisciplinary approach and very serious consideration of every patient on an individual basis by an unbiased team of specialists has performed well in our institution.

REFERENCES

1. Parodi JC, Palmaz JC, Barone HD. Transfemoral intraluminal graft implantation for abdominal aor-tic aneurysms. Ann Vasc Surg 1991;5:491-9.
2. Carpenter JP, Baum RA, Barker CF, Golden MA, Velazquez OC, Mitchell ME, et al. Durability of ben-efits of endovascular versus conventional abdomi-nal aortic aneurysm repair. J Vasc Surg 2002; 35:222-8.
3. Greenhalgh RM, Brown LC, Kwong GP, Powell JT, Thompson SG. Comparison of endovascular aneurysm repair with open repair in patients with abdominal aortic aneurysm (EVAR trial 1), 30-day operative mortality results: randomised con-trolled trial. Lancet 2004;364:843-8.
4. Prinssen M, Verhoeven EL, Buth J, Cuypers PW, van Sambeek MR, Balm R, et al. A randomized trial comparing conventional and endovascular repair of abdominal aortic aneurysms. N Engl J Med 2004;351:1607-18.
5. Hertzer NR, Mascha EJ, Karafa MT, O'Hara PJ, Kra-jewski LP, Beven EG. Open infrarenal abdominal aortic aneurysm repair: the Cleveland Clinic experi-ence from 1989 to 1998. J Vasc Surg 2002;35: 1145-54.
6. Le Bas JF. Endovascular aneurysm repair versus open repair in patients with abdominal aortic an-eurysm (EVAR trial 1): randomised controlled tri-al. Lancet 2005;365:2179-86.
7. Blankensteijn JD, de Jong SE, Prinssen M, van der Ham AC, Buth J, van Sterkenburg SM, et al. Two-year outcomes after conventional or endo-vascular repair of abdominal aortic aneurysms. N Engl J Med 2005;352:2398-405.
8. Dias NV, Ivancev K, Malina M, Resch T, Lindblad B, Sonesson B. Does the wide application of en-dovascular AAA repair affect the results of open surgery? Eur J Vasc Endovasc Surg 2003;26: 188-94.
9. Brewster DC, Jones JE, Chung TK, Lamuraglia GM, Kwolek CJ, Watkins MT, et al. Long-term outcomes after endovascular abdominal aortic aneurysm repair: the first decade. Ann Surg 2006;244:426-38.
10. Peterson BG, Matsumura JS, Brewster DC, Mak-aroun MS. Five-year report of a multicenter con-trolled clinical trial of open versus endovascular

treatment of abdominal aortic aneurysms. J Vasc Surg 2007.

11. Prinssen M, Buskens E, Nolthenius RP, van Sterkenburg SM, Teijink JA, Blankensteijn JD. Sexual dysfunction after conventional and endovascular AAA repair: results of the DREAM trial. J Endovasc Ther 2004;11:613-20.

12. Schermerhorn ML, Finlayson SR, Fillinger MF, Buth J, van Marrewijk C, Cronenwett JL. Life expectancy after endovascular versus open abdominal aortic aneurysm repair: results of a decision analysis model on the basis of data from EUROSTAR. J Vasc Surg 2002;36:1112-20.

13. Endovascular aneurysm repair and outcome in patients unfit for open repair of abdominal aortic aneurysm (EVAR trial 2): randomised controlled trial. Lancet 2005;365:2187-92.

14. Moore WS, Matsumura JS, Makaroun MS, Katzen BT, Deaton DH, Decker M, et al. Five-year interim comparison of the Guidant bifurcated endograft with open repair of abdominal aortic aneurysm. J Vasc Surg 2003;38:46-55.

15. Faries PL, Brener BJ, Connelly TL, Katzen BT, Briggs VL, Burks JA, Jr., et al. A multicenter experience with the Talent endovascular graft for the treatment of abdominal aortic aneurysms. J Vasc Surg 2002;35:1123-8.

16. Zarins CK. The US AneuRx Clinical Trial: 6-year clinical update 2002. J Vasc Surg 2003;37:904-8.

17. Chaikof EL, Blankensteijn JD, Harris PL, White GH, Zarins CK, Bernhard VM, et al. Reporting standards for endovascular aortic aneurysm repair. J Vasc Surg 2002;35:1048-60.

18. Katzen BT, Dake MD, MacLean AA, Wang DS. Endovascular repair of abdominal and thoracic aortic aneurysms. Circulation 2005;112:1663-75.

19. Diehm N, Schumacher H, Allenberg JR. Influence of morphological changes on midterm results of endovascular AAA therapy in selected patients. Gefaesschirurgie 2002;7:58-64.

20. CDC. United States life tables; http://www.cdc.gov/nchs/datawh/statab/unpubd/mortabs/lewk3_10.htm.

21. Hertzer NR. Current status of endovascular repair of infrarenal abdominal aortic aneurysms in the context of 50 years of conventional repair. Ann N Y Acad Sci 2006;1085:175-86.

22. Executive Summary of The Third Report of The National Cholesterol Education Program (NCEP) Expert Panel on Detection, Evaluation, And Treatment of High Blood Cholesterol In Adults (Adult Treatment Panel III). Jama 2001;285:2486-97.

23. Leurs LJ, Visser P, Laheij RJ, Buth J, Harris PL, Blankensteijn JD. Statin use is associated with reduced all-cause mortality after endovascular abdominal aortic aneurysm repair. Vascular 2006;14:1-8.

24. Lloyd GM, Newton JD, Norwood MG, Franks SC, Bown MJ, Sayers RD. Patients with abdominal aortic aneurysm: are we missing the opportunity for cardiovascular risk reduction? J Vasc Surg 2004;40:691-7.

Methods of fixation of endovascular aortic stent-grafts

Robert J. Hinchliffe

INTRODUCTION

Endovascular aortic stent-grafts are subject to many forces when placed in the infra-renal abdominal aorta. The major force acts distally on the stent-graft in the aortic neck. First generation stent-grafts were not designed to withstand these forces, resulting in a high incidence of failure. Gradually the nature of these forces has been elucidated and stent-graft design has been improved to deal with them.

The ideal stent-graft fixation mechanism should possess a number of important properties. It should resist the distal forces for a variety of stent-graft sizes and range of blood pressure. Fixation must not compromise the blood-tight seal required in the aortic neck. Any mechanism must be durable. It should not damage or degrade the aortic neck so as not to provoke dilatation.

Adaptation may be required to a hostile aortic neck which may be calcified or thrombus lined. It should not interfere with aortic side-branch flow or cause embolisation and not damage extra-aortic tissue.

MIGRATION AND THE FIXATION OF STENT-GRAFTS

There is clear consensus from the Society of Vascular Surgery (SVS) on the definition of migration. It is a movement of the stent-graft greater than 10 mm or any clinical event (secondary intervention or complication).[1]

The importance of the definition can be seen by examining in detail some of the published studies on migration. The incidence of migration with the AneuRx stent-graft varied widely in two studies from 6.1% at one year to 40% at 24 months.[2,3] The variation may be attributable to operator experience or pre-operative aneurysm morphology. However, the threshold for diagnosis migration is important. In the latter study, migration was defined as being a greater than 3 mm movement.

Many of the first generation stent-grafts were studied *in vitro*. The forces required to distract these stent-grafts from cadaveric aortas was small. In most cases, they were significantly less than the estimated *in vivo* forces (7-9N) predicted by mathematical modelling. Later, clinical studies of the long-term follow-up of first generation stent-grafts confirmed these concerns.[4] Many of the first generation stent-grafts have migrated.

There is insufficient healing of current graft materials and self-expanding stents in the aorta to provide a blood tight seal and the necessary fixation for aortic stent-grafts. A friable neo-intimal layer, covers the luminal aspect of stent-grafts.[6] Thus aortic stent-grafts require some form of mechanical fixation to prevent caudal migration and aid seal.

The importance of stent-graft fixation and prevention of migration to the success of EVAR was confirmed in a review of 2.464 patients enrolled in the EUROSTAR (European Collaborators on Stent-graft Techniques for Abdominal Aortic Aneurysm Repair) registry.[7] Migration was found to be a significant risk factor for subsequent aneurysm rupture. A study by Sampaio confirmed the association between migration and endoleak.[8] At a median follow-up of nine months, one-third of patients with migration required intervention for proximal endoleak. Additional analyses of the EUROSTAR data have demonstrated that migration was also a risk factor for trans-femoral and trans-abdominal secondary interventions.[9]

Migration is a time dependent phenomenon. In the very early stent-graft systems which did not have any method of fixation in the aortic neck, migration only started to appear at 18 months to two years post-operatively.[5]

When Zarins' analysed the migration rates of three commonly used EVGs, he found no difference at one year (AneuRx 2.2%, Excluder 2.3% and Zenith 2.3%).[10] However, at 2 years follow-up the migration rates were significantly higher for the AneuRx (5.3%) than the Excluder (1.4%) (Zenith not available).

After the first 18 months, the migration rates continue to rise. In one study they gradually increased from 7.2% at one year, 20.4% at 2 years, 42.1% at 3 years and 66.7% at 4 years.[11] It can be difficult to establish the resistance of a particular stent-graft because of the multi-factorial nature. It was not possible to compare migration rates between grafts in the large EUROSTAR registry because there were a variety of durations of follow-up from very short eg Zenith to longer Vanguard.[7]

However, any assessment of migration rates should report sufficient follow-up before meaningful comparisons can be made.

There are many patient specific and stent-graft variables which make it difficult to identify which patients are at greatest risk of stent-graft migration. The precise risk factors for migration remained elusive in small studies.[12] Using the large EUROSTAR registry and mathematical modelling, Mohan and co-workers attempted to establish clinical, morphological and stent-graft factors associated with migration. Smoking, hypertension, maximum aortic diameter, large proximal graft diameter, degree of diameter change of stent-graft and angulation of the iliac arteries were significantly associated with stent-graft migration in data from the registry. In the most recent review of 4,233 patients from the EUROSTAR registry, independent variables for migration were a wider neck and aneurysmal diameter, shorter necks, proximal endoleak, and absence of suprarenal fixation.[14]

The results of stent-graft registries, multi-centre and single centre studies appear to confirm the important role played by the infra-renal neck in stent-graft fixation. All adverse morphological features have reportedly been associated with migration. Many studies are biased. If a very small number of patients have pre-operative adverse morphological variables then the results may not be significant enough to draw meaningful conclusions. Similarly by performing EVAR in more complex anatomy complication and migration rates may be expected to be higher.

Albertini examined the risk factors for proximal endoleak and migration in a study of 184 patients (1994-1998).[15] All patients received a home-made aortouniiliac stent-graft (Dacron graft/Gianturco stents) with either infra- or supra-renal fixation. The only significant factor associated with migration was proximal neck angulation. Patients with proximal endoleak were more likely to have either neck angulation or wide neck diameter.

Although aortouniiliac stent-grafts are used less widely now, it is possible that they are subject to greater distraction forces than their bifurcated counterparts. This is a theoretical problem and increased rates of migration have not been recorded in later generations of aortouniiliac stent-grafts. However, this configuration is now reserved for a relatively small number of patients with specific indications.

Measuring Stent-Graft Migration

Assessment of stent-graft migration is conveniently and most commonly performed on contrast enhanced CT. The movement of the stent-graft can be assessed relative to aortic side-branches. In the presence of a supra-renal graft this may be done relative to the coeliac or superior mesenteric arteries. It is usually possible to differentiate the top of the graft from the supra-renal stent by identifying the markers on the top of the graft (changing the window setting on the CT scan). Infra-renal grafts are best compared to the renal arteries.

It is possible to assess stent-graft migration using plain abdominal radiographs. However, consistent centering of the radiograph is required.[16] MRA is also a valid tool to assess migration but requires the presence of a non ferro-magnetic stent-graft.

Alternative approaches to the assessment of migration are being developed including the use of stereotactic techniques.

Types of Stent-Graft Fixation

Stent friction, hooks and barbs

Currently there are two main types of fixation for aortic stent-grafts. These are fric-tion from the use of a self or balloon expandable stent and hooks or barbs designed to engage the aortic wall.

Early stent-grafts only had vestigial hooks or barbs to prevent migration. Some did not have hooks or barbs and relied completely on the radial force of the stents. In long-term studies of these designs, migration rates approached 60%.[5]

The length of apposition of the stent-graft with the neck is an important factor in the prevention of migration for stents of the self-expanding variety. Lambert was able to demonstrate that increasing the length of overlap of self-expanding stent-grafts in cadaveric aortas increased the friction forces resisting migration.[17] However, it has been difficult to confirm these in vitro findings in clinical studies. Papers attempting to correlate short neck length with migration have been confounded by the relatively small number of patients included with short necks and the presence of other forms of stent-graft fixation e.g. hooks or barbs. Cao's study was unable to demonstrate an association between the presence of a short neck and subsequent migration.[18] However, one study of the AneuRx stent-graft and another comparing the AneuRx and Zenith stent-grafts confirmed Lambert's results.[19] Tonnessen's study compared patients with migration (15) against non-migrators (115) in a study of the Zenith and AneuRx devices.[20] At just under 3 years follow-up, the aneurysm neck length was shorter in those patients developing migration (22 mm versus 31 mm P = 0.02).

The orientation of barbs and hooks on infra-renal stent-grafts is caudad to oppose migration. In some stent-grafts such as the Ancure they were orientated perpendicular to the aortic lumen. Different hooks and barbs have evolved during the development of aortic stent-grafts. A greater number and more robust hooks or barbs have been added to later generations of stent-grafts. Greenberg suggested that the barbs of early Zenith devices were, in some cases, insufficient to prevent migration.[21] In a multi-centre retrospective series, eight patients with the early generation devices were detected with migration at two years. The latest Zenith design (since 1998) were provided with a more robust 10-12 barbs to prevent migration. None of the latest generation migrated.

It is likely that the addition of these more robust and frequent barbs may have played a significant role in the reduction of migration in Greenberg's study and those published by others, however, it is difficult to be certain.[22] There have also been other improvements in stent-graft design and an increase in operator experience.

Veerapen compared a variety of stent-grafts with and without barbs in a cadaveric aortic pull-out study.[23] The barbed devices (Zenith and Ancure) required significantly higher ($p = 0.0004$) force (approximately 25%) to displace them than the other stent-grafts tested.

Hooks and barbs are designed to engage the full thickness of the aortic wall. An atherosclerotic aorta with calcified plaques may prevent successful hook or barb penetration, reducing fixation. In addition, if the hooks or barbs are located in the infra-renal aortic neck, the graft may be lifted away from the aortic wall, potentially compromising seal.

Penetration of the full thickness of aortic wall theoretically risks damage to extra-aortic tissues such as the inferior vena cava or duodenum. There have been isolated case reports of patients with an intact stent-graft presenting with aorto-enteric fistula.[24] However, reported cases of aorto-enteric fistula are usually the result of late graft leaks, migration or graft disintegration. In a number of instances there has been a suspicion of infection or fistulation prior to stent-graft insertion. There is little evidence to suggest that the hooks or barbs of stent-grafts have been primarily responsible for aorto-enteric fistulae.

The natural history of migration has always been assumed to be progressive and unremitting. Studies of migration rates would appear to confirm this. However, recent work by Zhou and co-workers from Liverpool suggested that migration in stent-grafts with barbs may occur in two distinct phases.[25] First, the barbs 'give' (up to 5 mm) as they fully engage the aortic wall. The second phase is the progressive dislodgement of the device. They concluded that the first phase of migration may result in compromise of seal in short aortic necks. The results of this study may not be applicable to all stent-graft designs. The Zenith (used in that study) has 5 mm long barbs. Barbs or hooks on other stent-grafts are shorter. In the case of the Excluder and Ancure they measure 2 mm in length.

The use of low pressure intra-aortic "molding" balloons may encourage the engagement of the hooks or barbs with the aortic wall. Whether they reduce the first phase of migration is uncertain. Resch was unable to demonstratre a consistently higher pull-out force following balloon inflation.[26] Some stent-grafts responded whereas others did not.

Stent fractures and hook/barb separation were a frequent occurrence during the long-term follow-up of first generation stent-grafts. They were sometimes associated with catastrophic failure and aneurysm rupture. Barb separation still remains a theoretical problem requiring surveillance. Although with more robust barbs it occurs much less frequently. It was reported in 1.7% of patients at 12 months in the US Zenith multicentre trial.[27] Migration is frequently asymptomatic. One patient had migration of 5mm but no secondary procedures were required and there were no ruptures (Figure 1).

Oversizing

The concept of stent-graft oversizing is now widely believed to be a relevant fac-

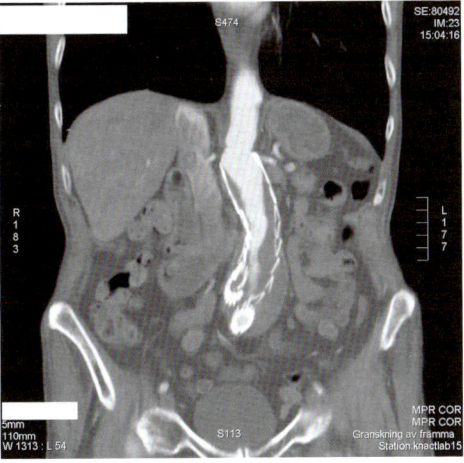

FIGURE 1: Migrated Zenith.

tor in stent-graft planning. First generation stent-grafts were not oversized. Oversizing of 10-20% in the aortic neck has been found to significantly reduce the incidence of endoleak.[28]

Although oversizing has been shown to prevent endoleak, its effect on the development of migration remains less certain. The practice of generous oversizing (>20-30%) has been widely adopted in treating patients with adverse proximal neck morphology. Concerns have been raised regarding the potential for neck dilatation due to oversizing, especially when greater than 20%. Sternbergh analysed the effect of device oversizing on outcomes from the US Zenith multi-centre study.[29] Of the 350 Zenith stent-grafts implanted, 88% (309) had standard oversize, whereas 12% (41) had >30% oversize. At 12 month follow-up, 5 mm migration had occurred in four (4/29) patients with oversizing >30% compared with two (2/232) in the standard oversizing group. There was a fourteen fold greater risk of migration in the greater oversizing group. One potential explanation for this observation was the tendency of surgeons to oversize to a greater degree in the presence of adverse neck morphology. Adverse morphology tended to

be encountered more often in the greater oversizing group but not statistically so. Interestingly, the percentage of oversizing did not correlate with aortic neck dilation at 12 months. However, endograft oversizing >30% was associated with a lower rate of sac shrinkage and higher expansion rates at 24 months post implantation. However, this data must be interpreted with caution. The number of patients with device migration was small (6) raising the possibility of a type II error. The threshold of 30% graft oversizing was chosen arbitrarily. There was a trend toward worse morphology in the large oversizing group, particularly conical neck and the duration of follow-up was relatively short (12 months).

Conners also examined the relationship of large (>20%) graft oversizing with subsequent migration. A total of 7/15 migrators had >20% oversizing.[11] He suggested, similarly that migration was not solely a consequence of oversizing but more likely a multifactorial complication (Figure 2).

SELF-EXPANDING AND BALLOON EXPANDABLE STENTS

It has been suggested that balloon expandable stents become better incorporated in to the aortic wall. Damage of the arterial internal elastic lamina by the balloon expandable stent results in intimal hyperplasia. However, studies of a variety of explanted stent-grafts seem to suggest that there is no difference in healing or incorporation between any of the currently available stent or graft materials.[30]

One of the major concerns about the use of stents in the infra-renal aortic neck is their potential to cause neck dilation and subsequent migration or endoleak. Singh-Ranger performed a detailed longitudinal CT analysis of aortic necks in patients with both self and balloon-expandable stent-grafts.[31] He found the two types

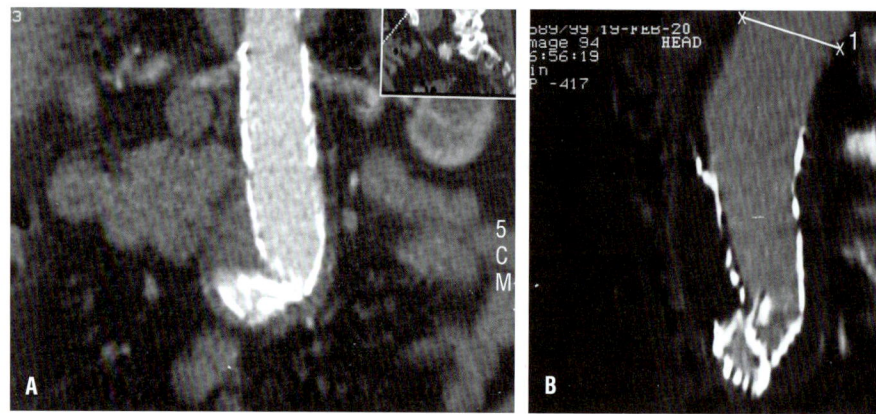

FIGURE 2: A. EVAR successfully deployed with supra-renal fixation. **B.** Post-operative neck dilatation results in migration.

of stents behaved differently. Self-expanding stents exerted a continuous steady force against the arterial wall, appearing to increase the diameter of the aortic neck up to six months after implantation but not thereafter. In contrast, the balloon expandable variety resulted in an immediate neck diameter increase which remained constant thereafter.

Others studies have confirmed the absence of continued neck dilatation post EVAR using balloon expandable stents. In a study of 41 patients with balloon expandable stent-grafts (Montefiore Endograft System) oversized 5% at implantation during a mean of 31 months followup, no patients developed significant neck dilation (>2.5 mm).[32] However, the median pre-operative neck diameter was narrow (23 mm), suggesting these patients may be a group who were less likely to develop neck dilation.

A number of studies report significant neck dilation after EVAR. Twenty percent of patients with the Ancure system had neck dilation (>2.5 mm) at three years.[33] These rates were similar to the early experiences with the Malmo aortouniiliac graft which used self-expanding Z-stents.[34] Interestingly there was only one case of migration in the Ancure series by Makaroun

whereas the migration rate was 45% at three years in the Malmo series.

Later generations of self-expanding stent-grafts have not been plagued by such high rates of neck dilation.[29] In some studies no neck dilation after insertion of stent-grafts with self-expanding stents was observed at all.[35] Studies have confirmed that pre-operative wide necks are more likely to dilate. The patients in the Malmo series had wide necks and more adverse morphological features and were possibly more likely to dilate.[36] Other possible explanations for the high rates of dilation include high rates of migration due to suboptimal graft fixation and low deployment of the graft in the aortic neck.

There have not been any studies directly comparing the migration rates of balloon and self-expanding stents. In vitro analysis suggests the median dislodgment force for patients with a variety of Palmaz stent-graft designs (8.1 N to 10.7 N) was similar to the force required to dislodge the Talent (8.1 N) and Ancure (10.7 N) devices.[23] In another, similar study, the Palmaz stent-graft required a median dislodgement force of 25 N, surpassing all other designs.[26] The difference in forces may be related to the size of aortas tested and degree of stent oversizing/dilation.

As previously stated, the cadaveric study by Resch suggested that balloon dilatation of self-expanding stent-grafts may increase fixation.[26] Large balloon expandable stents such as the Palmaz stent have been successfully used for a number of years in the endovascular treatment of proximal endoleak in patients with self-expanding stent-grafts. They improve graft-wall apposition and have been shown during in vitro studies to significantly augment the fixation of self-expanding stent-grafts.[23]

A study from Leicester suggested there were high rates of microembolisation in patients undergoing EVAR compared with open repair.[37] The clinically significant reates of peripheral embolisation are low following EVAR. Particular risk factors include thrombus lined aortic necks and a heavy load of thrombus within the aneurysm sac. The Leicester study used balloon expandable stent-grafts only. Balloon expandable and self-expanding stents were not compared. Although some of these emboli may be attributable to wire manipulation and early EVAR experience it is also possible that the balloon expandable stents were more likely to contribute to the production of microemboli.

However, Bockler was unable to demonstrate any differences between the rate of renal infarction between patients undergoing EVAR with balloon expandable and self-expanding stents.[61]

COLUMN STRENGTH

Some surgeons and manufacturers have used stiff stent-grafts to try and improve fixation and prevent migration. This has been termed "column strength".

In vitro experiments shed some light on the ability of sent-grafts to withstand the forces placed upon them in vivo. In one study, the pull-out force from the aortic neck was significantly greater in a first generation stent-graft (Vanguard, 9.0 N) than in one of the second-generation stent-graft systems with a supra-renal uncovered stent (Talent, 4.5 N).[26] The Vanguard was plagued by high rates of migration, whereas the Talent has not. This observation suggests the Talent possesses other properties which resist in vivo forces. The Talent is a rigid stent-graft (high column strength) which may be an explanation for its improved performance in vivo.

Claims that high columnar strength is an effective method in isolation at reducing migration have never been substantiated. Few studies have directly compared the in vivo migration rates of stiff and fully stented conventional grafts. A clinical study comparing a stent-graft with supra-renal fixation (Zenith) and one with high column strength (AneuRx) was unable to detect any migration in either group during follow-up.[38] Although high column strength has the potential to reduce migration, there are concerns that such stiff stent-grafts conform poorly to aortoiliac angulation and may be at increased risk of either endoleak or kinking. Some authors have also suggested that these very stiff stent-grafts may precipitate proximal migration during postoperative conformational change of the aneurysm sac.

In Kalliafas' review of the Nottingham-Malmo stent-graft, patients were analysed according to the use of a fully or partially stented design as well as supra –or infrarenal fixation.[39] The fully stented Nottingham-Malmo stent-graft does not have high column strength but is more rigid than the partially stented version. At a median follow-up of 19 months, the incidence of migration was similar in the partially stented group was at 10% (9/88) compared to 13% (5/40) with the fully stented design (p >0.05).

In an ovine model, Arko and colleagues assessed the effect of increasing iliac fixation length on the force required to produce migration in a stiff stent-graft without fixation (AneuRx).[40] They found that iliac fixation length was 31.0 +/- 0.3 mm in the maximum iliac fixation group and 11 +/- 0.25 mm in the minimum fixation group (P <.0001). Peak displacement force to initiate migration was 30.2 N in animals with maximum iliac fixation compared with 18.1 N (range, 13 to 21) in those with minimum fixation (P =.01). They concluded that the longitudinal in vitro force needed to displace a fully supported stent graft was significantly higher in the presence of maximum iliac fixation. The in vivo forces are more complex and are not simply compressive as was the case in Arko's experiment. It is possible that increasing the number of stents in the common iliac artery simply increased the resistance to compression.

A recent clinical study of the AneuRx device examined the factors, primarily morphological, associated with migration.[41] The authors concluded there was a significant role played by iliac fixation length in the prevention of migration. Particularly, the proximity of the stent-graft to the iliac bifurcation appeared to provide stability. Unfortunately, the results of the study may have been biased by patient selection, the duration of follow-up and evolving experience. Further studies are required to confirm these observations.

SUPRARENAL VERSUS INFRARENAL FIXATION

Early stent-grafts with fixation in the infra-renal neck had high rates of migration and endoleak. Neck dilation was thought to play a major role in a number of these failures. Lawrence-Brown suggested placing a top-anchor stent in the visceral aorta might provide a more secure and durable stent-graft fixation.[42] Long-term radiographic studies have confirmed that the visceral aorta is less prone to subsequent

dilatation than the infra-renal aortic segment.[43] The supra-renal aorta is also relatively disease free and there is little evidence to suggest that supra-renal stents are associated with neck dilatation.[36]

Cadaveric studies have demonstrated that supra-renal stents per se do not improve fixation strength without the use of hooks or barbs. The supra-renal stent graft does, however, separate the zone of fixation (supra-renal aorta) from that of seal (infra-renal aortic neck). Barbs or hooks of infra-renally fixated stent-grafts which fail to engage the aortic neck may encourage endoleak because of poor graft-wall apposition.

Adverse aneurysm neck morphology is the factor most responsible for patient unsuitability for EVAR. In one study almost 30% (44 of 154) of a population of patients with AAA were unsuitable for EVAR due to inadequate neck length.[44] Stent-grafts with supra-renal fixation can achieve aneurysm seal with shorter necks and potentially treat more patients.

There are few published comparisons of outcome following supra-renal and infra-renal fixation. Many observational studies have simply been too small or with insufficient follow-up to detect any difference between migration rates.[45] There are a number of major confounding factor with many of the retrospective studies comparing supra-renal and infra-renal fixation. The proximal neck morphology in patients with supra-renal stent-grafts is more likely to be adverse. Because the supra-renal stent concept is more recent, the experience of the operating surgeons is likely to be better and any follow-up period relatively shorter than in the infra-renal group.

The largest series of comparative data on migration comes from the EUROSTAR registry.[46] The data limitations include a lack of consistent reporting standards, retrospective data and evolving experience. A total of six stent-grafts (AneuRx, EVT/Ancure, Excluder, Stentor, Talent, Zenith) were compared against each other and a standard first generation design, the Vanguard. All the stent-grafts were less likely to migrate than the Vanguard. The outcome data was adjusted for a variety of demographic and clinical data. The Talent stent-graft was more likely to migrate than the Zenith (Hazard ratio 3.61, 95% confidence interval 2.1 - 6.4), underscoring the importance of hook or barb fixation even for stent-grafts with a supra-renal stent. All stent-grafts with hooks and barbs were less likely to migrate than those without these appendages, even when fixation was in the infra-renal aorta.

Migration rates were compared in patients with two generations of the Nottingham-Malmo stent-graft.[39] The migration rate in the infra-renal group was 10.9% (14/128) compared with 2.1% (1/48) in the supra-renal group. The difference did not quite reach statistical significance (p = 0.06). The outcomes may have been biased in favour of the supra-renal group. These patients were treated later in the centre's endovascular experience and had a slightly shorter duration of follow-up (19 and 12 months respectively).

In a small single centre study, Cowie directly compared the outcome of patients treated with supra- and infra-renally fixed Talent stent-grafts.[47] Pre-operative aneurysm morphology was not stated. Of the 38 patients, 31 were treated with supra-renal stents. There were two migrations, both of whom had infra-renal stent-grafts.

The AneuRx and Zenith device outcomes have been analysed in a comparative study.[20] The number of patients with migration of 10 mm was 14/77 in the AneuRx group and 1/53 in the Zenith group. When patients were included with 5 mm of migration, there were 22/77 and 4/53 respectively. The Zeniths were used to treat wider necks but the duration of follow-up was shorter (31 versus 39 months).

Stanley reviewed Zenith stent-grafts in

Australasia 1994-1998. By the end of the study period (1998), 69% of stent-grafts were placed outside the recommended morphological criteria. The authors were therefore well placed to examine the effects of adverse morphology on outcome of a stent-graft with supra-renal fixation. He found only 10 patients (4.2%) with migration at a median 13.4 months follow-up.[48] Interestingly, only a neck diameter of greater than 28 mm was associated with migration.

Supra-renal fixation may also provide improved stent-graft stability and a reduction in endoleak in patients with adverse neck morphology. It is possible that the supra-renal stent simply improves the conformability of the stent-graft in the aortic neck. Marin examined endoleak rates in the two stent groups (infra-renal fixated [16] stent-grafts with supra-renal [37]). He detected more proximal type I endoleaks in those with infra-renal grafts.[49]

Robbins compared outcome in patients grouped according to degrees of neck angulation.[50] All patients were treated with the Talent stent-graft. In contrast, at 12 month follow-up, there was no significant difference in proximal endoleak rate between groups. A quarter of patients had proximal endoleak in the group with angulation greater than 60 degrees, although unfortunately the number of patients was small (n = 8), limiting any conclusions drawn from the study. Albertini's study was too small to determine, using sub-group analysis, whether the factors associated with migration and endoleak were different for supra- and infra-renal stent-grafts.[15] Similarly it is important to state that the risk factors for migration and endoleak with this Gianturco stent-graft design may differ from others. Patients with supra-renal stent-grafts may not suffer migration as commonly as those with infra-renal fixation if the infra-renal neck dilates. A paper reviewing the experience of the AneuRx graft revealed that patients with late aortic neck dilation had a significant association with migration.[11] Whether the necks dilated prior to migration or as a result of migration is difficult to evaluate. The initial neck diameter did not seem to affect the rate of subsequent migration

Although the mid-term results of supra-renal stents are encouraging, they are not without late failures. One mode of failure is separation of the supra-renal stent from the stent-graft body (Figure 3). In a case from Perth, this resulted in late migration at four years and required insertion of a stent-graft extension.[51]

RENAL COMPLICATIONS OF INFRA- AND SUPRA-RENAL FIXATION

The severity of peri-operative renal injury is substantially reduced with EVAR compared to open repair. The degree of renal injury following EVAR is usually sub-clinical. Inexperienced endovascular manipulation, embolisation or large contrast volumes may contribute to the degree of renal injury.

Supra-renal stents have the potential to impair renal function by atherothrombo embolisation or impaired blood flow secondary to stent struts crossing the renal artery ostia. A number of studies have been performed in an attempt to identify the effect of trans-renal stents on renal artery blood flow and function.

Liffman and colleagues used *in vitro* experiments to assess the effect of 0.46 mm wire traversing renal artery ostia (3 mm and 7 mm). The stent wire was placed in a number of different positions or configurations relative to the renal artery ostia.[52] The effect on blood flow rate was minimal (decreasing by around 1%) for all configurations in arteries 3 mm diameter or larger. The smaller diameter artery had a larger reduction in flow rate. This reduction in blood flow may become clinically important in diseased renal arteries (renal artery stenosis) or in smaller diameter accessory renal arteries.

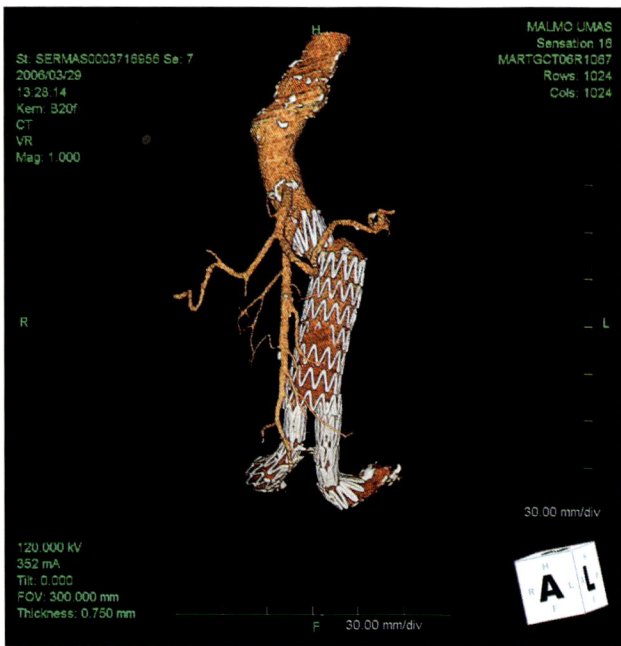

FIGURE 3: Top stent separation.

The presence of two stent wires across the renal artery ostia had a more marked effect than only partial coverage by one wire. However, when material was allowed to build up on the wires over time, blood flow decrease was more marked, up to 40%, but in most cases, did not exceed 10%.

A study by Birch of three transrenally placed stents in a porcine aorta suggested the potential for renal artery complications may be determined by stent type.[53] In the animals receiving nitinol Memotherm stents, a disorganised acellular matrix caused partial ostial occlusion in 12/13 ostia. In contrast, the stainless steel stents (Wallstent and Palmaz) were well tolerated with only one (of nine) of the renal artery ostia in the Palmaz stents suffering partial occlusion.

Desgrange's assessment of tantalum Strecker stents in the procine model was also unfavourable.[54] Of 18 renal arteries observed, one thrombosed and six stenosed due to neointimal formation on the stent struts. In a study of trans-renal stainless steel Gianturco stents in a canine model, no intimal hyperplasia or embolisation was found up to 35 weeks of follow-up.[55]

CT virtual intravascular endoscopy was recently used by investigators to calculate the percentage of patients who had stent struts crossing the renal artery ostia.[56] Twenty-nine percent of renal artery ostia were crossed by stent struts of the Talent stent-graft. In contrast, 90% of ostia were covered by the struts of the Zenith stent-graft.[57] The difference between the two stent-grafts presumably relates to the higher number of struts in the Zenith stent design.

One of the main issues when comparing data in patients with the supra- and infra-renal stent types is the heterogeneity of aneurysm morphology. Patients with supra-renal stents often have more challenging neck morphology, potentially increasing the risk of renal embolisation.

Many studies of renal function following EVAR have concentrated on serum creatinine levels. Evidence suggests that creatinine is more predictive of post-operative renal impairment in patients with aneurysms than measurements of creatinine clearance. Serum creatinine also appears more clinically relevant.[58,59] More sensitive methods of measuring glomerular and tubular function have only been performed in small numbers of patients with limited follow-up. Macierewicz assessed peri-operative glomerular filtration rate and whole kidney transit time measured by radionuclide 99 mTc DTPA renography, between a group of 11 patients undergoing infra-renal EVAR and 19 undergoing supra-renal repair.[60] He was unable to detect any difference in renal injury between infra- and supra-renal stent-grafts. In contrast, Bockler and co-workers found that supra-renal stents were significantly more likely to cause infarction.[61] Renal infarction was encountered in 19% of patients in the supra-renal group compared with 3.7% of the infra-renal patients. However, patients in the supra-renal group were more likely to have adverse proximal aneurysm neck morphology (neck diameter >30 mm, neck length <15 mm), which may be partly responsible for the adverse outcome not observed in other studies.

In Bockler's study the mean time to the detection of renal infarction was 12 days (mean follow-up 37 months), suggesting that renal infarction was a direct consequence of endoluminal instrumentation and stent deployment or proximal migration of the graft rather than late consequences of intimal hyperplasia.[61] Interestingly, the use of an aortic balloon to expand the stents did not appear to affect the rate of infarction.

The risk of renal and systemic embolisation in patients undergoing EVAR is likely to be related to aneurysm morphology. "Shaggy aortas" and thrombus lined aortic necks carry an increased risk. Ballooning of the aortic neck and stent-graft after deployment should probably be avoided in these cases to reduce the risk of emboli. Patients with thrombus at the level of the renal arteries or in the visceral aorta may be at increased risk of embolisation with supra-renal stents.

Alsac demonstrated no difference in renal outcome between a number of patients with a variety of supra- and infra-renal stent-grafts at one-year follow-up.[62] Pre-operative demographics were similar in both groups of patients. Longer-term outcomes also appear similar.[63,64] The only significant factor associated with post-operative renal impairment in patients with both supra- and infra-renal stent-grafts appeared to be the presence of pre-operative renal impairment.

Parmer compared the renal effects of supra- and infra-renal fixation in a multi-centre non-randomised study of a single stent-graft, the Powerlink.[65] A total of 192 patients received the infra-renal device and 91 the supra-renal. Unfortunately no data was presented on the morphology of the aneurysm neck and patients receiving the supra-renal stent-graft did so after a possible learning curve was established in the early infra-renal group (July 2000-October 2001). Follow-up was shorter in the supra-renal group commensurate with its later introduction. In every other aspect, patients were similar. There were no differences in terms of outcome with respect to renal function (biochemically), renal adverse events or blood pressure.

Renal emboli when they occur during or following EVAR are usually detectable on contrast CT scanning as punctate defects occurring in the renal cortex and usually measure <10% of the parenchymal volume.[66] Over follow-up these defects tend to shrink. Kramer's study suggested the majority (94%) of patients who suffer renal infarctions do so silently without any rise in creatinine. Patients who have a detectable deterioration of renal function are more likely to have pre-existing renal impairment. In that study there was no difference between the rate of renal infarction following both supra- and infra-renal stents.

DISEASED RENAL ARTERIES/ CHRONIC RENAL IMPAIRMENT

Progression of renal artery occlusive disease in patients with stent-grafts may reflect the natural history of the underlying occlusive disease with or without exacerbation from the stent. Renal atherosclerotic occlusive disease is progressive, with the majority of patients developing more advanced disease at five years follow-up.[67] Lau compared a group of 55 patients who underwent EVAR with infra-renal fixation (AneuRx) with 32 who received a supra-renal stent-graft (Zenith).[38] There were two patients in each group with unilateral renal artery stenosis (>50%). During a follow-up of 12 months, both patients in the supra-renal group developed renal artery occlusion. The authors suggested trans-renal stents may accelerate the progression of renal artery stenosis.

Sun recently studied 17 renal ostia using CT virtual intravascular endoscopy following Zenith stent-graft repair.[68] Ten of the renal ostia were significantly calcified. Nearly half (8 of 17) of the renal ostia were covered by two stent wires. However, there was no evidence of a decrease in renal ostial diameter in either the non-diseased or calcified ostia post-operatively. Patients were not followed-up and the longer-term effects of the stent wires on the configuration of the renal arteries remains to be determined.

Others have reported inconclusive results regarding the progression of renal artery stenosis after supra-renal stenting. Lobato found one patient (of five) with renal artery stenosis who subsequently developed progression of disease with hypertension at four months follow-up.[69] Marin's study of trans-renal placement of Palmaz stents was unable to detect any progression of renal artery stenosis up to 18 months follow-up.[49] There was no change in blood pressure or increased requirement for anti-hypertensive therapy in that study.

A more recent study has compared the effect of trans-renal stenting on renal artery patency and degree of stenosis.[70] In a total of 41 normal renal arteries, three developed stenoses and one occluded (progression rate of 10%). In 19 diseased renal arteries, the progression rate was 16%, although two patients with severe stenosis (>60%) underwent stenting. The authors were unable to conclude whether the progression rate in the diseased renal arteries reflected the natural history of the underlying atherosclerosis.

Alric demonstrated that the main risk factor for the development of renal impairment following EVAR was the presence of pre-operative renal impairment. However, there was no suggestion that patients treated with supra-renal stents were more likely to develop peri-operative or late renal impairment than their infra-renal counterparts.[63] Similarly, Mehta analysed patients with pre-operative chronic renal impairment. He found that renal dysfunction developed in 18.2% of the infra-renal group (19 months), and 17.1% of the trans-renal group (p = 0.95) at 19 and 17 months of follow-up respectively.

It is technically possible to perform renal artery stenting before, during and after EVAR, even in the presence of a supra-renal stent (Figure 4). The outcome data of renal artery stenosis after EVAR has also

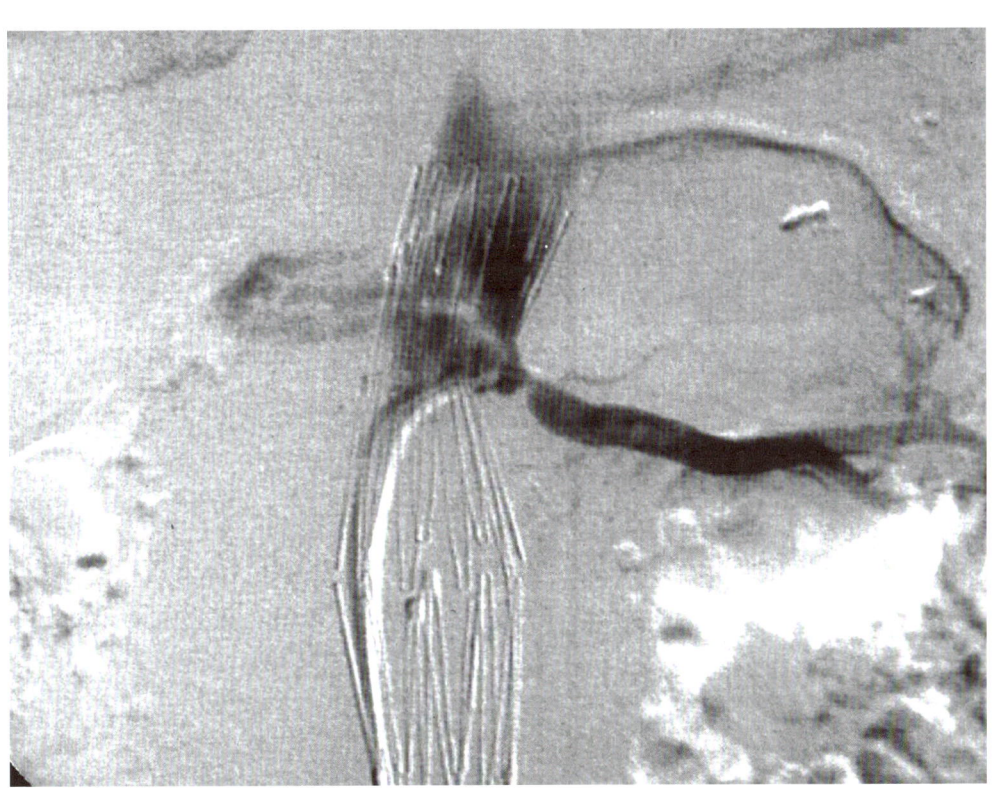

FIGURE 4: A.Tight renal artery stenosis following EVAR. *(continued)*

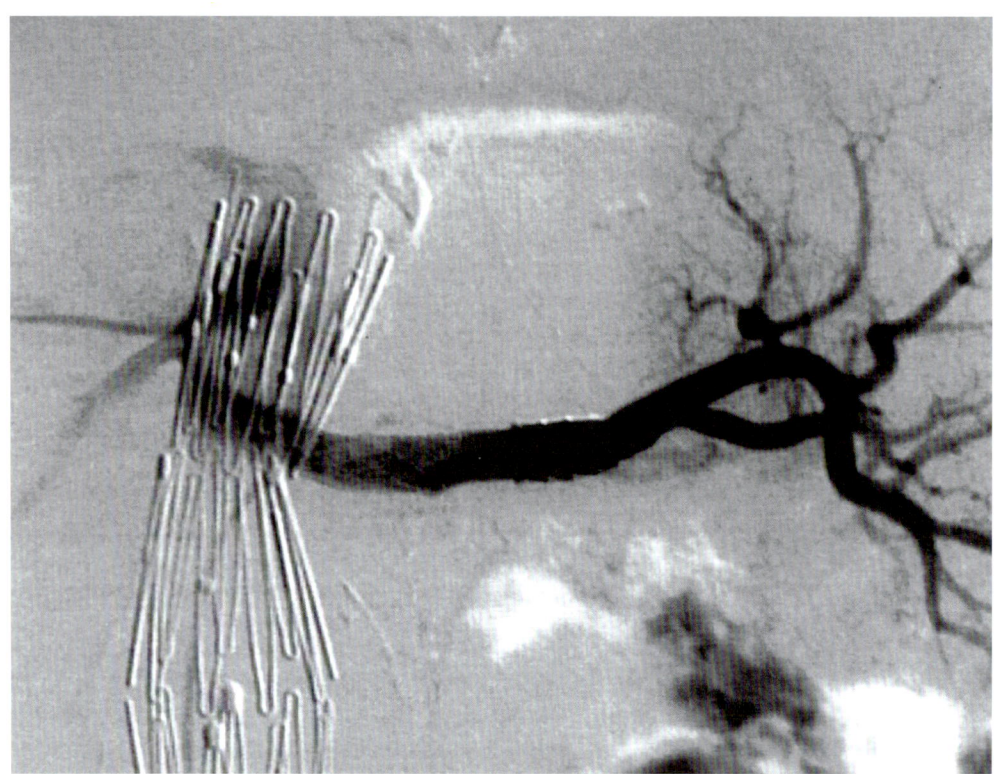

FIGURE 4: B. Renal artery stented post-op.

been clouded by a significant number of patients receiving pre or peri-operaive renal stenting. The correct indications and timing of renal interventions for atherosclerotic occlusive disease therefore remains a subject of debate. At present it is probably best to maintain the same indications as for patients without EVAR.

Many of the large supra-renal stents will traverse the visceral as well as the renal arteries. Marin's post-operative contrast CT review of supra-renal EVAR found that of the 97 Talent and Palmaz stents placed across the renal arteries, 95 crossed the visceral arteries (72 trans-SMA, 13 trans-coeliac).[72] However, during a mean follow-up of 25 (6-44) months, there was no evidence of atheroembolisation or ostial stenosis either clinically or radiologically. These results concur with the generally observed low rate of clinically manifest visceral ischaemia with supra-renal stents.

Duplex ultrasonography is a useful tool for screening and detecting high-grade renal artery stenosis following supra-renal stent placement but may not be so useful for the SMA.[73,74] Intrarenal color duplex ultrasonography was technically successful in 98% of patients in the former study. However, visualisation of the SMA was only possible in 76% of patients in the latter study (Figure 5).

FENESTRATED AND BRANCHED STENT-GRAFTS

An alternative approach to stent-graft fixation, especially in patients with short necks is the fenestrated or branched stent-graft. In a recent study in cadaveric aortas, Lin-

FIGURE 5: The supra-renal stent often crosses the visceral arteries. In this case the supra-renal stent crosses the SMA.

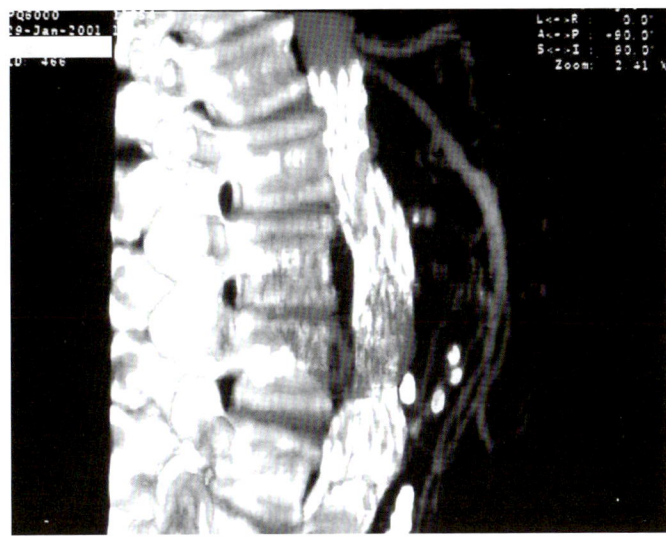

sen and colleagues found that the median distraction force for branched stent-grafts (16.95 N) was significantly higher than for either fenestrated (9.17 N) or conventional infra-renal (4.67 N) endografts.[75] The stent-grafts used did not have hooks or barbs and were tested under a continuous longitudinal force rather than pulsatile blood flow. In addition, the length of the aortic neck was 20 mm in all aortas. Consequently, the fenestrated graft had an attachment length of approximately 35mm compared to the 20 mm of the infra-renal graft. This greater length itself may have contributed to the improved fixation. In clinical practice, the length of the aorta is likely to be shorter in patients receiving fenestrated or branched stent-graft technology (hence the need for that technology). The effect of a shorter neck on the distraction force of a fenestrated or branched graft was not investigated.

Although fenesrated and branch stent-graft technology may require a greater distraction force and therefore have greater stability, the consequences of small movements on renal and visceral artery patency are considerable. The stability of the stent-graft must be balanced against the potential complications, particularly, renal, which are more likely when compared with infra-renal EVAR.[76]

Zhou also concurred that the forces required to distract fenestrated stent-grafts was greater than regular stent-grafts (in this case the Zenith).[25] He concluded that the two phase migration may result in compromise of seal in short aortic necks, especially in using regular stent-grafts where the force required to produce movement in the first phase is significantly inferior to the use of fenestrated stent-grafts.

FUTURE DEVELOPMENTS

Many of the early failures of stent-graft fixation required open surgery. A variety of procedures have been used including the placement of sutures through the aneurysm neck in to the stent-graft and peri-aortic ligatures/bands. Many of these procedures can now be performed endovascularly using stent-graft extensions and Palmaz stents. However, some patients will not respond to these endovascular techniques.

Animal studies have demonstrated the

possibility of laparoscopic banding to prevent aneurysm neck dilation.[77] It is possible that this technique could be used in patients to augment fixation of aortic stent-grafts. Kolvenbach has reported the feasibility of laparoscopically placed external sutures in the aortic neck of patients with stent-grafts to prevent migration.[78]

Preliminary reports have emerged on a variety of endovascular stapling devices. These devices are intended to attach stent-grafts to the aortic wall and be used in the prevention and treatment of endoleak and migration.

The endostaple developed by Trout and Tanner uses a coil shaped staple made from either stainless steel or shape memory alloy.[79] The delivery system comprises a laser fiber which "drills" a hole through the stent-graft and aortic wall. The endostaple is then delivered through the hole and acts as a rivet to secure graft/aortic wall apposition and fixation.

The Hopkinson endostaple developed in conjunction with Lombard Medical (Abingdon, Oxon, U.K.) comprises a nitinol staple in a pre-formed "seagull" shape (Figure 6). One of the advantages of this system is that the staple can be deployed, retrieved and re-deployed in order to be placed optimally. This is particularly useful in the heavily calcified aorta. Other designs are a "one-shot".[80] The Hopkinson endostaple has undergone successful *in vitro* and animal studies and is currently seeking appropriate regulatory approval for clinical trials.

One endovascular stapling system which is already being studied in patients is the Aptus AAA repair system (Aptus Endosystems Inc, Sunnyvale, CA). Patients have recently been enrolled in an FDA trial. The results of this system are awaited.

Other non-mechanical methods are in development to improve the healing and incorporation of stent-grafts in to the aortic wall. These include the use of growth factors.[81] It remains to be seen whether these novel techniques can be transferred from animal models to humans.

CONCLUSIONS

Self-expanding stents alone are insufficient to ensure stent-graft fixation. Robust barbs or hooks are sufficient to resist migration. In cadaveric experiments the force required to dislodge stent-grafts with these appendages is the same whether

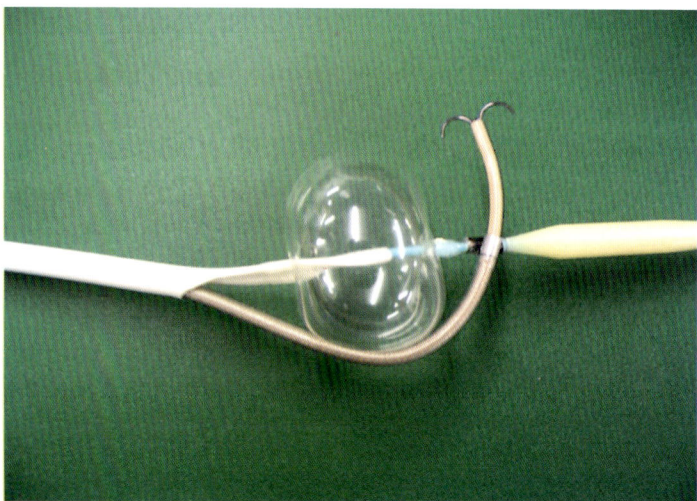

FIGURE 6: The endovascular delivery kit with the staple in the deployed position. The curved cannula holds the staple and the hinged flexed outer cannula allow the staple to approach the target area at right angles to the stent-graft surface. The balloon helps to stabilise the whole system during deployment.

placed in the infra- or supra-renal aorta. Clinical evidence suggests that endoleak and migration rates are lower with supra-renal stents with barb fixation. Infra-renal stents may be less successful in the presence of a diseased aortic neck or in patients who develop neck dilatation. Infra-renal stent-graft fixation is better suited to longer disease free aortic necks.

Supra-renal stents potentially increase the number of patients suitable for EVAR by expanding the proximal neck morphological criteria.

Studies comparing the renal complications of supra- and infra-renal stent-grafts have found little difference in complication rates, even in patients with chronic renal impairment and renal artery stenosis. In patients with high grade stenosis, renal artery stenting may be justified.

Stent-grafts without hooks and barbs rely on column strength to prevent migration. There is little compelling evidence to support this as a successful method of fixation in isolation.

There is no consistent data to support continued aortic neck dilation in balloon-expandable or self-expanding stents after the first six months following implantation. There does appear to be a sub-group of patients who will develop neck dilatation. These patients may be better served with stents which engage the supra-renal aorta which is less prone to dilate.

Gross oversizing in the aortic neck is associated with complications. Patient selection (adverse morphology) may be partly responsible for this observation. Consequently, gross oversizing should be avoided in such patients. In the presence of adverse neck anatomy, fenestrated stent-grafts may provide a more reliable method of fixation.

A variety of new endovascular techniques are emerging to improve stent-graft fixation and deal with its consequences. Most promising of these new techniques appear to be the endovascular staples.

REFERENCES

1. Chaikof EL, Blankensteijn JD, Harris PL, White GH, Zarins CK, Bernhard VM, Matsumura JS, May J, Veith FJ, Fillinger MF, Rutherford RB, Kent KC; Ad Hoc Committee for Standardized Reporting Practices in Vascular Surgery of The Society for Vascular Surgery/American Association for Vascular Surgery. Reporting standards for endovascular aortic aneurysm repair. J Vasc Surg 2002,35:1048-60.
2. Zarins CK, White RA, Schwarten D, Kinney E, Diethrich EB, Hodgson KJ, Fogarty TJ. AneuRx stent graft versus open surgical repair of abdominal aortic aneurysms: multicenter prospective clinical trial. J Vasc Surg. 1999;29:292-305.
3. Ebaugh JL, Eskandari MK, Finkelstein A, Matsumura JS, Morasch MD, Hoff FL, Pearce WH. Caudal migration of endoprostheses after treatment of abdominal aortic aneurysms. J Surg Res. 2002;107:14-7.
4. Liffman K, Lawrence-Brown MM, Semmens JB, Bui A, Rudman M, Hartley DE. Analytical modeling and numerical simulation of forces in an endoluminal graft. J Endovasc Ther. 2001;8:358-71.
5. Alric P, Hinchliffe RJ, Chuter TA, Whitaker SC, Wenham PW, Hopkinson BR. Lessons learned from the long-term follow-up of a first generation stent-graft. J Vasc Surg 2003;37:367-73.
6. Malina M, Brunkwall J, Ivancev K, Jonsson J, Malina J, Lindblad B. Endovascular healing is inadequate for fixation of Dacron stent-grafts in human aortoiliac vessels. Eur J Vasc Endovasc Surg. 2000;19:5-11.
7. Harris PL, Vallabhaneni SR, Desgranges P, Becquemin JP, van Marrewijk C, Laheij RJ. Incidence and risk factors of late rupture, conversion, and death after endovascular repair of infrarenal aortic aneurysms: the EUROSTAR experience. European Collaborators on Stent/graft techniques for aortic aneurysm repair. J Vasc Surg. 2000;32:739-49.
8. Sampaio SM, Panneton JM, Mozes G, Andrews JC, Noel AA, Kalra M, Bower TC, Cherry KJ, Sullivan TM, Gloviczki P. AneuRx device migration: incidence, risk factors, and consequences. Ann Vasc Surg. 2005;19:178-85.
9. Laheij RJ, Buth J, Harris PL, Moll FL, Stelter WJ, Verhoeven EL. Need for secondary interventions

after endovascular repair of abdominal aortic aneurysms. Intermediate-term follow-up results of a European collaborative registry (EUROSTAR). Br J Surg. 2000;87:1666-73.

10. Zarins CK, Heikkinen MA, Lee ES, Alsac JM, Arko FR. Short- and long-term outcome following endovascular aneurysm repair. How does it compare to open surgery? J Cardiovasc Surg (Torino). 2004;45:321-33.

11. Conners MS 3rd, Sternbergh WC 3rd, Carter G, Tonnessen BH, Yoselevitz M, Money SR. Endograft migration one to four years after endovascular abdominal aortic aneurysm repair with the AneuRx device: a cautionary note. J Vasc Surg. 2002;36:476-84.

12. Lee JT, Lee J, Aziz I, Donayre CE, Walot I, Kopchok GE, Heilbron M Jr, Lippmann M, White RA. Stent-graft migration following endovascular repair of aneurysms with large proximal necks: anatomical risk factors and long-term sequelae. J Endovasc Ther. 2002;9:652-64.

13. Mohan IV, Harris PL, Van Marrewijk CJ, Laheij RJ, How TV. Factors and forces influencing stent-graft migration after endovascular aortic aneurysm repair. J Endovasc Ther. 2002;9:748-55.

14. Leurs LJ, Stultiens G, Kievit J, Buth J; EUROSTAR Collaborators. Adverse events at the aneurysmal neck identified at follow-up after endovascular abdominal aortic aneursym repair: how do they correlate? Vascular. 2005;13:261-7.

15. Albertini J, Kalliafas S, Travis S, Yusuf SW, Macierewicz JA, Whitaker SC, Elmarasy NM, Hopkinson BR. Anatomical risk factors for proximal perigraft endoleak and graft migration following endovascular repair of abdominal aortic aneurysms. Eur J Vasc Endovasc Surg. 2000;19:308-12.

16. Hodgson R, McWilliams RG, Simpson A, Gould DA, Brennan JA, Gilling-Smith GL, Harris PL. Migration versus apparent migration: importance of errors due to positioning variation in plain radiographic follow-up of aortic stent-grafts. J Endovasc Ther. 2003;10:902-10.

17. Lambert AW, Williams DJ, Budd JS, Horrocks M. Experimental assessment of proximal stent-graft (InterVascular) fixation in human cadaveric infrarenal aortas. Eur J Vasc Endovasc Surg. 1999;17:60-5.

18. Cao P, Verzini F, Zannetti S, De Rango P, Parlani G, Lupattelli L, Maselli A. Device migration after endoluminal abdominal aortic aneurysm repair: analysis

of 113 cases with a minimum follow-up period of 2 years. J Vasc Surg. 2002;35:229-35.

19. Zarins CK, Bloch DA, Crabtree T, Matsumoto AH, White RA, Fogarty TJ. Stent graft migration after endovascular aneurysm repair: importance of proximal fixation. J Vasc Surg. 2003;38:1264-72

20. Tonnessen BH, Sternbergh WC 3rd, Money SR. Mid- and long-term device migration after endovascular abdominal aortic aneurysm repair: a comparison of AneuRx and Zenith endografts. J Vasc Surg. 2005;42:392-400.

21. Greenberg RK, Lawrence-Brown M, Bhandari G, Hartley D, Stelter W, Umscheid T, Chuter T, Ivancev K, Green R, Hopkinson B, Semmens J, Ouriel K. An update of the Zenith endovascular graft for abdominal aortic aneurysms: initial implantation and mid-term follow-up data. J Vasc Surg. 2001;33(2 Suppl):S157-64.

22. Resch T, Malina M, Lindblad B, Ivancev K. The impact of stent-graft development on outcome of AAA repair--a 7-year experience. Eur J Vasc Endovasc Surg. 2001;22:57-61.

23. Veerapen R, Dorandeu A, Serre I, Berthet JP, Marty-Ane CH, Mary H, Alric P. Improvement in proximal aortic endograft fixation: an experimental study using different stent-grafts in human cadaveric aortas. J Endovasc Ther. 2003;10:1101-9.

24. Sternbergh WC 3rd, Conners MS 3rd, Money SR. Explantation of an infected aortic endograft with suprarenal barb fixation. J Vasc Surg. 2003;38:1136.

25. Zhou SS, Brennan J, How TV, Gilling-Smith G, Harris PL. Comparison of the fixation strength of fenestrated and non-fenestrated stentgrafts for endovascular abdominal aortic aneurysm repair (EVAR). Br J Surg 2006, 93; (Issue S2):24.

26. Resch T, Malina M, Lindblad B, Malina J, Brunkwall J, Ivancev K. The impact of stent design on proximal stent-graft fixation in the abdominal aorta: an experimental study. Eur J Vasc Endovasc Surg. 2000;20:190-5.

27. Greenberg RK, Chuter TA, Sternbergh WC 3rd, Fearnot NE; Zenith Investigators. Zenith AAA endovascular graft: intermediate-term results of the US multicenter trial. J Vasc Surg. 2004;39:1209-18.

28. Mohan IV, Laheij RJ, Harris PL; EUROSTAR COLLABORATORS. Risk factors for endoleak and the evidence for stent-graft oversizing when undergo-

ing endovascular aneurysm repair. Eur J Vasc Endovasc Surg 2001;21:344-9.

29. Sternbergh WC 3rd, Money SR, Greenberg RK, Chuter TA; Zenith Investigators. Influence of endograft oversizing on device migration, endoleak, aneurysm shrinkage, and aortic neck dilation: results from the Zenith Multicenter Trial. J Vasc Surg. 2004;39:20-6.

30. McArthur C, Teodorescu V, Eisen L, Morrissey N, Faries P, Hollier L, Marin ML. Histopathologic analysis of endovascular stent grafts from patients with aortic aneurysms: Does healing occur? J Vasc Surg. 2001;33:733-8

31. Singh-Ranger R, Adiseshiah M. Differing morphological changes following endovascular AAA repair using balloon-expandable or self-expanding endografts. J Endovasc Ther. 2000;7:479-85.

32. Malas MB, Ohki T, Veith FJ, Chen T, Lipsitz EC, Shah AR, Timaran C, Suggs W, Gargiulo NJ 3rd, Parodi JC. Absence of proximal neck dilatation and graft migration after endovascular aneurysm repair with balloon-expandable stent-based endografts. J Vasc Surg. 2005;42:639-44.

33. Makaroun MS, Deaton DH. Is proximal aortic neck dilatation after endovascular aneurysm exclusion a cause for concern? J Vasc Surg. 2001;33 (2 Suppl): S39-45.

34. Resch T, Ivancev K, Brunkwall J, Nyman U, Malina M, Lindblad B. Distal migration of stent-grafts after endovascular repair of abdominal aortic aneurysms. J Vasc Interv Radiol. 1999;10: 257-64.

35. Walker SR, Macierewicz J, Elmarasy NM, Gregson RH, Whitaker SC, Hopkinson BR. A prospective study to assess changes in proximal aortic neck dimensions after endovascular repair of abdominal aortic aneurysms. J Vasc Surg. 1999;29: 625-30.

36. Cao P, Verzini F, Parlani G, Rango PD, Parente B, Giordano G, Mosca S, Maselli A. Predictive factors and clinical consequences of proximal aortic neck dilatation in 230 patients undergoing abdominal aorta aneurysm repair with self-expandable stent-grafts. J Vasc Surg. 2003;37:1200-5.

37. Thompson MM, Smith J, Naylor AR, Nasim A, Sayers RD, Boyle JR, Thompson J, Tinkler K, Evans D, Smith G, Bell PR. Microembolization during endovascular and conventional aneurysm repair. J Vasc Surg. 1997;25:179-86.

38. Lau LL, Hakaim AG, Oldenburg WA, Neuhauser

B, McKinney JM, Paz-Fumagalli R, Stockland A. Effect of suprarenal versus infrarenal aortic endograft fixation on renal function and renal artery patency: a comparative study with intermediate follow-up. J Vasc Surg. 2003;37:1162-8.

39. Kalliafas S, Albertini JN, Macierewicz J, Yusuf SW, Whitaker SC, Davidson I, Hopkinson BR. Stent-graft migration after endovascular repair of abdominal aortic aneurysm. J Endovasc Ther. 2002;9:743-7.

40. Arko FR, Heikkinen M, Lee ES, Bass A, Alsac JM, Zarins CK. Iliac fixation length and resistance to in-vivo stent-graft displacement. J Vasc Surg. 2005;41:664-71.

41. Heikkinen MA, Alsac JM, Arko FR, Metsanoja R, Zvaigzne A, Zarins CK. The importance of iliac fixation in prevention of stent graft migration. J Vasc Surg. 2006;43:1130-7.

42. Lawrence-Brown M, Sieunarine K, Hartley D, et al. Should an anchor stent cross the renal artery orifices when placing an endoluminal graft for abdominal aortic aneurysm? In: Greenhalgh RM, ed. Indications in vascular and endovascular surgery, London: WB Saunders, 1998; 261-269.

43. Sonesson B, Resch T, Lanne T, Ivancev K. The fate of the infrarenal aortic neck after open aneurysm surgery. J Vasc Surg 1998;28:889-894.

44. Armon MP, Yusuf SW, Latief K, Whitaker SC, Gregson RH, Wenham PW, Hopkinson BR. Anatomical suitability of abdominal aortic aneurysms for endovascular repair. Br J Surg. 1997;84:178-80.

45. Biebl M, Hakaim AG, Oldenburg WA, Lau LL, Klocker J, Neuhauser B, Paz-Fumagalli R, McKinney JM. Midterm results of a single-centre commercially available devices for endovascular aneurysm repair. The Mount Sinai Journal of Medicine 2005;72:127-35.

46. Van Marrewijk CJ, Leurs LJ, Vallabhaneni SR, Harris PL, Buth J, Laheij RJF, EUROSTAR collaborators. Risk-adjusted outcome analysis of endovascular abdominal aortic aneurysm repair in a large population: How do stent-grafts compare? J Endovasc Ther 2005;12;417-29.

47. Cowie AG, Ashleigh RJ, England RE, McCollum CN. Endovascular aneurysm repair with the Talent stent-graft. J Vasc Interv Radiol. 2003;14:1011-6.

48. Stanley BM, Semmens JB, Mai Q, Goodman MA, Hartley DE, Wilkinson C, Lawrence-Brown MD.

Evaluation of patient selection guidelines for endoluminal AAA repair with the Zenith Stent-Graft: the Australasian experience. J Endovasc Ther. 2001;8:457-64.

49. Marin ML, Parsons RE, Hollier LH, Mitty HA, Ahn J, Parsons RE, Temudom T, D'Ayala M, McLaughlin M, DePalo L, Kahn R. Impact of transrenal aortic endograft placement on endovascular graft repair of abdominal aortic aneurysms. J Vasc Surg. 1998;28:638-46.

50. Robbins M, Kritpracha B, Beebe HG, Criado FJ, Daoud Y, Comerota AJ. Suprarenal endograft fixation avoids adverse outcomes associated with aortic neck angulation. Ann Vasc Surg. 2005;19:172-7.

51. Ghanim K, Mwipatayi BP, Abbas M, Sieunarine K. Late stent-graft migration secondary to separation of the uncovered segment from the main body of a zenith endoluminal graft. J Endovasc Ther. 2006;13:346-9.

52. Liffman K, Lawrence-Brown MM, Semmens JB, Sutalo ID, Bui A, White F, Hartley DE. Suprarenal fixation: effect on blood flow of an endoluminal stent wire across an arterial orifice. J Endovasc Ther. 2003;10:260-74.

53. Birch PC, Start RD, Whitbread T, Palmer I, Gaines PA, Beard JD. The effects of crossing porcine renal artery ostia with various endovascular stents. Eur J Vasc Endovasc Surg. 1999;17:185-90.

54. Desgranges P, Hutin E, Kedzia C, Allaire E, Becquemin JP. Aortic stents covering the renal arteries ostia: an animal study. J Vasc Interv Radiol. 1997;8:77-82.

55. Lawrence DD Jr, Charnsangavej C, Wright KC, Gianturco C, Wallace S. Percutaneous endovascular graft: experimental evaluation. Radiology. 1987;163:357-60.

56. England A, Butterfield JS, Ashleigh RJ. Incidence and effect of bare suprarenal stent struts crossing renal ostia following EVAR. Eur J Vasc Endovasc Surg 2006;32(5):523-8.

57. Sun Z, Winder RJ, Kelly BE, Ellis PK, Kennedy PT, Hirst DG. Diagnostic value of CT virtual endoscopy in aortic stent-grafting. J Endovasc Ther 2004;11:13-25.

58. Powell RJ, Roddy SP, Meier GH, Gusberg RJ, Conte MS, Sumpio BE. Effect of renal insufficiency on outcome following infrarenal aortic surgery. Am J Surg. 1997;174:126-130.

59. Johnston KW. Multicenter prospective study of nonruptured abdominal aortic aneurysm. Part II. Variables predicting morbidity and mortality. J Vasc Surg 1989;9:437-447.

60. Macierewicz J, Walker SR, Vincent R, Wastie M, Elmarasy N, Hopkinson BR. Perioperative renal function following endovascular repair of abdominal aortic aneurysm with suprarenal and infrarenal stents. Br J Surg. 1999;86:69.

61. Bockler D, Krauss M, Mansmann U, Halawa M, Lange R, Probst T, Raithel D. Incidence of renal infarctions after endovascular AAA repair: relationship to infrarenal versus suprarenal fixation. J Endovasc Ther. 2003;10:1054-60.

62. Alsac JM, Zarins CK, Heikkinen MA, Karwowski J, Arko FR, Desgranges P, Roudot-Thoraval F, Becquemin JP. The impact of aortic endografts on renal function. J Vasc Surg. 2005;41:926-30.

63. Alric P, Hinchliffe RJ, Picot MC, Braithwaite BD, MacSweeney ST, Wenham PW, Hopkinson BR. Long-term renal function following endovascular aneurysm repair with infrarenal and suprarenal aortic stent-grafts. J Endovasc Ther 2003;10: 397-405.

64. Davey P, Rose JD, Parkinson T, Wyatt MG. The mid-term effect of bare metal suprarenal fixation on renal function following endovascular abdominal aortic aneurysm repair. Eur J Vasc Endovasc Surg. 2006;32:516-22.

65. Parmer SS, Carpenter JP; Endologix Investigators. Endovascular aneurysm repair with suprarenal vs infrarenal fixation: a study of renal effects. J Vasc Surg. 2006;43:19-25.

66. Kramer SC, Seifarth H, Pamler R, Fleiter T, Buhring J, Sunder-Plassmann L, Brambs HJ, Gorich J. Renal infarction following endovascular aortic aneurysm repair: incidence and clinical consequences. J Endovasc Ther. 2002;9:98-102.

67. Caps MT, Perissinotto C, Zierler RE, Polissar NL, Bergelin RO, Tullis MJ, Cantwell-Gab K, Davidson RC, Strandness DE Jr. Prospective study of atherosclerotic disease progression in the renal artery. Circulation 1998;98:2866-72.

68. Sun Z, Zheng H. Effect of suprarenal stent struts on the renal artery with ostial calcification observed on CT virtual intravascular endoscopy. Eur J Vasc Endovasc Surg 2004;28:534-42.

69. Lobato AC, Quick RC, Vaughn PL, Rodriguez-Lo-

pez J, Douglas M, Diethrich EB. Transrenal fixation of aortic endografts: intermediate follow-up of a single-center experience. J Endovasc Ther. 2000;7:273-8.

70. Bove PG, Long GW, Shanley CJ, Brown OW, Rimar SD, Hans SS, Kitzmiller JW, Bendick PJ, Zelenock GB. Transrenal fixation of endovascular stent-grafts for infrarenal aortic aneurysm repair: mid-term results. J Vasc Surg. 2003;37:938-42.

71. Mehta M, Cayne N, Veith FJ, Darling RC 3rd, Roddy SP, Paty PS, Ozsvath KJ, Kreienberg PB, Chang BB, Shah DM. Relationship of proximal fixation to renal dysfunction in patients undergoing endovascular aneurysm repair. J Cardiovasc Surg (Torino). 2004;45:367-74.

72. Burks JA, Faries PL, Gravereaux EC, Hollier LD, Marin ML. Endovascular repair of abdominal aortic aneurysms: Stent-graft fixation across the visceral arteries. J Vasc Surg 2002;35:109-13.

73. Kalliafas S, Travis SJ, Macierewicz J, Yusuf SW, Whitaker SC, Davidson I, Hopkinson BR. Intrarenal color duplex examination of aortic endograft patients with suprarenal stents. J Endovasc Ther. 2001;8:592-6.

74. Kalliafas S, Travis SJ, Macierewicz J, Yusuf SW, Whitaker SC, Davidson I, Hopkinson BR. Color duplex ultrasonography of the superior mesenteric artery after placement of endografts with suprarenal stents. Vasc Endovascular Surg. 2002;36:29-32.

75. Linsen MAM, Floris Vos AW, Diks J, Rauwerda JA, Wisselink W. Fenestrated and branched endografts: assessment of proximal aortic neck fixation. J Endovasc Ther 2005;12:647-53.

76. Haddad F, Greenberg RK, Walker E, Nally J, O'Neill S, Kolin G, Lyden SP, Clair D, Sarac T, Ouriel K. et al. Fenestrated endovascular stent-grafting: the renal side of the story. J Vasc Surg 2005;41:181-90.

77. Sonesson B, Montgomery A, Ivancev K, Lindblad B. Fixation of infrarenal aortic stent-grafts using laparoscopic banding –an experimental study in pigs. Eur J Vasc Endovasc Surg. 2001;21:40-5.

78. Kolvenbach R, Pinter L, Raghunandan M, Cheshire N, Ramadan H, Dion YM. Laparoscopic remodeling of abdominal aortic aneurysms after endovascular exclusion: a technical description. J Vasc Surg. 2002;36:1267-70.

79. Trout HH, Tanner HM. A new vascular Endostaple: A technical description. J Vasc Surg 2001;34:565-8.

80. Bolduc et al. United States Patent Application Publication. Pub No: US2005/0187613 A1.

81. van der Bas JM, Quax PH, van den Berg AC, Visser MJ, van der Linden E, van Bockel JH. Ingrowth of aorta wall into stent grafts impregnated with basic fibroblast growth factor: a porcine in vivo study of blood vessel prosthesis healing. J Vasc Surg. 2004;39:850-8.

Endograft fixation on the aortic bifurcation for better stability. Composite endoprosthesis

Theodossios P. Perdikides, Efthimios Avgerinos, Vasilios Tzilalis, Nikolaos Bessias, George Georgiades, Konstantinos Lagios

With the introduction of endovascular aneurysm repair (EVAR), the trusted durability of a conventional anastomosis was replaced by the questioned durability of endograft stability. Despite the favourable short and mid term results of standard endografts concern has been raised for endograft migration as this will be responsible for almost all late complications in EVAR, including secondary type I endoleak, AAA enlargement and rupture.[1,2] Midterm results for conventional endografts show migration rates varying from 0% to 13%[3-6] while long-term results may be disappointing.[7,8]

According to Mahan et al several aspects of aneurysm morphology (large proximal and terminal aortic diameters), while also the proximal endograft diameter are risk factors for stent-graft migration. A theoretical model of stent-grafts indicated that high pressure, angulated iliac arteries, large proximal graft diameter, and the degree of diameter-change along the endograft increase the displacement force exerted at the proximal fixation site for stent-grafts.[9]

It is nowadays clear that graft stability is more important, than just deploying it successfully. Although in the short term EVAR success is determined upon patient and physician related factors, the long term results are additionally based on factors related to the AAA anatomy and on the device's specific characteristics (fixation, hemodynamic seal, mechanical integrity and patency).[10-14] Early generation grafts used to have a short main body and long limbs with quite a lot disadvantages (e.g inability of deploying a proximal cuff). Even more, the short main body and the long limbs of these early endografts showed significant migration rates associated partly to the high, unsupported position of the endograft's bifurcation: blood-flow forces tend to push the device distally due to the significant diameter decrease at the level of the flow divider.[9]

Currently available endografts have enhanced their stability by using a long main body with short limbs and improved their fixation by radial forces, appendages such as hooks and barbs, and suprarenal bare stents. However, migration and the ensuing proximal type I leak are still encountered.

Until now, primary attention had been placed on the proximal graft stability (suprarenal struts and hooks), whereas the distal fixation was not that much appreciated. Recent studies reveal that it is the close proximity of the distal end of the stent graft to the iliac bifurcation that seems to provide the greatest stability against migration.[15]

These concerns on migration rates inspired the development of a new generation graft, derived from the double tube concept which involves the placement of a distal tube graft exactly into the aortic bifurcation and a proximal tube graft directly beneath the renal arteries.[16,17] Professor Wolf Stelter developed the multimodular composite concept to position a bifurcated stent-graft into the aortic bifurcation and to extend the stent-graft proximally with an aortic cuff. The Zenith Composite Endovascular graft (William A. Cook Australia, LTD) is extensively used by Stelter and colleagues in Frankfurt, since 2000. The endograft configuration uses a self expanding modular design with an uncovered Gianturco Z-Stent for proximal suprarenal fixation, while distal stability is enhanced by accommodation of the graft onto the patients' natural aortic bifurcation. Modifications of the graft preserve side branch perfusion by incorporating fenestrations (independently of the bifurcated component), successfully used during the last 7 years.

GRAFT DESIGN

The Zenith Composite Endovascular graft is a modular graft derived from the Zenith Trifab device. It is a three-part system, but additional elements can be added as required. The main body (distal body) is a caudad bifurcated segment that allows close apposition to the patient's natural aortic bifurcation. (Figure 1) The next component is a cephalad tube (proximal body) with an uncovered Z stent and 8mm flexible inter-stent gaps that facilitate precise infrarenal aortic placement, especially for kinked necks. (Figure 2) Its relatively short length facilitates accurate deployment. The graft is completed with one or two iliac limbs (Figure 3).

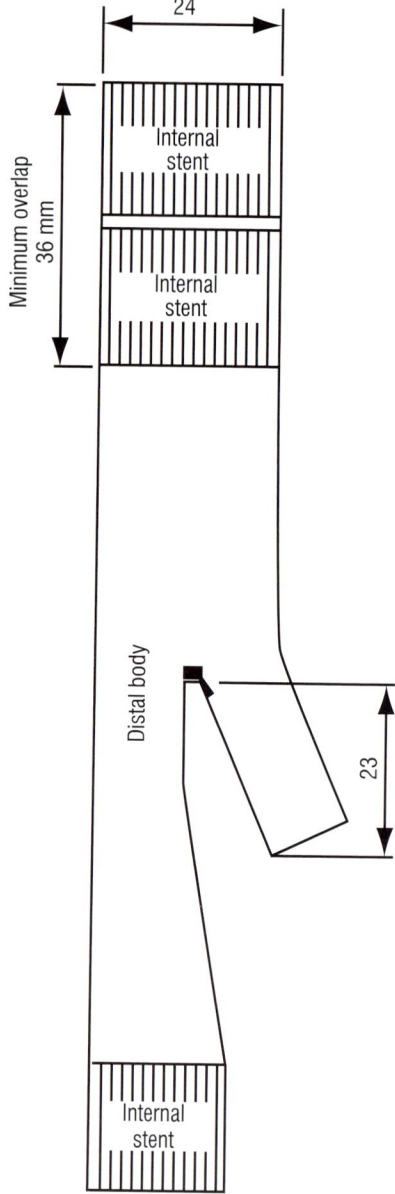

FIGURE 1: Bifurcated component (distal body).

The proximal body is available in a wide range of diameters (24-36 mm) and lengths (91-129 mm), while a variable length is also available for the distal body. The fixed ipsilateral limb of the distal main body component is available in 4 different distal diameters (12, 16, 20 and 24 mm)

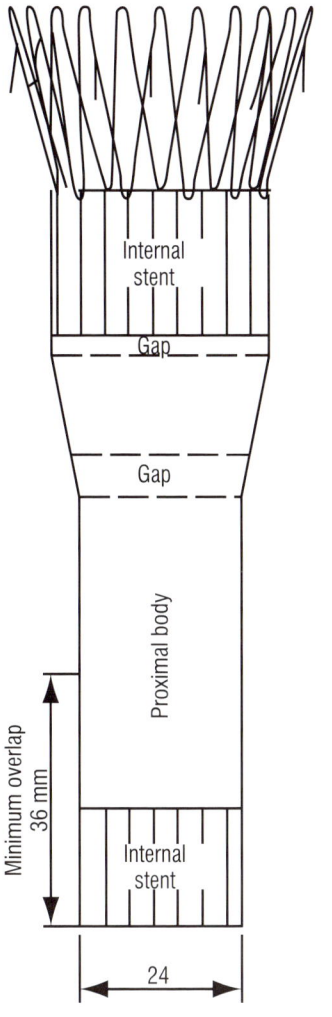

FIGURE 2: Tubular component (proximal body).

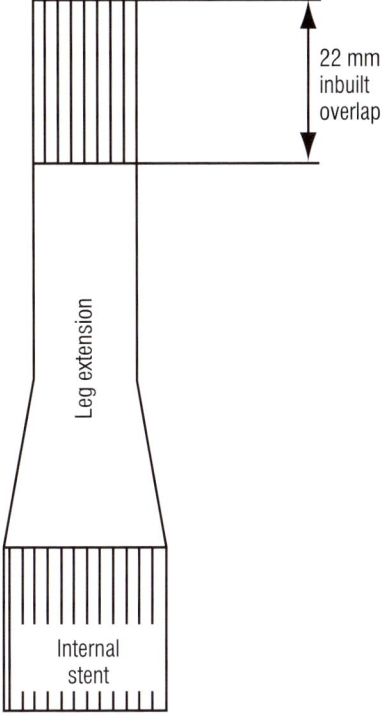

FIGURE 3: Leg extension.

and 3 different lengths (51, 68 and 85 mm). The modular contralateral limb ranges in diameters between 12 and 24 mm (2 mm size intervals) and in lengths between 37 and 105 mm (5 sizes available).

IMPLANTATION TECHNIQUE

Composite endograft deployment is carried out as previously described.[18] Briefly, the bifurcated part (distal body) is inserted first through the selected femoral artery and deployed till the contralateral stump is released. Following cannulation of the contralateral leg the proximal end of the distal body is released. A 12 mm x 4 cm angioplasty balloon is introduced into the contralateral leg and then inflated with 2/3 of its balloon length inside and its 1/3 remaining outside the stump. A simultaneous "pulling down manoeuvre" on the delivery system (un-deployed ipsilateral leg) from one side and on the inflated balloon from the other side guides the stump into the contralateral common iliac ostium, bringing down the distal body of the endograft onto the aortic bifurcation. The balloon is removed and the proximal body is inserted through the contralateral groin, while firmly holding the delivery system of the un-deployed ipsilateral leg to avoid its dislocation from the aortic bifurcation. The tubular graft is advanced and the ipsilateral leg is fully deployed. The body overlapping (proximal-distal body) needs to be a minimum of three stents to maximize column strength and stability. The proximal body is fully deployed, the top cap is released and the suprarenal stent deployed, while the remaining part of the procedure, including the contralateral leg insertion is carried out using the standard technique for Zenith devices. Figure 4 illustrates step by step the implantation technique.

DISCUSSION

Proximal fixation has been always the target parameter of endograft designers and users, while distal fixation was not that much appreciated until recently.[15] It seems that the strong pulsating forces that try to bring down the bifurcation of the graft and buldge out its long limbs have been underestimated. By accommodating the graft onto the natural aortic bifurcation the blood flow splits in the normal anatomical position, thus hemodynamics improve substantially. The proposed implantation can provide support to counteract the downward pulsatile forces and, ultimately, prevent downward migration (though not lateral/anterior migration).

The Composite configuration, and the proposed implantation technique, is extensively used in Frankfurt and is also favourable in Munster and Athens. An attempt to compare the outcomes of the the Trifab graft versus the Composite graft cannot be sufficiently supported, since the anatomies chosen for the Composite implantation were "by definition" more com-

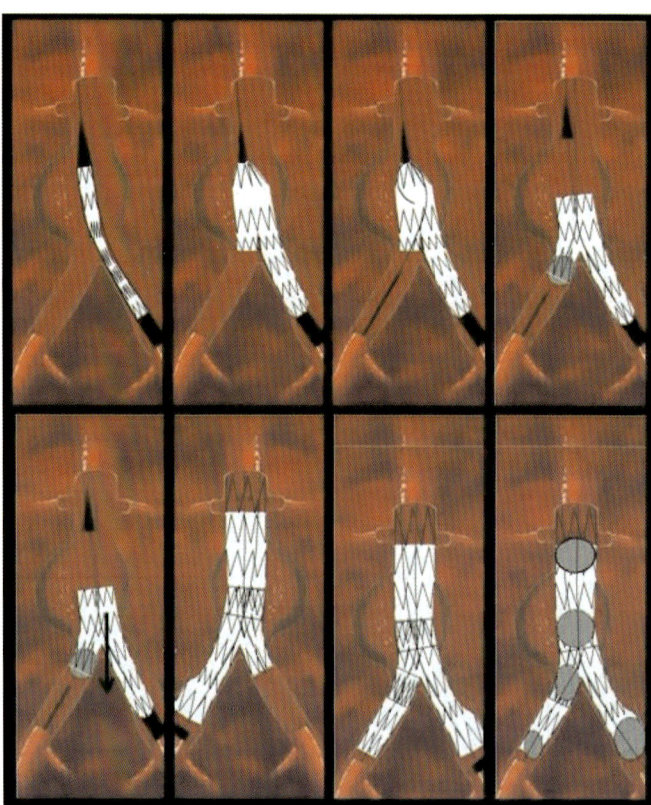

FIGURE 4: Implantation technique, step by step.

plex. Even so though, migration events appear to emerge in a lower rate with the Composite graft.[18]

Given our experience and the endograft's specific characteristics the Composite graft currently provides the best available concept for anatomically demanding cases of EVAR. It could be used as an alternative in the armamentarium of grafts, to ensure a high security index for difficult anatomies. The 8 mm gaps of Composite endografts are the key feature for angled necks (>60°), while the accommodation on the aortic bifurcation is the key feature for distal fixation when proximal stability is within borderlines as it is in short (10-15 mm), and conical necks. (Figure 5) In conical necks in particular, endograft oversizing on the largest diameter of the neck leads to excessive stretching of its narrower part, thus risking endograft wrinkling and type I endoleak. The use of the Composite config-

uration, in such cases, allows reduced oversizing, since fixation is already enhanced by resting on the aortic bifurcation. (Figure 6)

The specific contraindications of the Composite endograft implantation are governed by the concept of distal fixation. These include narrow distal aorta (<22 mm) and extreme angulation (>80°) of the common iliac arteries. Narrow bilateral common iliac arteries are also not favorable for the composite configuration due to an increased risk of limb occlusion and a potential risk of iliac rupture when applying the "pull down" maneuver.

Interestingly, the concept of the graft accommodation onto the aortic bifurcation has been also recently advocated by Raithel[19] using the Powerlink unibody bifurcated stent graft (Endologix, Inc, Irvine, CA). The encouraging results confirm the importance and the promising future of such a fixation concept.

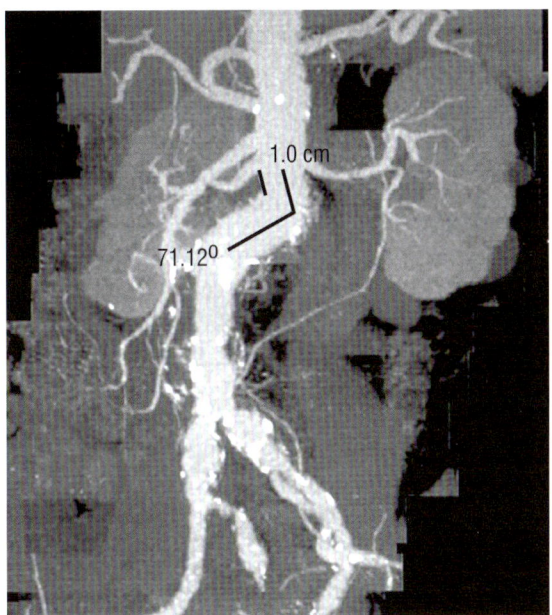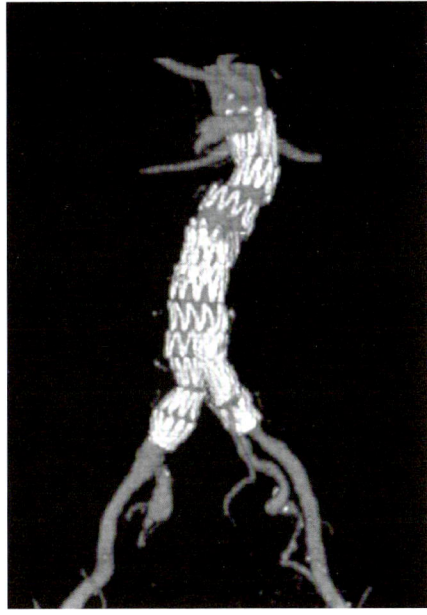

FIGURE 5: Preoperative CTA of an infra-renal AAA with a hostile short and angulated neck. Notice the postoperative result with the Composite Graft accommodated on the aortic bifurcation. The 8 mm gaps of the proximal main body have allowed a smooth accommodation and proximal attachment of the graft.

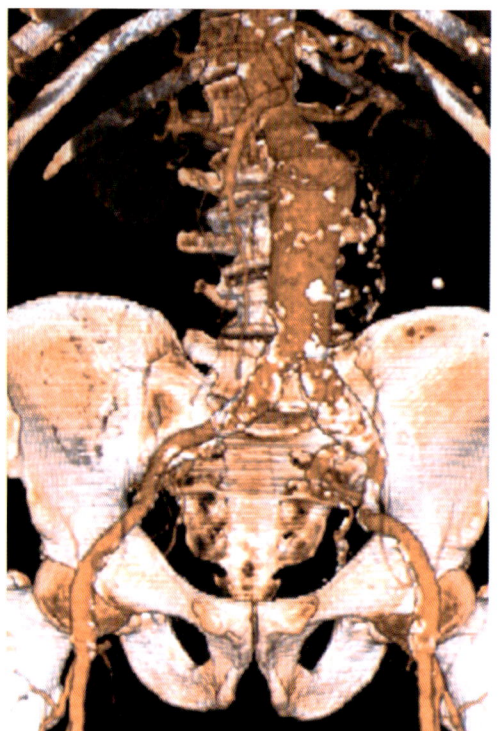
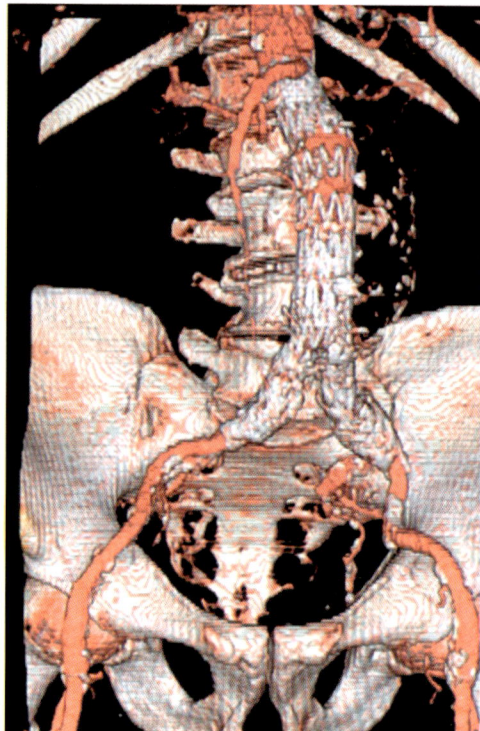

FIGURE 6: Preoperative CTA of an infra-renal AAA with a hostile conical neck. Notice the postoperative result with the Composite Graft accommodated on the aortic bifurcation.

REFERENCES

1. Harris PL, Vallabhaneni SR, Desgranges P, Becquemin JP, van Marrewijk C, Laheij RJ. Incidence and risk factors of late rupture, conversion, and death after endovascular repair of infrarenal aortic aneurysms: the EUROSTAR experience. J Vasc Surg 2000;32(4):739-749.

2. Tonnessen BH, Sternbergh WC, Money SR. Late problems at the proximal aortic neck: migration and dilation. Semin Vasc Surg 2004;17(4):288-293.

3. Greenberg RK, Chuter TA, Sternbergh WC, Fearnot NE, Zenith Investigators. Zenith AAA endovascular graft: intermediate- term results of the US multicenter trial. J Vasc Surg 2004;39(6):1209-1218.

4. Fairman RM, Velazquez OC, Carpenter JP, Woo E, Baum RA, Golden MA, Kritpracha B, Criado F. Midterm pivotal trial results of the Talent Low Profile System for repair of abdominal aortic aneurysm: analysis of complicated versus uncompli-

cated aortic necks. J Vasc Surg 2004;40(6): 1074-1082.

5. Kibbe MR, Matsumura JS, for the Excluder Investigators. The Gore excluder US multi-center trial: analysis of adverse events at 2 years. Semin Vasc Surg 2003;16(2):144-150.

6. Schmittling ZC, McLafferty RB, Danetz JS, Ramsey DE, Hodgson KJ. The AneuRx modular endograft device for the treatment of abdominal aortic aneurysms. Overview of 7 years of clinical use. J Cardiovasc Surg (Torino) 2004;45(4):301-306.

7. Cao P, Verzini F, Zannetti S, De Rango P, ParlaniG, Lupattelli L, Maseli A. Device migration after endoluminal abdominal aortic aneurysm repair: analysis of 113 cases with a minimum follow-up period of 2 years. J Vasc Surg 2002;35(2):229-235.

8. Zarins CK, Bloch DA, Crabtree T, Matsumoto AH, White RA, Fogarty TJ. Stent graft migration after endovascular aneurysm repair: importance of proximal fixation. J Vasc Surg 2003;38(6):1264-1272.

9. Mohan IV, Harris PL, van Marrewijk CJ, Laheij RJ, How TV. How factors and forces influencing stent-graft migration after endovascular aortic aneurysm repair. J Endovasc Ther 2002;9(6):748-755.

10. van Marrewijk CJ, Leurs, LJ, Vallabhaneni SR, Harris PL, Buth J, Laheij RJ; Eurostar Collaborators. Risk-Adjusted Outcome Analysis of endovascular Abdominal Aortic Aneurysm Repair in a Large Population: How Do Stent-Grafts Compare? J Endovasc Ther 2005;12(4):417-429.

11. Buth J, Laheij RJ. Early complications and endoleaks after endovascular abdominal aortic aneurysm repair: report of a multicenter study. J Vasc Surg. 2000;31(1 pt 1):134-147.

12. Laheij RJ, van Marrewijk CJ, for the EUROSTAR group. The evolving technique of endovascular stenting of abdominal aortic aneurysm: time for reappraisal. Eur J Vasc Endovasc Surg 2001; 22(5):436-442.

13. Ouriel K, Clair DG, Greenberg RK, Lyden SP, O'Hara PJ, Sarac TP, Srivastava SD, Butler B, Sampram ES. Endovascular repair of abdominal aortic aneurysms: device-specific outcome. J Vasc Surg 2003;37(5):991-8.

14. Brewster DC, Jones JE, Chung TK, Lamuraglia GM, Kwolek CJ, Watkins MT, Hodgman TM, Cambria RP. Long-term outcomes after endovascular abdominal aortic aneurysm repair. The first decade. Ann Vasc Surg 2006;244(3):426-438.

15. Heikkinen MA, Alsac JM, Arko FR, et al. The importance of iliac fixation in prevention of stent graft migration. J Vasc Surg 2006;43(6):1130-7.

16. Stelter WJ. Use of Aortic Bifurcation for Better Graft Stability: A New Generation Concept. [abstract] XV International Congress on Endovascular Interventions, Phoenix, Arizona, USA, Feb 2002, Abstract IV-2.

17. Stelter WJ. New concepts for graft stability in EVAR. Suprarenal and/or bifurcation fixation. [abstract] Veith Symposium, New York, USA, Nov 2002, Abstract V4.1.

18. Theodossios P Perdikides, Efthimios D. Avgerinos, Konstantinos Lagios, Peter Ziegler, Wolf J. Stelter. Improving Endograft Stability by Accommodation onto the Aortic Bifurcation. J Endovasc Ther 2007;14:634-8.

19. QU L, Hetzel G, Raithel D. Seven years' single center experience of Powerlink unibody bifurcated endograft for endovascular aortic aneurysm. J Cardiovasc Surg 2007;48:13-9.

Multibranched endografts for complex anatomy

Timothy A.M. Chuter, David E. Hartley

THE TWIN GOALS OF COMPLEX ENDOVASCULAR RECONSTRUCTION: ANEYRYSM EXCLUSION AND BRANCH PERFUSION

Most aortic stent-grafts exclude flow to some intercostal and lumbar arteries without diret consequences. These segmental arteries are usually well collateralized and dispensable, as is the inferior mesenteric artery. Indispensable arteries that take origin within the field of endovascular exclusion have to be supplied with blood, either through a branch of the stent-graft, or through a conventional surgical bypass. Problem areas include the great vessels of the aortic arch, the visceral branches of the the thoracoabdominal aorta, the common iliac branches of the aorta, and the internal and external iliac branches of the common iliac artery.

EXPERIENCE WITH EARLY BIFURCATED STENT-GRAFT DESIGNS

Bifurcated stent-grafts have become so commonplace it is easy to forget that the aortic bifurcation is a prime example of aneurysm encroachment on the origin of a vital aortic branch, the common iliac artery. In the absence of a distal aortic implantation site, the alternatives for endovascular repair are the implantation of a bifurcated stent-graft, or the implantation of a uni-iliac stent-graft in combination with femoro-femoral bypass.

Branched stent-grafts fall into two groups, unibody and modular. Unibody stent-grafts are inserted whole, while modular stent-grafts are assembled in-situ for two, or more, components. Commercial unibody bifurcated designs at one time included the Ancure, Trivascular, and Endologix stent-grafts, of which only the Endologix is still available. The fate of the other two stent-grafts is an example of evolution in action. The unibody approach limits the range of readily available combinations of length and diameter, and introduces unique failure modes related to the mechanisms of contralateral limbs deployment. Modular bifurcated stent-grafts have proven to be simpler, safer, and more versatile. Their one disadvantage, the potential for component separation,[1] has been largely eliminated through changes in stent-graft design and implantation technique that increased the length of the inter-component overlap zone. The lessons of the bifurcated stent-graft experience also apply to other branched stent-grafts. The addition of each branch, produces an exponential increase in the complexity of a unibody stent-graft. The problems that plagued unibody bifurcated designs render multi-branched versions all but undeliverable. If an overlap zone is important for the stability of a bifurcated modular stent-graft, it is even more important for the stability of a multi-branched modular stent-graft, where every additional component represents an additional opportunity for component separation.

THERAPEUTIC OPTIONS FOR ANEURYSMS WITH INDISPENSIBLE BRANCHES

Bifurcated stent-graft insertion benefits from easy access to downstream arteries in the groin. None of the vital branches of the thoracoabdominal aorta run through such accessible locations. The celiac, superior mesenteric and renal arteries originate high in the retroperitoneum and their branches never exit the abdominal cavity. The combination of visceral bypass and endovascular exclusion is a formidable operation. Compared to conventional direct repair, the combined procedure may reduce aortic exposure, visceral ischemia, and hemodynamic instability, but the operation is hardly minimally invasive.[2,3] The lack of downstream access is also a problem for multi-branched stent-grafts of unibody design, because catheters cannot be used to pull the pre-attached branches of the stent-graft into the branches of the aorta. Instead, the branches have to be pushed into position, which is far more difficult and far less reliable. Although the first stent-graft with any kind of visceral branch was of a unibody design,[4] the irreducible complexity of this approach has limited application to a handful of cases, using single and double branch devices.[5] The only vi-

able multi-branched stent-grafts for pararenal and thoracoabdominal aortic aneurysms employ a the modular approach, which allows an otherwise complicated procedure to be broken up into bite-sized pieces.

The multi-branched approach also offer a mean of internal iliac artery preservation offers in cases of bilateral common iliac aneurysm. Cross pelvic collaterals generally provide adequate flow so long as one of the two internal iliac arteries remains patent, but collaterals from the deep femoral and mesenteric arteries are not such a reliable source of pelvic flow and there is some debate as to the safety of bilateral internal iliac artery occlusion. Like the branches of the thoracoabdominal aorta, the internal iliac artery is far from readily accessible. Surgical bypass to the internal iliac artery is one option,[6] but the necessary exposure can be difficult to obtain in the presence of obesity, prior surgery or irradiation.

Implantation of a mult-branched stent-graft is one possible way to treat an aneurysm of the arch, but it may not be the safest way. The arch of the aorta is wide and its branches feed an organ, the brain, with no tolerance for ischemia. Besides, one cannot long interrupt the rapid flow of blood, or stop the constant movement produced by the beating heart. Any air or dislodged fragments of atheroma or thrombus can find their way to the cerebral circulation and cause stroke. In the presence of these factors, that the safest endovascular intervention will be the quickest and the simplest. Fortunately, this is an achievable goal, because the great vessels are readily accessible in the neck for the creation of surgical bypass grafts, which supply all the branches from a single source, the innominate artery.[7] The arch then becomes a bifurcation, susceptible to endovascular repair using a bifurcated stent-graft.[8] As such, this technique falls outside the scope of the current chapter on "multi-branched endoprostheses". However, the underlying development work[9] does serve as a good illustration of how the accessibility of vital branches can alter the risk-benefit analysis between multi-branched and combined surgical/endovascular approaches to the repair of an aneurysm.

FENESTRATED VERSUS CUFFED MULTI-BRANCHED STENT-GRAFTS

At this point, all the widely used branched stent-grafts are derived from a single design, the Zenith (Cook, Inc., Bloomington, IN). The reasons are many: the Zenith delivery system allows partial deployment for trans-graft catheterization and precise placement, the Zenith stent-graft is stable in shape, structure and position, Cook (through subsidiaries outside the United States) has supported development efforts, and most of the innovators in this field have extensive experience with the original Zenith stent-graft. These Zenith-based modular multi-branched stent-grafts fall into two groups, based on the type of connection between the primary aortic stent-graft and the covered stents, which form its branches. A fenestration is just a wire-reinforced hole in the wall of the primary stent-graft. The only contact between the covered stent, that forms the branch, and a fenestrated stent-graft occurs at the margin of this hole. In contrast, the cuffed approach provides an inter-component overlap zone within short, longitudinally-oriented branches (cuffs) sewn into the wall of the primary stent-graft.

Whether the primary stent-graft is cuffed or fenestrated, the basic implantation technique is the same. Catheters are introduced through the end of the primary stent-graft, out through the cuffs or fenestrations, across the perigraft space and into the target arteries. These catheters are then exchanged over stiff guidewires for covered stent delivery systems. Finally,

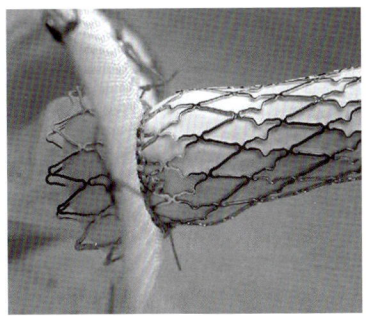

FIGURE 1: The slightly overdilated covered stent flares both inside and outside the Nitinol reinforced fenestration in the wall of the primary aortic stent-graft.

the covered stents are deployed with their proximal ends in the primary stent-graft and their distal ends in the target arteries.

Differences between the cuffed and fenestrated approaches to the construction of a multi-branched stent-graft

Fenestrated stent-grafts rely upon overdilation of a balloon-expanded covered stent just inside and just outside the margin of the fenestration to secure the inter-component connection and improve the seal (Figure 1). Cuffed stent-grafts rely upon the overlap zone for contact between the inner surface of the cuff and the outer surface of the covered stent (Figure 2). Since the cuffs tend to be inelastic, and balloon-expanded covered stents recoil with balloon deflation, more intimate inter-component contact is achieved using slightly oversized self-expanding stents.

In fenestrated designs, the covered stents generally lie at right angles to the longitudinal axis of the primary stent-graft. In cuffed designs, the covered stents curve through the aneurysm from longitudinally-oriented cuffs proximally to the orifices of target arteries distally. The curved path from a cuffed primary stent-graft to a target artery is longer, more variable and

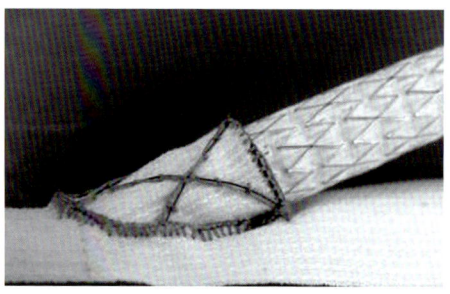

FIGURE 2: The self-expanding covered stent has 18 mm of contact with the inner surface of the simple "inside/outside" cuff sutured into the wall of the primary aortic stent-graft.

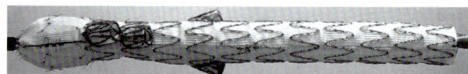

FIGURE 4: The proximal tapering of this cuffed stent-graft is apparent, even with the constraining ties in place.

less acutely angled than the trans-axial path of the fenestrated approach.

Since most cuffs are caudally-oriented, their covered stents can only be inserted through a brachial approach, following full deployment of the primary stent-graft. Although fenestrations have no direction, their balloon expanded covered stents are usually inserted from a femoral approach through the partially-deployed primary stent. This state of partial deployment (Figure 3) limits stent-graft diameter and provides the necessary perigraft space for catheter manipulations. In the case of cuffed stent-grafts, the perigraft space is provided by limiting the diameter of the central, cuff-bearing, segment (Figure 4).

The effects of differences between fenestrated and cuffed stent-grafts on planning and implantation

The curved path from an axially-oriented cuff can accommodate variations in the

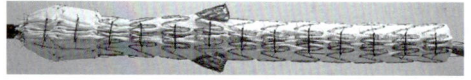

FIGURE 3: Diameter reducing ties contract the back of the stent-graft around a removable control wire.

relative positions of the cuff and target artery, which reduces the likelihood of failure and allows standardization of stent-graft design and implantation, despite variable arterial anatomy.

The differences between fenestrated and cuffed stent-grafts also affect long-term stability. The overlap zone of the cuffed approach helps prevent leakage and component separation. Furthermore, the self-expanding stents of the cuffed approach should be are more robust than the balloon-expanded stents of the fenestrated approach, which can deform, and stay deformed, with movement every time they move (with respiration or pulsation). Finally, the axially oriented branches of the cuffed approach serve as props, which protect the stent-graft from caudally-oriented displacment force. On the other hand, the tapered shape of the cuffed stent-graft probably generates more displacement force than the more cylindrical shape of the fenestrated stent-graft.

MODULAR BRANCHED STENT-GRAFTS FOR PARARENAL AND THORACOABDOMINAL AORTIC ANEURYSMS

The first stent-graft with branches to the celiac, superior mesenteric and renal arteries was implanted for contained rupture of a thoracoabdominal aortic aneurysm.[10] The homemade device used in this case had all the features of the current cuffed stent-graft: axially-oriented cuffs, a barbed stent for proximal attachment, and a tapered shape. The first fenestrated stent-grafts emerged at roughly the same time.[11] They were used to treat cases of juxtarenal aortic aneurysm. Trans-graft insertion of bridging catheters and flared bridging stents helped ensure accurate alignment of the fenestrations and renal arteries. The substitution of balloon-expanded covered stents for balloon-expanded uncovered stents was a minor technical modification, but the practical consequences were huge.[12] While the uncovered stent could only help maintain a seal between the stent-graft around the margin of the fenestration and the aorta around the orifice of the renal artery, the covered stent could carry blood across a gap between the two, extending the indications to include pararenal and thoracoabdominal aortic aneurysms (TAAA). The commercial availability of fenestrated stent-grafts outside the United States has led to the rapid adoption of this technique.[13] However, the largest experience worldwide has been at the Cleveland Clinic where fenestrated stent-grafts were implanted under a single-center investigational device exemption.[14]

Fenestrated multi-branched stent-grafts

Commercially available fenestrated stent-grafts employ a "composite" approach whereby one aortic stent-graft has all the fenestrations and another the bifurcation. This allows the operator to focus on one task at a time, while varying the overlap between components to achieve optimal position both proximally and distally. A secondary effect is to free the fenestrated component from caudally-directed hemodynamic forces, which act mainly on the bifurcation.[15]

The main body of the fenestrated stent-graft is oversized by at least 10% relative to the outer diameter of the implantation site. However precisely the findings of preopertive imaging delineate aortic anatomy, the ultimate postitions of the fenestrations can only approximate the sizes and positions of the target arteries (usually the renals) because fenestrations are confined to the spaces between stent struts.

The delivery system resembles that of the Zenith stent-graft with the addition of constraining ties, which maintain a state of partial deployment to allow some degree of positional adjustment during bridging catheter insertion. Stent-graft deployment involves the removal of three trigger wires. The first releases the constraining ties, the second releases the uncovered proximal stent from the top cap, and the third releases the distal stent from the central shaft of the delivery system. The caliber of the Flexor sheath varies from 18-24 French, depending on the diameter of the stent-graft, which may be as large as 46 mm.

In most cases, the bridging catheters, bridging sheaths and covered stents are delivered through the contralateral femoral artery. Some surgeons insert them all through multiple punctures of a single large sheath, others prefer multiple separate punctures of the femoral artery. In either case, one should insert the sheath into the stent-graft before trying to guide a catheter through a fenestration into the target artery. It can be difficult to advance make a sheath or covered stent delivery system when there is a long path to traverse the long path through the perigraft space of a large aneurysm, especially when caudal angulation of when the target artery induces additional tortuosity tortuosityanother bend by running in a caudal direction. The change indirection from an axial stent-graft to a trans-axial covered stent also complicates the creation of the necessary flange on either side of the fenestration. Even a short angioplasty balloon tends to align itself with the primary stent-graft, despite attempts to push it into a horizontal flatter position. As soon as the balloons, catheters and wires are removed, the branch stent inevitably descends, changing the geometry of the inter-component connection. The possible resulting leakage can be difficult to eliminate.

Cuffed stent-grafts

Cuffed and fenestrated stent-grafts are constructed from the same materials, and employ the same multi-component (composite) approach. In addition, they both undergo staged deployment, using the same delivery system with the same control mechanisms. But there the similarities end (see "modular multibranched stent-grafts").

Cuffs can be short or long, internal or external, outside the stent-graft or inside, curved or straight, and oriented caudally or cranially. All these alternatives have been tried alone, or in combination with fenestrations, and each has particular advantages and disadvantages, depending on arterial anatomy. However, the simplest, most versatile and most predictable cuff appears to be a short stent-supported cylinder sutured into the wall of the primary stent-graft with one end on the inside and one end on the outside (Figures 2 and 4), the "inside/outside cuff". Cuff orientation is usually chosen to match the orientation of the corresponding target artery. Since most visceral arteries run in a caudal direction (down-going), most cuffs do likewise. These cuffs are only accessible from above through brachial artery access. Up-going cuffs, for patients with up-going renal arteries, are accessible from a femoral approach, while the stent-graft remains in a partially expanded state. Covered stent delivey through the partially-expanded stent-graft can be an advantage when the pararenal aorta is non-dilated, but a combination of up-going and down-going cuffs does complicate stent-graft design and delivery (see below). Moreover, the presence of up-going cuffs may

disrupt flow patterns within the narrow central segment of the stent-graft. Our preferred approach involves 4 inside/outside cuffs, all down-going (Figures 4 and 5). The cuffs for the celiac and superior mesenteric arteries measure 8x18 mm and the cuffs for the renal arteries measure 6x18 mm.

Each stent-graft is custom made, based on pre-operative peroperative imaging of arterial anatomy. The arrangement of cuffs on the narrow central segment of the primary stent-graft attempts to replicate the distribution of branch arteries. However, cuff position is not critical, as so long as the outer end of a down-going cuff is located a short distance (10-20 mm) comes to lie above (cranial to) the corresponding arterial orifice. When all the cuffs are down-going, this goal can be assured by moving the cuffs up the stent-graft, or moving the stent-graft up the aorta. When some of the cuffs are up-going, gross changes in stent-graft position are limited by the width of the gap between up-going and down-going orifices. If the gap is narrow and the stent-graft is

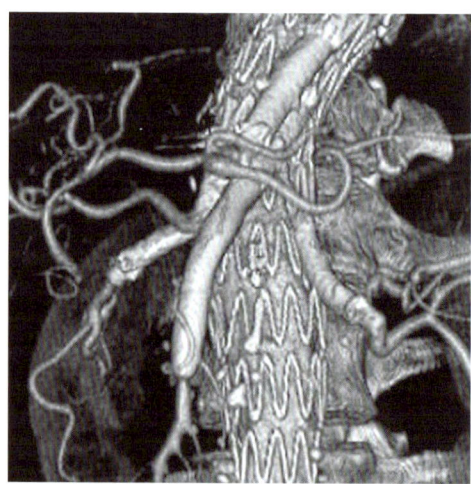

FIGURE 5: Postoperative CT views (the same stent graft as figure 4), showing 4 down-going branches, extending from 4 down-going cuffs.

implanted too far upstream, the up-going cuffs will come to lie upstream from their renal targets, which will then be impossible to catheterize. Variations in the gap between cuff and target artery are accommodated by variations in the length of the covered stents, or the combined lengths of overlapping covered stents, which form the branches of the stent-graft.

The implantation of the usual 4-branch stent-graft has two distinct stages. The Zenith-based aortic, and aorto-iliac, stent-grafts are inserted through the femoral or iliac arteries,. The and then the self-expanding covered stents (Fluency, Bard Inc., Murray Hill, NJ) are inserted through a brachial artery, usually the left.

The use of a conduit to the common iliac artery depends on the relative sizes of the external iliac artery and stent-graft delivery system. In most cases, the delivery system is small enough, and the external iliac artery large enough, for trans-femoral insertion. This determination is best made through CT-based assessments of arterial anatomy during the planning and sizing phase, rather than through trial and error at the time of operation. The creation of a conduit, or external iliac artery bypass, provides an opportunity for surgical re-routing of flow to an iliac artery, in cases of common iliac aneurysm. We work hard to preserve both internal arteries in cases of TAAA, because pelvic collaterals to the anterior spinal artery may help prevent paraplegia.

Spinal catheters are inserted for CSF pressuring monitoring and drainage. The spinal catheter also provides a route for spinal anesthesia during the trans-femoral portion of the operation. Broad spectrum antibiotics are administered 4-hourly throughout the operation. Heparin is given at even shorter intervals to maintain activated clotting time (ACT) above 300 seconds. The aortic stent-grafts are placed by reference to angiographically located visceral aortic branches. Whenever possible, selective catheterization is substituted for flush aortagram to conserve contrast. Once the aortic and aorto-iliac stent-grafts are in place, all the catheters and sheaths are removed, the femoral arteries repaired, and unimpeded flow to the lower extremities restored. The groin wounds are packed with antibiotic sponges and dressed. They are not closed until the end of the whole operation when clotting function is restored using protoamine. Otherwise, slow oozing throughout the second half of the operation accumulates in the groins forming hematomas.

The trans-brachial portion is performed under local anesthesia. The path from the brachial artery to the primary stent-graft is long and tortuous. The combined effects of multiple, co-axial, wire wrapped sheaths (Flexor, Cook, Inc., Bloomington, IN) help minimize loop formation and kinking at the junction between the subclavian, or innominate, artery and the aorta. A short (40 cm) 12 French sheath also isolates the aortic arch from multiple on going catheter manipulations, that might otherwise dislodge fragments of clot or atheroma, causing embolic stroke. A long (70-80 cm) 10 French sheath smooths the path through the primary stent-graft, and provides a route for contrast injection around the 9 French delivery system of the Fluency covered stent.

Covered stents are inserted one-by-one from each cuff on the primary stent-graft to each target artery, starting with the most distal renal and ending with the celiac. For any given covered stent, the combined length of the proximal and distal overlaps varies inversely with the distance between the corresponding cuff and arterial orifice. The wider the gap the shorter the overlap. However, we We generally use 60mm long bridging stents and apply a lower limit of 15 mm for the length of overlap at both the proximal and distal ends of the covered stent. When the gap is greater than 30 mm, multiple overlapping covered stents are sometimes needed. However, under these circumstances, we prefer to use a single longer (80 mm-long) covered stent. The additional bulk of two or more overlapping covered stents can compromize the lumen, causing graft occlusion. Besides, the additional connection adds a potentially site for component separation and/or type 3 endoleak.

In most cases the celiac and superior mesenteric branches are formed using 9x60 mm Fluency covered stents, while the renal branches are formed using 7 x 60 mm Fluency covered stents. All branches are lined with additional stents to increase stiffness, provide attitional pull-out resistance, and prevent kinking. We have found that Wallstents (Boston Scientific, Natick, MA) are well suited this purpose, but we have occasionally used others, such as the Zilver (Cook, Inc., Bloomington, IN). Balloon expanded covered stents could also be used at the ends of the bridging covered stent. These "lining" stents are oversized, both in length and diameter, so that they protrude from both ends of the covered stent. At the proximal end, the inner stent (Wallstent) creates a funnel shaped bulge, that is difficult to pull out through the cuff. At the distal end, the inner stent is in direct contact with 5-10 mm of the arterial lumen. We assume that this exposed portion of the stent will become incorporated into the wall of the artery, as it does in occlusive disease applications, thereby anchoring the downstream end of the covered stent. The short segment of bare stent also keeps the wall of a tortuous target artery away from the end of covered stent, thereby preventing occlusion. Our sole case of total branch occlusion occurred when the distal end of the covered stent abutted the bifurcation of a tortuous renal artery and there was no space for protruding Wallstent.

Covered stent delivery systems sometimes track poorly along the tortuous path from the brachial artery to the visceral artery. Long kink-resistent sheaths and stiff guidwires help, but stenosis, angulation, or early branching of the target artery and tortuosity of the thoracic aorta all impede the control of these over-the-wire systems. Additional preliminary maneuvers include balloon dilatation, stent-placement, and zig-zag wire techniques. The chief risk is small scale renal arterial injury in the setting of prolonged anticoagulation. This complication was resposibe for the only case of renal failure, paraplegia and death in our series of cuffed TAAA repairs. We have adopted various preventative measures, such as the substitution a round-tipped Rosen guidewire for the hydrophilic guidewire that we previously used during covered stent insertion, which seem to have eliminated this problem. However, were it to happen again, we would coil embolize the injured artery, terminate the procedure, and restore normal coagulation, with the intention of returning another day.

BRANCHED STENT-GRAFS FOR BILATERAL ILIAC ANEURYSMS

The aorto-iliac multi-branched stent-grafts used in cases of bilateral iliac aneurysm arborize by serial bifurcation, (like an oak tree), unlike the thoracoabdominal multi-branched stent-grafts, which arborize by serial radiation (like a pine tree). As a result, the components of the aorto-iliac stent-graft are relatively simple; each stent-graft has only one bifurcation. The aortic part of the repair is performed using standard Zenith stent-grafts and delivery systems. The technique becomes multi-branched with the substitution of a bifurcated iliac stent-graft for the standard unbifurcated iliac stent-graft (limb). The short axially oriented cuff of the bifurcated iliac component provides a proximal implantation site for a covered stent to the internal iliac artery. Whether this cuff is short and straight, or long and curved, the insertion procedure and net result are the same.[16]

The order of (Zenith-based) stent-graft insertion depends on the route of covered stent insertion. If the aneurysm is long enough, it is usually best to insert the covered stent from the contralateral femoral access point, using a cross-femoral wire to hold the cross-femoral sheath in place. But this is no longer feasible once the bifurcated aortic stent-graft (main body, TFB) has been inserted. In this technique, the bifurcated iliac stent-graft is placed first, followed by the covered stent, then the bifurcated aortic stent-graft, and finally a bridging stent-graft between the cuff of the bifurcated aortic stent-graft and the trunk of the bifurcated iliac stent-graft.

If the aneurysm is short, the cross-femoral route is difficult to navigate, or bilateral bifurcated iliac reconstruction is planned, the covered stent can be inserted from the arm. Under these circumstances, the procedure follows the normal proximal to distal sequence of stent-graft insertion, and the covered stents are the last components to be deployed. Long sheaths (>100 cm) and covered stent delivery systems (>110 cm) are required. The covered stents can be introduced from above using more readily available 90cm long sheaths through an axillary/subclavian access site

The goal in positioning the bifurcated iliac stent-graft is to place the distal orifice of the cuff just above the orifice of the internal iliac artery. The manufactured version of the bifurcated iliac stent-graft comes packaged with an indwelling catheter and wire traversing the cuff, from outside (distal) to inside (proximal). This catheter and wire are snared for femoro-femoral or brachio-femoral guidewire control, which aids in the passage of a sheath all the way to the orifice of the internal iliac artery. Although the common iliac bifurcation is one of the least mobile parts of the arterial tree, there have been reports of balloon-expanded covered stents kinking or collapsing. We generally prefer Fluency self-expanding covered stents, lined with Wallstents. The distal end of the covered stent is placed in a non-dilated segment of the internal iliac artery, preferrably the trunk. When the cross-femoral route is used to insert the covered stent, and the bifurcated iliac stent-graft is inserted before the bifurcated aortic stent-graft, the degree of overlap between the covered stent and the trunk of the bifurcated iliac stent-graft becomes an issue. Any more than 10-15 mm of overlap encroaches on the distal implantation site for the bridging stent-graft, because the bridging stent-graft and covered stent end up competing for space within the trunk of the bifurcated iliac stent-graft.

The bifurcated reconstruction of a common iliac aneurysm provides an opportunity to practice gain experience in the techniques of multi-branched repair, before attempting multi-branched thoracoabdominal aortic stent-graft implantation, where the consequences of failure may be dire. Internal iliac artery preservation is desirable, but not as important as superior mesenteric artery preservation, for example. If bifurcated common iliac artery reconstruction fails, one can always implant a stent-graft limb across the orice of the cuff, thereby excluding the aneurysm from direct perfusion (endoleak, types II and III). Embolization of the internal iliac artery may also be feasible, in which case the aneurysm will also be excluded from indirect perfusion (endoleak, type II). The most likely result will be self-limited buttock claudication. Colon necrosis, lumbosacral plexopathy, and spinal ischemia are less likely.

CONCLUDIONS AND PREDICTIONS

Multi-branched stent-grafts are starting to extend the scope of endovascular aneurysm repair to include the aortic arch, thoracoabdominal aorta and common iliac artery bifurcation. Early results have already shown short-term safety and effectiveness in selected high-risk patients. More widespread application will depend on the long-term durability of the stent-grafts, expanded access to the necessary technology (regulatory approval), and dissemination of the necessary skills. Some components of contemporary multi-branched stent-grafts have a long track record of use in similar applications. They can be expected to withstand the rigors of the endovascular environment. Others, such as the various covered stents, were not designed to be used in combination with cuffed and fenestrated stent-grafts, nor were they designed to be used inside aneurysmal arteries. Their long-term fate is more uncertain performance is less predictable.

Most of the techniques involved in the placement of a modular multi-branched stent-graft, visceral catheterization for example, are part of standard interventional practice. Experienced vascular surgeons, cardiologists, and interventional radiologists should be able to adapt their skill sets to the demands of this new category of procedures, thereby shortening the learning phase.

Although multi-branched endovascular repair will become quicker and easier as the technology develops, these operations will always be longer and more complex than conventional unbranched stent-graft implantation. Yet they offer the only minimally invasive alternatives to the maximally invasive operations that would otherwise be required to treat aneurysms involving branched segments of the aorta. These operations are painful, expensive, debilitating, and potentially fatal.[17,18] The persistently high mortality and morbidity rates of conventional surgery will probaly continue to spur developments in the field of multi-branched endovascular aneurysm repair for years to come.

REFERENCES

1. Beebe HG, Cronenwett JL, Katzen BT, et al. Results of an aortic endograft trial: Impact of device failure beyond 12 months. J Vasc Surg 2001; 33: S55-63.
2. Black SA, Wolfe JHN, Clark M, Harmady M, Cheshire NJW, Jenkins MP. Complex thoracoabdominal aortic aneurysms: Endovascular exclusion with visceral revascularization. J Vasc Surg 2006;43:1081-9.
3. Zhou W, Reardon M, Peden EK, Lin PH, Lumsden AB. Hybrid approach to complex thoracic aortic aneurysms in high-risk patients: Surgical challenges and clinical outcomes. J Vasc Surg. 2006;44:688-93.
4. Inoue K, Iwase T, Sato M, Yoshida Y, Ueno K, Tamaki S, et al. Transluminal endovascular branched graft placement for a pseudoaneurysm: reconstruction of the descending thoracic aorta including the celiac axis. J Thorac Cardiovasc Surg 1997; 114-61.
5. Saito N, Kimura T, Toma M, Watanabe S, Imai M, Hamaguchi Y, Kita T, Inoue K. Endovascular repair of a thoracoabdominal aortic aneurysm involving the celiac artery and the superior mesenteric artery. Ann Vasc Surg 2006. e-pub ahead of print.
6. Parodi JC, Ferreira M. Relocation of the iliac artery bifurcation to facilitate endoluminal treatment of abdominal aortic aneurysms. J Endovasc Surg. 1999;6:342-7.
7. Criado FJ, Barnatan MF, Rizk Y, Clark NS, Wang CF. Technical strategies to expand stent-graft applicability in the aortic arch and proximal descending thoracic aorta. J Endovasc Ther 2002; 9:II32-8.
8. Schneider DB, Curry TK, Reilly LM, Kang JW, Messina LM, Chuter TA. Branched endovascular repair of aortic arch aneurysm with a modular stent-graft system. J Vasc Surg. 2003;38:855.
9. Chuter TA, Schneider DB, Reilly LM, Lobo EP, Messina LM. Modular branched stent graft for endovascular repair of aortic arch aneurysm and dissection. J Vasc Surg. 2003;38:859-63.
10. Chuter TA, Gordon L, Reilly LM, Pak LK, Messina LM. Multi-branched stent-graft for type III thoracoabdominal aortic aneurysm. J Vasc Interv Radiol 2001;12:391-2.

11. Stanley BM, Semmens JB, Lawrence-Brown MM, Goodman MA, Hartley DE. Fenestration in endovascular grafts for aortic aneurysm repair: new horizons for preserving blood flow in branch vessels. J Endovasc Ther 2001: 8:16-24.

12. Anderson JL, Adam DJ, Berce M, Hartley DE. Repair of thoracoabdominal aortic aneurysms with fenestrated and branched endovascular stent-grafts. J Vasc Surg 2005;42:600-7.

13. Muhs BE, Verhoeven EL, Zeebregts CJ, Tielliu IF, Prins TR, Verhagen HJ, van den Dungen JJ. Midterm results of endovascular aneurysm repair with branched and fenestrated endografts. J Vasc Surg. 2006;44:9-15.

14. Greenberg RK, West K, Pfaff K, Foster J, Skender D, Haulon S, et al. Beyond the aortic bifurcation: Branched endovascular grafts for thoracoabdominal and aortoiliac aneurysms. J Vasc Surg 2006; 43:879-86.

15. Liffman K, Lawrence-Brown MMD, Semmens JB, Bui A, Rudman M, Hartley DE. Analytical Modeling and Numerical Simulation of Forces in an Endoluminal Graft. J Endovasc Ther 2001; 8: 358-371.

16. Abraham CZ, Reilly LM, Schneider DB, Dwyer S, Sawhney R, Messina LM, Chuter TA. A modular multi-branched system for endovascular repair of bilateral common iliac artery aneurysms. J Vasc Endovasc Ther 2003;10:203-7.

17. Rigberg DA, McGory ML, Zingmond DS, Maggard MA, Agustin M, Lawrence PE, Ko CY. Thirty day mortality statistics underestimate the risk of repair of thoracoabdominal aortic aneurysms: A statewide experience. J Vasc Surg 2006;43:217-23.

18. Cowan JA Jr, Dimick JB, Henke PK, Huber TS, Stanley JC, Upchurch GR Jr. Surgical treatment of intact thoracoabdominal aortic aneurysms in the United States: hospital and surgeon volume-related outcomes. J Vasc Surg 2003;37:1169-74.

Endovascular treatment of aortoiliac aneurysms using side branched iliac endografts

Peter Ziegler, Efthimios Avgerinos, Theodossios P. Perdikides, Thomas Umscheid, Wolf Stelter

Currently, an increase in the number of patients presenting with both aortic aneurysms and enlarged iliac arteries is encountered frequently. Combined aortic and common iliac artery aneurysms (CI-AA), encountered in 20-30% of cases,[1-2] pose a barrier for a solitary EVAR procedure. Though small CIAA (18-24 mm) might often be treated by the "bell bottom" technique, our experience proved it to be a questionable concept. In longer follow up, further vessel dilatation and/or distal leak due to retrograde migration usually emerge, necessitating some kind of secondary intervention. According to our experience, when iliac diameter exceeds 24 mm safe endograft landing proximal to the internal iliac artery (IIA) is impossible.

The endovascular challenge is even higher when bilateral CIAA are involved and the concerns of severe pelvic ischemia are profound.[3,4] Traditionally, extension of the endograft's iliac leg to the external iliac artery has been used, excluding the hypogastric artery, occasionally accompanied by coil embolization.[5] Measures to preserve internal iliac flow such as

aortouniliiliac endografts, external to internal iliac endografts and IIA revascularization techniques (transposition or bypass to the external iliac or femoral artery) followed by femoro-femoral bypass have been adopted.[5-9]

Clinically, an IIA unilateral occlusion may range from asymptomatic occlusion to the development of buttock claudication and impotence and less frequently of colon and spinal ischemia, all symptoms summing up to 12%-45%.[10-13]

Bilateral occlusion of the hypogastric circulation may be associated with increased risk and severity of ischemic symptoms and associated morbidity and mortalirty.[11-13] Most authors agree that flow in at least one IIA should be maintained and this is of significant importance if bifurcated endografts are used, since these occlude the IMA, which would otherwise have the potential for recruitment of collateral vessels to the pelvic region.

Since branched endograft devices are already used successfully, modular iliac bifurcated devices (IBD) are an appealing alternative to avoid IIA occlusions or complicated surgical procedures.[14-16]

FIRST GENERATION ILIAC BIFURCATION DEVICES

The previously gained experience using composite grafts for aortic aneurysms[17] was the initial benchmark to try its concept for the iliac bifurcation. The caudal segment (distal body) of the composite graft is a bifurcated component with one long limb for the ipsilateral and a short stump for the contralateral iliac artery. This component could be easily and successfully pulled into the aortic bifurcation - common iliac arteries, so we figured we would do the same for the iliac bifurcation.

The first generation unibody IBD was a two branch stent graft consisting of common (12 mm diameter, 45 mm length), external (10 mm diameter, 37 mm length) and internal iliac portions (12 mm distal diameter, 29 mm length). The internal portion was planned to be introduced into the

IIA. A preloaded catheter passed through the external into the common segment from where it curved back into the internal portion like a shepherd-hook catheter. Its metallic rounded tip formed the tip of the constricted internal branch.

SECOND GENERATION ILIAC BIFURCATION DEVICE

The early attempts with the first generation devices had not all been successful, especially for tortuous iliacs. The use of a fixed sidearm was not the ideal solution, and modifications such as the modular bifurcation component brought up the second generation devices.

The new generation IBD is modular. (Figure 1) It consists of a two branch vessel graft featuring the common iliac portion (12 mm diameter, 44 mm length), the

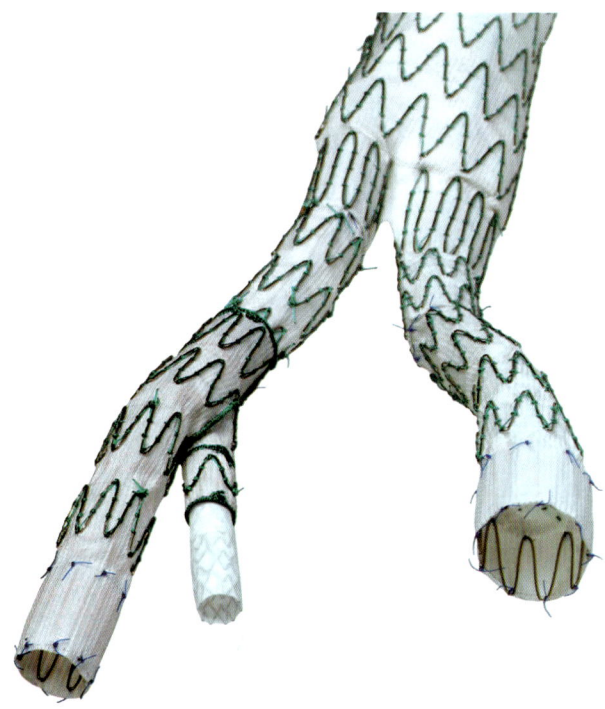

FIGURE 1: Iliac bifurcation device built in a Zenith platform.

external iliac portion (10, 12 or 14 mm diameter, 54 or 71 mm length) and the reinforced stump (8 mm diameter, 12 mm length) for the hypogastric side branch.

Markers are placed on the branch to facilitate fluoroscopic orientation. The graft is preloaded, with proximal and distal fixation, into a 20 F introducer sheath. A preloaded catheter passes through the introducer, enters the branch in a retrograde manner exiting through the proximal end of the common iliac segment. Two release strings on the handle are controlling proximal and distal attachment.

ILIAC BIFURCATION DEVICE IMPLANTATION TECHNIQUE

The first generation unibody iliac bifurcation device's implantation technique belongs in the past and the technique has been described elsewhere.[18]

With the second generation IBD graft it is significantly easier to access the internal ilac artery: the sidebranch is a modular stent-graft, available in different lengths and diameters, therefore easier to adapt to the individual anatomical situation. To introduce the rigid side branch of the first generation IBD into the IIA was much more difficult than to advance a flexible 8 F cross-over sheath with the help of a partially inflated balloon, which subsequently allows to deploy the modular stent graft in the intended position. Introducing the side - branch was even more difficult in the presence of a narrow ostium of the IIA and/or a steep offspring of more than 50° angle. An additional problem with the first generation graft was a narrow lumen of the common iliac artery in case of present thrombus and a kinked external iliac artery (present in most cases of CIAA). In these cases adjustments of the rotational graft position led to torsion of the fixed sidebranch, often ending up with a sidebranch stuck between wall and iliac graft.

The second generation modular iliac bifurcation device's implantation technique has been recently described, by three teams following the same principles.[16,18,19] In brief, with the aid of the gold radiopaque markers the IBD is advanced over a guide wire until the side branch is just proximal to the origin of the internal iliac artery. Following withdrawal of the delivery sheath until the distal end of the side branch is exposed a thin wire through the indwelling catheter is advanced into the aorta and snared from the contralateral iliac artery. An 8 F cross-over-sheath is passed from the contralateral groin over the thin through-and-through wire into the origin of the common iliac component into the branch limb, terminating in the distal aspect of the branch. Alternatively, the thin wire of the preloaded catheter can be snared through the longer brachial access. Through the cross-over-sheath the hypogastric artery is cannulated and after retrieval of the thin wire the sheath is further advanced into the hypogastric artery using a partially inflated low diameter (4-5 mm) balloon catheter. The selected extension stent-graft is advanced into the internal iliac artery and after withdrawal of the crossover sheath deployed in such a manner that there is at least a 2 cm seal within the IIA and within the branch limb. (Figure 2) An angiography through the crossover sheath confirms the adequate positioning of the side branch (Figure 3). Figure 4 illustrates a preoperative 3D CT angiography of a giant left common iliac aneurysm and the postoperative result.

DISCUSSION

To our knowledge the iliac bifurcation device is extensively used by three teams and currently the technique is spreading by proctoring to other vascular centers: the team of Greenberg in Cleveland, USA,[15,19] the team of Malina in Malmo,

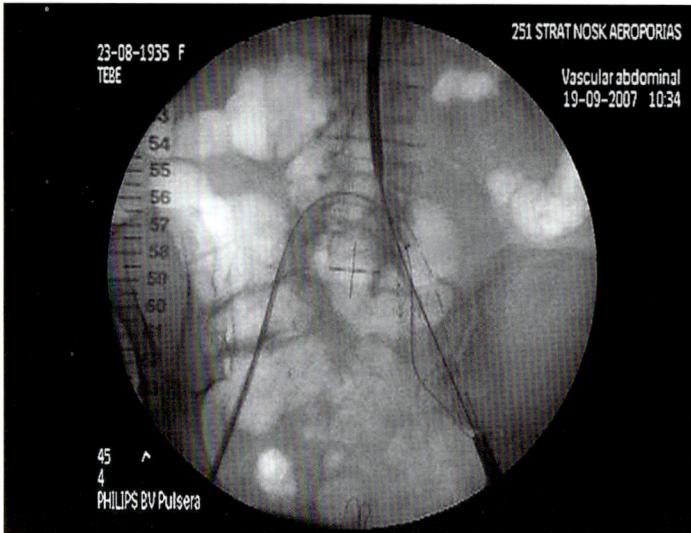

FIGURE 2: A stent-graft has been deployed within the internal iliac artery.

Sweden, 16 and the team of Stelter in Frankfurt, Germany.[18] The only five (to our knowledge) published works[15,16,18,19,20] depict favourable initial and mid-term results and are summarized in Table 1. Excluding the old IBD, the technical success rate ranges between 85-100%, while the mid-term follow up shows an IIA occlusion rate 11-12%. Notably, all vessel loses happened during the first year period and no side branch occlusions have been reported during the longer term follow up.

The iliac bifurcation devices, along with the fenestrated and branched endografts seem to break the barriers of "non-eligible" for endovascular repair anato-

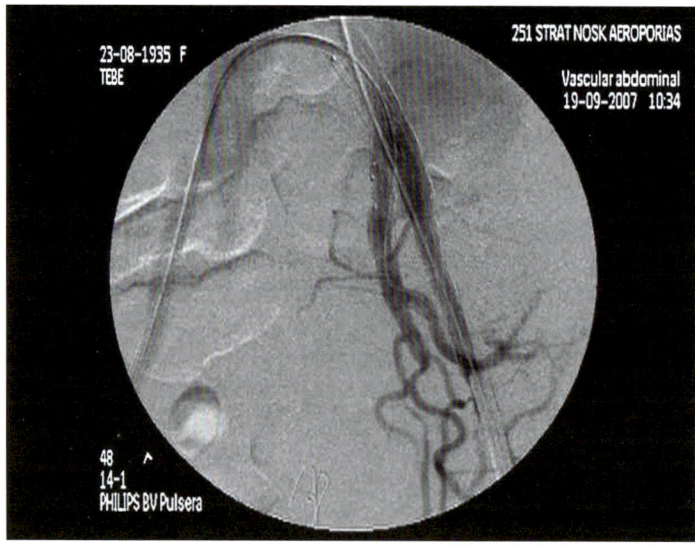

FIGURE 3: Final angio depicting the patency of the hypogastric branch.

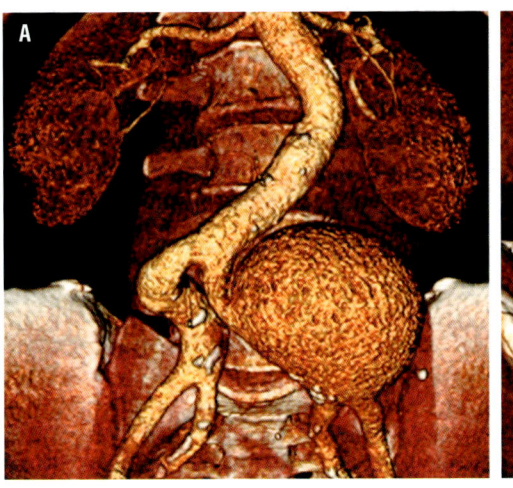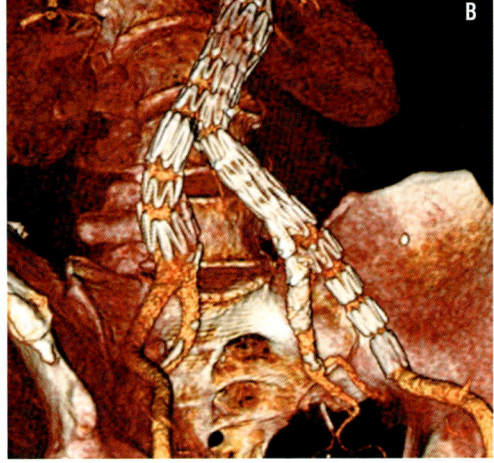

FIGURE 4: A. A preoperative CTA indicating a giant left common iliac artery aneurysm. **B**. The postoperative CTA indicating aneurysm exclusion and a patent internal iliac artery.

TABLE 1

DATA AND OUTCOMES OF THE CURRENT PUBLISHED WORKS

	Patients/ Iliacs	Technical success	Mean follow up (months)	Late vessel loss
Frankfurt, Germany (old device)[18]	26/31	18/31 58%	36.6	4/35 11.4%
Frankfurt, Germany (new device)[18]	20/20	17/20 85%	11.3	
Cleveland, USA & Lille, France*[19]	52/53	49/52 94%	14.2	6/49 12.2%
Cleveland, USA* [15]	21/21	18/21 86%	11	2/18 11.1%
Malmo, Sweden [16]	10/10	9/10 90%	6	1/9 11.1%
Newcastle, Australia [20]	8/8	8/8 12.5%	6	1/8

* Greenberg's team uses a slightly different device, also based on a Zenith (Cook) platform. Unlike the IBD as herein described, the internal iliac side branch arises from the side lateral to the internal iliac artery and foilows a helical path around the device. The junction between the helical limb and the tubular common iliac portion is a bevelled anastomosis.

mies. Fenestrated grafts have already shifted the proximal sealing zone from the infrarenal to the suprarenal aortic segment (for -juxta, -para and -suprarenal AAA), while the IBDs extent distal endograft fixation beyond the iliac bifurcation (for common iliac aneurysms) preserving internal iliac flow and permitting a solitary endovascular procedure. Of course, target patients still remain those, selected ones, considered as high risk for an open repair.

Meticulous planning and expert catheterization skills are of utmost importance. However, experience has showed that careful patient selection is the cornerstone of technical and long-term success, especially when choosing the first patients. Candidate anatomies would be those with no extreme iliac kinking, efficient thrombus-free iliac lumen, sufficiently wide - open, angled 30°-50°, IIA ostium, and no large IIA aneurysm.[18] In case of bilateral CIAA, attempting implantation of two IBDs is not recommended for inexperienced users since it would increase the need for fluoroscopy time, the increased usage of contrast media, the longer anaesthesia time, as well as the the risk of the procedure, possibly outweighing the benefits. In these cases, coil embolization and overstenting of the one IIA or bell bottom technique (if applicable) would be a fair solution. The IBD should be implanted on the side with the larger and "easier" iliac bifurcation.

Concluding, the IBD enables the exclusion of aorto-iliac aneurysms in a safe manner, but also less complex than previous endovascular or hybrid methods that attempted to exclude these aneurysms whilst maintaining pelvic blood flow. The results of the current published works are encouraging and promising for the future of endovascular management of common iliac aneurysms. The high costs of the device will potentially be outweighed by the short and long-term benefits.

REFERENCES

1. Armon MP, Wenham PW, Whitaker SC, Gregson RH, Hopkinson BR. Common iliac artery aneurysms in patients with abdominal aortic aneurysm. Eur J Vasc Endovasc Surg 1998;15:255-7.
2. Henretta JP, Karch LA, Hodgson KJ, Mattos MA, Ramsey DE, McLafferty R, et al. Special iliac artery considerations during aneurysm endografting. Am J Surg 1999;178:212-8.
3. Karch LA, Hodgson KJ, Mattos MA, Bohannon WT, Ramsey DE, McLafferty RB. Adverse consequences of internal iliac artery occlusion during endovascular repair of abdominal aortic aneurysms. J Vasc Surg 2000;32:676-83.
4. Yano OJ, Morrissey N, Eisen L, Faries PL, Soundararajan K, Wan S, et al. Intentional internal iliac artery occlusion to facilitate endovascular repair of aortoiliac aneurysms. J Vasc Surg 2001;34:204-11.
5. Cynamon J, Lerer D, Veith FJ, Taragin BH, Wahl SI, Lautin JL, et al. Hypogastric artery coil embolization prior to endoluminal repair of aneurysms and fistulas: buttock claudication, a recognized by possibly preventable complication. J Vasc Interv Radiol. 2000; 11:573-577.
6. Bergamini TM, Rachel ES, Kinney EV, Jung MT, Kaebnick HW, Mitchell RA. External iliac artery-to-internal iliac artery endograft: a novel approach to preserve pelvic inflow in aortoiliac stent grafting. J Vasc Surg. 2002;35:120-124.
7. Woo EY, Lombardi JV, Carpenter JP. Endovascular external-to-internal iliac bypass as an adjunct to endovascular aneurysm repair for patients with extensive common iliac artery aneurysmal disease. J Vasc Surg. 2004;39:470.
8. Delle M, Lonn L, Wingren U, Karlstrom L, Klingenstierna H, Risberg B, et al. Preserved pelvic circulation after stent-graft treatment of complex aortoiliac artery aneurysms: a new approach. J Endovasc Ther 2005;12:189-195.
9. Faries PL, Morrissey N, Burks JA, Gravereaux E, Kerstein MD, Teodorescu VJ, et al. Internal iliac artery revascularization as an adjunct to endovascular repair of aortoiliac aneurysms. J Vasc Surg 2001;34:892-899.
10. Mehta M, Veith FJ, Ohki T, Cynamon J, Goldstein D, Suggs WD, et al. Unilateral and bilateral hypogastric artery interruption during aortoiliac aneu-

rysm repair in 154 patients: a relatively innocuous procedure. J Vasc Surg 2001;33:S27-32.

11. Razavi MK, DeGroot M, Olcott C III, Sze D, Kee Ssemba CP, Dake MD. Internal iliac artery embolization in the stent-graft treatment of aortoiliac aneurysms: analysis of outcomes and complications. J Vasc Interv Radiol 2000;11:561-6.

12. Karch LA, Hodgson KJ, Mattos MA, Bohannon WT, Ramsey DE, McLafferty RB. Adverse consequences of internal iliac artery occlusion during endovascular repair of abdominal aortic aneurysms. J Vasc Surg 2000;32:676-83.

13. Yano OJ, Morrissey N, Eisen L, Faries PL, Soundararajan K, Wan S, et al. Intentional internal iliac artery occlusion to facilitate endovascular repair of aortoiliac aneurysms. J Vasc Surg 2001;34: 204-11.

14. Semmens JB, Lawrence-Brown MM, Hartley DE, Allen YB, Green R, Nadkarni S. Outcomes of fenestrated endografts in the treatment of abdominal aortic aneurysm in Western Australia (1997-2004). J Endovasc Ther 2006;13:320-9.

15. Greenberg RK, West K, Pfaff K, Foster J, Skender D, Haulon S et al. Beyond the aortic bifurcation: Branched endovascular grafts for thoracoabdominal and aortoiliac aneurysms. J Vasc Surg 2006; 43:879-86.

16. Malina M, Dirven M, Sonesson B, Resch T, Dias N, Ivancev K. Feasibility of a branched stent-graft in common iliac artery aneurysms. J Endovasc Ther 2006;13:496-500.

17. Perdikides T, Avgerinos ED, Lagios K, Ziegler P, Stelter WJ. Improving Endograft Stability by Accommodation onto the Aortic Bifurcation. J Endovasc Ther 2007, in press.

18. Ziegler P, Avgerinos ED, Umscheid T, Perdikides T, Erz K, Stelter WJ. Branched Iliac Bifurcation: 6 Years Experience with Endovascular Preservation of Internal Iliac Artery Flow. J Vasc Surg 2007;46: 204-10.

19. Haulon S, Greenberg RK, Pfaff K, Francis C, Koussa M, West K. Branched grafting for aortoiliac aneurysms. Eur J Vasc Endovasc Surg 2007; 33:567-574.

20. Serracino-Inglott F, Bray AE, Myers P. Endovascular abdominal aortic aneurysm repair in patients with common iliac artery aneurysms - Initial experience with the Zenith bifurcated iliac side branch device. J Vasc Surg 2007;46:211-7.

The management of the "wide neck" aneurysm

Marcel Goodman, James B. Semmens

INTRODUCTION

Extensive experience over many years have enabled us to identify features of aortic aneurysm morphology which predict successful exclusion following endoluminal grafting.[1,2] Of these, neck diameter and length are paramount.[3] We have been able to confidently recommend this technique for aneurysms with neck diameter of 28 mm or less, and neck length greater than 15 mm. However, when the aneurysm neck was wider, exceeding 30 mm in diameter, the patient was usually advised to undergo open surgery or accept conservative management.[4] This approach took into account the risk of progressive neck dilatation, similar to the progressive enlargement of the infra-renal segment following open surgery. Adverse literature reports as well, reinforced negative perceptions of the endoluminal treatment of complex aneurysms such as those with wide necks.[5] However, the prevailing pessimistic attitude was by no means universal. Clinicians and development consultants in Perth considered that the extensive experience they had gained in basic planning and device design could be directed towards these aneurysms to permit cautious endoluminal treatment.

The case against endografting wide neck aneurysms was strong.[5] One of the most cogent arguments was knowledge gained from the open surgery model. The majority of vascular surgeons had experienced dilatation and frank aneurysmal progression in an excessively long residual infrarenal segment. This is more likely to have occurred when the original surgery was emergent or where the operating conditions were sub-optimal. Extreme obesity, hostile abdomen and surgeon inexperience are classical examples. Facing this clinical problem years later, we assume the residual neck has dilated significantly. However, we cannot be sure that in some of these patients a wide neck was not already present at the original operation. In these circumstances, leaving a moderately long aortic cuff was a judicious and safe surgical technique to avoid clamping an oversize neck immediately distal to the renal arteries. Thus in these cases, the degree of aneurysmal progression may not have been so great, although they still served to confirm the potential for a wide infra-renal aorta to expand. This concern not unnaturally carried into the endoluminal era.

One of the concerns in endoluminal grafting was that even a "normal" aneurysm neck would dilate in response to the radial force of the apposed stent. This was more of a controversial issue in the early days of endoluminal grafting. Most accept that neck remodelling occurs and that the calibre of the endograft is probably the most critical factor determining the endpoint. The extent to which a well apposed endograft protects the aneurysm from dilatation is also an issue.

In routine aneurysm endografting, there is little evidence that modest neck dilatation adversely affects aneurysm exclusion. However, a wide neck may be considered already pathological. The mean aortic diameter is 21.4 mm for a 65 year old Caucasian male.[6] Therefore, a neck of 30 mm or more may be considered already aneurysmal. Accordingly if we accept that radial force induced expansion of the neck may develop over time, it may occur sooner and to a greater degree in these patients with "pathological" necks.

Reports in the literature of graft failure, proximal endoleak and migration, attributed to progressive dilatation of a wide neck would naturally reinforce concerns.[4,5,7] In some of these cases factors other than dilatation of the wide neck, may have contributed to the poor outcome. Graft selection may not have allowed optimal oversizing or the endograft may not have been deployed immediately distal to the lowest renal artery. Alternative explanations for some of these poor results may be relevant. However, concern persists that a pathological neck will further dilate, leading to migration, Type 1 endoleak and graft failure. This concern receives further support from a review of 238 patients who had undergone endoluminal grafting in Western Australia between 1994-8. In this series, Stanley et al showed that when the diameter of the aortic neck exceeded 28 mm and particularly if it was flared, the incidence of endoleak and migration increased significantly.[3]

Studies of computational fluid dynamics have made an enormous contribution to understanding the complex forces acting on endografts and thus, the potential causes of failure.[8,9] These studies demonstrated that the downward displacement forces normally acting on a bifurcate graft would be significantly increased on an over-size device such as could be used to seal in a wide aneurysm neck. These forces would theoretically increase the risk of migration and combine with neck dilatation to become a potent cause of graft failure in these wide neck aneurysms.

Fenestrated endoluminal grafting has been shown to address many of the potential causes of failure in complex aneurysms especially those with wide, flaring necks.[10-12] The obvious advantage would be to achieve a seal above the wide neck. Here the aorta tends to be narrow and straight and less likely to dilate. Unfortunately fenestrated grafting is far from a universal solution. Problems such as lack of operator experience, increased costs, and the risk of adverse events restrict its potential application.

As clinicians, we continued to be exposed to patients with wide neck aneurysm who were either unable or unwilling to accept non-operation or open surgery both prior and subsequent to the fenestration era. There has thus existed an on-going stimulus to provide a solution for these patients and to design a routine endograft which would seal within a wide neck. The added challenge was whether the theoretical and historical evidence presented above was correct in predicting a poor outcome.

EARLY AUSTRALASIAN EXPERIENCE

In Australia during the late 1990's, routine endografting was well established as the procedure of choice for the majority of vascular surgeons. In response to frequent requests for an endoluminal solution for wide neck aneurysms, a modification of the then current "Zenith Tri-Fab" endograft was produced. The body component was expanded to provide adequate oversizing.

From the latter part of 1999, surgeons experienced in endografting, were able to request the 36 mm "custom" graft to treat patients with aneurysm neck diameters ranging from 28 to 34 mm. Potential graft recipients were evaluated by members of the Zenith Planning Service using "real size" scaled drawings derived from computerized technology to confirm that the use of this device was appropriate and would ensure adequate oversizing and seal. Early experience using this oversized graft was remarkably free of adverse reports. Both deployment and aneurysm exclusion appeared satisfactory. This was the incentive for further development.

In 2002, the "Zenith" 36 mm x 12 mm bifurcate endograft was introduced in Australia. This was the largest body size in the "Flex" range. Over-sized grafts were then available "off-the-shelf", greatly facilitating patient management. Members of the "Zenith" Planning Service continued to provide advice and assistance to potential users. The 36 mm endograft differed from the "custom" models that preceded it and from smaller grafts in the "Flex" range. The sealing Z-stent was longer at 22 mm compared to 17 mm in the previous model. The longer stent provided stability and was an advantage when the neck was irregular. Also, the increased length appeared to reduce the tendency to guttering or in-folding when the endograft was constricted in a narrow portion of neck. The steel used to construct the longer, larger stent was stronger (20 G v 18 G) to maintain optimum radial force. The anchor stent has 12 crowns and barbs. Apart from the very earliest models, there was double-loop suturing between the anchor stent and the endograft body to counter the large downward distraction forces. There was a 6 mm gap between the sealing stent and body to accommodate to angled or tortuous necks.

THE "ZENITH" 36 mm GRAFT – EARLY AND MEDIUM TERM EXPERIENCE

In 2005, an initial retrospective review was carried out on patients who had received the Zenith 36 mm endograft (William Cook Australia, Brisbane, Queensland). The operating surgeons were approached to provide information on their "36 mm graft" patients. Clinical records of 67 patients were available for analysis. The review was carried out in all cases by the operating surgeon who had undertaken follow-up, according to the "Zenith" protocol. This consisted of plain abdominal X-ray and abdominal CT at six weeks and six months. Thereafter a CT or duplex ultrasound was undertaken annually to confirm aneurysm exclusion and to assess aneurysm sac size.

With the patient's permission, the treating surgeon responded to a questionnaire and provided information on endograft deployment and follow-up. Data was requested on complications such as device migration, endoleak and the need for secondary interventions. Information relating to patient deaths was sourced from patient records or the State Death Registry. This included the date and cause of death and whether the death was related to the endovascular repair procedure.

Retrospective review of 36 mm grafts from 1999-2004 in Australia and New Zealand
N = 67 (males 62, females 5); mean age: 76.6yrs

Deployment
Failure to deploy: 0
Proximal endoleak
   (intra-operative):   2 - treated by covered
                               extension +
                               Palmaz stent
Technical success: 100%

Early follow-up: 30 days
Proximal endoleak: 1

Distal endoleak:	3
Iliac occlusion:	2
Mortality (non graft related)	2
Procedural success	88%

Proximal endoleaks were observed in two patients during deployment. They were successfully controlled by deploying a combination of graft body extension and Palmaz stent. It is gratifying that only two patients had deployment problems. These were patients with complex aneurysms and wide flaring necks. More technical problems would have been anticipated.

CT imaging during early follow-up revealed one further patient with a proximal endoleak. This was treated at nine days from deployment. Again, aneurysm exclusion was achieved by using a combination of covered body extension and a Palmaz stent.

Three patients had distal endoleaks and these were controlled by extending the iliac limb into the external iliac artery. Two patients suffered occlusion of an iliac limb. Both were symptomatic and were treated by extra-anatomic bypass. This was unsuccessful in one patient and he underwent below knee amputation. Two patients died from cardio-respiratory causes within 30 days. Neither patient had experienced a complication related to graft deployment.

Medium term follow-up of these patients was relatively free of major complications. However, the mean period of surveillance was only 13 months. This was too short a period for any meaningful conclusion on treatment efficacy of the 36 mm graft. The treating vascular surgeons were then approached 15 months later to provide further follow up information. Their co-operation in providing this data has extended the mean duration of surveillance to 27 months.

Medium term follow-up:

Mean surveillance period	27 months (range 20 - 75 months)

Complications

Mortality	20
Graft related mortality	1 (CVA)
Body Migration/ Proximal Endoleak (graft disruption)	1
Conversion/Explantation (peri-graft sepsis)	1
Distal Endoleak	1
Type 2 Endoleak - IMA ligation	2

During this period, a further 18 patients died. Only one death could be related to the endograft. This patient developed peri-aortic sepsis which did not respond to antibiotic. Imminent disruption of the affected aortic wall appeared likely and he underwent urgent graft ex-plantation. This procedure was complicated by major blood loss, hypotension and renal failure requiring dialysis. Some months later, while apparently recovering, he sustained a fatal CVA.

The separating of the endograft body from the anchor stent occurred very early in the series. The resulting downward migration and large proximal endoleak re-pressurized the aneurysm sac. Fortunately the leak was fairly easily controlled by deploying a graft body extension to reseal below the renal arteries. That repair has remained durable. This was the stimulus for double-loop suture between the anchor and sealing stent.

The overall incidence of complications appeared low for this potentially high risk group. However, considering the natural concerns, the critical issue is the durability of aneurysm exclusion. This can be evaluated indirectly by reference to endoleaks. The incidence was low. In addition, both proximal and distal leaks were controlled by endovascular intervention. Based on endoleak numbers, aneurysm exclusion may be considered satisfactory.

This is not sufficient as endoleak incidence alone fails to address the possibility of endotension. In theory, neck dilatation or graft migration may have been in progress during the period of surveillance resulting in a defective seal allowing pressurizaton via laminated thrombus of the aneurysm sac. Contraction of the aneurysm sac can be considered reliable evidence of satisfactory seal. Some aneurysm walls are rigid. Therefore, a sac which is stable may also be considered, with some reservation, to be adequately excluded.

Aneurysm sac dimensions (N = 47)

Contracted	27
Unchanged	18
Enlarged	2

Analysis of sac dimensions was performed only on those patients who survived to the time of the second review. Contraction of the sac was recorded in 57% of those studied. There was no sac enlargement in 95%. In the two cases where there was sac enlargement at the time of review, one was associated with a Type 2 leak and the other, a treated distal endoleak.

The separation of the endograft body from the anchor stent occurred very early in the series. The complication was consistent with the computational fluid dynamic data. Calculations from this data demonstrated that at an inlet systolic blood pressure of 150 mmHg, the 36 x 12 mm endograft is subjected to downward drag forces of 16.0 N. compared to 4.8 N on a 24 x 12 mm endograft. The separation and proximal endoleak were corrected by deploying a suitable body extension. To prevent reoccurrence of this problem, the endograft was modified by strengthening the suture ligature between the components. Since this was carried out, there has been no recurrence of the problem. The above calculations also highlight the critical function of the anchor stent barbs in resisting the very significant downward drag forces. In doing so, these barbs maintain the graft/sealing zone apposition which is so critical to durable aneurysm exclusion.

The higher than anticipated mortality in this group of patients, predominantly of cardio-respiratory causes, suggest significant co-morbidity. Patient selection relating to age and co-morbidity was entirely in the hands of the treating vascular surgeon. It is conceivable that a large aneurysm neck may be a marker for increased susceptibility to cardio-respiratory complications. It may be therefore advisable that any patient who is a candidate for this oversized device be assessed critically. Those patients with indifferent cardiovascular status and life expectancy may be better managed by conservative treatment.

The patient whose endograft was explanted reflects the insidious nature of endograft infection. In this case it became apparent at 15 months. This case raises the question as to whether the infection occurred at implantation or whether it was an acquired prosthetic infection. It also raises the question as to whether the mortality should be considered endograft related. Many weeks had elapsed since the ex-plant operation during which he was recovering well.

These medium term results indicate that the 36 mm endograft has been very effective in the management of a potentially difficult group of aneurysms. We consider they reflect the successful adaptation of basic concepts and techniques to more complex situations. The overwhelming majority of the endograft users were experienced and busy vascular surgeons with well established follow-up regimes who co-operated to provide the information required.

This review represents a comprehensive follow-up of the majority of 36 mm "Zenith" Endografts, manufactured and deployed during the period under review.

THE ANEURYSM NECK

The practice in the Zenith Planning Service in Perth has been to use CT derived "real size" scaled drawing for all graft planning. Information was also available from these planning records. The normal practice is to measure neck diameters every 5 mm as shown in a typical record. This information has been extremely valuable in evaluating the neck sealing zone (Figure 1).

These are the mean diameters for the 67 patients who were studied. We define the proximal sealing zone at the level of the most caudal renal artery. The distal sealing zone diameter is at 20 mm from this point.

Proximal Sealing zone	27.2 mm +/- 2.5 mm
Distal Sealing Zone	31.9 mm +/- 1.7 mm
Neck Flare	4.6 mm +/- 2.6 mm
Neck Flare >3 mm	76%

The degree of neck flaring is very significant and exceeds that considered by Stanley et al as a marker for concern.[3] These figures highlight the dual potential hazards of endografting this category of patients, namely a neck that may expand and which cannot offer uniform oversizing, even at the time of deployment.[4]

It is customary to refer to the calibre of the infra-renal neck by a single measurement. The accepted reference point is the most caudal renal artery. Provided the infrarenal segment is cylindrical, it is not critical whether the measure is taken at this or one of the alternate levels such as 5 or 10 mm distal to the lowest renal artery. However, if the neck is not strictly cylindrical, and particularly if it is flaring as in the majority our patients, a single diameter measurement may not accurately describe the morphology of this immediate infrarenal segment. Accurate information is absolutely vital to optimal graft selection.

There is uniform agreement that an endograft should be planned so that it is oversized in the neck by at least 10 to 15%. Equally important, this oversizing must extend across the full length of the proximal sealing zone. We have recommended the term "proximal sealing zone" to define accurately the infrarenal aorta extending 20 mm caudal to the lowest renal artery. This concept becomes critical in discussion of complex anatomy such as wide necks because of their tendency to flare.

It is extremely unlikely that the long accepted term "aneurysm neck" will be replaced by the more precise one. We con-

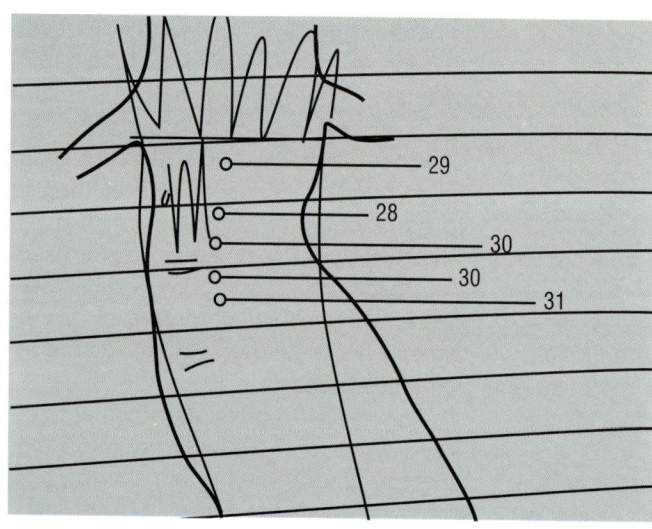

FIGURE 1: Typical planning study for an oversized endograft.

sider this concept is important in evaluating other clinicians experience with wide neck aneurysms. In some cases where adverse results are reported, the optimum size endograft may not have been selected. The necks may also have been flaring, resulting in undersizing in the more distal neck and a poor seal.

The issue of neck dilatation is a complex one.[4] We frequently see the narrower part of a proximal sealing zone become "ironed out" and the sealing stent become more uniform in calibre. We have evidence in this group of patients of a modest but uniform enlargement of the sealing zone. We consider the calibre of the graft will be the limiting factor in this expansion, provided it is closely apposed to the aortic wall in this sealing zone. Provided there has been no other complication such as a distal or high pressure Type 2 endoleak, we have not observed progressive neck enlargement.

There is another factor which must be considered. The graft fabric and stent, closely applied across the full length of the proximal sealing zone, may in fact be protecting the infrarenal aorta from the dilating influence of the aortic pulse. In the open surgery model to which we have referred, infra-renal aortic dilatation may result from years of exposure to these forces. These direct forces may be a greater stimulus to dilatation than the continuous radial force of an endograft stent.

OVERSIZING FOR FLARING NECKS

In our series, the mean diameter at the level of the lowest renal artery was 27.2 mm. Using the 36 mm device, we thus have an oversizing ratio close to 25%. The mean diameter in the distal sealing zone was 31.9 mm. The distal oversizing ratio here was 11%. Thus, in this group of patients, the 36 mm endograft fulfills the obligation of providing adequate oversizing along the sealing zone.

We have shown significant flaring in the majority of wide neck aneurysms in this series. Lee et al also reported distal flaring in a series of wide neck aneurysms.[13] Interestingly, the incidence in his patients was lower than ours (30% v 76%). Commenting on their satisfactory outcomes, the authors also stressed the importance of their addressing neck morphology.

It is obvious that ensuring adequate oversizing distally in the flared section, may lead to significant proximal oversize. This has the theoretical potential to induce instability and "guttering". However, this has not been the case and our experience has been more consistent with the example below (Figures 2 and 3). In the proximal sealing zone, the metal of the sealing stent could not be more tightly compressed, yet no infolding is observed at 40% oversizing!

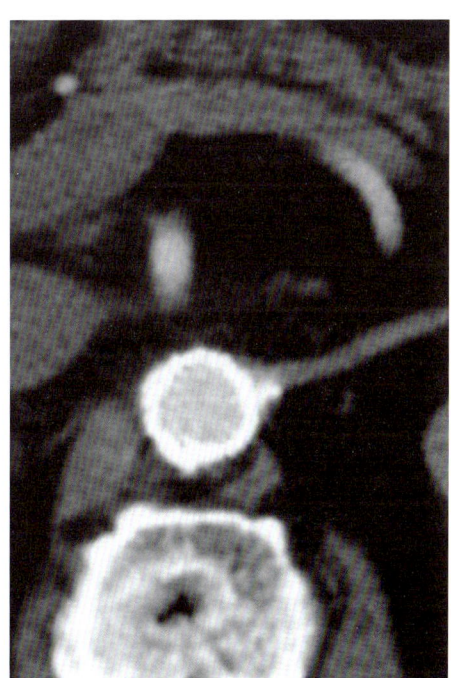

FIGURE 2: 36 mm graft at the proximal sealing zone- neck diameter is 26 mm = 40% oversizing.

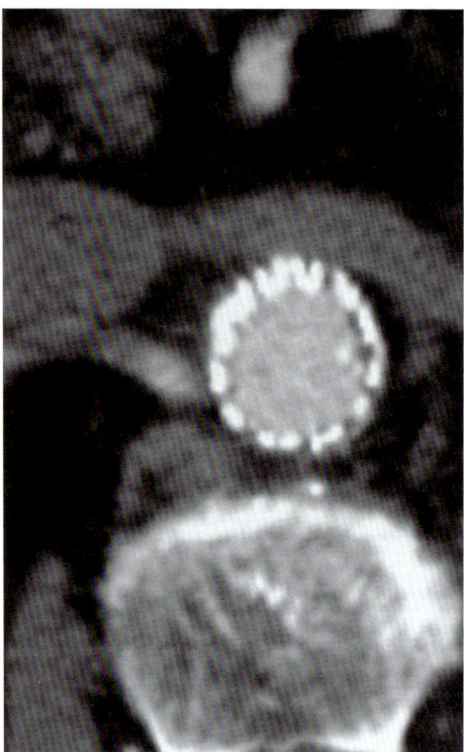

FIGURE 3: 36 mm graft at the distal sealing zone-neck diameter is 34 mm = 7% oversizing.

This example demonstrates endograft stability at extremes of oversizing as well as the wide range of oversizing ratios along a typical wide flaring neck. This example also emphasizes the importance of planning to take into account the widest sealing zone diameter. The 7% distal oversizing ratio above is barely adequate for a good seal in spite of such gross proximal oversize.

In the example below of a typical distal flaring neck, use of the lowest renal artery as reference diameter, invites selection of a 26 mm graft (Figure 4). However, it will contact only 12 mm of the proximal sealing zone. A 34 mm graft is more appropriate for the distal portion of the sealing zone, although it will result in proximal oversizing of over 50%.

As stated, this degree of oversizing is the typical situation which may predispose

to graft instability with infolding or "guttering". We believe that the lengthening of the sealing stent from 17 to 22 mm contributes to the stability we have consistently observed. If proximal infolding did occur with the use of an oversize device, correction should be achievable with a combination of covered extension and Palmaz stent. The wide calibre of the sealing zone makes the Palmaz stent alone much less effective. Reluctance to choose a large graft due to concern about infolding may lead to undersizing. This is a greater potential problem. Migration or proximal endoleak resulting from undersizing can only be corrected by graft removal, neck banding or fenestration grafting.

Adverse reports in the literature from Sternbergh et al have indicated that generous oversizing (>30%) is associated

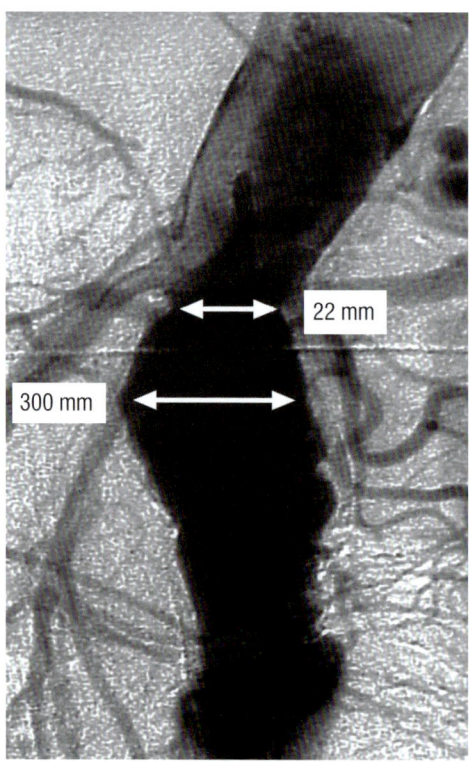

FIGURE 4: Typical flaring aneurysm neck graft selection must reflect distal sealing zone.

with a poor outcome with a significant increase in device migration and sac expansion. The device they used also had proximal barb fixation which should have countered the tendency to migrate as in our series. Conners et al also reported adverse outcomes with oversizing >20%.[14] The devices used in their series did not have barbs and they report satisfactory results. This fact must confirm the importance of optimal oversizing.

The incorporation of fenestrated grafting into the mainstream endovascular armamentarium has been very significant. This technique would then represent the optimal approach to the wide neck especially one that flares significantly. In theory this approach is correct. The para-renal sealing zone is likely to be stronger, narrower and not flared and is thus, a superior sealing zone for a fenestrated graft. These properties alone should guarantee durable aneurysm exclusion.

However, we must accept that fenestrated grafting is not possible for all situations and great judgment is often required. Fenestrated grafting involves greater complexity and costs. We must deploy stents, often covered, within renal and visceral arteries which are then at risk for occlusion. Many patients with wide-neck aneurysms have significant co-morbidities such as renal insufficiency or reduced life expectancy and would not tolerate complex procedures. In addition, cost and population restrictions will result in some surgeons lacking exposure to sufficient cases to gain optimum experience to be competent in fenestrated grafting. The availability of a non-fenestrated alternative maintains our graft selection flexibility.

IMAGING AND WIDE NECKS

Improvements in CT imaging with faster and more powerful machines facilitating the use of very sophisticated reformatting software enables the extraction of data which provide a most accurate assessment of parameters such as neck morphology. The ability to view the various aneurysm components "in-line" may indicate that an aneurysm neck, initially considered suitable only for fenestration was in fact long enough for routine endografting. This presumed of course provided that adequate oversizing could also be achieved.

As the use of dedicated workstations become more widely accepted, surgeons and their patients will benefit from intuitive selection of the most appropriate device. From our experience with image manipulation techniques in wide neck aneurysms, we can identify an intermediate group for which both routine oversize and fenestrated grafting are equally acceptable. In this "grey zone", the final decision may be made on criteria such as age, co-morbidity, iliac access etc.

Many factors combine to provide a spectrum of endovascular treatment options. There is a definite role for over-size grafts to treat aneurysms with wide necks. There may be circumstances where both open surgery and oversize grafts appear equally acceptable and a more subtle "grey zone" between oversize and fenestrated graft. As imaging and reformatting techniques become even more sophisticated, we will be better placed to select the most appropriate device and technique for these complex anatomies.

The challenge is whether the less complex oversize graft can provide durable aneurysm exclusion. Our follow up is still fairly modest at a mean of 27 months. Prior to completing further patient review, we can report no evidence of late graft failure. Confirmation of continued success will be critical in these high risk aneurysm patients.

CONCLUSION

The Zenith 36 mm endograft has performed successfully in the short and medium term. It is considered that as well as calibre, design features of the endograft, including sealing stent length and proximal fixation barbs have contributed to this success. This combined with sophisticated imaging and intuitive planning increases our confidence in managing complex aneurysms.

The 36 mm Zenith endograft has the potential to fill an intermediate role in endografting between standard and fenestrated endografting. In situations where the transition to aneurysm is less abrupt and the sealing zone diameter, irrespective of profile, does not exceed 32-33 mm, an off-the-shelf 36 mm graft may be an alternative and satisfactory solution. This device will have an obvious cost and availability advantage and is also appropriate where operators will neither have the financial nor logistic capacity to advance to more complex procedures such as fenestration grafting. This concept is consistent with the principle of exploring the most simple, efficient and effective means of excluding aneurysms.

ACKNOWLEDGEMENTS

I am indebted to the following surgeons who kindly permitted their patients to be included in this study and who performed the clinical and imaging review.
- Drs. M Lawrence-Brown, K Sieunerine, J Chleboun, S Baker, P Norman, F Prendergast, Dr. B. Stanley (Perth, West Australia).
- Drs. A Johnston, M Denton, G Fels (Melbourne, Victoria).
- Drs. P Colman, K Hahnel, R Lusby (New South Wales).
- Dr. T Vasudevan (New Zealand).

I am also indebted to the following for expert and technical assistance with this study.

- Statistic analysis: Professor J. Semmens and Dr M. Rosenberg.
- Data collection: A. Bartlett and E Allen.
- David Hartley, Design and Development Consultant for the 36 mm "Zenith" Endograft.

REFERENCES

1. Lawrence-Brown M.M.D., Hartley D, MacSweeny S, Kelsey P, Ives F, Holden A, Gordon M., Goodman M.A., Sieunarine K. The Perth Endoluminal Bifurcated Graft System-Development and Early Experience. Journal of Cardiovascular Surgery 1996; 4:706-712.
2. Chuter TAM, Parodi JC, Lawrence-Brown MMD. The management of abdominal aortic aneurysm: a decade of progress. Journal of Endovascular Therapy (In press - December Edition)
3. Stanley B, Semmens JB, Mai Q, Goodman M, Hartley D, Wilkinson C, Lawrence-Brown MMD. Evaluation of patient selection guidelines for endoluminal AAA repair with the Zenith stent-graft: the Australasian experience. Journal of Endovascular Therapy. 2001; 8:457-464.
4. Goodman M, Lawrence-Brown MMD, Hartley D, Allen YB, Semmens JB. The Treatment of Infrarenal Abdominal Aortic Aneuryms with Oversized (36mm) Zenith Endografts. Journal of Endovascular Therapy. 2007;14:23-29.
5. Greenberg RK, Clair D, Srivastava S, Bhandari G, Turc A, Hampton J, Popa M, Green R, Ouriel K. Should patients with challenging anatomy be offered endovascular aneurysm repair? Journal of Vascular Surgery. 2003;38:990-6
6. Lawrence-Brown MMD, Norman PE, Jamrozik K, Semmens JB, Donnelly NJ, Spencer C, Tuohy R. Initial results of ultrasound screening for aneurysm of the abdominal aorta in Western Australia: Relevance for endoluminal treatment of aneurysm disease. Cardiovascular Surgery 2001;9:234-240.
7. Fearn S, Lawrence-Brown MMD, Semmens JB, Hartley D. Follow-up after endovascular aortic aneurysm repair: The plain radiograph has an essential role in surveillance. Journal of Endovascular Therapy 2003;10:894-901.
8. Liffman K, Lawrence-Brown MMD, Semmens JB, Bui A, Rudman M, Hartley D. Analytical modelling

and numerical simulation of forces in an endoluminal graft. Journal of Endovascular Therapy 2001; 8:358-371.

9. Liffman K, Sutalo I, Lawrence-Brown MMD, Semmens JB, Aldham B. Movement and dislocation of modular stent-grafts due to pulsatile flow and the pressure difference between the stent-graft and the aneurysm sac. Journal of Endovascular Therapy 2006; 13:51-61.

10. Anderson JL, Berce M, Hartley DE. Endoluminal aortic grafting with renal and superior mesenteric artery incorporation by graft fenestration. Journal of Endovascular Therapy 2001; 8: 3-15

11. Stanley B, Semmens JB, Lawrence-Brown MMD, Goodman MA, Hartley D. Fenestration in endovascular grafts for aortic aneurysm repair: new horizons for preserving blood flow in branch vessels. Journal of Endovascular Therapy 2001;8:16-24.

12. Semmens JB, Lawrence-Brown MMD, Hartley DE, Allen YB, Green R, Nadkarni S. Outcomes of fenestrated endografts in the treatment of abdominal aortic aneurysm in Western Australia (1997 - 2004). Journal of Endovascular Therapy 2006;13: 320-329.

13. Lee JT, Lee J, Aziz I, Donayre CE, Walot I, Kopchok GE, Heilbron M Jr, Lippmann M, White RA. Stent-graft migration following endovascular repair of aneurysms with large proximal necks: anatomical risk factors and long-term sequelae. Journal of Endovascular Therapy. 2002;9:652-64.

14. Conners MS 3rd, Sternbergh WC 3rd, Carter G, Tonnessen BH, Yoselevitz M, Money SR. Endograft migration one to four years after endovascular abdominal aortic aneurysm repair with the AneuRx device: a cautionary note. Journal of Vascular Surgery 2003; 37(4):916.

Managing angulated necks and tortuous iliacs during endovascular repair of abdominal aortic aneyrysms

Jan Nöel Albertini, Isabelle Javerliat, Jan Macierewicz,
Chee V. Soong, C. Capdevilla, Claude Clement, Brian R. Hopkinson

INTRODUCTION

Endovascular repair (EVAR) is now considered as a viable alternative to open repair of abdominal aortic aneurysms. Postoperative mortality and morbidity is very low in good risk patients with selected anatomy. However, it has long been recognised that adverse anatomical features of proximal neck and iliac arteries may increase the probability of technical failure. Amongst the various anatomical features increasing technical difficulties during EVAR, proximal neck angulation and iliac tortuosities may well represent the most challenging. The aim of this review is 1) to explain the mechanisms by which aortic and iliac angulation may lead to failure of EVAR and 2) to describe how to prevent and/or deal with the corresponding complications.

ANGULATED PROXIMAL AORTIC NECKS

Proximal neck angulation (PNA) may be defined as the angle between longitudinal axis of the infra-renal neck and longitudinal axis of the aneurysm lumen. It has long been recognised from clinical studies that PNA was a major risk factor for proxi-

mal type I endoleak and stent-graft proximal end migration.[1,2] Untreated proximal type I endoleak results in AAA rupture in most patients. Bench-test study allowed to elaborate on the mechanism of proximal type I endoleak when using Gianturco Z stented grafts.[3] Stiff Z stents do not comply with the angulation, therefore the graft fabric does not apply properly against the aortic wall which subsequently results in direct leakage to the aneurysm sac. Further clinical studies identified that adverse events were increased in patients with neck angulation equal or greater than 60 degrees.[4,5]

Selection of patients with PNA less than 45 degrees allows to prevent type I endoleak and associated adjunctive procedures in most patients.

When using Gianturco Z stented grafts the planning of a wider gap (of about 10 mm) between the first two covered stents may enhance the seal at the level of the first covered stent (Figure 1).

Positioning the graft exactly at the level of the renal arteries is of paramount importance when dealing with short and angulated necks. Proper orientation of the C-arm according to neck angulation allows to avoid parallax errors that usually result in low deployment.

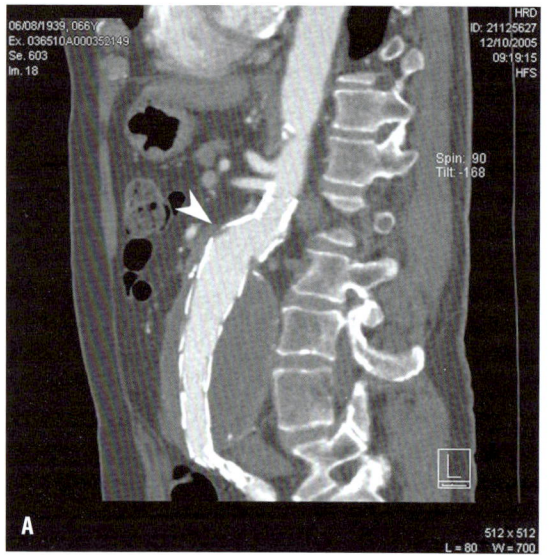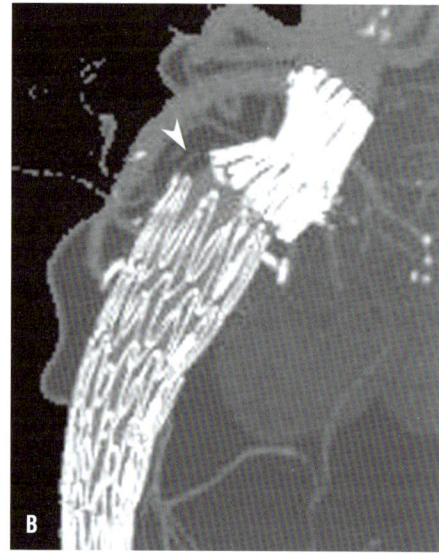

FIGURE 1: Gianturco Z-stented aorto-uni-iliac graft with 10 mm gap (*arrow*) between first and second covered stent. This technique allows better alignment of the first covered stent along the axis of the neck above the top of the angle.

Difficulties may be encountered when the delivery system reaches the top of the neck angulation. Using the stiffest wires is of paramount importance (Backupmeier (Boston Scientific, Natick,MA) or Lunderquist (Cook Europe, Bjaerverskov,Denmark)) to facilitate the passage of the delivery system at the level of the angulation. Choosing the side of introduction opposite to the inside of the bend may also facilitate this maneuver. However, in patients with very tight angulations, realignment of the neck along the axis of the sac may be necessary. This may be accomplished by a simple hand push maneuver in thin patients, or, if necessary, by reaching the aneurysm sac retroperitoneally through an extension of the groin incision.

When proximal type I endoleak is identified on intraoperative angiography, various additional maneuvers may be attempted. Dilatation with aortic balloon at the level of the neck may be sufficient to realign the stent-graft within the neck and seal the leak. If not, insertion of a giant Palmaz stent (P4014 or P5014, Cordis, Miami FL) allows a more rigid fixation and is successful in most patients.[6,7] Care must be taken in positioning a large sheath up to the level of the renal to prevent the Palmaz stent from jamming within the stent-graft during insertion. If Palmaz stent is not successful, peri-aortic ligatures may be applied at the level of the proximal neck through laparotomy[8] or laparoscopically.[9] Conversion to open repair may be the ultimate solution, but it carries a high mortality and morbidity, particularly in the high-risk patient.

Although these additional procedures have proven to be efficient in a number of patients, they seriously increase operative time and therefore the risk of post-operative complications, especially in frail patients. Furthermore, their outcome may be particularly hazardous in patients with severe PNA of 60 degrees or more. In order to overcome these issues a research program was started to design and manufacture a more flexible stent-graft. This program lead to the development of the Aorfix stent-graft (Lombard Medical, Didcot, UK). This stent-graft consists in a Dacron fabric supported by a succession of concentric circular nitinol wires[10] (Figure 2). This circular frame gives to the Aorfix stent-graft its flexibility. A bench-test study suggested better performance in terms of seal with high PNA of the Aorfix compared to other commercial stent-graft.[11] These results were confirmed by a preliminary clinical study of 29 patients with PNA greater than 45 degrees which showed 96 % technical success and 3% post-operative mortality rates.[12] In this series, twenty-three patients (79%) had PNA greater than 60 degrees. The patient who died postoperatively developed multiorgan failure following groin wound revision for hemorrhage. Seven patients had type I proximal endoleak detected on intraoperative angiography. In five patients the cause of the proximal endoleak was low deployment of the endograft. Proximal extension was successful in four patients and failed in one (for this latter patient, no Palmaz stent was available and the procedure was terminated; he had later another proximal extender that failed to seal the leak; conversion to open repair was considered but not undertaken because the patient was a poor surgical candidate). In the two other patients proximal leak occurred despite the stent-graft was properly deployed at the level of the renal arteries. Balloon dilatation alone was successful in one patient and placement of P4014 Palmaz stent was necessary in the last patient. It is noteworthy that patients with PNA greater than 60 degrees would have been precluded from EVAR if a flexible stent-graft had not been available. Indeed, 60 degrees is the usual limit beyond which EVAR is not recommended for currently available manufactured stent-grafts. Figure 3 gives an example of patient with severely angulated proximal neck treated with a bifurcated stent-graft who developed proximal end migration with large type I endoleak. Insertion of an aorto-iliac Aorfix stent-graft allowed to treat this patient successfully.

TORTUOUS ILIAC ARTERIES

Tight angulation of iliac arteries may lead to intraoperative or early/late postoperative complications in a number of patients. It may be useful to distinguish difficulties with stent-graft delivery and/or retrieval of delivery system from stent-graft limb stenosis or thrombosis.

The effect of iliac tortuosity on either difficulty is directly related to the amount of calcification of the artery. The less calci-

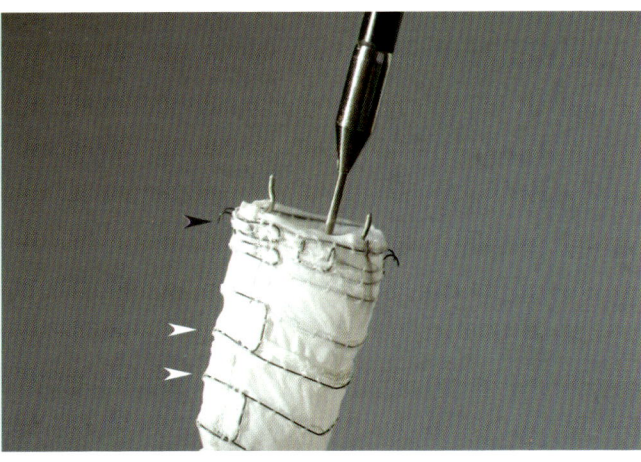

FIGURE 2: Detail of the proximal end of an Aorfix stent-graft showing circular nitinol rings (*white arrow*) and double fixation hooks (*black arrow*).

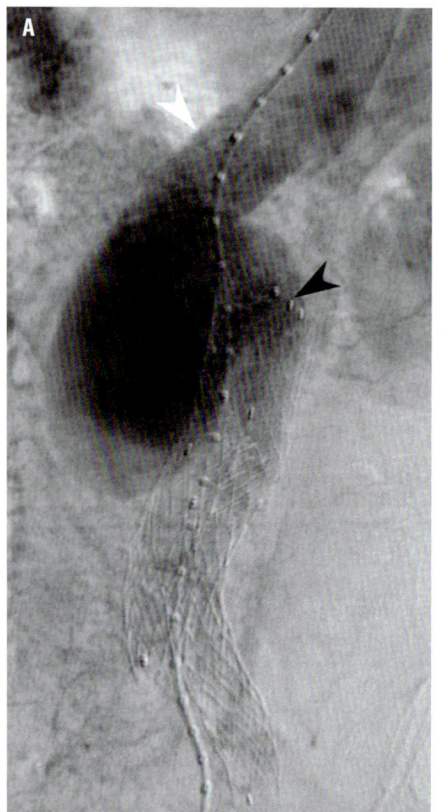

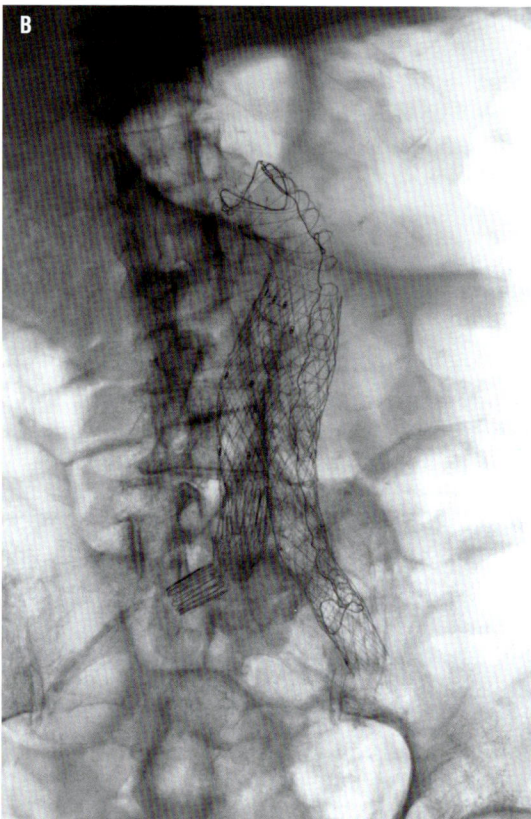

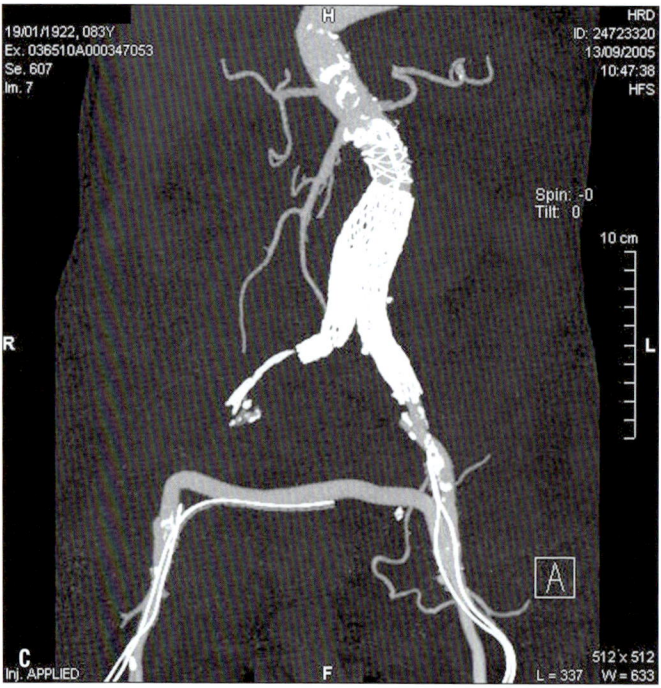

FIGURE 3: Patient previously treated with bifurcated stent-graft who developed proximal migration. Note the severe angulation at the proximal neck (*black arrow*) and the top end of the stent-graft which has migrated at the back of the aneurysm sac (**A**). Aorto-uni-iliac Aorfix stent-graft allowed to treat the patient successfully. Note the even curvature of the stent-graft along the aneurysm neck (**B**) and the absence of endoleak (**C**).

fied the artery the less the effect of tortuosity and vice-versa.

Difficulty in introduction of the delivery system may occur in case of tortuous iliac system. Using ultra-stiff guide-wires as described above is effective in the vast majority of patients. Brachio-femoral stiff wires have been described but their use is very rare. Stretching the iliac artery by a "pull-down maneuver" from the groin have been described by Parodi,[13] but again, in our practice this maneuver is usually not required. When it is not possible to get the delivery system through the external iliac arteries, a Dacron ilio-femoral bypass may be performed and used as a conduit to introduce the stent-graft delivery sheath.

Limb stenoses due to iliac angulation have been observed with most current stent-grafts. They may lead to claudication and/or acute ischemia in case of limb occlusion. They are usually treated with additional iliac stenting (Figure 4). Again, flexible stent-graft may reduce the incidence of kinking at the level of tight angulations.

Introduction of large delivery sheath (>20 F) in small diameter and tortuous external iliac arteries (<7 mm) may result in dissection. These are treated by using uncovered stent as soon as the diagnosis is made.

Severe tortuosities of common iliac arteries may have an impact on the accuracy of stent-graft limb positioning at the level of the iliac bifurcation. Inaccurate positioning of the C-arm regarding to the axis of the artery may lead to parallax errors. A very tortuous artery usually concertina when straightened by a stiff guide wire. Improper placement of the distal end of the iliac limb may lead to inadvertent coverage of internal iliac artery or distal type I endoleak. Such complications may be avoided by proper C-arm orientation. Also, the use of 4 F straight catheters positioned in common iliac arteries just above the iliac bifurcation allows to check the position of the iliac bifurcation while the delivery sheath is inserted and while the limb is deployed.

As for any type of iliac related anticipated difficulty, it is most often possible to perform aorto-uni-iliac stent-graft opposite to the tortuous iliac together with contralateral iliac occlusion and femoral crossover graft.

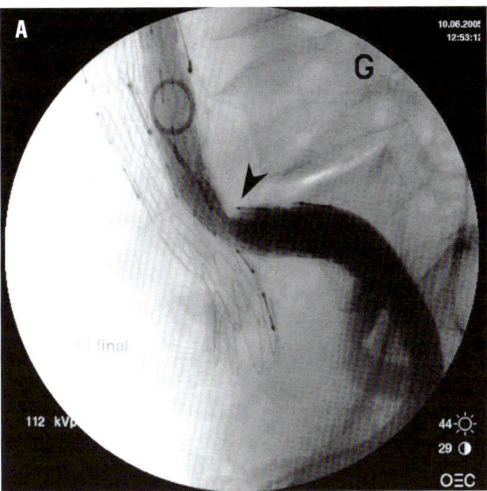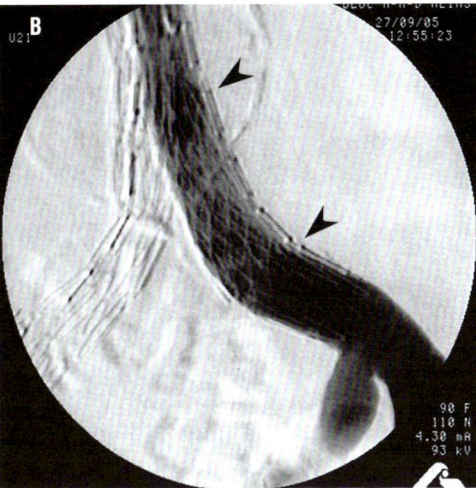

FIGURE 4: Gianturco-stented bifurcated stent-graft with kinking of the middle portion of the left iliac limb (**A**). This lesion was treated successfully with a balloon expandable stent (**B**).

Conclusion

Angulated proximal aneurysm neck remains a challenge as it carries a major risk of type I endoleak. Tortuous iliac arteries may lead to difficulties in introduction of delivery sheath and kinking of endograft limb. Careful preoperative evaluation allows to identify these features and prevent the potentially severe associated complications. Flexible stent-grafts may improve the feasibility and outcome of EVAR in patients with such difficult anatomy.

References

1. Rockman CB, Lamparello PJ, Adelman MA, et al. Aneurysm morphology as a predictor of endoleak following endovascular aortic aneurysm repair: do smaller aneurysm have better outcomes? Ann Vasc Surg 2002; 16:644-51.
2. Albertini JN, Kalliafas S, Travis S, et al. Anatomical risk factors for proximal perigraft endoleak and graft migration following endovascular repair of abdominal aortic aneurysms. Eur J Vasc Endovasc Surg 2000; 19:308-12.
3. Albertini JN, Macierewicz JA, Yusuf SW, et al. Pathophysiology of proximal perigraft endoleak following endovascular repair of abdominal aortic aneurysms: A study using a flow model. Eur J Vasc Endovasc Surg 2001; 22:53-6.
4. Sternbergh WC 3rd, Carter G, York JW, et al. Aortic neck angulation predicts adverse outcome with endovascular abdominal aortic aneurysm repair. J Vasc Surg 2002; 35:482-6.
5. Choke E, Munneke G, Morgan R, et al. Outcomes of endovascular abdominal aortic aneurysm repair in patients with hostile neck anatomy. CardioVasc Intervent Radiol 2006; 29:975-80.
6. Dias NV, Resch T, Malina M, et al. Intraoperative proximal endoleaks during AAA stent-graft repair. Evaluation of risk factors and treatment with Palmaz stents. J Endovasc Ther 2001; 8:268-73.
7. Cox DE, Jacobs DL, Motaganahalli RL, et al. Outcomes of endovascular AAA repair in patients with hostile neck anatomy using adjunctive balloon-expandable stents. Vasc Endovasc Surg 2006;40:35-40.
8. Kalliafas S, Albertini JN, Macierewicz J, et al. Incidence and treatment of intra-operative technical problems during endovascular repair of complex abdominal aortic aneurysms. J Vasc Surg 2000;31: 1185-92.
9. Kolvenbach R, Lin J. Combining laparoscopic and endovascular techniques to improve the outcome of aortic endografts. Hybrid techniques. J Cardiovasc Surg 2005; 46:415-23.
10. Hinchliffe RJ, Macierewicz JA, Hopkinson BR. Early results of a flexible bifurcated endovascular stent-graft (Aorfix). J Cardiovasc Surg 2004; 45:285-91.
11. Albertini JN, De Masi MA, Macierewicz JA, et al. The Aorfix stent-graft for abdominal aortic aneurysms reduces the risk of type I endoleak in angulated necks: a bench test study. Vascular 2005; 13:321-6.
12. Albertini JN, Perdikides T, Soong CV, et al. Endovascular repair of abdominal aortic aneurysms in patients with severe angulation of the proximal neck using a flexible stent-graft: European multicenter experience. J Cardiovasc Surg 2006.
13. Parodi JC. Endovascular repair of abdominal aortic aneurysms and other arterial lesions. J Vasc Surg 1995; 21:549-57.

When to use the aortouniiliac configuration

*Nikolaos Melas, Nikolaos Saratzis, Athanasios Saratzis
Dimitrios Kiskinis*

INTRODUCTION

It is now well established that endovascular repair (EVAR) of abdominal aortic aneurysms (AAA) is feasible (EVAR Trial I[1] and DREAM[2]), efficacious and has considerable short-term benefits over conventional open surgery (duration of operation, blood loss, length of hospital and internal care unit stay, QOL, 30-day mortality and morbidity).[1-5,25] Moreover, mid-term results of EVAR are sufficiently encouraging to justify the choice of the procedure, especially in patients at high surgical risk[24-27,43-46] (as far as the long term results are concerned, the verdict is still unclear).[23,47-50] In certain cases, though, endografting with a bifurcated endoprosthesis is contraindicated due to various anatomical restrictions.[9,10] In those patients, the deployment of an aortouniiliac endograft –followed by a femorofemoral crossover bypass, could overcome the anatomical limitations and successfully exclude the aortic pathology.[6,7,11,18-21]

DEFINITIONS

An aortouniiliac (AUI) endograft is a tapered unibody stent-graft with a gradually decreasing diameter from the top to the bottom. It is proximally attached in a manner that allows free blood flow to both renal arteries. The covered distal end is inserted into a single common iliac artery, excluding blood flow to the opposite iliac vessel. In order to avoid type II endoleak from the contralateral axis towards the aneurysmal sac, the contralateral common iliac artery must be obliterated with a short occluding graft (occluder). In order to provide blood flow to both lower limbs, an extra-anatomical femoro-femoral or ilio-femoral cross-over bypass follows the grafting procedure.

INDICATIONS

The indications for EVAR using the AUI configuration are the following:

1. **Narrow terminal aorta** (diameter <15 mm), since in such a narrow space the contralateral leg of a bifurcated endograft would lack adequate space for safe deployment with sequential narrowing and future thrombosis of one leg. Moreover catheterization of the contralateral leg through a narrow space would be very difficult).
2. **Contralateral common iliac artery angle >90°** from the longitudinal axis of the aneurysm.[42] This anatomy could

cause kinking of the contralateral leg of a bifurcated endograft and future thrombosis (Figure 1).

3. **Heavily calcified contralateral external iliac artery**, which could cause difficulty in advancing and deploying the contralateral leg of a bifurcated endograft and probably lead to leg thrombosis. On the contrary, the sheath of the occluder is usually smaller in diameter, enabling easier passage. (Relative indication).

4. **Narrow contralateral common iliac artery** (diameter <5 mm with or without PTA). The sheath of the occluder (usually smaller in diameter) is advanced only up to the common iliac artery and not across the terminal aorta. (Relative indication).

5. **Obstructed contralateral common iliac artery**.

6. **Concomitant ecstatic or frankly aneurysmal common iliac arteries**. In such circumstances the AUI graft could land in the less aneurysmal common iliac artery, while the occluder could be deployed in the ecstatic one (diameter of the occluder comes up to 25 mm.[22] (Relative indication).

7. **Isolated infrarenal abdominal aortic dissections**. The AUI endograft is deployed in the true lumen while the occluder obstructs the contralateral iliac axis (Figure 2).

8. **A combination of the previous indications**.

9. **Conversion of a bifurcated endograft to AUI** due to impossible contralateral limb catheterization.

10. **Ruptured AAA (emergency EVAR)**, the AUI configuration is easier and considerably less time consuming (Figure 3).

CONTRAINDICATIONS

The contraindications for AUI graft implantation are the following:

1. Proximal neck <10 mm in length (device depended).
2. Proximal neck >32 mm in diameter (device depended).
3. Proximal neck thrombus >30% of the perimeter.
4. Bilateral common iliac arteries >18 mm in diameter with indispensable internal iliac arteries (device depended).
5. Excessive bilateral iliac artery tortuosity greater than 90° (Figure 4).
6. Excessive bilateral iliac artery calcification.
7. Indispensable IMA.
8. General contraindications for every endovascular procedure: age <18, allergy to contrast medium, coagulopathy, pregnancy-lactation, creatinine level >1.7 mg/dl, groin infection and connective tissue disease.

Whenever a bifurcated endograft is implantable the AUI configuration should be avoided, as it involves an extra-anatomical by-pass.

PREOPERATIVE MANAGEMENT

Preoperative abdominal iv-contrast enhanced computed tomography (CT) scan (aortography) with 3D reconstruction including groin slices, is the standard practice. The exact anatomical measurements of the proximal and distal landing zones (diameter and length), the aortic and iliac arteries tortuosity and the inner diameters of the access vessels should be determined in all cases. In patients with impaired renal function (creatinine level ≥1.7 mg/dl), a pre operative magnetic resonance angiography (MRA) scan should be obtained instead of contrast enhanced CT.

PROCEDURE

The patient is set on supine position on a

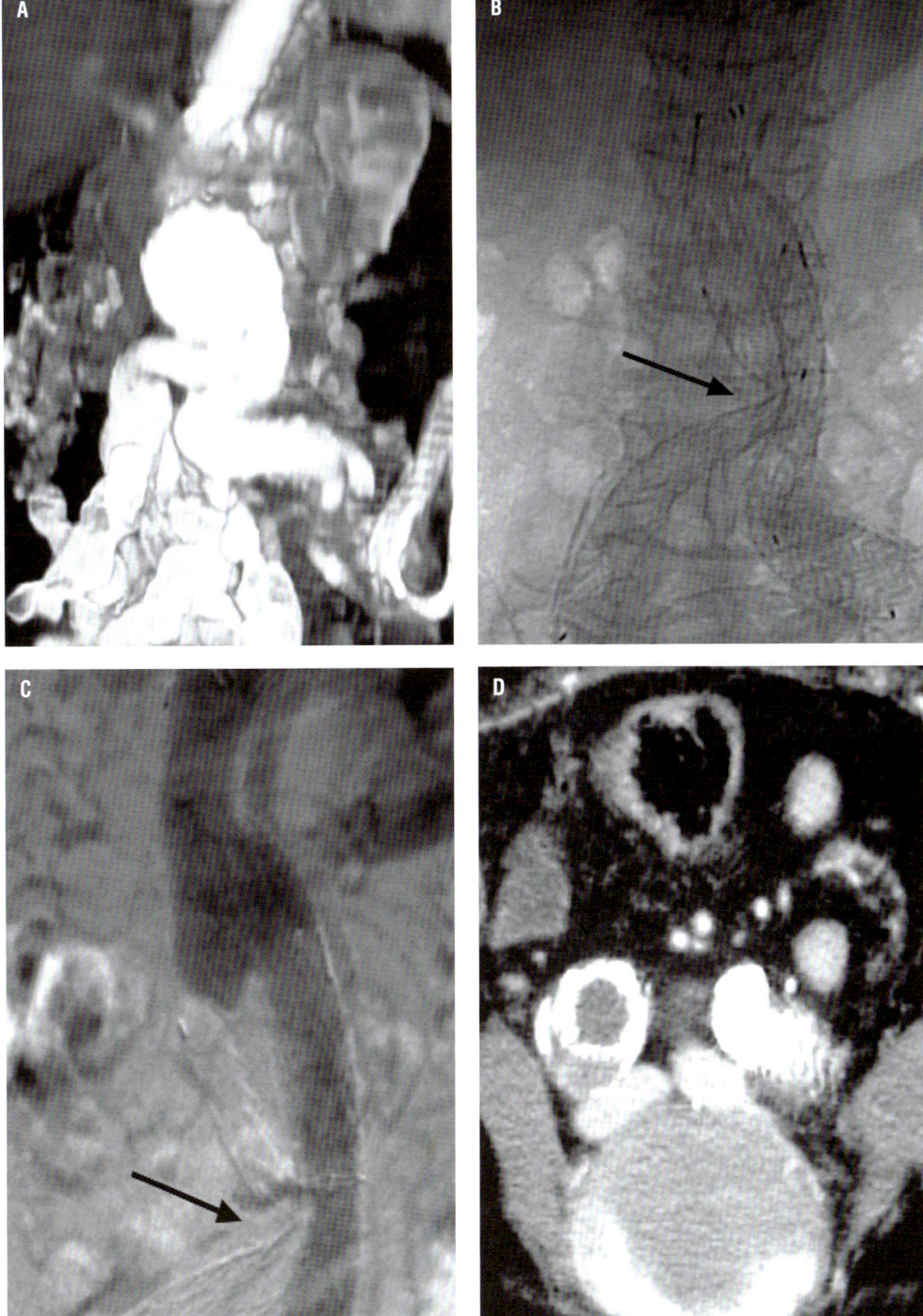

FIGURE 1: Right iliac leg thrombosis of a bifurcated endograft. The morphology of the AAA includes narrow terminal aorta and high degree iliac tortuousity (**A**). The previous morphology caused kinking of the right leg (**B**) and subsequent thrombosis (**C**, **D**). The complication probably could be avoided if a left AUI was implanted.

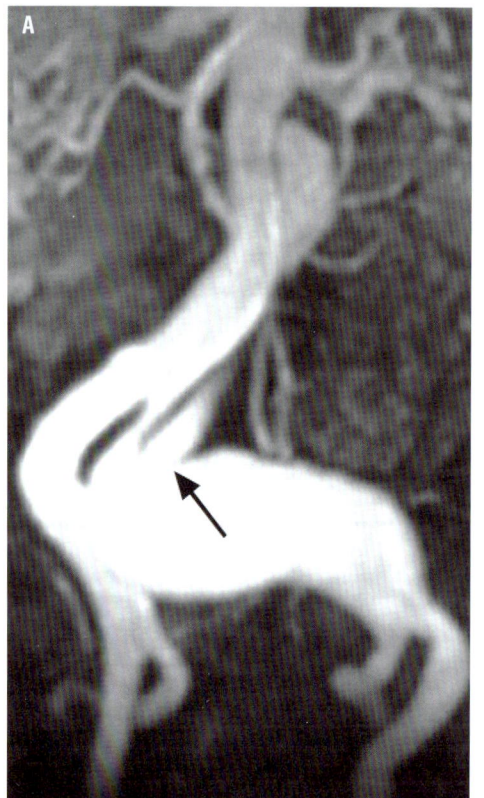

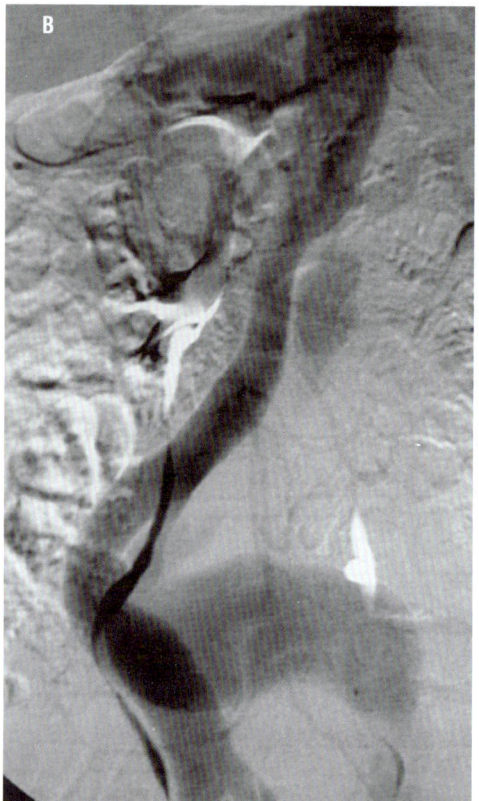

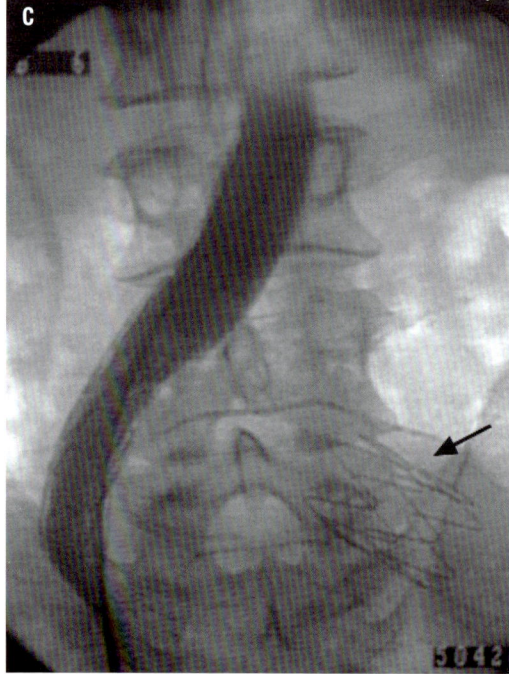

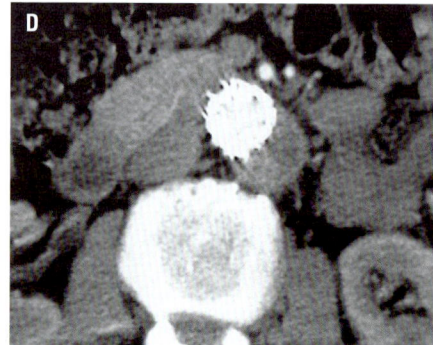

FIGURE 2: Isolated infrarenal abdominal aortic dissection repaired with a right AUI. (**A**) Preoperative MRA, (**B**) initial intraoperative angiography, (**C**) Completion angiography, the black arrow shows the occluder, (**D**, **E**) postoperative CT showing thrombosis of the false lumen and (**F**) patency of left external iliac artery.

(continued to next page)

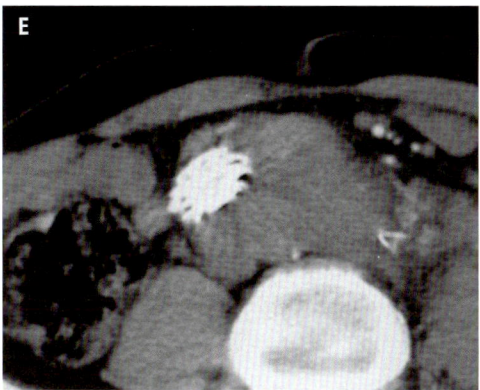
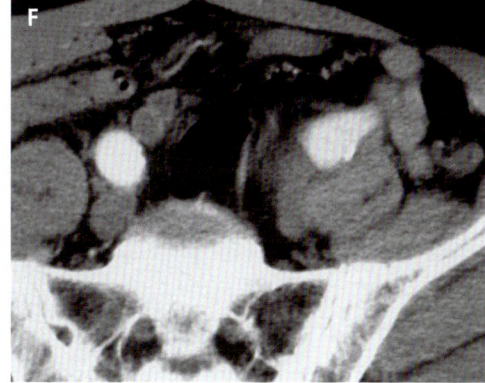

FIGURE 2: *(continued)*

radiolucent floating surgical table, in an operating room equipped with a portable C-arm. Standard patient monitoring, include ECG and pulse pressure should be available. All manipulations are carried out under regional or general anesthesia. The femoral arteries are bilaterally exposed in standard fashion. The ipsilateral common femoral artery is catheterized using a Seldinger needle and a 7 or 8 Fr short sheath is introduced into the vessel. Heparin (100 IU/Kg) is administered intravenously. A hydrophilic guide wire is advanced, under fluoroscopic control, in order to track the iliac axis. A guiding catheter is inserted over the guide-wire and the latter is ex-

changed for a stiff 0.035″, 260 cm long guide-wire. The contralateral common femoral artery is catheterized and the initial guide-wire is advanced beyond the renal arteries. A long (45 cm) 7 Fr sheath is then introduced over the wire. An initial angiogram (20 cc contrast medium) confirms the exact orifice of the lower renal artery. An additional angiogram obtained from the ipsilateral short sheath (20 cc contrast medium) confirms the position of the ipsilateral internal iliac artery. The ipsilateral short sheath is removed and the 18-22 Fr introducer sheath (with the preloaded endoprosthesis) is advanced, under fluoroscopic control. The bare proxi-

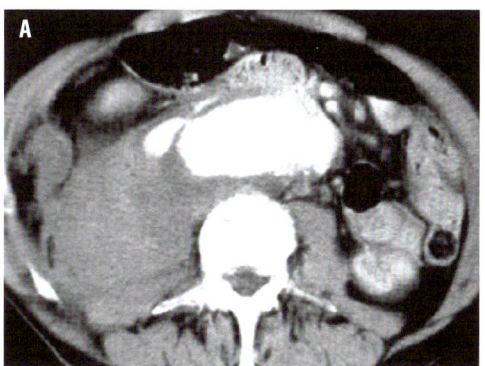
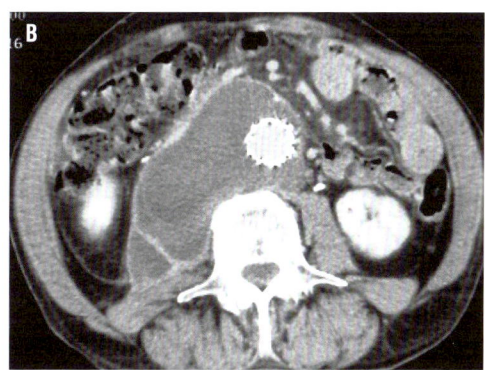

FIGURE 3: Ruptured AAA repaired successfully with an AUI Endofit stentgraft.

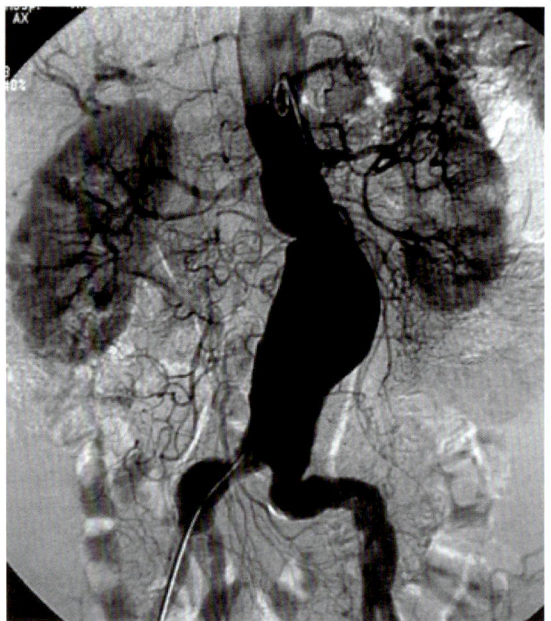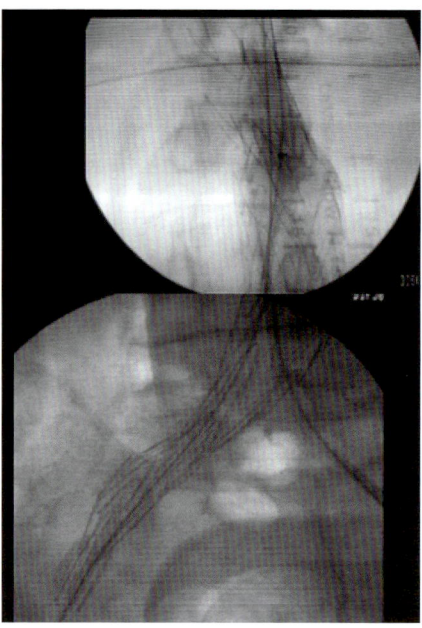

FIGURE 4: From left to right: Initial angiogram (note the excessive left common iliac tortuosity), AUI graft deployment.

mal stent is positioned precisely above the orifice of the lower renal artery. The graft is deployed upon withdrawal of the introducer sheath. During deployment, angiography is obtained from the contralateral axis through the contralateral sheath, which is withdrawn precisely below the aneurismal neck – inside the aneurysmal sac. The systemic blood pressure is lowered to 90 mmHg during deployment to ensure accurate positioning.

The graft is distally sealed upon a non-aneurysmal segment of the ipsilateral common iliac artery. In case the orifice of the ipsilateral hypogastric artery is involved in the aneurysm, the occlusion of the vessel is unavoidable. The graft is then distally attached into the external iliac artery, usually by interposing an extension. In some cases, preoperative coil embolization of the aneurysmal internal iliac artery is necessary in order to avoid a type II endoleak after the deployment of the AUI graft. In order to increase proximal and distal affixation, balloon inflation of the attachment or

the overlapping zones should follow the grafting procedure in selected cases. An angiography through the contralateral femoral artery (20 cc contrast medium) reveals the exact configuration of the contralateral iliac axis. Once the initial sheath has been removed, a 12-18 Fr introducer sheath is inserted and the "occluder" is advanced to the contralateral common iliac artery under fluoroscopic control. A new angiography through the contralateral femoral artery should confirm the absence of endoleak from the occluder. A completion angiogram (20 cc contrastmedium) from the ipsilateral axis should be performed to confirm the absence of endoleak, migration, stenosis, kinking or other procedure-related complication.

Upon completion of the procedure, the sheaths and wires are removed and an 8 mm ring re-inforced PTFE graft is sutured from the ipsilateral to the contralateral common femoral artery in standard fashion, to provide blood flow to the contralateral axis.

Aspirin is administered the same day, clopidogrel is added on the 1st postoperative day and the patient is mobilized on the 2nd postoperative day. A plain abdominal radiogram is performed to image the graft integrity and positioning. The patient is usually released on the 3rd postoperative day. The post-operative follow-up should include plain chest radiograms (assesed for frame integrity and possible graft migration) and iv contrast enhanced computed tomography scans which should be compared to the pre-operative slices in terms of sac diameter and volume. In case of endoleak, digital subtractive angiography should be performed in order to clarify the type and the extent of the endoleak.

ADVANTAGES AND DISADVANTAGES OF THE PROCEDURE

The aorto-uni-iliac configuration was initially reported by May et al,[6] Parodi et al,[56] and Marin et al[57] using a balloon-expandable stent-graft (proximal graft affixation) and a distal anastomosis of the graft to the iliac artery.

Recognized advantages of the AUI configuration include the ease of device deployment and the absence of modular interface requirements and their potential pitfalls. The AUI configuration is favored in patients presented with ruptured aneurysms[62] as the rapid exclusion of the aneurismal sac is of great importance. The AUI graft is deployed in considerably less time as there is no need for contralateral catheterization and deployment of the contralateral leg of the graft. The disadvantages of this configuration include the potential drawbacks of the femoro-femoral bypass (poor late patency and infection), and the development of thigh or buttock claudication when the pelvic blood flow has been affected. Further oc-

casional difficulties with therapeutic contralateral iliac occlusion, e.g. endoleak, may occur.

COMPLICATIONS OF THE PROCEDURE

Patency of the femoro-femoral crossover by-pass

Some authors were reluctant concerning the applicability of the technique, claiming that the femoro-femoral crossover bypass patency rates are quite poor, influencing the durability of the endo-graft. Various publications referring to femoro-femoral crossover by-pass demonstrated a 5-year patency rate ranging from 35%[12] to 92%.[13,14,28-35] Moreover, aorto-bifemoral bypass was considered to be the gold standard for aortoiliac occlusive disease, showing patency rates that greatly exceeded those of the femoro-femoral bypass configuration.[12,14,36,37] AUI endografting, though, followed by femoro-femoral crossover bypass is usually applied in patients with aneurysmal disease who are typically not presented with occlusive peripheral arterial disease (PAD). A series of publications[16-22] evaluating the patency rates of femoro-femoral crossover bypass adjunctive to AUI endografting, report increased patency, ranging from 91% at 3 years[15] to 99% at 4 years.[41]

The patency of femorofemoral crossover bypass may be affected by the occlusion of the superficial femoral artery[12,38] and the poor runoff in the infrapopliteal arteries.[39,40]

Hinchliffe RJ et al[15] reported that 10 patients with a femoro-femoral bypass occlusion were presented with a coexistent occlusion of the aortic endograft. The poor in-flow from the kinked or stenotic AUI graft is a primary cause for femorofemoral graft thrombosis. The iliac limb of the endograft was deployed in the external iliac artery in 5 of those 10 patients. In a report of the failure of endovascular aortic limbs, the aortouniiliac grafts (97%) appeared to have superior patency rates at 18 months compared with the bifurcated grafts (90%); however, the results did not reach statistical significance.[63] Fully stented endograft limbs appear to offer improved patency over unsupported limbs, a result that may be related to superior kinking resistance.[63] Bifurcated endografts may be susceptible to occlusion of one iliac limb when both limbs compete for space in the presence of a narrow distal aorta. Graft limb thrombosis for bifurcated stent-grafts has been reported at the following rates: 7% at a mean of 11 months of follow-up by Stelter et al[64] and 5% at 7 months of follow-up by Faries et al.[65] The in-flow problems leading to early graft occlusion in the Hinchliffe et al[15] group were either due to instrumentation damage of the external iliac artery, a low flow state created by an unrecognized kinking of the endograft, or deployment of the endograft in a narrow external iliac artery. Carroccio et al[66] suggested that deployment of endografts in narrow external iliac arteries should be avoided. Occlusion of endografts extending into the external iliac arteries may be related to a number of factors, including gross graft-oversizing with inadequate deployment or crowding of graft material in the relatively narrow external iliac artery, low flow within a narrow external iliac artery or kinking of the endograft at the level of the angulation between the common and external iliac artery. Late occlusions were primarily associated with caudal migration and endograft kinking.[15]

Hinchliffe et al[15] demonstrated that there is no relationship between the incidence of complications and the type of graft material used for fem-fem by-pass, which corresponds to the findings of a recent large prospective randomized study of Dacron and PTFE bypass grafts.[67]

Conclusively, the patency rates of femoro-femoral bypass grafting for aneurysmal disease are generally superior to the rates that have been reported for arterial occlusive disease and comparable to aortobifemoral or bifurcated endovascular repair of AAA over the medium and long term. The patency of the femorofemoral bypass graft is ultimately related to the performance of the aortouniiliac endograft. Occlusion of the crossover graft may be prevented by paying particular attention to avert the damage caused by arterial sheaths and guidewires to the external iliac or common femoral artery, by preventing or treating the possible kinking of the iliac limbs, and by avoiding the deployment of endografts in narrow external iliac arteries.[15]

Local wound complications, graft infection and morbidity

Local wound complications, e.g. hematoma, seroma and superficial wound infection, are not necessarily related to the femorofemoral bypass and can just as easily be related to dissection of the common femoral artery. The reported rate of local groin complications after the deployment of a bifurcated endoprosthesis is 8.4%,[65] similar to the rate (11%) reported by Hinchliffe et al for AUI grafting.[15]

Yilmaz et al demonstrated that ever since they adopted the oblique incision for surgical exposure of the femoral arteries, they have performed 139 repairs without a single wound-related or graft-associated infection.[16]

It is interesting that infections of the femoro-femoral bypass grafts have not been associated with direct or indirect spread of the infection to the endograft.[15]

In conclusion, perioperative morbidity associated with aortouniiliac endovascular aneurysm repair and femorofemoral crossover is similar to that reported for bifurcated endovascular repair.[15]

PERSONAL EXPERIENCE

A wide variety of AUI endografts are currently commercially available in Europe and the US. Some incorporate stainless steel Gianturco Z-stents and others feature nitinol self-expanding stents. The grafts are tapered and some feature a bare proximal stent that enhances proximal affixation. In our department, we have gained noteworthy experience with the EndoFit AUI self-expanding stent-graft (Le Maitre Vascular, USA) which consists of a nitinol frame "sandwiched" between two layers of PTFE fabric and a proximal suprarenal bare stent. The device is either preloaded on the introducer sheath or it can be loaded on an empty sheath from its cartridge during the procedure.

During a period of two years, (January 2002-February 2004) we have treated 39 patients (36 males, mean age: 74 years; range: 68-84) at high surgical risk (ASA III+) with an AAA (33) or an AAA and a common iliac artery aneurysm (6), using the AUI configuration.[68] The mean aneurysmal diameter was 6.7 cm (range: 5-11 cm).The mean follow up was 14 months. The EndoFit (Le Maitre Vascular, USA) AUI device was deployed in all cases (size of the grafts deployed: 26-16 x 16 mm to 36-22 x 18 mm). An 8 mm PTFE ring reinforced graft was always used for the femoro-femoral cross-over by-pass [GORE ringed GoreTex graft (W.L. Gore & Associates Inc, Sparrow Av., Flagstaff, AZ, USA) in 6 cases, Seal ePTFE ringed Vascutek (Vascutek, Scotland) in 22 cases and Impra ePTFE ringed vascular graft (Bard Peripheral Vascular Inc., Tempe AZ) in 11 cases]. The contralateral iliac axis was obstructed using an endoluminal occluder. Patient selection and measurements were based on pre-op spiral iv contrast-enhanced CT angiography with 3d reconstrustion.

The exclusion of the AAA and the common iliac artery aneurysm was feasible in all cases (100% technical success). Eleven (28%) extensions were used, either for landing in the external iliac artery (the hypogastric artery was occluded in 6 cases) or when the main graft body was too short to reach the distal landing zone (5 cases). 35 procedures were conducted under regional anesthesia and 4 were conducted under general anesthesia. The mean operative time was 124 min (92-243 min) and the mean fluoroscopy time was 13 min (9-38 min). The mean amount of contrast medium used was 155 cc (100-280 cc) and the mean blood loss was 350 cc (180-670 cc). The mean pre-op serum creatinine level was 1.15 mg/dl while the mean post-op serum creatinine level was 1.22 mg/dl. The length of the hospital stay ranged from 4 to 11 days (mean 6 days) and the length of the ICU stay ranged from 12 to 72 hours (mean 20 hours). The ipsilateral internal iliac artery was intentionally occluded in 6 cases (15%) in order to accomplish safe distal attachment and sealing (a common iliac artery aneurysm was present in all cases). No deaths were reported during the follow-up. Endoleak occurred in three cases (7.7%-1 proximal type I endoleak, identified on the 1st month, treated with the deployment of a proximal cuff, 2 type II endoleaks currently under surveillance). Femorofemoral graft thrombosis occurred in one case during the immediate postoperative period, due to insufficient inflow caused by a residual stenosis of the endograft (the primary patency was 97.5%). The deficit was treated immediately with thrombectomy of the PTFE graft and balloon dilatation of the endograft (the secondary patency was 100%). A tunnel hematoma occurred in 2 cases and was treated conventionally (5.1%). Superficial infection and lymphorrhea were identified in 2 cases (5.1%), treated conventionally. Graft migration, graft infection, paraplegia, distal embolization or any other serious complications were not observed.

During the 5 year period from 2002 to 2007, 70 selective patients were treated with the AUI configuration, with a mean follow up 36 months. 18 patients were treated for a ruptured AAA. The results are still under evaluation. Primary clinical findings are promising.

CONCLUSION

AUI endografting followed by a femoro-femoral crossover bypass is feasible, efficacious and has proven high mid-term patency rates. It should be applied in high risk patients and when the deployment of a bifurcated endoprosthesis is contraindicated, as it utilizes an extra-anatomical bypass (with potential complications) and because long-term results are yet to be confirmed.

REFERENCES

1. Comparison of endovascular aneurysm repair with open repair in patients with AAA (EVAR trial 1), 30-day operative mortality results: randomized control trial: The Lancet Sep 4, 2004 (364):843-848.
2. Frank A. Lederle, M.D. Abdominal Aortic Aneurysm - Open versus Endovascular Repair. New England Journal of Medicine October 14, 2004 Volume 351 Number 16:1677-1679.
3. Chuter TA et al. Endovascular aneurysm repair in high risk patients. JVS 2000;31(1 pt 1):122-33
4. Carpenter JP et al. Durability of benefits of endovascular versus conventional AAA repair. JVS 2002;35:222-8.
5. Faries PL et al. A multicenter experience with the Talent endovascular graft for the treatment of AAA. JVS 2002;35:1123-8.
6. May J, White G, Waugh R et al. Treatment of complex aortic aneurysms by a combination of endoluminal and extraluminal aortofemoral grafts. JVS 1994;19:924-33.
7. Parodi JC, Palmaz JC, Barone HD. Transfemoral intraluminalgraft implantation for AAA. Ann Vasc Surg 1991.
8. Treiman GS et al. An assessment of the current aplicability of the EVT endovascular graft for treatment of patients with infrarenal AAA. JVS 1999;30:68-75.
9. Carpenter JP et al. Impact of exclusion criteria on patient selection for EVAR. JVS 2001;34:1050-55
10. Arko FR, et al. How many patients with infrarenal aneurysms are candidates for endovascular repair. The Nothern California experience. JEVT, 2004;11: 33-40.
11. Chuter TA et al. Aortouniiliac endovascular grafting combined with femorofemoral by-pass: an acceptable compromise or a preferred solution? Semin Vasc Surg 1999;12:176-81.
12. Piotrowski JJ et al. Aortobifemoral by pass: the operation of choice for unilateral iliac occlusion ? JVS 1988;8:211-8.
13. Lamerton AJ et al. The femorofemoral graft: hemodynamic improvement and patency rate. Arch Surg 1985;120:1274-8.
14. Plecha F et al. Femorofemoral by grafts: ten-year experience. JVS 1984;1:555-61.
15. Hinchliffe RJ et al. Durability of femorofemoral bypass grafting after AUI endovascular aneurysm repair. JVS 2003;38(3):498-503.
16. Yilmaz PK et al. Is cross femoral bypass grafting a disadvantage of AUI endovascular aortic aneurysm repair? JVS 2003;38(4):753-7.
17. Walker SR et al. Early complications of femoro-femoral crossover bypass grafts after AUI endovascular repair of abdominal aortic aneurysms. JVS 1998;28:647-50.
18. Yusuf SW et al. Early results of endovascular aortic aneurysm surgery with AUI graft, contralateral iliac occlusion and femorofemoral bypass. JVS 1997;25:162-172.
19. Thompson MM et al. AUI endovascular grafting: difficult solutions to difficult aneurysms. J Endovasc Surg 1997;4:174-181.
20. Rehring TF, Brewster DC, Cambria RP, et al. Utility and reliability of endovascular Aortouniiliac with femorofemoral crossover graft for aortoiliac aneurysmal disease. JVS 2000;31:1135-1141.
21. Moore WS et al. AUI endograft for complex aortoiliac aneurysms compared with tube bifurcated endogrsfts: results of the EVT trials. JVS 2000;33 (suppl):S 11-20.
22. Clouse WD et al. Durability of aortouniiliac endo-

grafting with femorofemoral crossover: 4-year experience in the EVT/Guidant trials. JVS 2003;37: 1142-1150.

23. Harris P, Vallabhaneni SR, Desgranges P, et al. For the EUROSTAR Collaborators. Incidence and risk factors of late rapture and death after endovascular repair of infrarenal aortic aneurysm: the EUROSTAR experience. JVS 2000;32:739-49.

24. Brewster DC, Cronenwett JL, Hallett JW, et al. Quidelines for treatment of AAA. JVS 2003;37: 1106-17.

25. Lee AW, Carter JW, Upchurch G, et al. Perioperative outcomes after open and endovascular repair of intact AAA in the USA during 2001. JVS 2004; 39:491-6.

26. Rutherford RB, Krupski WC. Current status of open versus endovascular stent-graft repair of abdominal aortic aneurysm. JVS 2004;39:1129-39.

27. Carpenter JP, Baum RA, Barker CF, et al. Durability of benefits of endovascular versus conventional AAA repair. JVS 2002;35:222-8.

28. Flaningan DP, Pratt DG, Goodreau JJ, et al. Aortofemoral or femorofemoral revascularization? Aprospective evaluation of the papaverine test. Arch Surg 1978;113:1257-62.

29. Eugene J, Goldstone J, Moore WS. Fifteen year experience with subcutaneous bypass grafts for lower extremity ischemia. Ann Surg 1977;186: 177-83.

30. Brief DK, Brener BJ. Extra-anatomic bypasses: femorofemoral crossover grafts in Wilson SE, Veith FJ, Hobson RW, William RA (eds): Vascular surgery Principals and practice. New York, Mc Graw-Hill, 1987, pp 415- 418.

31. Dick LS, Brief DK, Alpert J, et al. 12- year experience with femorofemoral crossover grafts. Arch Surg 1980;115:1359-65.

32. Mosley JG, Marston A: long term results of 66 femorofemoral bypass grafts: 9-year follow up. Br J Surg 1983;70:631-634.

33. Maini BS, Mannick JA: Effect of arterial reconstruction on limb sulvage: a ten - year appraisal. Arch Surg 1978;113:1297-1304.

34. Criado E, Burnhum SJ, Tinsley EA, et al. Femorofemoral bypass grafts: analysis of patency and factors influencing long term outcome. JVS 1993;18:495-505.

35. Mingoli A, Sapienza P, Feldhaus RJ, et al. Femo-

rofemoral bypass grafts: factors influencing long term patency rate and outcome. Surgery 2001; 129:451-8.

36. Sneider JR, Besso SR, Walsh DB et al. Femorofemoral versus aortobifemoral bypass: outcome and hemodynamic results. JVS 1994;19:43-57.

37. Self SB, Rchardson JD, Klamer DW et al. Utility of femorofemoral bypass. Comparison of results with indications for operations. Am Surg 1991; 57:602-6.

38. Komori K, Okadome K, Funahashi S, et al. Correlation of long-term results of extra-anatomic bypass and flow wave-form analysis. Eur J Vasc Surg 1993;7:479-82.

39. Tomson - Fawcett M, Moon M, Hands L, et al. The significance of donor leg distal runoff in femorofemoral bypass grafting. Aust NZ J Surg 1998;68;493-97.

40. Farber MA, Hollier LH, Eubanks R, et al. Femorofemoral bypass: a profile of graft failure. South Med J 1990;83:1437-43.

41. Lipsitz EC, Ohki T, Veith FJ, et al. Patency rates of femorofemoral bypass associated with endovascular aneurysm repair surpass those performed for occlusive disease. JEVT 2003;10:1061-65

42. Stanley BM, Semmens JB, Qun Mai BM, et al. Evaluation of patient selection guidelines for endoluminal AAA repair with the Zenith stent-graft: The Australian experience. J Endovasc Ther 2001; 8:457-464.

43. Moore WS, Kashyap VS, Vescera CL, et al. Abdominal Aortic Aneurysm: A 6-year comparison of endovascular versus transabdominal repair. Ann Surg 1999;230:298-308.

44. Zarins CK, White RA, Moll FL, et al. The AneuRX stent graft: 4-year results and worldwide experience 2000. JVS 2001;33:S135-45.

45. Dattilo JB, Brewster DC, Fan C-M, et al. Clinical failures of endovascular Abdominal Aortic Endograft repair: incidence, causes and management. JVS 2002;35:1137-44.

46. Clouse WB, Brewster DC, Marone LK, et al. Durability of Aortouniiliac endografting with femorofemoral crossover: 4-year experience in the EVT/Guidant trials. JVS 2003 in press.

47. Holzenbein TJ, Kretschmer G, Thurner S, et al. Midterm durability of Abdominal Aortic endograft repair: a word of caution. JVS 2001;33:S46-54.

48. Zarins CK, White RA, Fogarty TJ, et al. Aneurysm rupture after endovascular repair using AneuRX stent graft. JVS 2000;31:960-70.

49. Ohki T, Veith FJ, Shaw P, et al. Increasing incidence of midterm and longterm complications after endovascular graft repair of AAA: a note of caution based on a 9-year experience. Ann Surg 2001;234:323-35.

50. Bernhard VM, Mitchell RS, Matsumura JS, et al. Ruptured abdominal aortic aneurysm after endovascular repair. JVS 2002;35:1155-62.

51. Cardon JM, Cardon A, Joueux A, Vidal V, Noblet D. Endovascular repair of iliac artery aneurysm with endoprosystem I: a multicentric French study. J Cardiovasc Surg 1996;37:45-50.

52. Michel C, Laffy PY, Leblanc G, Angel CY, Riuou JY. Traitement Percutane d' anevrismes iliaques par endoprothese couvert. Jradiol 1996;77:433-436.

53. Mc Cready RA, Paizolero PC, Gilmore JC, et al. Isolated iliac artery aneurysm. Surgery 1983;93:688-93.

54. Richardson JW, Greenfield LJ. Natural history and management of iliac aneurysms. J Vasc Surg 1988;8:165-171.

55. R Mofid, P Otal, L Boyer, A Ravel, JM Garcier, H Rousseau. Common iliac aneurysms with short or absent proximal necks: Endoluminal repair with a covered endoprosthesis. Eur J Vasc Endovasc Surg 2003;26:334-336.

56. Parodi JC. Endovascular repair of abdominal aortic aneurysms and other arterial lesions. J Vasc Surg 1995;21;549-57.

57. Marin M L, Veith FJ, Cynamon J. Initial experience with transluminally placed endovascular grafts for the treatment of complex vascular lesions. Ann Surg 1995;22:449-69.

58. Treiman GS, Lawrence PF, Edwards WH Jr, Galt SW, Kraiss LW, Bhirangi K. An assessment of the current applicability of the EVT endovascular graft for treatment of patients with an infrarenal abdominal aortic aneurysm. J Vasc Surg 1999;30:68-75.

59. Armon MP, Yusuf SW, Latief K, Whitaker SC, Gregson RH, Wenham PW, et al. Anatomical suitability of abdominal aortic aneurysms for endovascular repair. Br J Surg 1997;84:178-180.

60. Balm R, Stokking R, Kaatee R, Blankensteijn JD, Eikelboom BC, van Leeuwen MS. Computed tomographic angiographic imaging of abdominal aortic aneurysms: implications for transfemoral endovascular aneurysm management. J Vasc Surg 1997;26:231-237.

61. Brewster DC. Do current results of endovascular abdominal aortic aneurysm repair justify more widespread use? Surgery 2002;131:363-367.

62. Ohki T, Veith F, Sanchez L, et al. Endovascular graft repair of ruptured aortoiliac aneurysms. J Am Coll Surg 1999;189:102-112.

63. Carpenter JP, Neschis DG, Fairman RM, et al. Failure of endovascular abdominal aortic aneurysm graft limbs. J Vasc Surg 2001;33:296-302.

64. Stelter W, Umscheid T, Zeigler P. Three year experience with modular stent-graft devices for endovascular AAA treatment. J Endovasc Surg 1997;4:362-9.

65. Faries PL, Brener BJ, Connelly TL, et al. A multicentre experience with the Talent endovascular graft for the treatment of abdominal aortic aneurysms. J Vasc Surg 2002;35:1123-8.

66. Carroccio A, Faries PL, Morrissey NJ, et al. Predicting iliac limb occlusions after bifurcated aortic stent grafting: anatomic and devicerelated causes. J Vasc Surg 2002;36:679-84.

67. Prager M, Polterauer P, Bohmig HJ, et al. Collagen versus gelatincoated Dacron versus stretch polytetrafluoroethylene in abdominal aortic bifurcation graft surgery: results of a seven-year prospective, randomized multicenter trial. Surgery 2001;130:408-14.

68. Saratzis N, Melas N, Lazaridis J, et al. Endovascular AAA Repair With the Aortomonoiliac EndoFit Stent-Graft: Two Years' Experience. J Endovasc Ther 2005;12:280-287.

Chapter 16

177

16. ENDOVASCULAR TREATMENT OF AAA WITHOUT AN ADEQUATE SEALING ZONE. FENESTRATED ENDOGRAFTS. SPECIFIC COMPLICATIONS AND MANAGEMENT

Endovascular treatment of AAA without an adequate sealing zone. Fenestrated endografts. Specific complications and management

Joseph F. Dowdall, Qingsheng Lu, Roy K. Greenberg

INTRODUCTION

Randomized-controlled trials such as the EVAR 1 trial and DREAM trials have established the safety and efficacy of endovascular repair using commercially available devices.[1-3] However, up to 50% abdominal aortic aneurysms may not be suitable for conventional endoluminal grafting, often for anatomical reasons.[4] The commonest of these is compromised proximal neck anatomy. The proximal neck is often dilated or conical indicating that it is part of the aneurysmal process. In most trials of endovascular aneurysm repair an increase in aortic diameter of 10% signifies the end of the proximal neck. Placing commercial endovascular devices into aneurysms with necks shorter than 15 mm may lead to increased risk of migration and type 1 endoleak.[5,6] The use of supra-renal stenting has been advocated to enhance proximal fixation, particularly when coupled with barbs,[7] and has been shown to have no detrimental effect on renal function.[6] However, an adequate region of proximal sealing is still required and must occur in the infrarenal position. If aneurysms in proximity to or involving impor-

tant branches are to be treated, clearly the branch vessels have to be preserved. Options include open repair with bypass/re-implantation of involved branches, hybrid procedures with preliminary bypasses to involved branches followed by endovascular stent placement[8] or finally the use of fenestrated or branched endografts to preserve the involved branches by endovascular stenting.

The concept of fenestration is to create holes in a stent-graft and line these up with branch vessels thus allowing the proximal fixation site of the graft to be moved upwards into a more healthy section of the aorta. This improves security of attachment and hemostatic sealing while maintaining perfusion of the branch vessels. Fenestration allows the technology of endovascular grafting to be applied to juxta-renal aneurysms, an area previously only amenable to open surgery, which often involved significant risk of renal failure and mesenteric ischaemia.[9,10]

HISTORY OF THE PROCEDURE

The first reports of fenestrated endografting

emerged in 1999 and were in animal models using home-made devices.[11,12] Shortly afterwards, there were initial human experiences of fenestrated grafting. These were small but successful. Anderson reported thirteen cases and 33 branch vessels.[13] Procedural success was 100%. No conversion to open operation or graft-related complications occurred. It was associated with no acute loss of branch vessels, and periprocedural mortality at 30 days was nil. At follow-up only one renal vessel had occluded. Stanley et al reported a series of three patients also without vessel loss or death.[14] The initial experience from the Cleveland Clinic[15] included 32 cases with a total of 83 visceral vessels stented. One patient died within 30 days following device implantation coupled with an attempted retroperitoneal internal to external iliac artery bypass, as a result of of aspiration pneumonia. Additional data have been published by group in Groningen, The Netherlands, where eighteen fenestrated grafts were implanted with 46 target vessels.[16] Forty-five of the intended branches were patent at the end of the procedure with only one possible proximal type I endoleak. Fenestrated grafts have also been employed to treat juxta-renal para-anastomotic aneurysms.[17] These and other early series indicated that successful fenestrated endovascular repair was possible in the hands of a limited number of skilled endovascular interventionalists but obviously did not indicate whether this may be possible on a more widespread basis.

An alternative technique of fenestrated grafting have been described. The Liverpool group has described a method of in-situ fenestration for the subclavian artery in a thoracic graft, whereby the graft is punctured with the back end of a guidewire, enlarged serially with cutting balloons and than stented.[18] Further data has been published regarding the use of fenestrations within thoracic endovascular grafts.[19]

The relative complexity of device planning and deployment execution has led to some skepticism about the dissemination of such a procedure. This, coupled with the fact that the devices are available on a restricted basis in Europe, Australia, and Canada and remain investigational in the United States, has resulted in experience concentrated in centers of excellence. However, the world experience with these devices is substantial, with greater than 1500 reported implants, by over 150 physicians. Detailed data is not available for most these implants, and the reports of intermediate-term results have been excellent, but restricted to a few ceneters.[4,16,19-21]

The primary issues with the use of these technologies are highlighted below. Much like other endovascular procedures employed to treat aortic pathology, close surveillance is mandatory. The early identification of visceral or branched vessel stenosis, device stability, inter-component relationships, and endoleaks are a few of the critical areas that need to be defined to determine long-term success. However, based on the data to date, failure, whether due to death, secondary interventions, device integrity, branch vessel patency issues, and complications seem to occur most commonly during the first year and then level off.[22] As the procedure matures, long-term results and randomized clinical trials will ultimately be required to determine the safety, efficacy, and stability of the procedure itself as well as devices. The other key question is whether this technique will achieve the same success outside the relatively small number of centers in which it has so far been performed. Device modifications which simplify the deployment process are likely to assist with this.

TECHNICAL ISSUES

The only fenestrated endograft at present

is the Zenith device (Cook, Bloomington, Ind). Currently in the USA the device is limited to investigational use but it was awarded a CE mark in 2005, and it is now available as a commercial device for sale in the European Union, Canada, Australia and New-Zealand. The design is similar to the standard Zenith device with stainless steel Gianturco stents sewn on to a woven polyester graft. There are two main components – a tubular component which contains the fenestrations and a bifurcate component which is similar to the standard Zenith device, with a variety of limb extensions (Figure 1). The device comes loaded in the familiar H & LB™ introducer

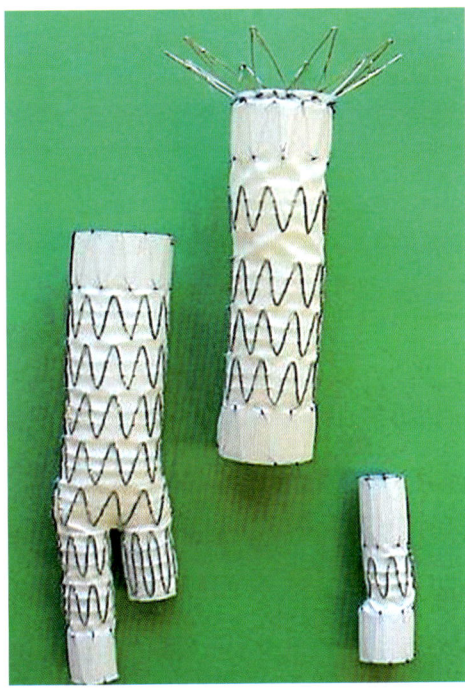

FIGURE 1: Fenestrated device. Reprinted with permission. This figure was published in Journal of vascular Surgery, Vol. 39; Roy K. Greenberg, Stephan Haulon, Sean P. Lyden, Sunita D. Srivastava, Adrian Turc, Matthew J. Eagleton, Timur P. Sarac, Kenneth Ouriel, Endovascular management of juxtarenal aneurysms with fenestrated endovascular grafting, pages 279-87. Copyright Elsevier (2004).

system with some significant modifications. On initial unsheathing of the stent-graft it remains constrained by posterior diameter-reducing ties (Figure 2), which allows the device to be manipulated partially deployed in the aorta so that the fenestrations can be accurately placed and canulated. There are also anterior and posterior gold markers as well as gold markers around the fenestrations and scallops to aid in orientation of the device (Figures 3a and b).

A small fenestration, with dimensions of 6 mm in width and 6 to 8 mm in height can be created a minimum of 15 mm inferior to the proximal aspect of the graft (Figure 3a). This type of fenestration has no crossing struts from the sealing stent and is intended to be used in conjunction with an additional balloon-expandable stent. Alternatively, a larger fenestration with a diameter between 9 and 12 mm can be created at least 10 mm below the top of the fabric. A portion of the large fenestration may be traversed by one or two of the struts of the proximal sealing Z-stent and, thus, is not typically used with an additional visceral vessel stent. Finally, a scallop, allowing the incorporation of one or more vessels, can be carved out of the proximal end of the fabric with a nominal width of 10 mm and a height ranging from 6 to 12 mm (Figure 3b). The location of the fenestrations and scallops are customized to fit individual patient anatomy.

Today, fenestrations are reinforced circumferentially with a nitinol ring. This helps to provide support such that a seal may be established between a balloon expandable stentgraft and the aortic device (Figure 4). This concept has provided a segway to treating aneurysms that involve (thoracoabdominal aneurysms), rather then aneurysms that simply abut the renal vessels (juxtarenal aneurysms). Alternative designs have been proposed to address aneurysms involving the visceral vessels. These focus on directional branches,

179

16. ENDOVASCULAR TREATMENT OF AAA WITHOUT AN ADEQUATE SEALING ZONE. FENESTRATED ENDOGRAFTS. SPECIFIC COMPLICATIONS AND MANAGEMENT

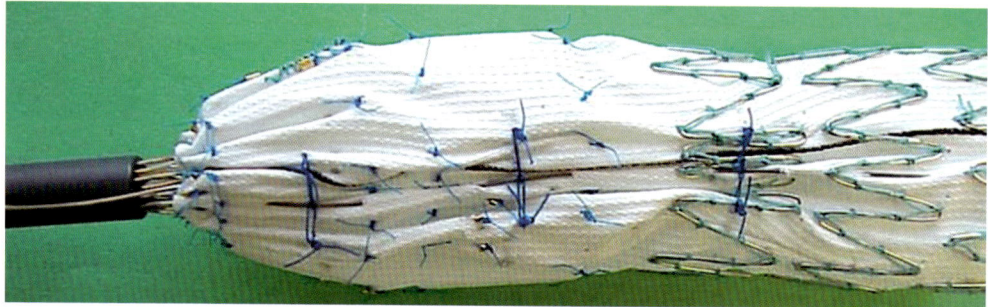

FIGURE 2: Posterior diameter-reducing ties. Reprinted with permission. This figure was published in Journal of vascular Surgery, Vol. 39; Roy K. Greenberg, Stephan Haulon, Sean P. Lyden, Sunita D. Srivastava, Adrian Turc, Matthew J. Eagleton, Timur P. Sarac, Kenneth Ouriel. Endovascular management of juxtarenal aneurysms with fenestrated endovascular grafting, pages 279-87. Copyright Elsevier (2004).

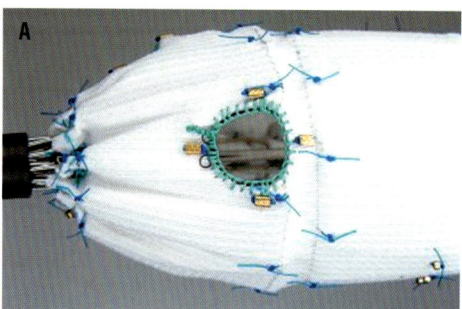

FIGURE 3: A. Small fenestration. **B**. Scallop.

where a portion of the graft material is formed into a branch in the direction of the target vessel. In such circumstances, the gap between the branch and the target vessel is crossed with a balloon expandable stent graft, rather than a simple uncovered stent. More complex designs have also been described[19,23] but are beyond the scope of this manuscript.

INDICATIONS

The generally accepted indications for fenestrated grafts are aneurysms with short, but not absent, necks (3-15 mm), i.e. juxtarenal aneurysms. It is important that the fenestrated vessels emerge from non-dilated aorta as the graft must be apposed to the aortic wall at the branch point to prevent leak. Necks that are heavily diseased in the region of the mesenteric vessels are generally felt not to be suitable for fenestrated grafts and are usually selected for branched grafts using reinforced fenestration or for directional branches.

SIZING

Each endograft is customized to accommodate for the patient specific anatomy as

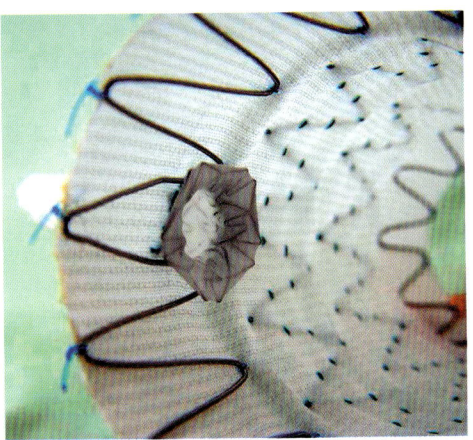

FIGURE 4: Reinforced fenestration with stent in-situ. Reprinted with permission. This figure was published in Journal of vascular Surgery, Vol. 43; Roy K. Greenberg, Karl West, Kathryn Pfaff, James Foster, Davorin Skender, Stephan Haulon, Jamie Sereika, Leslie Geiger, Sean P. Lyden, Daniel Clair, Lars Svensson, and Bruce Lytle. Beyond the aortic bifurcation: Branched endovascular grafts for thoracoabdominal and aortoiliac aneurysms, pages 879-86. Copyright Elsevier (2004).

assessed from the pre-operative high resolution CT scans. Angiography, magnetic resonance imaging, and intravascular ultrasound scanning may be used in selected patients but are not used routinely. Standard measurements are obtained (proximal and distal neck lengths and diameters, angulation, and aneurysm morphology). The use of a workstation with the availability of centerline of flow analysis (e.g. AquariusWS; Terarecon, San Francisco, CA) simplifies the planning process to such a degree that it is almost compulsory.

Anatomical inclusion guidelines include a neck diameter from 19-31 mm, angulation of less than 45 degrees, a 30 mm distal sealing zone on each side and access vessels of 7.5 mm or greater for delivery of the device. The configuration of the device comprising a proximal tubular component containing the fenestrations and a distal bifurcate component has several advantages. The tubular component

is easier than a bifurcate component to manipulate into accurate apposition with the branch vessels. The modular design also ensures that forces on the bifurcate component are uncoupled from the tubular component and the fenestrations by separation of the components, thus protecting the fenestrations from the effects of device migration.

As with conventional devices the outer diameter of the proximal component is oversized by 10-25% relative to the proximal implantation site. Next the fenestrated/seal zone must be planned. Clearly it is here that accuracy is of paramount importance (otherwise the fenestrations will not line up with their corresponding branches). The lowest aortic segment which will provide an adequate seal is chosen. The parallel sealing zone must be greater than 50% (preferably greater than 100%) of the proximal stent (21 or 26 mm in length depending on graft diameter) to create a parallel configuration of the sealing stent. Next the number of internal stents is chosen. There can be one or two – the advantage of the latter is to improve increase the potential seal as well as allow for later problem solving by providing a longer straight segment in the proximal neck prior to any device taper. However, this design lengthens the main body and, depending on overall infrarenal aortic length, may decrease the amount of overlap between the proximal and distal bifurcate components. This overlap is important in maintaining the integrity of the joint between the proximal tubular component and the distal bifurcate component. Next, the design of the fenestrated zone is chosen. Small fenestrations are generally used for the lowest vessels in a short neck (usually the renals). Scallops and large fenestrations are used for more proximal vessels. The ostial diameters of each vessel, their relative distances from the superior mesenteric artery, and orientations from which they arise from an aortic cross-section are recorded. Device design is intended to maximize the proximal sealing zone, accommodate native arterial angulation, and provide durable fixation. The areas of overlap between the tubular and bifurcate sections are intentionally long, preferably greater than 4 stents in length. The remainder of the design is similar to that for a conventional device.

OPERATIVE TECHNIQUE

After femoral artery exposure, patients are heparinized to maintain activated clotting times greater than 300 seconds for the duration of the procedure. A stiff wire is advanced into the aortic arch through the femoral artery on the intended side of delivery. Two sheaths are inserted through separate puncture sites into the contralateral femoral artery. A flush catheter is positioned immediately above the celiac artery through the contralateral femoral artery. An angled catheter is placed through the second sheath on the contralateral side and left at the level of the aortic bifurcation. The first (tubular) component is oriented, using radio-opaque markers, to accommodate the incorporated renal and visceral ostia and inserted over the stiff wire. Partial expansion of the device is then accomplished by sheath withdrawal, to reveal the first 2 covered stents (Figure 5). A further angiogram is performed at this point and the device is more accurately oriented. The graft is then fully exposed by complete withdrawal of the sheath. Diameter reducing ties cause posterior tethering and prevent complete expansion of the prostheses after sheath withdrawal. This allows additional adjustment of fenestration position by rotational and longitudinal movement.

Access to the partially expanded endograft is achieved through both of the contralateral femoral sheaths with the use of steerable catheter-guidewire systems. A

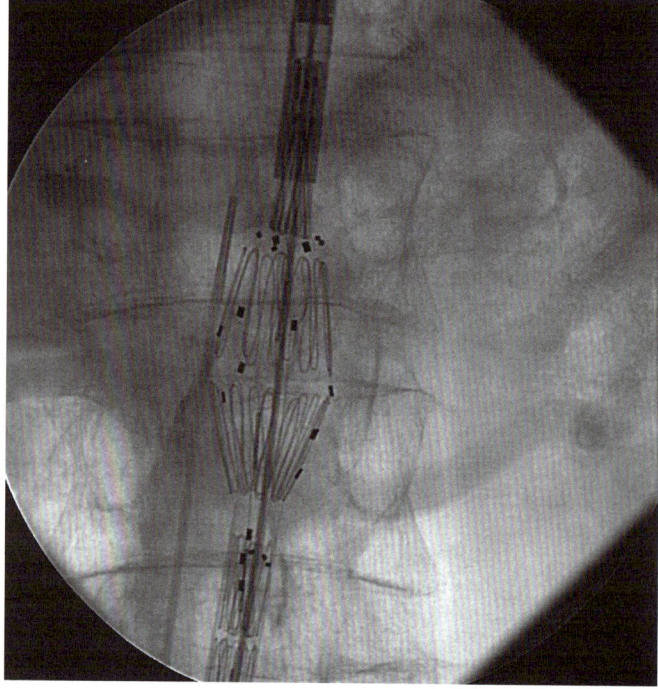

FIGURE 5: Partial expansion of the device. The left renal fenestration is perpendicular to the image intensifier and the markers overlie each other whereas the right renal fenestration can be seen to be oblique to the image intensifier.

minimum of two visceral vessels are then cannulated through the respective fenestrations from within the prosthesis. Guiding catheters or sheaths (8F Multipurpose B Lumex Guiding Catheter; Cook Inc or 6 or 7F Ansel Sheaths - Cook Inc.) are inserted over Rosen wires into both of the accessed fenestrations (Figure 6). The graft material is then fully expanded by removing the wire tethering the posterior aspect of the prosthesis. Relatively long (17- 24mm) balloon-expandable stents (Double Strut, EV3) or stentgrafts (Jomed, Abbott Labs, CA or Atrium, Boston Ma) are then used to stent the branch vessels. This is done such that approximately 2-3 mm of stent extends out into the aorta (Figure 7a). The visceral and renal stenting technique is modified to account for early bifurcations, ostial stenoses, and severe angulation. The aortic component of the balloon-expanded visceral stents is flared by further dilatation with a 10-12 mm balloon and then selectively flared with a compliant latex balloon. This maneuver 'rivets' the stent-graft to the aortic wall (Figure 7b). The top cap is retrieved while access to both stented vessels is maintained with the guiding catheters. The guiding catheters are removed after further angiography. The second (bifurcate) component of the system is then inserted through the ipsilateral femoral artery, oriented, and deployed such that the contralateral limb expands immediately above the aortic bifurcation. Contralateral access is then obtained through the most proximal of the contralateral sheaths, and the remainder of the deployment sequence is similar to the standard Zenith system. Compliant balloon inflation at all joints and distal sealing zones precede completion angiography. Routine CT scan prior to discharge is used to confirm device position, branch patency and absence of endoleak (Figure 8).

Cleveland Clinic Data

From 2001 onwards high-risk patients in

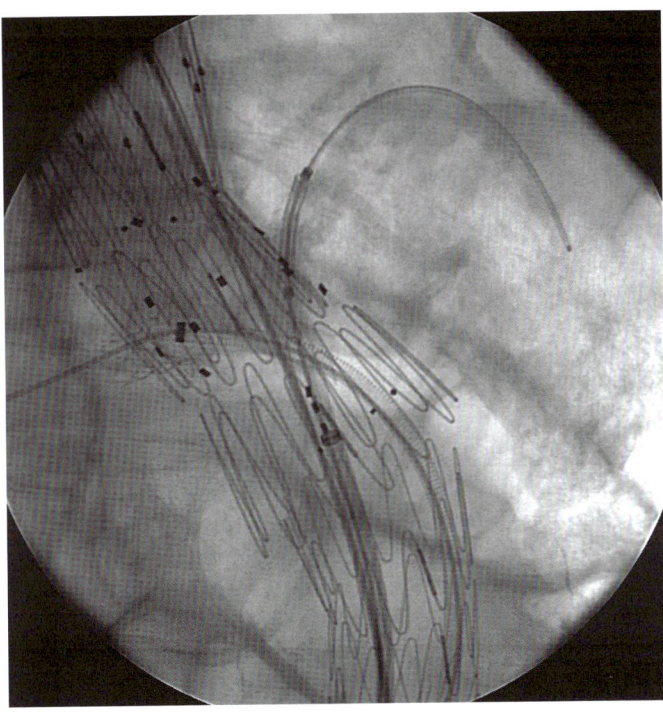

FIGURE 6: Deployed fenestrated tubular component with guiding catheters in position. Note the parallel orientation of the sealing stent indicating a seal in healthy aorta (*arrow*).

183

16. ENDOVASCULAR TREATMENT OF AAA WITHOUT AN ADEQUATE SEALING ZONE. FENESTRATED ENDOGRAFTS. SPECIFIC COMPLICATIONS AND MANAGEMENT

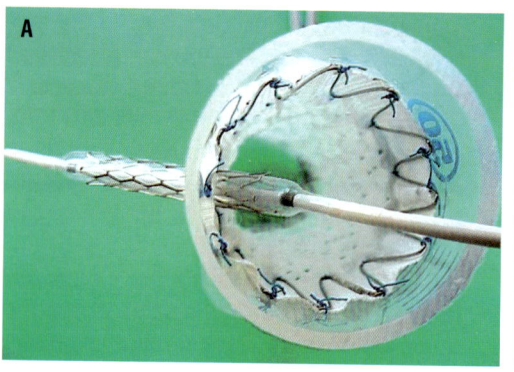
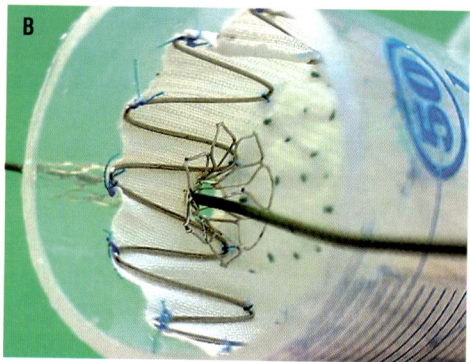

FIGURE 7: A. Visceral stent in position, expanded. **B.** Visceral stent in position flared (Reprinted from European Journal of Vascular and Endovascular Surgery, S. O'Neill, R.K. Greenberg, F. Haddad, T. Resch, J. Sereika and E. Katz, A Prospective Analysis of Fenestrated Endovascular Grafting: Intermediate-term Outcomes, 115-23, Copyright (2006), with permission from Elsevier Ltd).

the Cleveland Clinic with compromised neck morphology have been studied in a trial of the Zenith fenestrated device (Cook Inc, Bloomington, IN). The studies are prospective and non-randomized in nature and have been reported previously.[4,15,21,24] Follow-up studies include clinical, laboratory, and imaging studies at 1 month, 6 months, 12 months and annually thereafter. Helical CT scans, duplex ultrasound (with the exception of the discharge time

point), creatinine assessment, and flat plate radiography are obtained. Secondary interventions are performed in the setting of a suspected type I or III endoleak, selectively for type II endoleaks, compromised visceral vessel flow, or aneurysmal growth. When appropriate, outcome analyses were conducted in accordance with the reporting standards for endovascular aneurysm repair.[25] Duplex determined end systolic and diastolic velocities are collected for each visceral vessel treated at each follow-up visit. For the purposes of this report patient enrollment ended on December 30th 2005 and follow-up ended on November 30th 2006. The complete inclusion and exclusion criteria have been published elsewhere.[4]

In a manner similar to the EVAR trials,[1,2] the definition of 'high risk' was left to the treating physician, with some guidelines regarding anesthetic risk, cardiopulmonary dysfunction, and renal insufficiency provided. As well as physiologic factors, patients with multiple prior abdominal or aortic surgeries, inflammatory aneurysms, and other situations which may have resulted in unfavorable open surgical results were potentially considered high-risk. Pre-operative, intra-operative and post-operative data col-

FIGURE 8: Completed fenestrated graft.

lection was extensive, particularly in relation to risk factors and other physiologic information. Post-procedural complications were stratified into those that occurred within the first 30 days and those that occurred after the first 30 days. The complications were also categorized by body systems as follows: cardiac, respiratory, vascular, neurologic, renal, and gastrointestinal and those complications related to cancer and diabetes. Survival data was supplemented by querying the Social Security Death Index on a quarterly basis.

Results

The most recent CCF fenestrated experience was reported in 2006.[21] This included total of 119 patients. There were 98 men and 21 women with a mean age of 75 years. They were a high risk group with 49% having significant coronary artery disease and 26% having renal insufficiency. Although we have made several attempts to categorize these patients into their relevant high-risk factors, many patients had specific issues that did not lend themselves to grouping. The technical success rate was 100%. Conduits were used for access in 6 patients. In addition to proximal fenestrations 8 patients also had hypogastric branch devices inserted to preserve antegrade internal iliac flow in at least one internal iliac artery.[19,26]

Mortality

The mean follow-up was 19 months (range 0-48 months). Sixteen patients died during the follow-up period, one within 30 days, seven within the first year, and eight patients after 12 months of follow-up. Kaplan-Meier estimates of survival at 1, 12, 24, and 36 months are 0.99, 0.92, 0.83 and 0.79, respectively. There were no late aneurysm related deaths and no conversions to open procedures.

Endovascular Outcomes

The mean diameter of the proximal neck was 26 mm (range, 17-34 mm). The mean proximal neck length was 8 mm (range, 3-18 mm). The proximal neck length was <10 mm in 70 patients, and between 10 and 18 mm in 49 patients, all of which had morphologic factors implying compromised sealing or fixation. A total of 302 visceral vessels were incorporated in the prosthesis design. One patient died within 30 days of the initial procedure (previously discussed). Four of six patients with proximal type I endoleaks underwent post-operative secondary procedures prior to hospital discharge. There were no mortalities associated with secondary procedures.

DISCUSSION

Endovascular repair has been embraced by vascular surgeons since its introduction in 1991. The main criticisms of the technique have been the potentially inferior durability of endovascular repair compared to open repair and the requirement for more assiduous follow-up. However, despite the increased requirement for secondary intervention, most of these procedures can be performed endoluminally with minimal morbidity, and a very low risk of late conversion.[27,28] Fenestrated endografting is an extension of the technique, and it is likely that the mortality risk-reduction benefit achieved with endovascular repair of large or small infrarenal aneurysms (approximately 3% absolute risk reduction in "fit" patients)[1] will pale in comparison to the potential risk reduction were more proximal aortic aneurysms treated in an analogous manner. The mortality associated with the conventional treatment of juxtarenal aneurysms is higher than that for infrarenal aneurysms in our institution (5.1% vs 2.8%).[29] Traditional open repair is also associated with a number of potential major complications, including renal impairment and failure, especially if supra-visceral clamp is required. The application of evolving endovascular technologies to this patient group could change the face of aortic surgery. Endograft technology has the potential to even eliminate the majority of complex open procedures thus limiting mortality and providing a treatment option to patients who have long been deemed inoperable.

In spite of a good device design, the implantation procedure can be demanding and is associated with a learning curve. Challenging anatomic factors include visceral vessel stenoses, iliac tortuosity or calcifications that reduce the rotational freedom of the device, and proximal neck angulation. When implanting a fenestrated device, the longitudinal position must be accurate. In addition there is a need for precise rotational orientation (to allow access into the visceral vessels). It is the rotational positioning, which is frustrated by atheroma within the proximal neck (resulting in embolic issues) and severe aortic tortuosity (which limits torque that may be applied to the proximal graft). Data from our institution noted fewer renal complications as greater experience with the devices have been attained.[30]

While considerable technical success can be achieved with a fenestrated endovascular device, there remain some significant risks. Repair of juxtarenal aneurysms with an open or fenestrated graft approach is associated with a risk for adverse renal events.[29,30] Following fenestrated grafting, the incidence of worsening renal function is about 16% in those without baseline renal dysfunction (although none developed a creatinine >2 mg/dL), and 39% for patients with preoperative renal dysfunction, with 6% requiring hemodialysis. Following open surgical repair, 28% percent of patients had worsening renal function, and 6% required hemodialysis. Clearly, all patients following open or endovascular repair, must be carefully evaluated to assess for worsening renal dysfunction. When renal artery stenosis is

suspected or diagnosed, aggressive approach might be warranted to limit the extent of late renal dysfunction.[30]

The fenestrated endograft is a modular device with a tubular proximal component containing the fenestrations and a bifurcate distal component. Cross sectional area reduction at the bifurcation may result in caudad forces on the bifurcate component. The joint between tubular and bifurcate components acts to uncouple the caudad forces on the bifurcate component from the tubular component where even minor degrees of migration could have catastrophic effects on branch vessels. The capacity for the device to allow component separation may be advantageous in this respect. It is certainly preferable to the alternative which is to have a more rigid joint – in this situation the same caudad forces acting at the bifurcation would displace the entire graft (including the fenestrated component) downwards. Displacement by even a few millimeters may lead to branch vessel occlusion or compromise – we have observed this in two cases where a giant Palmaz stent (Cordis Endovascular, NJ) was used to strengthen the joint, thereby preventing component separation with resultant branch vessel compromise after only minor amounts of graft migration (far less than those defined as migration in the SVS reporting standards[31]). The importance of this phenomenon is that it is taken into account in the primary repair by maximizing the amount of overlap between the components. If sufficient overlap is not created at the primary procedure, graft component separation can occur to such a degree that complete disruption occurs (Figure 9a and b). This phenomenon should be routinely examined for at follow-up CT scanning as secondary procedures may be required to prevent complete component uncoupling with re-pressurization of the sac.

The definition of complications also

187

16. ENDOVASCULAR TREATMENT OF AAA WITHOUT AN ADEQUATE SEALING ZONE. FENESTRATED ENDOGRAFTS. SPECIFIC COMPLICATIONS AND MANAGEMENT

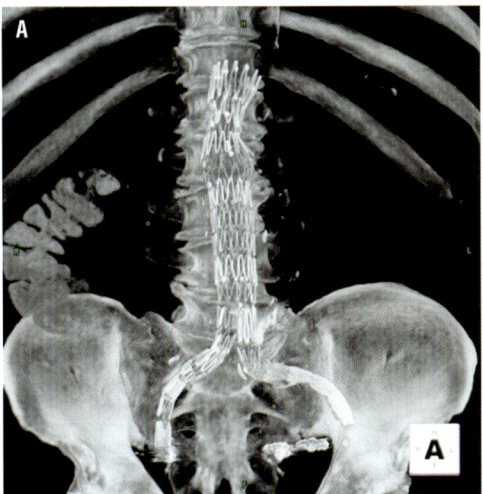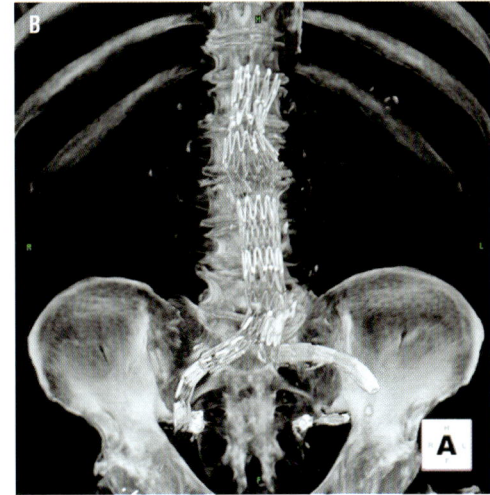

FIGURE 9: A. Fenestrated graft in 2003 with four stent overlap. **B**. Fenestrated graft 3 years later with only 3 stent overlap.

merits discussion. In the CCF series there were 29 endoleaks in total.[21] Those that underwent secondary intervention all had it carried out endoluminally, without mortality. Historically, most type 2 endoleaks do not require intervention. When they do, the procedures are done with a miniscule incidence of morbidity and mortality, thus it is debatable whether type II endoleaks should be classified as complications of endovascular repair. Secondary interventions have long been considered the bane of EVAR. However all of the interventions in our series of complex grafts were achieved by endovascular means without recourse to open surgery. The magnitude of the intervention and its associated morbidity is more important than its mere existence. In EVAR 2 (a high risk group similar to ours but undergoing conventional engrafting) there were 32 secondary interventions out of 178 patients, including 3 conversions to open surgery. It is clear that secondary interventions did not contribute to the mortality rate in our series or in EVAR 2 as the 30 day mortality rate following secondary intervention was zero in both series. One might expect an excess

of certain complications that are unique to fenestrated endografting. The multi-modular nature of the system results in more joints in the system, thus more potential for component separation and the creation of type 3 endoleaks. There were 4 type 3 endoleaks in 119 patients in our series.

Some would suggest that the EVAR 2 trial should give one pause to regard how broadly this technology should be disseminated. Elective aneurysm repair, whether open or endovascular is a prophylactic procedure. Many of these high-risk patients have a relatively short life expectancy, but need to live long enough to benefit from aneurysm repair if this new procedure is to be beneficial. Few would doubt that there are some patients who have such extensive co-morbidity that peri-operative mortality is prohibitive and others who do not benefit from repair even if they survive the initial procedure because their overall longevity related to their co-morbidities is diminished. The peri-operative mortality in EVAR 2 was 9%. If the intervention can be accomplished with low peri-operative mortality then maybe the EVAR 2 results do not apply. There are studies which suggest that EVAR can be achieved with acceptable morbidity and mortality in patients who were previously considered unfit for treatment,[32,33] including a multicenter trial where patients were preoperatively segregated according to physiologic risk.[6] The peri-operative mortality in this group of patients was 1%. Yet the conclusions of the various publications remain conflicting, leaving clinicians with more questions than answers with regard to the proper management of the high-risk patient. Clearly, EVAR 1 and 2 trials have altered the paradigm by which patients with aneurysms >5.5 cm are treated. However, information gleaned from the presented data must be interpreted within the context of the abilities of physician and hospital system embarking on treatment, in addition to specific patient factors. Thus, patient selection will become even more crucial in this patient cohort, where anatomic evaluation will obviously be more challenging than for conventional endografts. At least in the near future, this highly complex technology needs to be developed under the strict scrutiny of well-documented clinical trials sponsored by manufacturers or centers of expertise.

FUTURE PERSPECTIVES

As the methods and materials technology mature, fenestrated and branched endografts for more complex thoracoabdominal aortic aneurysms will likely expand to a relatively small number of centers in the context of clinical trials. Many abdominal aortic aneurysms are unsuitable for conventional endografting, most frequently as a result of compromised neck anatomy. Recent history and results from experienced centers as well as simplification of the sizing and deployment processes makes it seem likely that fenestrated endograft technology will disperse widely to these patients.

In a thoracoabdominal aneurysm, by definition the branch vessels are emerging from aneurysmal aorta. In this case formal branch grafts are clearly required. There are 2 basic types of branch – reinforced fenestrations and directional branches. In reinforced fenestrations, a fenestration is reinforced with a nitinol ring such that a covered stent-graft can be used to traverse the gap between the device and the branch. Directional branches are used to provide more favorable flow dynamics in aneurysms with large lumens, particularly when the aortic prosthesis will be situated a significant distance from the branch ostia. These can emerge from the body of the graft in a variety of configurations and at transverse and longitudinal orientations. One novel concept is to pre-load the branch with a wire and catheter, thus giving relatively easy access to the branch by simply snaring the pre-loaded wire.

Branch device implantation can be made more difficult by tortuosity and limited space around branches. Forces at branch points, analogous to the situation at bifurcations result in displacement forces on the entire graft with possibility for migration and failure. Helical branches are employed in an attempt to negate these factors (Figure 10). The helical design has a larger orifice (similar to a standard vascular end-side anastomosis) and a gentle curve both of which contribute to reducing the forces on the device. The helical design was created to provide a long overlap zone between the device and mating self-expanding stent graft, as well as alter the direction of the branch in an effort to diminish the tortuosity and risk of kinking.

One might ask why this technology has taken so long to disseminate. There are several reasons why this may be so. First as the devices are not yet FDA approved, each patient must be part of an investigational device exemption in the USA. There is also a perception that the

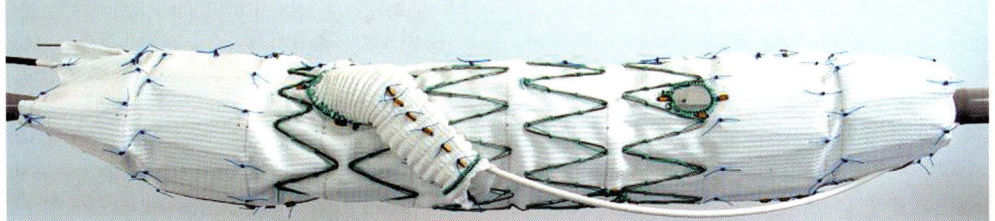

FIGURE 10: Helical branch with preloaded catheter and wire.

technical aspect of inserting a fenestrated endovascular graft is very complex. There is no doubt that it is technically more demanding than conventional endografting. Designing and implanting a device that will accommodate the visceral vessels of the aorta is an intricate task, and one that should only be attempted by an experienced interventionist. The prosthesis must be able to accommodate branches to the visceral segment of the aorta, and maintain the perfusion of critical end organs. These will be dependent on accurate design and precise deployment of the device. Thus, device-related complications that may occur following infrarenal aneurysm repair, such as migration or component separation, will have catastrophic implications if encountered following a repair that incorporates critical aortic branches. Therefore, treatment of aneurysms of the more proximal aorta is optimally performed with a device that has proven to be stable in the infrarenal segment and will require proficiency of the interventionalist in planning, sizing, and in technical issues with implantation of aortic endografts. In addition, experience with visceral and supra-aortic vessel stenting, and in troubleshooting is necessary. Despite the obstacles for development of such technologies, successful early and intermediate term results have been achieved in a number of centers using endovascular means to treat aneurysms of juxtarenal and thoracoabdominal aorta. Assiduous follow-up is vital as late complications, such as component separation can occur. The expense of the endograft itself may also be prohibitive in some regions.

Conclusions

Available data today suggest that fenestrated endovascular grafting is relatively safe and feasible with a low morbidity and mortality. It is clearly an option for the high risk patient with compromised proximal neck morphology, particularly in high risk patients who undoubtedly have high morbidity and mortality associated with complex aortic repair. The relative proportion of aneurysms involving the renal arteries is small, yet up to 40% of all AAA are precluded from conventional endovascular repair. It is likely that fenestrated techniques will allow for endovascular repair to be conducted in these patients.

Reference

1. Greenhalgh RM, Brown LC, Kwong GP, Powell JT, Thompson SG. Comparison of endovascular aneurysm repair with open repair in patients with abdominal aortic aneurysm (EVAR trial 1), 30-day operative mortality results: randomised controlled trial. Lancet 2004;364:843-8.
2. Endovascular aneurysm repair and outcome in patients unfit for open repair of abdominal aortic aneurysm (EVAR trial 2): randomised controlled trial. Lancet 2005;365:2187-92.

3. Prinssen M et al. A randomized trial comparing conventional and endovascular repair of abdominal aortic aneurysms. N Engl J Med 2004;351:1607-18.

4. Greenberg RK et al. Endovascular management of juxtarenal aneurysms with fenestrated endovascular grafting. J Vasc Surg 2004;39:279-87.

5. Leurs LJ, Kievit J, Dagnelie PC, Nelemans PJ, Buth J. Influence of infrarenal neck length on outcome of endovascular abdominal aortic aneurysm repair. J Endovasc Ther 2006;13:640-8.

6. Greenberg RK, Chuter TA, Sternbergh WC, III, Fearnot NE. Zenith AAA endovascular graft: intermediate-term results of the US multicenter trial. J Vasc Surg 2004;39:1209-18.

7. Greenberg RK. Abdominal aortic endografting: fixation and sealing. J Am Coll Surg 2002;194:S79-S87.

8. Black SA et al. Complex thoracoabdominal aortic aneurysms: endovascular exclusion with visceral revascularization. J Vasc Surg 2006;43:1081-9.

9. West CA et al. Factors affecting outcomes of open surgical repair of pararenal aortic aneurysms: a 10-year experience. J Vasc Surg 2006;43:921-7.

10. Sarac TP et al. Contemporary results of juxtarenal aneurysm repair. J Vasc Surg 2002;36:1104-11.

11. Browne TF et al. A fenestrated covered suprarenal aortic stent. Eur J Vasc Endovasc Surg 1999;18:445-9.

12. Faruqi RM et al. Endovascular repair of abdominal aortic aneurysm using a pararenal fenestrated stent-graft. J Endovasc Surg 1999;6:354-8.

13. Anderson JL, Berce M, Hartley DE. Endoluminal aortic grafting with renal and superior mesenteric artery incorporation by graft fenestration. J Endovasc Ther 2001;8:3-15.

14. Stanley BM, Semmens JB, Lawrence-Brown MM, Goodman MA, Hartley DE. Fenestration in endovascular grafts for aortic aneurysm repair: new horizons for preserving blood flow in branch vessels. J Endovasc Ther 2001;8:16-24.

15. Greenberg RK, Haulon S, O'Neill S, Lyden S, Ouriel K. Primary endovascular repair of juxtarenal aneurysms with fenestrated endovascular grafting. Eur J Vasc Endovasc Surg 2004;27:484-91.

16. Verhoeven EL et al. Treatment of short-necked infrarenal aortic aneurysms with fenestrated stent-grafts: short-term results. Eur J Vasc Endovasc Surg 2004;27:477-83.

17. Adam DJ, Berce M, Hartley DE, Anderson JL. Repair of juxtarenal para-anastomotic aortic aneurysms after previous open repair with fenestrated and branched endovascular stent grafts. J Vasc Surg 2005;42:997-1001.

18. McWilliams RG, Murphy M, Hartley D, Lawrence-Brown MM, Harris PL. In situ stent-graft fenestration to preserve the left subclavian artery. J Endovasc Ther 2004;11:170-4.

19. Greenberg RK et al. Beyond the aortic bifurcation: branched endovascular grafts for thoracoabdominal and aortoiliac aneurysms. J Vasc Surg 2006;43:879-86.

20. Anderson JL, Adam DJ, Berce M, Hartley DE. Repair of thoracoabdominal aortic aneurysms with fenestrated and branched endovascular stent grafts. J Vasc Surg 2005;42:600-7.

21. O'Neill S et al. A prospective analysis of fenestrated endovascular grafting: intermediate-term outcomes. Eur J Vasc Endovasc Surg 2006;32: 115-23.

22. Muhs BE et al. Mid-term results of endovascular aneurysm repair with branched and fenestrated endografts. J Vasc Surg 2006;44:9-15.

23. Chuter TA, Buck DG, Schneider DB, Reilly LM, Messina LM. Development of a branched stent-graft for endovascular repair of aortic arch aneurysms. J Endovasc Ther 2003;10:940-5.

24. Haddad F et al. Fenestrated endovascular grafting: The renal side of the story. J Vasc Surg 2005;41: 181-90.

25. Chaikof EL et al. Reporting standards for endovascular aortic aneurysm repair. J Vasc Surg 2002;35:1048-60.

26. Haulon S et al. Branched Grafting for Aortoiliac Aneurysms. Eur J Vasc Endovasc Surg 2007.

27. Becquemin JP et al. Outcomes of secondary interventions after abdominal aortic aneurysm endovascular repair. J Vasc Surg 2004;39:298-305.

28. Verhoeven EL et al. Frequency and outcome of re-interventions after endovascular repair for abdominal aortic aneurysm: a prospective cohort study. Eur J Vasc Endovasc Surg 2004;28:357-64.

29. Sarac TP et al. Contemporary results of juxtarenal aneurysm repair. J Vasc Surg 2002;36:1104-11.

30. Haddad F et al. Fenestrated endovascular grafting:

The renal side of the story. J Vasc Surg 2005;41: 181-90.

31. Chaikof EL et al. Identifying and grading factors that modify the outcome of endovascular aortic aneurysm repair. J Vasc Surg 2002;35:1061-6.

32. Chuter TA et al. Endovascular aneurysm repair in high-risk patients. J Vasc Surg 2000;31:122-33.

33. Zannetti S et al. Endovascular abdominal aortic aneurysm repair in high-risk patients: a single centre experience. Eur J Vasc Endovasc Surg 2001;21: 334-8.

16. ENDOVASCULAR TREATMENT OF AAA WITHOUT AN ADEQUATE SEALING ZONE. FENESTRATED ENDOGRAFTS. SPECIFIC COMPLICATIONS AND MANAGEMENT

Endografting and independent transmural fixation: Implications for design, surveillance and endograft utilization

David H. Deaton

HISTORICAL BACKROUND

The history of aortic reconstruction has its earliest roots in the 19th century with various reports of aortic ligation but saw little real progress until the latter half of the 20th century. Bigger's summary of surgical therapy for aortic aneurysms at the 1940 American Surgical Association meeting summarized the consensus of the era: "Judging from the literature, only a small number of surgeons have felt that direct surgical attack upon aneurysms of the abdominal aorta was justifiable, and it must be admitted that the results obtained by surgical intervention have been discouraging".[1]

The early part of the 20th century saw a wave of enthusiasm for rigid prostheses for replacement of the aorta. While this period lasted for nearly two decades it became clear that the thrombotic complications of rigid prostheses would prevent any real possibilities for widespread use or further development. A similar but shorter wave of enthusiasm occurred for the use of homografts between 1945 and 1955. Again, the promise of favorable acute outcomes was tarnished by early failure and the realization that homografts

were susceptible to a myriad of degenerative effects that led to early thrombosis and failure.[2]

The advent of fabric prostheses and the realization that these prostheses required permanent mechanical fixation to the aorta produced a true revolution in aortic reconstruction over the latter half of the 20th century. Voorhees early development of fabric vascular prostheses[3] and the iterative progress of suture technology leading to the development of permanent monofilament suture as a desired technique for the vascular anastomosis have allowed the technical facility of vascular surgeons throughout the world to advance aortic and vascular reconstruction in general to levels unimagined a generation prior.

The development of endovascular aortic reconstruction has followed, to a remarkable degree, the development of open aortic reconstruction. Early endovascular grafts incorporated rigid designs that simplified the technology for deployment and the technical facility required for implantation. The designers of these rigid endografts touted the concept that their "columnar strength" would supplant the proven requirement for permanent transmural fixation so amply demonstrated in the evolution of open aortic reconstruction technique. While some more compliant endografts that employed transmural fixation were developed, the technical complexity of their deployment and the large catheter diameters required to incorporate both a radial stent and a transmural hook resulted in a steep learning curve and frequent technical misadventures at implantation. In a technology predicated on diminished acute morbidity and mortality there was little appetite for the possibility of acute conversion to open surgical reconstruction.

While the popular adoption of transmural fixation by the clinical community was diminished in the early development of endografts, the improved chronic integrity of endograft technologies that employ transmural fixation is now widely accepted.[4] The ability of endografts to harness elements of transmural fixation has been limited by the constraints of catheter delivery and the acceptable diameter of those catheters to incorporate all three requirements for endovascular grafts: radial stents, graft prosthesis and hooks or barbs. Current endograft designs incorporate either a lesser degree of transmural fixation in the infrarenal segment of the graft or a more robust transmural element positioned in the suprarenal segment on bare stent from which the endograft is suspended. Both of these strategies are challenged by the requirements for long-term aortic graft success. A paucity of transmural fixation increases the risk of late migration[5] while the suprarenal technique risks the disjunction of the suprarenal and infrarenal segments.[6]

The concept of endostaples as a necessary adjunct to endovascular grafts is akin to the development of suturing techniques in the development of all surgical procedures and vascular reconstruction in particular. For 2000 years the only surgical technique applied with any degree of success in vascular reconstruction was ligation. The realization of effective sutured

vascular anastomosis made possible the development of vascular surgery as a routine in surgical practices and gave birth to the development of vascular surgery as a specialty over the last 50 years. Endovascular staples have the possibility of giving the surgeon the same freedom of creativity and confidence in outcome that early pioneers created with suturing techniques in the development of open vascular reconstruction.

DESIGN CONSIDERATIONS

From a design standpoint, staples delivered to an endovascular graft as separate components allow an entirely different approach to the design of the primary endograft. The primary advantage comes in the form of a markedly reduced catheter diameter for the endograft enabled by the absence of any primary fixation elements. Secondary benefits are realized in the ability of the surgeon to apply as many staples as desired and in the locations desired. This allows the surgical creativity that is often taken for granted in open surgical reconstruction but which is severely limited in the minimally invasive technique of endovascular reconstruction. Other benefits include the ability to address Type I endoleak with staples, to implant staples at a later time and the potential to facilitate graft positioning, graft-graft attachments and novel endograft designs.

While the concept of endovascular stapling has existed for some time, the development and execution necessary to advance the concept to a clinical reality has only recently occurred. There are currently four endovascular staple designs in some degree of active development and testing. Three of these designs are independent of any particular endograft system while the fourth is paired with an endograft developed specifically to utilize the advantages of an independent fixation system and the features of that particular endostaple design.

The EVA staple

In 2001, Trout and Tanner[7] described a staple intended for use in the wide variety of endografts being developed and deployed at the time. The system described employed a flexible catheter that delivered either a stainless steel or nitinol coil that resumed a coiled shape after deployment to "rivet" the graft to the aorta (Figure 1 and 2).

The catheter used to deliver this staple incorporates and optical fiber that transmits a laser to form a hole through the graft, aorta and any of the disease states commonly found in the aorta. The staple is deployed through this hole in a straight configuration before reforming into its coiled configuration. While the innovation and novelty of this approach is intriguing, there are no published results from this system of endostaple application in either a laboratory or a clinical setting.[7] The current status of the development of this technology is unknown.

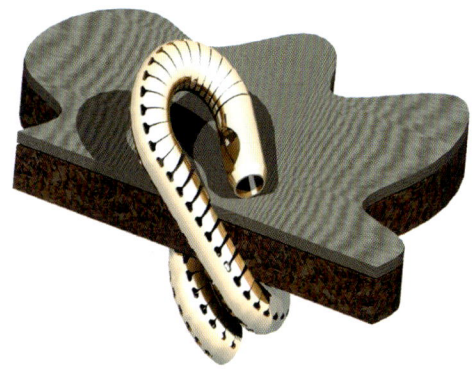

FIGURE 2: Schematic diagram of EVA staple deployed transmurally.

The Edrich staple

A patent for an endovascular staple and the catheter intended to deliver the staple was filed in July of 2004. Little is known in the public domain regarding this device or its delivery component other than what can be gleaned from patent filings. The device is assigned to Edrich Vascular Devices, Inc. (95 Madison Avenue, Suite 103, Morristown, NJ 07960). An exhibit at the 2006 Endovascular Congress in Scottsdale, AZ demonstrated a prototype of the device. This showed a U-shaped staple that penetrated the intended target(s) with two points that curled back towards the crossbar of the intraluminal portion of the staple. The end result of stapling is a crossbar on the inner lumen connected by two points of penetration. The extraluminal portion curves back towards the vessel after penetration presenting only a curved metal surface on the outside rather than a sharp point.

Anson Refix – Lombard Medical

Lombard Medical (Oxfordshire, UK) has developed a vascular stapler to be used in open procedures (Anson Refix™) and an

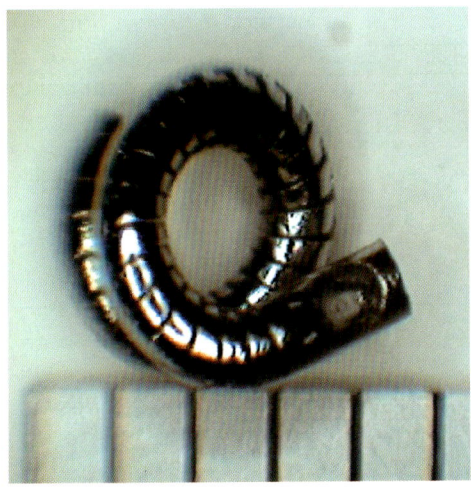

FIGURE 1: The EVA staple in deployed configuration on a millimeter scale.

endovascular device (EndoRefix™) to be used percutaneously to apply staples to new or previously implanted endografts. The staple in each of these devices is a nitinol device that has two piercing arms that wrap back towards the vessel after penetration. The details of this device, its development and current clinical status will be covered in another chapter in this text authored by Dr. Brian Hopkinson, one of the developers of the device.

Aptus EndoStapling System

Aptus Endosystems was founded in 2002 to develop a novel endograft system that incorporated both an aortic endograft (Aptus™ Endovascular AAA Repair System) and an endovascular stapling system (Aptus™ EndoStapling System) each specifically designed to complement each other and to function as a system. The main body of the endograft is a bifurcated device with two modular limbs that physically lock on to the main body (Figure 3). The proximal portion of the endograft has a short sealing stent. The main body of the graft is unsupported to allow implantation into tortuous anatomy[8] and to accommodate aortic remodeling after aneurysm exclusion. The modular limbs of the device have robust radial support with longitudinal flexibility to accommodate tortuous anatomy and provide radial support to prevent limb stenosis in tortuous iliac anatomy. The graft material is manufactured using a low porosity woven polyester and the endograft delivery system is in a 16 French outer diameter catheter for smaller diameters and an 18 French outer diameter catheter for larger sizes.

The Aptus™ endostaple is a helical screw that is deployed via a 16 French outer diameter steerable guide sheath.

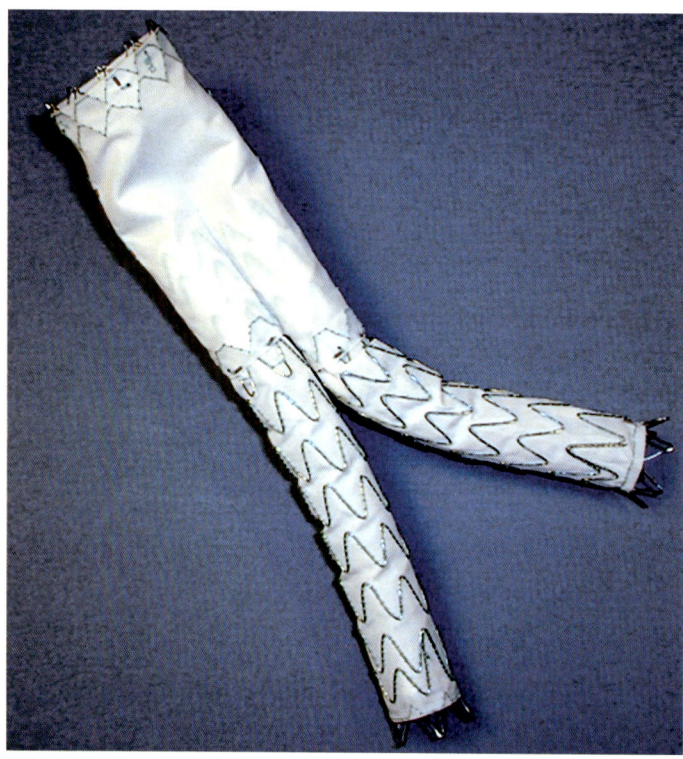

FIGURE 3: The Aptus Endograft with two modular limbs locked into main body.

(Figure 4 and 5) This is inserted through the contralateral limb after the main body is initially deployed but still attached to the primary delivery catheter. The main body is stabilized by both its proximal sealing stent and its attachment to the endograft delivery catheter prior being affixed to the aortic wall with the staples. Each staple is 4 mm in length and designed to incorporate a cylinder of aortic tissue equal to the width of the helical screw to the level of the adventitia. The strength of this attachment has been tested in a silastic tube model at twenty newtons per staple. The in vivo strength will obviously be dependent on the integrity of the tissue in which the staple is deployed. The discrete nature of each staple will allow the operator to deploy as many staples as desired into locations felt to provide the most robust and least diseased aortic tissue.

The staple applier is delivered through the steerable guide sheath and each staple is deployed with an electronically controlled torque motor (Figure 6). The staple applier deploys the staple halfway in its initial step. At this point the operator can either fully deploy the staple or reconstrain the staple to its original position. The rotational quality of deployment, close application of the device to the wall and sharp

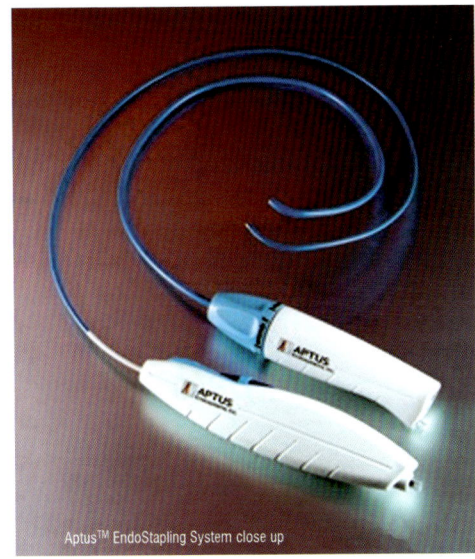

Aptus™ EndoStapling System close up

FIGURE 5: The Aptus steerable endoguide and stapler delivery catheter.

tip of the staple has allowed penetration across a wide variety of aortic pathologies in pre-clinical work done in human cadavers. The Phase I clinical study of the Aptus EndoStapler did not record any incident where a staple could not be deployed once in position at the desired location in the aorta.[9]

Early clinical results of the Aptus System

The first human implants with the Aptus™ Endovascular AAA Repair System were performed in July of 2005 on two patients in Venezuela by Drs. David Deaton, Takao Ohki and Jose Condado.[10] Both cases were initially successful and at two years follow-up both of these patients have shrinking aneurysms with no evidence of any migration or other device malfunction. Of note, the first of these implants was noted to have a large Type I endoleak on completion imaging after the desired number of four staples had been implanted to secure the graft. Examination of the

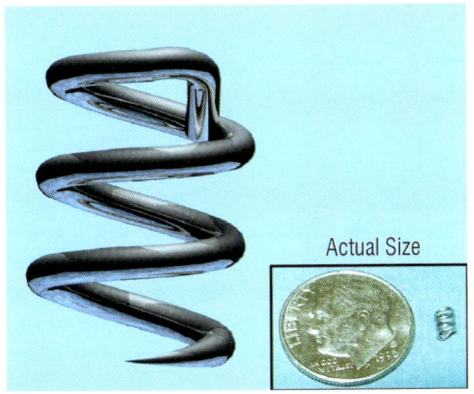

Actual Size

FIGURE 4: The Aptus staple made from MP35N LT™, an alloy similar to Elgilloy.

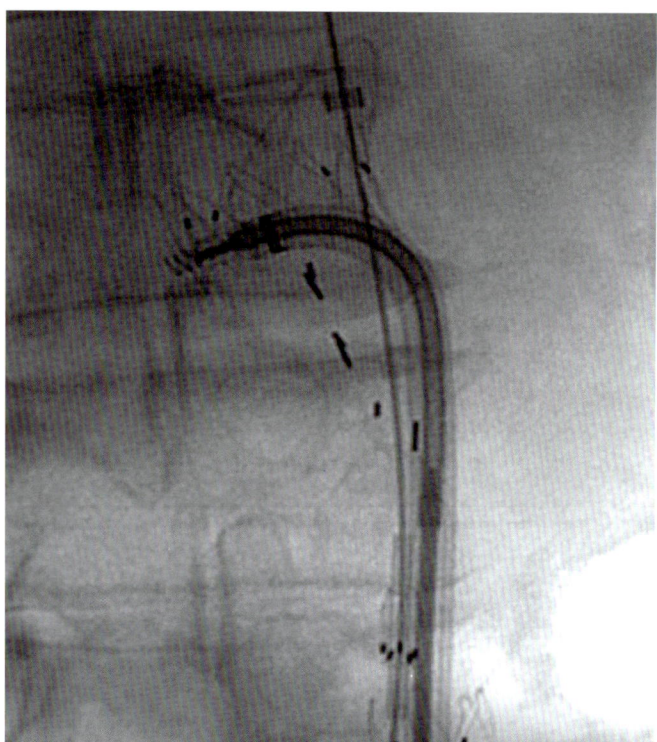

FIGURE 6: Fluoroscopic image of staple deployment illustrating staple penetration past proximal sealing stent and into the aortic wall.

preoperative CT reconstructions and the images in the OR indicated some proximal neck irregularity and lack of proximal stent apposition. Additional staples were applied in this area to tack down the stent into the irregular area resulting in ablation of the Type I endoleak. This patient never exhibited any evidence of postoperative endoleak and has demonstrated aneurysm exclusion and shrinkage at every point in follow-up through two years.

The FDA approved Phase I trial of the Aptus™ Endovascular AAA Repair System in the United States began with the first implant at Georgetown University Hospital on July 25, 2006. Twenty-one patients were enrolled at five institutions over the ensuing[10] months through May of 2007. All endograft components were successfully deployed, including a total of 93 EndoStaples. The range of EndoStaples implanted was 2 to 10, with a median of 4 per patient. There were no Type I, III, or IV endoleaks at 30 days. Device related adverse events included two limb thromboses, at nine and thirty days. Adjunctive devices used were two proximal cuffs and one limb extension. There were no Endo-Staple-related adverse events.[9]

POTENTIAL BENEFITS OF ENDOSTAPLING

Irrespective of the design, any endostapling technology that allows the operator to securely attach a graft or other device to the load-bearing portion of the vascular wall, the adventitia, has the potential to change the nature of endovascular aortic grafting and potentially a variety of other endovascular procedures and devices. In addition to the secure attachment of the graft to the wall, endostaples have the potential to secure the aortic wall to the graft preventing one of the most insidious late complications of aortic aneurysm repair, namely continued aortic dilation at the proximal attachment site.[11] The discrete nature of staples allows their use to treat focal defects including the effective address of Type I endoleaks by creating apposition in an irregular area not sealed by the uniformity of a radial stent. The independence of an endovascular stapling device from the primary graft also allows staple application at a time other than primary graft implantation allowing future issues of fixation or other degenerative changes in the aorta to be addressed with an endovascular procedure rather than conversion to open surgery. While the benefits of endovascular stapling are well demonstrated in the application of endograft fixation, there may well be other applications for independent and discrete fixation in a variety of vascular pathologies and new treatment paradigms made possible by this new endovascular modality.

DISCUSSION

The foundations of successful vascular reconstruction are based on the development of viable conduits and reliable techniques for vascular anastomosis. While many endovascular therapies represent alternative methods to achieve revascularization (i.e. endoluminal recanalization vs. bypass), aortic endovascular graft therapy is a reproduction of open aortic grafting with the exception of endovascular delivery. The early success of endovascular aortic grafts satisfied the requirements for reductions in acute morbidity and mortality relative to the open procedure[12] but the inability to reproduce the transmural fixation and control of the open procedure resulted in long term outcomes clearly inferior to open repair.[13] The potential for endovascular aortic grafting to surpass both the acute and chronic outcomes of open reconstruction rest on development of technologies that effectively reproduce the principles of open reconstruction.[14] While the graft materials of both open and endovascular grafts are similar, the fixation technologies are radically different. Enabling the surgeon to apply staples that represent the functional equivalent of sutured anastomosis and the control inherent in that technique holds promise for a significant advance in both the acute and chronic success of aortic endografting. Such advances might well allow the endovascular technique to equal and surpass the chronic performance of open surgical reconstruction and reduce or eliminate the current requirements for postoperative imaging. The capability to deliver a discrete fixation technology independent of the primary device will also allow medical device design a new level of creativity for aortic endografts and, potentially, a host of other devices and therapies.

REFERENCES

1. Friedman SG. A History of Vascular Surgery. 2nd ed. Oxford, UK: Futura/Blackwell Publishing, 2005.
2. Thompson JE. Early history of aortic surgery. J Vasc Surg 1998;28(4):746-52.
3. Voorhees AB, Jr. The development of arterial prostheses. A personal view. Arch Surg 1985; 120(3):289-95.
4. Tonnessen BH, Sternbergh WC, 3rd, Money SR. Mid- and long-term device migration after endovascular abdominal aortic aneurysm repair: a comparison of AneuRx and Zenith endografts. J Vasc Surg 2005;42(3):392-400; discussion 400-1.
5. Sampaio SM, Panneton JM, Mozes G, et al. AneuRx device migration: incidence, risk factors, and consequences. Ann Vasc Surg 2005;19(2):178-85.
6. Ghanim K, Mwipatayi BP, Abbas M, Sieunarine K. Late stent-graft migration secondary to separation of the uncovered segment from the main

body of a Zenith endoluminal graft. J Endovasc Ther 2006;13(3):346-9.

7. Trout HH, 3rd, Tanner HM. A new vascular Endo-staple: a technical description. J Vasc Surg 2001;34(3):565-8.

8. Fulton JJ, Farber MA, Sanchez LA, et al. Effect of challenging neck anatomy on mid-term migration rates in AneuRx endografts. J Vasc Surg 2006;44 (5):932-7; discussion 937.

9. Deaton D, Neville R, Mehta M, et al. Discrete Fixation for Endovascular Aortic Grafting: Interim Results of the Phase I Multicenter Trial of the Aptus™ Endovascular AAA Repair System. Society for Vascular Surgery Annual Meeting. Baltimore, MD, 2007.

10. Ohki T, Deaton D, Condado J. Aptus Endovascular AAA Repair System Report of the 1-year fol-low-up in a first-in-man study. Endovascular Today 2006:29-36.

11. Dalainas I, Nano G, Bianchi P, et al. Aortic neck dilatation and endograft migration are correlated with self-expanding endografts. J Endovasc Ther 2007;14(3):318-23.

12. Sicard GA, Zwolak RM, Sidawy AN, White RA, Siami FS. Endovascular abdominal aortic aneurysm repair: long-term outcome measures in patients at high-risk for open surgery. J Vasc Surg 2006; 44(2):229-36.

13. Becquemin JP, Allaire E, Desgranges P, Kobeiter H. Delayed complications following EVAR. Tech Vasc Interv Radiol 2005;8(1):30-40.

14. Lee WA. Infrarenal aortic devices: failure modes and unmet needs. Semin Vasc Surg 2007;20 (2):75-80.

Endostaplers for short necks

Brian R. Hopkinson

INTRODUCTION

The basic principle of the surgical management of aortic aneurysms is to replace the weakened, expanding and threatening to rupture area by a tough graft, joining normal arterial wall above to normal arterial wall below. In the case of an abdominal aortic aneurysm the object is to place the reinforcing graft as near as possible to the renal arteries in normal aorta and to fix the distal end of the graft into either normal aorta below the aneurysm or, in the case of a bifurcated graft, place the distal ends into normal iliac vessels. Traditionally this is done through a relatively large laparotomy incision. It was first performed in France by Dubois in the 1950s using freeze dried homografts of the aorta.[1] Soon these were replaced by polyester grafts championed by Debakey in Houston, Texas. From the 1950s to the present time the polyester graft has been widely employed and is still the most common material used to replace aortic lesions throughout the world. Long-term results of open surgical repair of abdominal aortic aneurysms have proved to be extremely good after 10, 20 or even 30 years. Unfortunately the traditional open repair is a fairly severe procedure for the patient and really should only be performed on the fittest of people.

During the 1990s less traumatic ways of dealing with abdominal aortic aneurysms were developed using either smaller incisions, retroperitoneal incisions or a truly minimal access technique associated with laparoscopy and endovascular repair.[2] One of the problems with the laparoscopic repair of abdominal aortic lesions is that the suturing techniques required are quite time consuming and difficult to master but they can give extremely good results that are quite comparable to those for open surgical repair. Currently work is in progress to develop suturing machines and various stapling devices that will help to make the anastomosis between the polyester graft and the normal vessels quicker and safer. Unfortunately for most stapling techniques an anvil is required on one side of the vessel and graft to be joined while the staple is passed from the other side. Although this can be relatively easily achieved by laparoscopic means with a clamp and open aorta and graft, it is of course not reasonable when considering a truly endovascular stapling device. Endovascular repair of the aorta is commonly achieved through minimal access surgery via the femoral vessels either via a cut down or a percutaneous technique and this has proved to be a very minimally traumatic way of getting an endovascular graft in place to isolate a life threatening aneurysm.

Although the immediate and short-medium results of endovascular repair of abdominal aortic aneurysms have been very good the earlier results were marred by leaking at the joints, called endoleak, or by disruption of the joints by migration of the graft from the attachment points. Hooks and barbs are placed either infra-renally or supra-renally in order to provide fixation and appropriate oversizing of the stent-graft to the native aorta along with a radial force from the stent-graft to the sealing area of aorta providing a good seal. Probably the best long-term results for endovascular repair have been achieved with supra-renal fixation passing uncovered stents above the renals and fixing them in place to the relatively normal area of aorta found above the renals with appropriate barbs. As a general rule the more barbs the better for fixation and the stronger the barbs the better they resist fracture and subsequent migration.

Despite improvements in hooks, barbs and other forms of fixation such as Palmaz stents there is still a problem associated with graft migration. This is particularly a risk to those devices which do not have hooks or spikes to hold them in place. Attempts to correct the migration and threat of endoleak have been made using extension pieces to reline the aorta and the slipping stent-graft but unfortunately experience shows that unless the extension piece is firmly fixed onto the aorta and to the slipping stent-graft the migration story can start all over again. It seemed to the author that there would be a place for an endovascular stapling device that could fix the extension piece to the aortic wall and the extension piece to the slipping endovascular graft. There may well be a place for primary stapling of stent-grafts in situations where it is recognised that there is a high risk of migration.

FACTORS THAT LEAD TO MIGRATION OF AORTIC STENT-GRAFTS

Length of normal neck available

Most stent-grafts require a normal length of the neck below the renals to be of the order of 20 mm to get a good sound seal. If the neck length is less than 10 mm or even 5 mm the risk of migration and leakage is very high. There may well be a place here for stapling a graft firmly into position to stop it migrating.

Diameter

The wider the diameter of the neck the more likely the graft is to migrate and leak. Generally speaking neck diameters >30 mm are probably already aneurysmal and the risk of further dilatation and graft slippage is high. There could well be a place for stapling the stent-grafts in place so as to prevent the dilatation of these diseased vessels and to maintain position and seal.

Irregularity

An irregular shape of neck is not conducive to fixation or seal with straight sided Gianturco stents. If the neck is barrel shaped, or curved, straight parts of the Gianturco type stent will not fit comfortably and seal. This is where a more flexible or less stented graft, such as the flexible Aorfix produced by Lombard Medical Technologies, or the ballooning associated with unfixed PTFE material of the Endologix device may get a better seal. It is still possible that these devices would benefit from the additional security of a series of staples. Irregularities in the neck surface due to atheroma or thrombus may provide good short-term sealing but do not provide good long-term fixation as the relatively short barbs on some devices may not actually reach the more firm aortic wall and simply slip through the softer atheroma with time. It could be here, again, that a staple could drive straight through the cloth and out through to the tougher aortic wall.

Angulated necks

Early experience with Gianturco stent based grafts[3-6] show that migration was quite common after grafts had been put into necks that were angulated by >60°. Unless the Gianturco type stents happened to fit with their junctions exactly at the point of angulation, it was likely that there would be an early endoleak as well as a risk of later migration. Probably the most serious risk of migration and endoleak is the patient with not only an angulated but a widening conical shaped neck. It is in these situations again where endostapling may well have a place, at least to fix the graft into position and to prevent migration and possibly to improve apposition between the stent-graft and aortic wall and get a better seal.

Although some manufacturers have gone on to make stronger hooks and barbs to prevent fracture and migration, there are still quite a lot of endografts in the world that have been placed without good fixation and will be at risk to migrate and leak. It is for these that the impetus arose to develop an endovascular staple that could fix them back into place and keep them there along with any necessary extension pieces to cover areas of seal in the neck.

THE REQUIREMENTS OF AN ENDOVASCULAR STAPLE

1. It should be capable of being delivered from femoral access to any part of the aorta or the iliac system where it is required.
2. It should be placed accurately within 2/3 mms of a target zone-at the back, front or sides of a stent graft.
3. A retractable and replaceable staple would have great advantages over a single shot staple. Vascular surgical experience has shown that a vascular surgical needle does not always go precisely where the surgeon would wish it to when being placed through calcified areas. It seems that an endovascular stapler should be retractable and replaceable as many times as is necessary to achieve correct positioning for the best fixation possible. A single shot staple that did not fix in properly could be at risk for embolising and causing peripheral problems.
4. The pull out strength of a stapled stent-graft to aorta should be of the order of at least 12 Newtons. Individual staples should have 5 or more Newtons pull out strength per staple, therefore, 2, 3 or 4 staples maybe required to get adequate fixation.

DEVELOPMENT OF A RETRACTABLE, REPLACEABLE VASCULAR STAPLING DEVICE

The device that is currently marketed as the Refix was developed by the engineers at Lombard Medical Technology in the UK, formerly known as Anson Medical. We had to have a staple that would be loaded into a small 2 mm cannula, pushed out so that it would fix in place and yet be pulled back into the deploying cannula by an appropriate loop of thread. We chose Nitinol for the wire for its super elastic properties and, to a certain extent, for its thermal memory properties. The earlier staples involved welding, which proved to be difficult, but after many configurations were tried we ended up with a "seagull" shaped piece of wire. The points of the wings were made very sharp and curved to lie around the outside of the aorta. The body of the "seagull" was a loop in the wire through which the retaining thread loop could be passed. By pulling on the loop the staple could be pulled back into its loading cannula and by pushing on an inner cannula the staple could be deployed. We soon found that it was best to deploy the staple after pushing firmly on the site to be stapled so that it tented it and then the wings of the staple would come out quickly, laterally, outside the aorta and inflict minimum risk of damage to surrounding structures. The staple and its deploying retaining loop is shown in Figure 1.

The simplest design of the stapling device was a hand held version intended for use in open surgery where the deploying end of the delivery tube could be placed firmly against the area to be stapled and the staple fired through and retracted as necessary. It proved to be perfectly possible to withdraw and redeploy the staple many times until the operator was satisfied that a good position had been obtained. Because the wire is extremely thin and sharp, minimum damage was done to the stapled stent-graft or the vessel wall (Figure 2). During the course of development we made many different sizes of staple, going from 3 mm up to 15 mm in distance between the deployed points at the ends of the wings. The smaller sizes were intended for fixing smaller vessels but for aortic work we found that 12 mm diameter staples worked the best.

BENCH WORK TESTING

Durability of the Nitinol staples was tested in a rapidly vibrating situation that could simulate up to 10 years heart beats. It was found that the retaining thread snapped long before the Nitinol, suggesting that in human deployment the wire should be strong enough for at least 10 years.

IN VIVO TESTING OF THE STAPLE

In order to test for any adverse reaction in the arterial situation an ovine model was used. At open laparotomy the aorta was opened using the hand held stapling device. A small patch of polyester fabric was stapled to the posterior wall of the ovine abdominal aorta. After multiple patches and staples had been inserted the aorta was closed. The animals recovered for 3

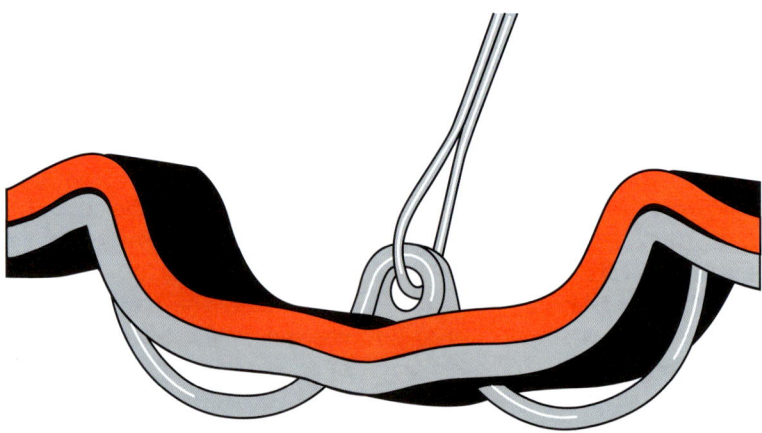

FIGURE 1: Shows the staple placed with the loop on the inside of the graft and 2 arms holding the outside of the aorta. The thread loop passing through the endostaple loop is used to retract and reload it in the delivery tube.

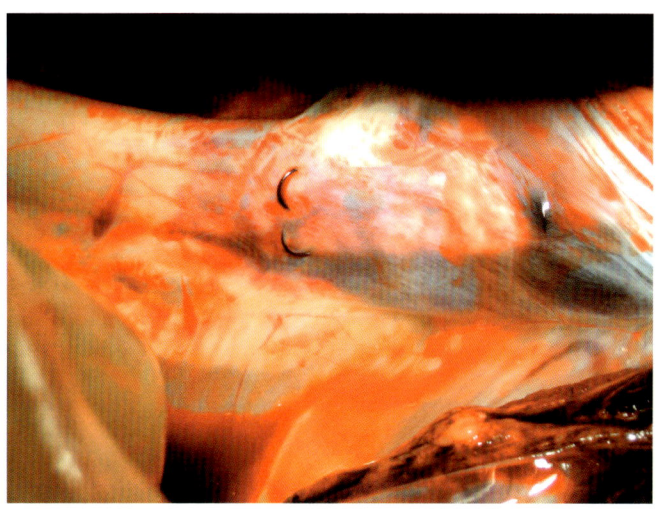

FIGURE 2: Shows the 2 arms of the endostaple on the outside of the aorta. There is very little evidence of haematoma.

months and then the aortas and patches were harvested. All the aortas were patent and histological examination showed no adverse features at the site of the staple or the polyester graft.

DEVELOPMENT OF AN ENDOVASCULAR STAPLER (ENDOREFIX)

The staple and loop are situated inside a small cannula, about 60-70 mm long, and attached to a hand held stapling device with a handle that can be squeezed to push the staple out and pull back to pull on the thread and pull the staple back in. The compressed staple in its loaded position can be pushed out with a very positive action and deploys extremely rapidly. The loaded staple cannula is passed up a slightly larger braided cannula. The outer braided cannula is threaded up a slightly larger cannula that is hinged at the aortic end, by pushing the braided catheter towards the patient it can be made to curve to assist the direction of aim and to get the staple to the position required. It is quite possible for the curve to be >90° and so allow the staple to be fired back-

wards, for instance in an angulated neck. There is also a balloon that is used to stabilise the device within the aorta. Three radiopaque markers on the braided hinged tube are used for orientation and another radiopaque marker can be seen at the staple end of the deploying cannula (see Figure 3). These radiopaque markers can be easily seen on fluoroscopy and act as a very good guide when directing the staple to the desired area (Figures 4 and 5).

BENCH TESTING OF THE ENDOSTAPLE

In order to practice and become skilled at deploying the staple we used a bench rig with either a silicone rubber aorta or bovine aorta. We first demonstrated that the staple could pass easily and equally well through these 2 structures and then proceeded to deploy a commercially available stent-graft within the artificial or bovine aorta and then passed the staple up the lumen to staple the stent-graft to the aorta. All this was done under direct vision. We perfected the techniques of deploying, retracting and redeploying the staple within the various stent-grafts over many times. We soon dis-

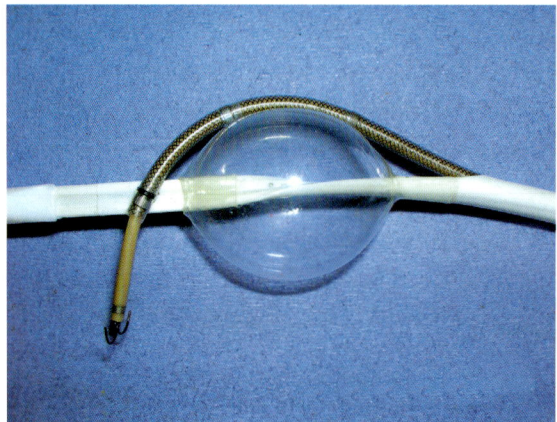

FIGURE 3: Shows the endovascular delivery kit with the staple in the deployed position. The curved cannula holds the staple and the hinged flexed outer cannula allow the staple to approach the target area at right angles to the stent-graft surface. The balloon helps to stabilise the whole system during deployment.

covered that when the staple was in its correct position the 2 wings were on the outside of the aorta and gentle traction on the delivery device would make the wings of the staple flap symmetrically. If one wing was not deployed properly through the aortic wall the wings would flap asymmetrically and this was an indication to retract the staple and redeploy it. There was no visible damage done to the commercial stent-graft cloth or to the artificial or bovine aorta by repeated deployment and retraction and redeployment of the staple (Figures 2, 4 and 6).

PULL OUT TESTS

The pull out test rig is illustrated in Figure 7. For this particular test we used 2 com-

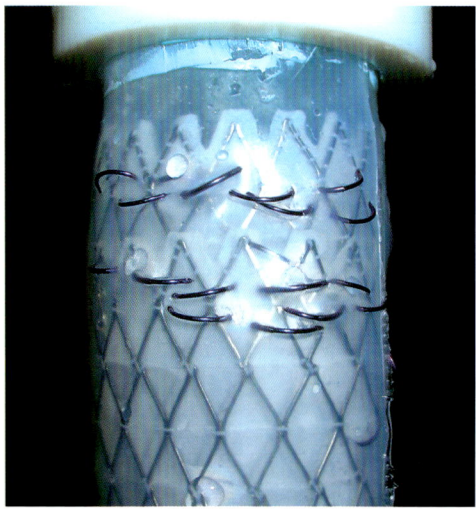

FIGURE 4: Shows multiple endostaples fixing a stent graft to a silicone rubber "aorta". Note how the arms lie circumferentially around the "aorta" to encourage seal.

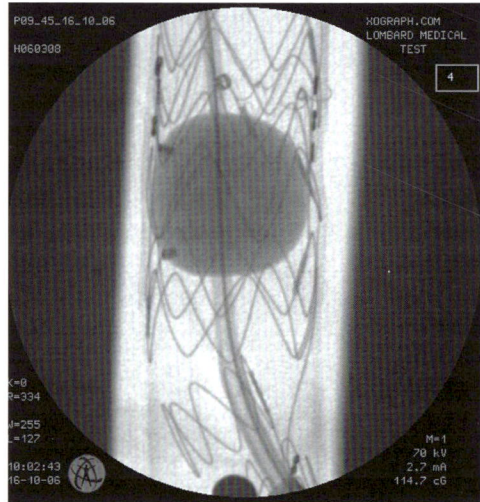

FIGURE 5: Showing inflated balloon, 3 radiopaque markers on the delivery cannulae and a staple in place on the top left close to a target marker.

FIGURE 6: Showing a stent graft after the "pull test". There is no visible staple damage to the opened aorta.

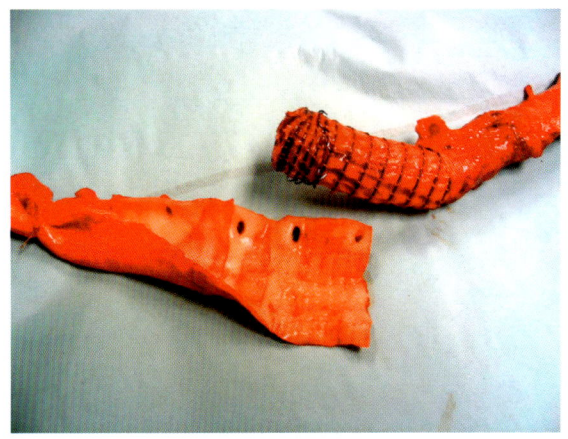

mercially available stent-grafts, the Medtronic Talent and AneuRx, deployed them in a bovine aorta of an appropriate size with no fixation and when fixation was assisted by 3 or 5 refix clips. These tests showed that the Talent graft pull out force with no clips was on average 1.9 Newtons. With 3 clips in place the average pull out force was 15 Newtons and with 5 clips in place the average pull out force was 24 Newtons. Using the AneuRx stent-graft the pull out force with no clips in place was 0.3 Newtons, with 3 clips in place was 17 Newtons and with 5 clips in place was 24 Newtons.

In Vivo Testing in the Porcine Aorta

These were all acute experiments, done with animals under a general anaesthesia and euthanaised at the end of the session. The femoral arteries were exposed and guidewires were introduced up from the femoral to the thoracic aorta. The endovascular stapling device was passed up over the wire to deploy the staples within the thoracic or abdominal aorta. The target zones were marked on previously placed endovascular stents. We found it was perfectly possible to recognise the staple on fluo-

roscopy and the positioning markers on the guiding cannulae and it was possible to rotate the whole device and to advance and to pull it back. We found the balloon stabilised the device and enabled the staple to be pushed firmly against the stent-graft and aortic wall so as to tent it before deployment. We soon learnt to recognise by general traction on the device when the staple was correctly deployed and when it was not. When correctly deployed it was possible to pull on the stapling device and the whole graft and aorta would move synchronously with it and the wings on the staple would move symmetrically. At this point we would cut the threat and release the stapler. It could then be seen that there was a clear radiolucent gap between the graft and the staple wings that represented a thickness of aortic wall. With suitable practice we found that we could place the staples within 2-3 mm of a previously marked target (Figure 5).

At the end of the procedure we euthanaised the animals, removed the aorta and photographed it. We could see the wings of the staples on the outside of the aorta with remarkably little haematoma present (Figure 2). We then cut away the aorta up to the stapled zone and found that a 10-15 mm cuff of aorta was very firmly held to the stent-graft by the staples. The pull out

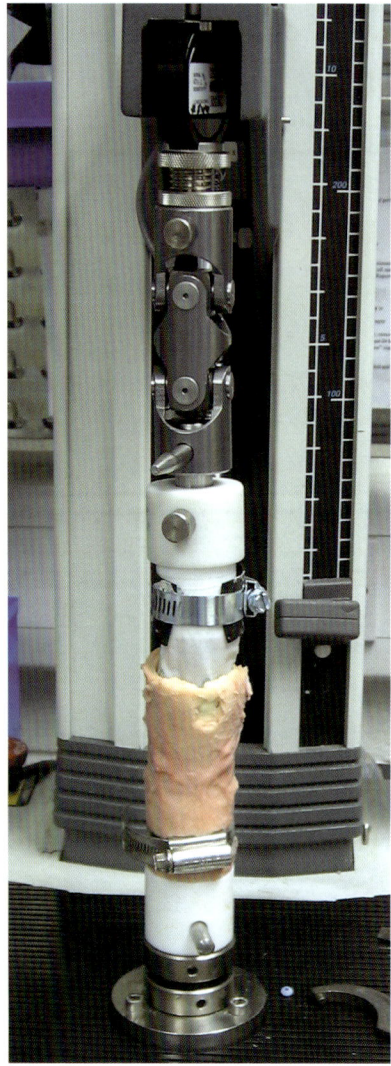

FIGURE 7: Test set up.

upper graft into the surrounding aorta and then to deploy 4 staples into the junction between the 2 stent-grafts overlapping each other and the aorta. This seemed to provide a very good pull out strength, again of the order of 20-30 Newtons between the various joins of graft to aorta and graft to graft. One such case, using an Aorfix graft (Figure 6) after the aorta has been opened to reveal very little damage at the site of the staple insertion but note that the intima has snapped above the stapled area during the course of the pull test, showing that the lining of the aorta gives way before the staples.

CADAVER TESTING UNDER X-RAY CONTROL

This was done in the laboratories at the University of Baltimore using fresh cadavers straight from the refrigerator. The arterial system was artificially pressurised to approximately 100 mm of mercury using warm water so as to encourage the thermal memory properties of the staples. Under standard C-Arm fluoroscopy we found it quite possible to deploy the staples in the abdominal aorta or the thoracic aorta. We then placed Talent or AneuRx stent-grafts within the abdominal or thoracic aorta and showed that we could staple them in place and, in addition, that we could join overlapping grafts firmly together, simulating the fixation of an extension piece put above a migrating graft. Again we found that we could deploy the staples within 2-3 mm of previously placed target zones on the stent-grafts and that it was perfectly easy to recognise not only the staple but also the various markers on the cannula and that we were able to deploy, retract and redeploy the staples as many times as was necessary to get them right. We confirmed that we knew when the staples were in the correct position by the movements that occurred when we pulled

forces were of the order of 20-30 Newtons when using devices such as the Talent or AneuRx or in a version of the Aorfix from which the upper hooks had been removed (Figures 6 and 7).

We then went on to try to join 2 pieces of stent-graft together so as to simulate the situation where an extension piece had been added above a migrating stent-graft. These again proved very satisfactory. We were able to deploy 4 staples through the

gently on the delivery device. When we were satisfied with the position of the staple we could cut the retaining thread and release the staple and remove the staple carrying cannula, replacing it with another staple carrying canula ready to fire the next staple.

This time we did not do a pull test with the intact aorta because we wanted to see the inside of the stent-graft and the appearance of the loops that form the body of the staple. To do this we split the aorta with the enclosed stent-grafts longitudely. We found it very difficult to see the wire body curls on the inside of the grafts because they were so nicely embedded and covered with a small layer of clot. The pull out tests we did were with the opened out flat aorta and stent-grafts. This naturally compromised that strength of the join but still we were able to get pull out forces between the graft and the aorta alone of the order of 20 Newtons between the 2 layers of graft and the aorta of 25-35 Newtons. We felt that the greater force of the graft to graft deployment strength was probably due to the close apposition of the 2 cloth materials and the relatively softer elastic nature of the natural aorta. Again, it was very difficult to see any damage done to the inside of the aorta when the staples and grafts were pulled out.

DISCUSSION

So far we have described the development and application of an endovascular stapling device. Previous stapling devices for vascular or general surgical use have used either stainless steel or Nitinol wire. Most of them require an anvil outside the structures to be stapled in addition to the working stapling part on the inside. Clearly this is not suitable for endovascular work but may find a place in general surgical or laparoscopic work. When dealing with aneurysmal vessels we find that they are inconsistent in the way they take sutures. Calcified areas may not allow sutures through at all but in soft weakened areas needles go through very easily and the vessel can be readily torn. Any stapling design that does not allow for repositioning of the staple will have difficulty in dealing with these vessels. Systems have been devised whereby a preliminary hole is punched using a laser, hot wire or sharp needle but the retractable refixable staple described in this article does not require preliminary holes to be made.

So far there have no reports of the EndoRefix being used in living humans to prevent migration or to correct it by stapling but now that the device has been awarded a CE mark we look forward with interest to its possible application in man. It could be used for fixing stent-grafts into short or angulated necks or for joining extension pieces together in the abdominal or in the thoracic aortic position.

The Aptus system has been developed in parallel and employs a spiral spring-like wire which is driven through the graft and the aortic wall with a drill-like motion, driven by an electric motor. This has been used in man, as reported in Phoenix in 2007 at the International Congress XX by DH Deaton. This device has been previously described.[7,8,9] There are other stapling devices being developed with C-shaped clips but like the EndoRefix they have only been used so far in the experimental situation and not actually placed in man.

The first clinical use of the Endorefix has been published from Munster (Germany).[10]

CONCLUSION

In conclusion, the concept of a retractable replaceable staple such as the EndoRefix has many attractive features and it is hoped that it will find a useful place in the treatment and prevention of stent-graft migration, so as to enable a wider range of patients to be suitable for endovascular repair of abdominal and thoracic aortic aneurysms. It may find a useful place in joining together several sections of stent-grafts that are overlapping each other so as to prevent them from separating. We anticipate that the first clinical use in man of this device will be for patients who have had a graft in place for 2-3 years and which is slowly migrating downwards. An extension piece could be placed to lie just below the renals, stapled in place there and the overlap between the extension and the migrating original endograft can be stapled together.

ACKNOWLEDGEMENTS

This project was conceived in conjunction with Prof Tony Anson and Dr Peter Phillips. Without their support and engineering "know how" it would never have got off the ground. The original concept arose from conversations with Waquar Yusuf who made the early drawings and took part in the necessary experimental laboratory work. Jan Macierewicz and Rob Hinchliffe also took part in the laboratory work.

I acknowledge the tremendous amount of engineering work done for this project by Duncan Keeble and Anthony Jones, engineers at Lombard Medical Technology and also for the use of the research facilities at the University of Nottingham, UK and Edwards Laboratories in Irvine, USA and the Department of Anatomy at the University of Baltimore, USA and at the Charles Rivers Laboratories.

REFERENCES

1. Dubost C, Allary M, Oecomomos N. Resection of an aneurysm of the abdominal aorta: Re-establishment of the continuity by a preserved human arterial graft with results after 5 months. Arch Surg 1952;64:405-8.
2. Parodi J, Palmaz J, Barone H. Trans-femoral intra-luminal graft implantation for abdominal aortic aneurysms. Ann Vascular Surgery 991;5:491-9.
3. Albertini JN, Kalliafas S, Travis S, Yusuf SW, Macierewicz JA, Whitaker SC, Elmarasy NM, Hopkinson BR: Anatomical risk factors for proximal perigraft endoleak and graft migration following endovascular repair of abdominal aortic aneurysms. Eur J Vasc Endovasc Surg 2000;19:308-312.
4. Dillavou ED, Muluk SC, Rhee RY, Tzeng E, Woody JD, Gupta N, Makaroun MS: Does hostile neck anatomy preclude successful endovascular aortic aneurysm repair? J Vasc Surg 2003;38: 657-663.
5. Albertini JN, DeMasi MA, Macierewicz J, El Idrissi R, Hopkinson BR, Clement C, Branchereau A: Aorfix stent graft for abdominal aortic aneurysms reduces the risk of proximal type 1 endoleak in angulated necks: bench-test study. Vascular 2005;13: 1-6.
6. Robbins M, Kritpracha B, Beebe HG, Criado FJ, Daoud Y, Comerota AJ: Suprarenal endograft fixation avoids adverse outcomes associated with aortic neck angulation. Ann Vasc Surg 2005;19:172-177.
7. Bolduc et al. United States patent Application Publication US 2005/0187613.A1.
8. Trout HT, Tanner HM. A New Vascular Endostaple: A Technical Description; Journal of Vascular Surgery Oct 2001.
9. Deaton DH. The Aptus system presented at International Congress XX 2007, Phoenix Arizona USA.
10. Donas et al. J Endovasc Ther 2008;15:499-503.

The "visceral hybrid" procedure: another option for the treatment of complex abdominal aortic lesions

Nikolaos Zarmpis, Karl Heinz Orend

If we wanted to summarize it all in a word, the visceral hybrid procedure is the "bridge" between the time honored "cut and sew" Crawford technique (where the diseased part of the abdominal aorta is replaced by a graft and the crucial aortic branches are preferentially reimplanted or bypassed) and the newly evolved totally endovascular treatment of abdominal aortic lesions utilizing fenestrated and/or branched stent grafts. In the visceral hybrid procedure, the abdominal aortic branches (i.e. Celiac Axis, Superior Mesenteric Artery, Renal Arteries and less common Inferior Mesenteric Artery) are individually and preferentially bypassed through an open procedure and the diseased abdominal aorta is treated by the endovascular implantation of a straight or bifurcated stent graft.

It is not in the scope of this chapter to condemn any of the aforementioned methods or to prove the superiority of any one of them. That will be judged by time. It is intended only to provide the reader with some late information concerning the prerequisites, the technical aspects and the results of the visceral hybrid procedure and if possible to shed some light on

some gray areas (such as post operative paraplegia), thus providing one more treatment option for the ever "challenging" patient with abdominal aortic disease. After all, the physical course of an aneurysm (whether abdominal or thoracoabdominal) is towards rupture, with only a 25% of the conservatively treated patients reaching the two years.[1]

Since the publication of Quinone[2] in 1999, more and more centers worldwide report their experiences with this technique[3-24] and commend on its' usage. Practically the visceral hybrid procedure can be applied to any thoracoabdominal aneurysm involving the celiac axis,[3] but on this chapter we will confine ourselves in its' application on Crawford type III and IV thoracoabdominal aneurysms (TAA), juxtarenal and suprarenal aneurysms,[22,24] pseudoaneurysms of the visceral arteries[21] and abdominal aortic dissections and anastomotic aneurysms that require suprarenal or supravisceral (either above the SMA or above the CA) cross-clamping. As juxtarenal aneurysms are considered those starting close to the renal artery or having an inadequate infrarenal neck for a "safe" infrarenal cross-clamping. As TAA III are considered aneurysms arising from the sixth intercostal space tapering to just above the infrarenal abdominal aorta to the iliac bifurcation and as TAA IV those from the 12th intercostal space tapering to the iliac bifurcation. The TAA V (from sixth intercostal tapering to just above the renal arteries) is also within the field of the visceral hybrid procedure.

Usually the above lesions come into consideration for intervention when they present with symptoms (rupture, impending rupture, pressure to neighboring organs), when they show signs of rapid expansion (>5-10 mm change over a 6-12 month period) and finally when the diameter of the aneurysm exceeds 5 cm for infrarenal aneurysms, 5.5 for pararenal and 6 cm for TAAs.[25,26]

TAA III and IV account for 16-32% and 10,4-24% of all TAAs respectively[4,11,27-30] and Visceral Aortic Aneurysms (VAA) for about 30% of all open repaired Abdominal Aortic Aneurysms.[25] According to Back[25] patients with VAA tend to be older, are more frequently females, have larger aneurysms and are more likely to have their aorta already operated upon in the past, compared to patients with simple AAA.

Most commonly in the visceral hybrid procedure the transperitoneal exposure is preferred, no aortic cross-clamping is applied and hence no additional adjuncts to counteract distal hypoperfusion and ischemia are utilized, each aortic branch is individually bypassed and finally a radiology suite or an adequately equipped Operating Room is required for the implantation of the stent graft. Of course deviations from this general description exist and will be discussed further down.

On the other hand, in the Crawfords' inclusion technique, after left thoracotomy and thoracoabdominal-transdiafragmatic-retroperitoneal exposure (Figure 1) the aorta is cross-clamped at a desired level, the diseased aorta is replaced by a tube

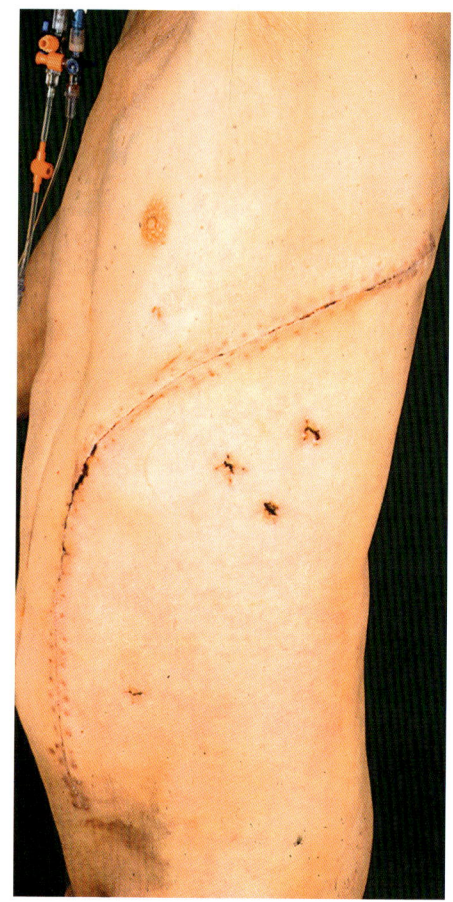

FIGURE 1: The thoracoabdominal-transdiafragmatic-retroperitoneal exposure of the Crawford procedure.

graft using the "cut and sew" technique and finally the aortic branches are either included in the remaining part of the aorta to be sewn to the graft (Figure 2) or are reimplanted individually or as "islands" to the graft (Figure 3). Several adjuncts have been developed and applied over the years to prevent or at best limit spinal cord and visceral ischemia and ameliorate the devastating effects of aortic cross-clamping to the circulatory system.

From these fundamental differences between the two techniques offspring the possible advantages and disadvantages that we present in Table 1.

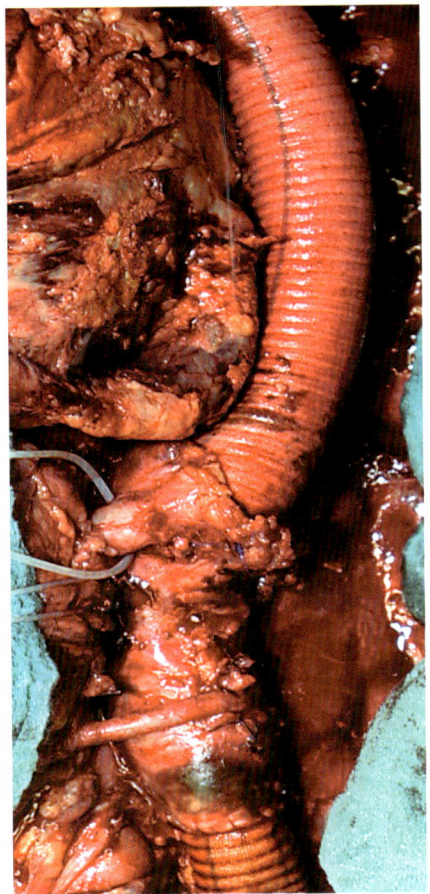

FIGURE 2: The aortic branches are included in the remaining part of the aorta to be sewn to the graft.

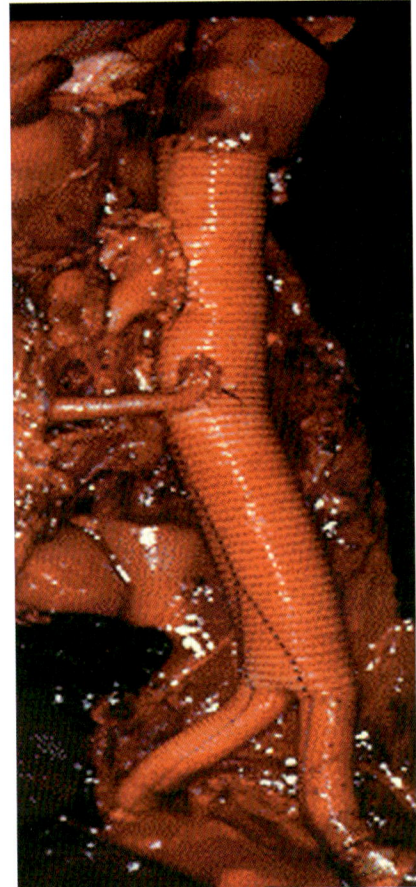

FIGURE 3: The aortic branches are reimplanted individually or as "islands" to the graft.

We left intentionally the comparison of the results of each technique out of the previous table. The unbiased evaluation of results is complicated by the mixing of urgent, emergent and elective repairs, by dissecting and non dissecting aneurysms and finally by the differences in treatment strategy applied for the same type of disease. Instead we provide in Table 2 the so far published results concerning the open repair of TAA III and IV.

As we can see, despite the progress in surgical techniques, anesthesia, post op. care and use of adjuncts of any kind the 30-day mortality ranges from 4 to 17%, renal impairment from 9 to 24% and paraplegia/paraparesis from 0 to 4%.

Unfortunately there are no publications of results from large series (the largest consists of 29 patients over a 3-year period)[4] concerning the visceral hybrid procedure. On Table 3 we provide the results of four series found in English literature and that of our own experience.

Nonetheless, gathering all the available data, published in the English literature, from centers applying the visceral hybrid procedure in complex abdominal aortic lesions[3-24] we could report a 30-day mortality of 0-26%, renal impairment 0%

Visceral hybrid procedure	Crawfords' procedure
Advantages	
1. Avoidance of thoracotomy and retroperitoneal exposure 2. Avoidance of aortic cross-clamping 3. Avoidance of adjuncts against distal hypo perfusion 4. Avoidance of traumatic preparation of the aorta 5. Avoidance of CardioPulmonary Bypass, with all its' consequences 6. Lesser amounts of Heparin given 7. None or minimal Visceral Ischemia Time 8. Attractive option for patients with marginal cardiac, respiratory and/or renal reserves 9. Attractive option in "redo" operations 10. Reduced blood loss[17,23] 11. Less straining anesthesia[23]	1. Time honored - Long term results available 2. Numerous published reports of large series 3. Widely applied 4. Reimplantation of dominant intercostals arteries possible
Disadvantages	
1. Rather new. Results of more than 9 years unavailable 2. Expertise in EVAR techniques required 3. No published reports from large series 4. Irradiation exposure 5. Contrast medium required 6. Risk of emboli, due to endovascular manipulations 7. Skepticism about the retrograde perfusion of the grafts 8. Potential aortoenteric erosion or fistula due to the extra anatomic routing of the grafts 9. Concerns for the long term durability and behavior of the stent grafts	1. Technically demanding 2. Results volume dependent (upon center and surgeon)[26,28,30,43,44] 3. Possible spinal cord and visceral ischemia despite the use of adjuncts 4. Devastating effects on the cardio respiratory system 5. 0.6 L/sec reduction in FEV1 caused only by the thoracoabdominal incision[27]

and paraplegia/paraparesis 0%.[4,11,17,30] In calculating these percentages though, urgent, emergent and elective repairs were included.

Back et al,[25] among others, showed that cross-clamp level and Visceral Ischemia Time clearly affect perioperative and long term survival. Thus, an advantage of the visceral hybrid procedure can be pre-

sumed, since cross-clamping is avoided and VIT is minimized.

TECHNIQUE

It is not in the scope of this chapter to go into a detailed description of the visceral hybrid procedure. We refer the reader to

TABLE 2

PUBLISHED SERIES ON OPEN REPAIR OF TAA III AND IV

Author	TAA type	No of patients	Length of study (years)	30-day mortality %	Renal failure %	Paraplegia/ para paresis %	Time period
Svenson[46]	IV	346	31	6	24	4	'60-'91
Coseli[29]	III	291	15	4.8	7	2.8	'86-
	IV	329	15	3.6	6.8	2.1	2000
Chiesa[28]	III	57	10	12.3	NR	5.3	'93-
	IV	39	10	7.7	NR	2.6	2003
Cina[30]	III	22	11	18.8	50	7.5	'90-
	IV	42	11	7.1	37.5	0	2001
Eide[42]	III	10	15	14.8	14.8	7.4	'85-
	IV	17	15				2000
Schepens[26]	III	93	22	15.1	6.9	10	'81-
	IV	42	22	7.1	6.1	4.8	2003
Bicknel[26]	IV	130	7	17.	15	4	93-2000
Lemaire[26]	IV	207	12	4	5	1	'86-'96
Martin [26]	IV	38	11	11	12	0.53	'89-'98
Schwartz[26]	IV	58	17	5	9	3	'77-'94
Gilling-Smith[26]	IV	55	10	15	14	0	'83-'93

NR = not reported

the selected literature at the end of this chapter.[2-4,11,17,22,23,31,32,47] But we would like to point out some aspects and some particularities of it.

a. General considerations

Thus far the visceral hybrid procedure is being reserved by the centers performing it for patients exhibiting one or more of the conditions described below, with the exception of Wolfe et al.[4] who tend to adopt this technique completely in treating TAAs.
- Elderly patients with cardiorespiratory co-morbidities.
- Patients who had another aortic operation in the past, especially for TAA.
- Patients with prior left chest or left retroperitoneal surgery.
- Patients with renal failure, COPD or Coronary Artery Disease.[3]
- Patients with TAA aneurysm and simultaneous aneurysms of the origins of each of the visceral vessels, thus precluding the Crawford inclusion technique.[2]
- Patients with recurrent HIV/AIDS-related TAAs and pseudoaneurysms.[48]
- Patients in which the proximal "neck" of the aneurysm is less than 15mm or is angulated more than 45 degrees or a thrombus is covering more than 50% of the aortic circumference, thus precluding the sole EndoVascular Repair.[11]

Author	TAA type	No of patients	Length of study (years)	30-day mortality %	Renal failure %	Paraplegia/ para paresis %	Time period
Orend	All types	15	7	26.6	0	0	99-2006
Schumacher[23]	All types	22/12 VAA	3.5	14.4	0	0	NM
Black[4]	All types	29/8 type III, IV	3	13	0	0	2002-2005
Fulton[11]	III, IV	10	3	0	0	0	2000-2003
Gawenda[47]	All types	6	8	0	0	0	98-2006

Easily we can understand that careful patient selection and preoperative planning is of paramount importance.[34]

Preoperative Pulmonary and Renal Function Tests, as well as evaluation of cardiac reserves are not to be forgotten.

Detailed imaging of the aorta with CT and 1 mm slices after the induction of contrast medium followed by aortic reconstruction is also imperative for a good outcome. The aim is to preserve or revascularize as many collateral pathways as possible, in order to limit the potential of post operative complications.

Careful selection of the stent graft (cross sectional size, extent of aortic coverage, straight vs. bifurcated, flexibility) is also a major determinant of the outcome. In our institution over the 8 years that we are using this technique we have utilized 3 different stent grafts: the TAG (W.L. Gore & Associates, Putzbrunn, Germany), the Talent (Medtronic World Medical, Sunrise, Fl, USA) and the Zenith (Cook Incorporated, Bloomington, IN, USA). The major determinant in deciding which to use each time, was the availability of each stent graft regarding the length of the aneurysm and the cross sectional size of its' proximal and distal neck. The flexibility of each specific stent graft played also an important, but secondary to availability in sizes, role.

We chose to cover only as much descending thoracic aorta as it was necessary according to the proximal extent of the aneurysm or the dissection and by securing a free-of-disease landing zone of at least 2,5 cm. We never needed to go beyond the Left Subclavian Artery and in most cases the greater part of the descending thoracic aorta was left uncovered, thus minimizing the risk of neurological complications.

Finally, familiarity and expertise in the endovascular techniques is a must on behalf of the surgeon who is about to undertake a "hybrid" operation. Here the saying "a good surgeon does it all", does not apply.

b. Technical notes

The transperitoneal approach is the one usually used, but the high risk patient, in an effort to minimize potential pulmonary and gastrointestinal complications, could benefit from a retroperitoneal approach, provided that full revascularization is not jeopardized and other contraindications (e.g. previous retroperitoneal operation) do not exist.

All anastomosis should function as they were end-to-end. A Doppler flow meter can be utilized to prove the adequacy of the bypasses before the insertion of the stent graft. If not satisfied with the results, that is the time to correct the problem.

PolyTetraFluoroEthylene (Figure 4) is an excellent material for the bypass conduits, with excellent long term results and low complication rates.[11] Woven Dacron (Figure 5) is an equally good alternative and a matter of preference. Autologus grafts, such as saphenous vein, have also been described.[5]

The CA and SMA should be both bypassed, if feasible each one independently, to deter short or long term complications, as many studies have shown[4,17,31] and we are afraid that we have to disagree with Gaweda et al.[47] who bypass only the SMA when the retrograde perfusion of the celiac trunk through the gastroduodenal collaterals is angiographically demonstrated.

The same principle applies to the renal arteries. Every effort should be made to bypass each one of them separately. Post op. renal impairment is one of the major factors affecting morbidity and mortality.[2,21,25,26,28] Adequate renal function is of paramount importance and should be insured regardless of surgeons discomfort.

The "visceral octopus technique" is the most widely used (Figure 6). In this, a tri- or more-furcated graft is constructed and through its' limbs the CA, SMA, and the RAs are revascularized through a transperitoneal exposure. The inflow for this complex graft should be obtained from the largest and healthiest vessel possible. Usually that vessel is a common or external iliac artery (more often of the left side) (Figures 7 and 8) but the infrarenal aorta can be used as well (Figure 9), provided the distal landing zone of the stent graft is not compromised and there is enough healthy aortic wall for an optimal anastomosis. Fulton[11] suggests also the descending thoracic aorta as inflow site of TAA IV, as this vessel is relatively free of atherosclerotic disease. He also proposes the external iliac to renal artery bypass

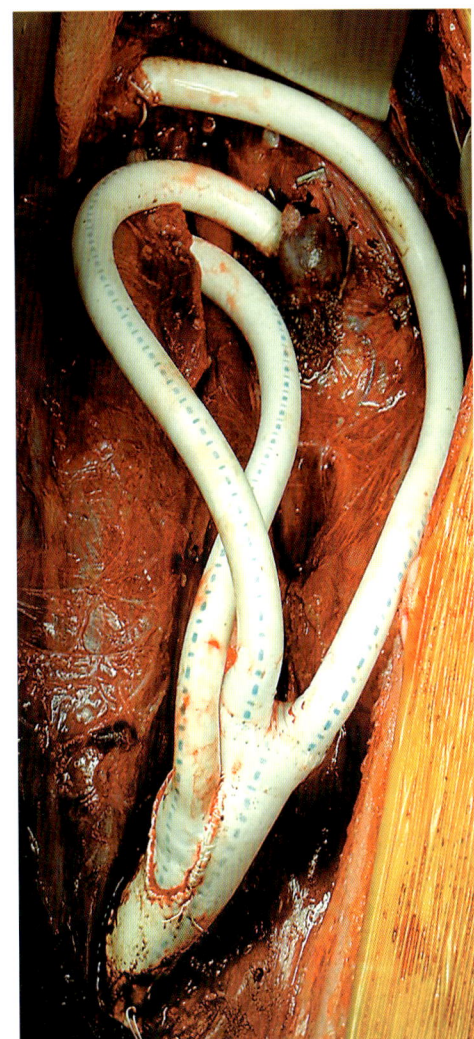

FIGURE 4: PolyTetraFluoroEthylene is an excellent material for the bypass conduits.

through minimal bilateral retroperitoneal exposures under local anesthesia. Further on, in cases with severe aortoiliac occlusive disease or with "high-riding" left RA or "low-lying" right RA, he advocates the construction of a splenorenal or a hepatorenal bypass, respectively. If an infrarenal synthetic graft is already in place, the bypass grafts can be anastomosed directly to it in an end-to-side fashion. The limb feeding the CA is usually tunneled in front

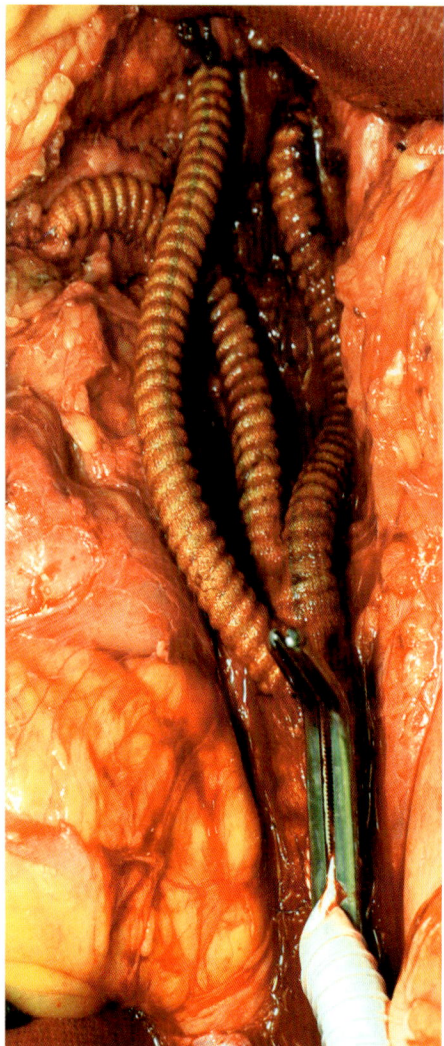

FIGURE 5: Woven Dacron is an equally good alternative for the bypass conduits.

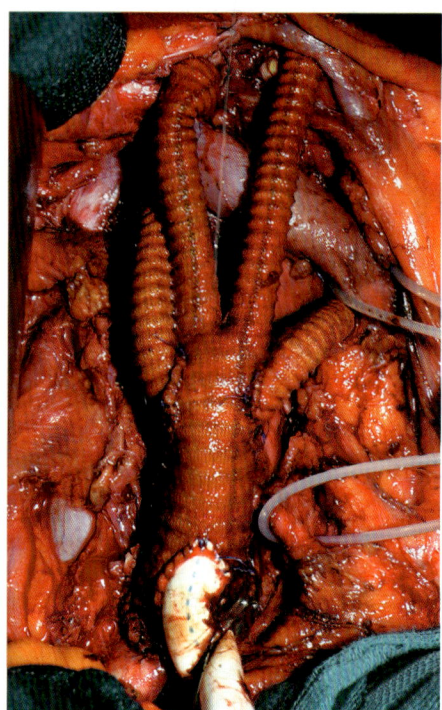

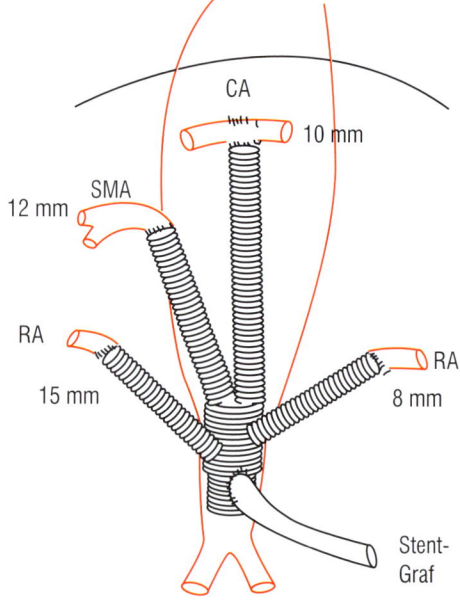

FIGURE 6: The "visceral octopus technique" is the most widely used. In this, a tri-or more-furcated graft is constructed and through its' limbs the CA, SMA, and the RAs are revascularized through a transperitoneal exposure.

of the renal vein and behind the pancreas to find its' target. By the end of the anastomoses every effort should be made to protect the extra anatomic grafts with surrounding tissue or omental flaps, in the fear of potential aortoenteric erosions or fistulas. Another point that should be emphasized is the imperative ligation of the origins of the recipient vessels, in order to prevent latter endoleaks.

After completion of all bypasses the

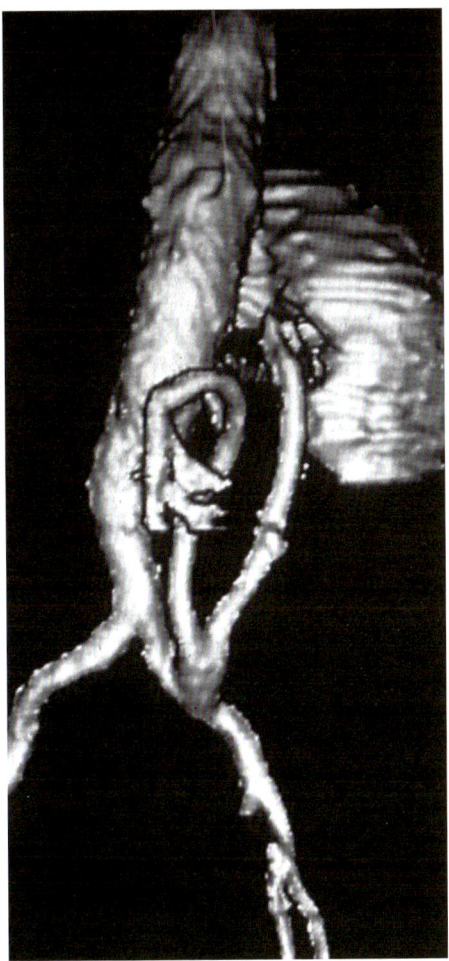

FIGURE 7: The common iliac artery (more often of the left side) is chosen as the donor vessel for the conduit.

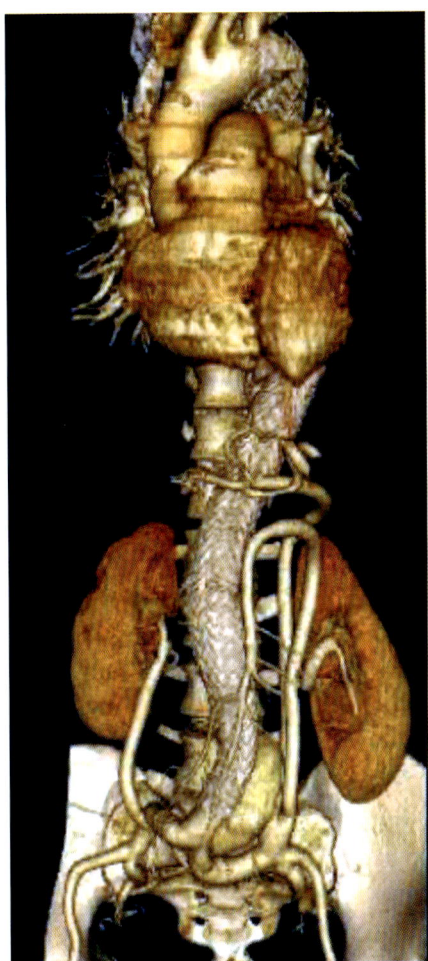

FIGURE 8: The common or external iliac artery (more often of the left side) is chosen as the donor vessel for the conduit.

endovascular stent is deployed, preferentially delivered through a formerly created conduit (Figure 10) instead of passing it through the femoral artery, in order to avoid complications from vessel tortuosity. Here an interesting variation should be mentioned. Black etal. treat patients with TAA II secondary to chronic dissection by first stenting the true lumen of the thoracic aorta and proceed to a visceral hybrid procedure at a separate operation. The logic in that is to increase the flow in the infrarenal aortic true lumen.

In the unfortunate case that some part of the stent graft is collapsed (usually the proximal), documented during the completion angiography after the deployment of all stents, balloon dilation of that part can and should be attempted. If that fails to produce reliable results a second stent graft should be utilized, in order to provide support to the problematic region. The minimum overlapping of the stent grafts is 2,5 cm. The same rule applies if a proximal type I endoleak is detected after the deployment of the stent. If the stent mi-

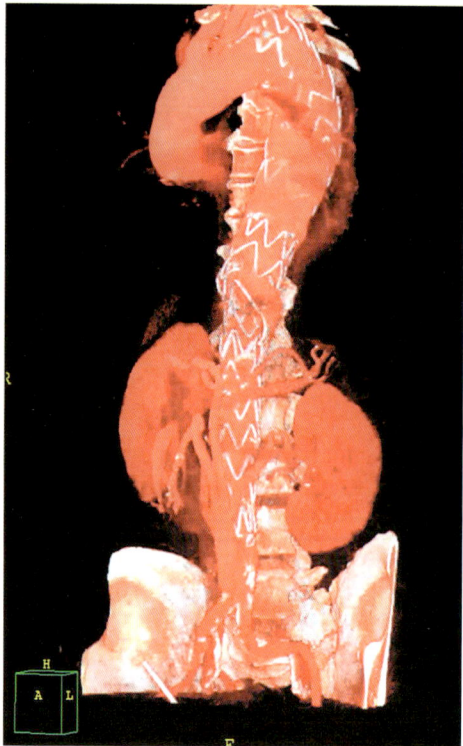

FIGURE 9: The infrarenal aorta can be used as well as the donor vessel for the conduit, provided the distal landing zone of the stent graft is not compromised and there is enough healthy aortic wall for an optimal anastomosis.

grates from the optimal preplanned position during its' deployment, the surgeon should assess the damage done. If a critical vessel (eg. a renal artery) is occluded then he/she should make every effort to revascularize that vessel, usually by bypassing it. If the diseased aorta is left uncovered, or if an endoleak appears he/she should utilize one or more stent grafts to correct the problem. But in no case, and that is our suggestion, should he/she try to move the migrated graft. Perhaps in the near future the "graft industry" will produce stent grafts that will allow us to instantly correct such problems by simply repositioning the stent graft, but we have to wait till then.

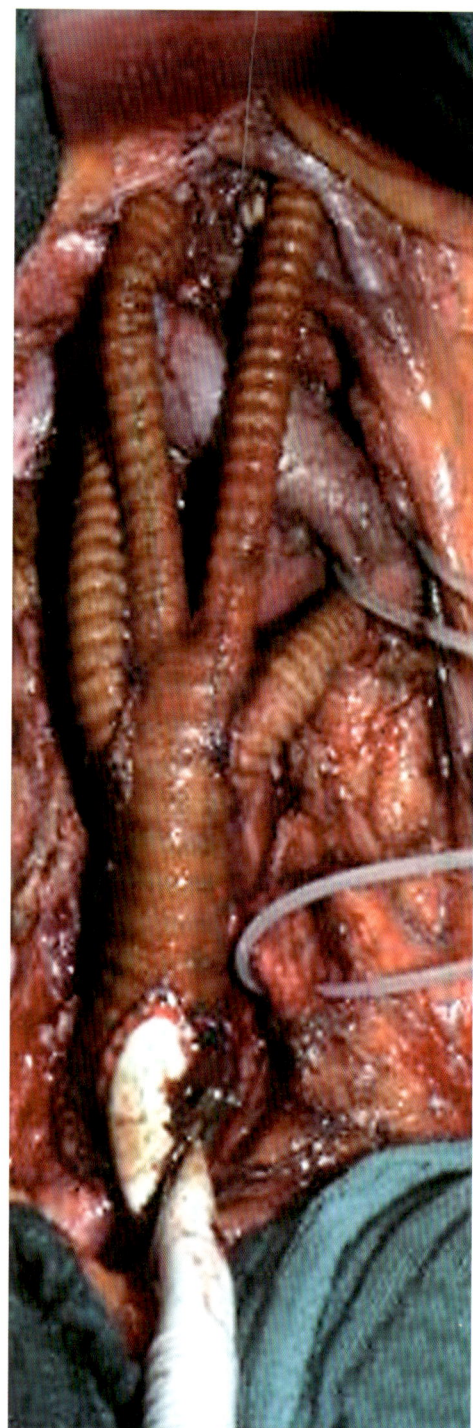

FIGURE 10: After completion of all bypasses the endovascular stent is deployed, preferentially delivered through a formerly created conduit.

Skepticism exists still about the safety and durability of the retrograde bypasses. According to numerous studies[2,4,11,24] this does not seem to be a real problem and graft patency is much more affected by routing and graft length (the latter should be as short as possible) rather than by direction of flow.

The median ischemia times, reported so far, are ca 15 minutes for the CA, SMA and RAs.[4,17,23]

Duration of the operation ranges, according to our experience, from 4 to 6 hours and irradiation time from 10 to 30 min. depending on type and number of stent grafts used (ie. straight, bifurcated, more than one piece, etc.).

c. Potential complications

Potential post op. complications include respiratory insufficiency, prolonged ventilation, renal failure (transient or permanent), neurological deficit, stroke, peripheral emboli, MI, wound infection, coagulopathies, arrhythmias, gastrointestinal complications,[33] SIRS and visceral ischemia.

d. Endoleaks

As a rule of thumb, any type I endoleak that is discovered should be repaired instantly or as soon as possible. The way to do that was analyzed before.

For type II and III endoleaks it is advisable to wait for a period of 3 months. If the aneurysmal sac increases in size or the pressure within it is such that impairs the proper function of the stent graft, then coil embolization should be attempted as a first step. If the result is unsatisfactory then endoclips or open suture ligation of the involved vessel/s could be undertaken.

e. Follow up

Almost all centers follow the same pattern –ie. the EUROSTAR protocol 49– and fol-low their patients with contrast medium enhanced CT and plain chest x-ray 3 days, 1 month, 6 months, 12 months, 18 months after operation and then yearly.[4,11,17,23,31] The structural integrity of the stent, its' position, the presence of endoleaks of any kind and the patency of the grafts are some of the things that are evaluated. The longest follow up time reported so far is 3 years,[3,18,19] though anecdotally, from our experience, we could report a patient who received two separate Dacron bypass grafts (iliac-SMA & iliac-CA) and a Medtronic Talent 34-99 stent graft in 1999 for a recurrent type IV TAA and is alive and well today, 8 years after, following a yearly follow up.

If during the follow up exams an abnormality is detected, the plan is modified accordingly.

Long Term Results

The technique was first reported in 1999 and thus far the longest reported follow up is 3 years. A single patient with a 8 year follow up from our experience was previously mentioned. Therefore very little credible data are available.[4,11,17,23,24] According to these, the 30 month survival is reported above 86%, comparable to the 70% of the Crawford procedure as reported by Svenson[46] and Cambria,[45] graft patency rate above 98% and endoleak prevalence ca 20,6%. No major complication have been reported.

Spinal Cord Ischemia

It is rather surprising to see that all the published reports of the visceral hybrid procedures applied for TAA III and IV, as well as for VAA, report zero incidence of paraplegia or paraparesis and most of them utilize no adjuncts to protect the spinal cord such as cerebrospinal fluid

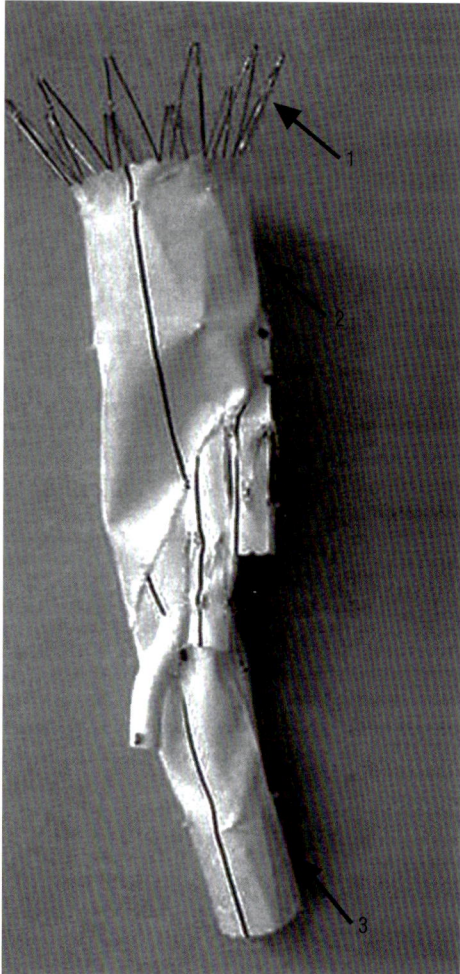

FIGURE 11: A commercially available branched graft.

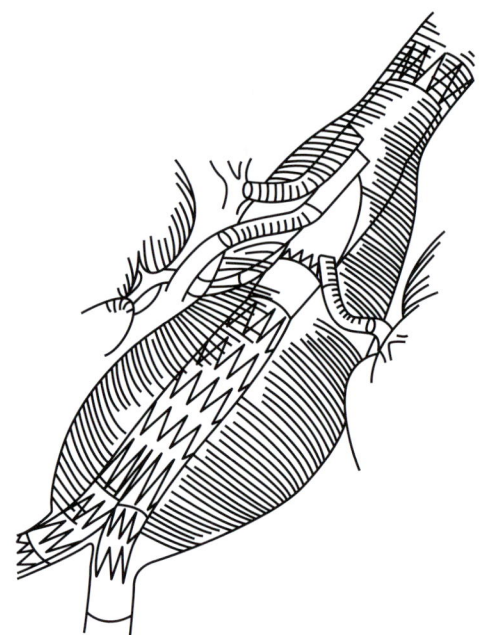

FIGURE 12: A schematic representation of the application of a branched graft.

drainage, shunts, spinal cooling or continuous neurological monitoring. Taking a look on table 2, we find only two reports that could match this number and only for TAA IV. Moreover, Weigang etal 35 report a 3% to 12% risk of spinal cord ischemia after endovascular thoracic or thoracoabdominal aortic repair and propose the use of spinal cord protective measures with motor- and somatosensory-evoked potential monitoring, cerebrospinal fluid drainage, and prevention of hypotension in order to reduce the incidence of spinal cord ischemia and improve the neurological outcome in patients undergoing endovascular thoracic or thoracoabdominal aortic repair. But their results incorporate the treatment of all thoracic and thoracoabdominal lesions.

The most obvious reason for this low paraplegia/paraparesis incidence would seem to be that for the treatment of TAA III or IV and VAA only a small portion of the thoracic aorta has to be overstented, thus a great deal of collaterals for the perfusion of the spinal cord are preserved. That is true to a certain extent, as the perplex anatomy of the aorta in certain patients mandates the overstenting of the whole descending thoracic aorta –even of the left subclavian– in order to achieve a secure fixation and/or avoid type I endoleak.

Another possible explanation could be that collateral arterial blood supply perfuse the spinal cord despite the overstenting of intercostals vessels, or that the overstenting does not necessarily lead to intercostal arteries occlusion. Equally convincing seems to be the assumption that avoidance of visceral ischemia and visceral embolization deters the cytokine release which evokes secondary cord ischemia through the "no reflow" phenomenon.[23]

Regardless what the reason might be, the early results are favorable for the visceral hybrid procedure. For sure the prolonged ischemia, the intraoperative hypotension, the injuries to the aorta from the surgeons' manipulations and finally the "reperfusion syndrome" that follows aortic cross-clamping, don't help in minimizing neurological complications.

VISCERAL HYBRID PROCEDURE AND TOTALY EVAR

Who of as wouldn't welcome the totally endovascular treatment of abdominal aortic lesions, utilizing branched and/or fenestrated grafts[36-38,40,41] (Figures 11 and 12). After all the visceral hybrid procedure is not an opponent of totally EVAR, rather an adjunct to it. There will always be a patient with extraordinary anatomy in which the aid of an open procedure would be warranted.[21,22]

But for the time being there are several aspects that limits its' use. Increased irradiation time, increased operating time, increased contrast-medium and heparin administration, increased cost, increased delivery (of the custom made stent graft) time, increased required surgical expertise coupled with requirement of sophisticated equipment, unknown long term results, frequent graft rotation during deployment leading to occlusion or dissection of vital arteries and lack of standardized industrial production are some of the limitations presenting nowadays.[39] As each one of these will be resolved in the not too distant future, so clearer the indications of it and the visceral hybrid procedure will evolve.

REFERENCES

1. Crawford ES, DeNatale RW. Thoracoabdominal aortic aneurysm: observations regarding the natural course of the disease. J Vasc Surg 1986;3:578-82.
2. Quinones-Baldrich WJ, Panetta TF, Vescera CL, Kashyap VS. Repair of type IV thoracoabdominal aneurysm with a combined endovascular and surgical approach.J Vasc Surg. 1999 Sep;30(3): 555-60.
3. Lawrence-Brown M, Sieunarine K, van Schie G, Purchas S, Hartley D, Goodman MA, Prendergast FJ, Semmens JB. Hybrid open-endoluminal technique for repair of thoracoabdominal aneurysm involving the celiac axis.J Endovasc Ther. 2000 Dec;7(6):513-9.
4. Black SA, Wolfe JH, Clark M, Hamady M, Cheshire NJ, Jenkins MP. Complex thoracoabdominal aortic aneurysms: endovascular exclusion with visceral revascularization.J Vasc Surg. 2006 Jun;43(6): 1081-9; discussion 1089.
5. Yoshida M, Mukohara N, Shida T, Fukuda T. Combined endovascular and surgical procedure for recurrent thoracoabdominal aortic aneurysm.Ann Thorac Surg. 2006 Sep;82(3):1099-101.
6. Ruppert V, Salewski J, Wintersperger BJ, Sadeghi-Azandaryani M, Allenberg JR, Reiser M, Steckmeier B. Endovascular repair of thoracoabdominal aortic aneurysm with multivisceral revascularization.J Vasc Surg. 2005 Aug;42(2):368.
7. Minami H, Mukohara N, Obo H, Yoshida M, Fukuda T, Shida T, Combined stent-graft and surgical treatment for a thoracoabdominal aortic aneurysm in a high risk patient.Jpn J Thorac Cardiovasc Surg. 2005 Aug;53(8):448-51.
8. Castelli P, Caronno R, Piffaretti G, Tozzi M, Lomazzi C, Lagana D, Carrafiello G, Cuffari S. Hybrid treatment for thoracic and thoracoabdominal aortic aneurysms in patients unfit for open conventional repair.Acta Chir Belg. 2005 Nov-Dec; 105(6):602-9.
9. Tachibana K, Morishita K, Kurimoto Y, Fukada J, Hachiro Y, Abe T. Endovascular stent-grafting for thoracoabdominal aortic aneurysm following bypass grafting to superior mesenteric and celiac arteries: report of two cases.Ann Thorac Cardiovasc Surg. 2005 Oct;11(5):335-8.
10. Gregoric ID, Gupta K, Jacobs MJ, Poglajen G, Su-

vorov N, Dougherty KG, Krajcer Z. Endovascular exclusion of a thoracoabdominal aortic aneurysm after retrograde visceral artery revascularization.Tex Heart Inst J. 2005;32(3):416-20.

11. Fulton JJ, Farber MA, Marston WA, Mendes R, Mauro MA, Keagy BA. Endovascular stent-graft repair of pararenal and type IV thoracoabdominal aortic aneurysms with adjunctive visceral reconstruction.J Vasc Surg. 2005 Feb;41(2):191-8.

12. Bonardelli S, De Lucia M, Cervi E, Pandolfo G, Maroldi R, Battaglia G, Gargano M, Matheis A, Stefano MG. Combined endovascular and surgical approach (hybrid treatment) for management of type IV thoracoabdominal aneurysm.Vascular. 2005 Mar-Apr;13(2):124-8.

13. Rubin BG. Extra-anatomic visceral revascularization and endovascular stent-grafting for complex thoracoabdominal aortic lesions.Perspect Vasc Surg Endovasc Ther. 2005 Sep;17(3):227-34; discussion 234-5, author reply 236.

14. Chiesa R, Melissano G, Civilini E, Setacci F, Tshomba Y, Anzuini A. Two-stage combined endovascular and surgical approach for recurrent thoracoabdominal aortic aneurysm.J Endovasc Ther. 2004 Jun;11(3):330-3.

15. Lundbom J, Hatlinghus S, Odegard A, Eide TO, Lange C, Aasland J, Aadahl P, Myhre HO. Combined open and endovascular treatment of complex aortic disease.Vascular. 2004 Mar;12(2):93-8.

16. Rimmer J, Wolfe JH. Type III thoracoabdominal aortic aneurysm repair: a combined surgical and endovascular approach. Eur J Vasc Endovasc Surg. 2003 Dec;26(6):677-9.

17. Kotsis T, Scharrer-Pamler R, Kapfer X, Liewald F, Gorich J, Sunder-Plassmann L, Orend KH. Treatment of thoracoabdominal aortic aneurysms with a combined endovascular and surgical approach. Int Angiol. 2003 Jun;22(2):125-33.

18. Iguro Y, Yotsumoto G, Ishizaki N, Arata K, Sakata R. Endovascular stent-graft repair for thoracoabdominal aneurysm after reconstruction of the superior mesenteric and celiac arteries.J Thorac Cardiovasc Surg. 2003 Apr;125(4):956-8.

19. Iguro Y, Yotsumoto G, Ishizaki N, Arata K, Sakata R. Endovascular stent-graft repair for thoracoabdominal aneurysm after reconstruction of the superior mesenteric and celiac arteries. J Thorac Cardiovasc Surg 2003;125:956-8.

20. Flye MW, Choi ET, Sanchez LA, Curci JA, Thompson RW, Rubin BG, et al. Retrograde visceral vessel revascularization followed by endovascular aneurysm exclusion as an alternative to open surgical repair of thoracoabdominal aortic aneurysm. J Vasc Surg 2004;39:454-8.

21. Juvonen T, Biancari F, Ylonen K, Perala J, Rimpilainen J, Lepojarvi M. Combined surgical and endovascular treatment of pseudoaneurysms of the visceral arteries and of the left iliac arteries after thoracoabdominal aortic surgery.Eur J Vasc Endovasc Surg. 2001 Sep;22(3):275-7.

22. Macierewicz JA, Jameel MM, Whitaker SC, Ludman CN, Davidson IR, Hopkinson BR. Endovascular repair of perisplanchnic abdominal aortic aneurysm with visceral vessel transposition.J Endovasc Ther. 2000 Oct;7(5):410-4.

23. Schumacher H, Bockler D, Bardenheuer HJ, Allenberg JR. Hybrid endovascular reconstruction for complex thoracoabdominal lesions. In: Thoracic Aorta Endografting, A Multidisciplinary approach, Amor M, Bergeron P, Castriota F, Cremonesi A, Mathias K and Raithel D.eds, 2004 p.187-196.

24. Hosokawa H, Iwase T, Sato M, Yoshida Y, Ueno K, Tamaki S, Inoue K. Successful endovascular repair of juxtarenal and suprarenal aortic aneurysms with a branched stent graft.J Vasc Surg. 2001 May;33(5):1087-92.

25. Back MR, Bandyk M, Bradner M, Cuthbertson D, Johnson BL, Shames ML, Bandyk DF. Critical analysis of outcome determinants affecting repair of intact aneurysms involving the visceral aorta.Ann Vasc Surg. 2005 Sep;19(5):648-56.

26. Wahlgren CM, Wahlberg. Management of thoracoabdominal aneurysm type IV. Eur J Vasc Endovasc Surg. 2005 Feb;29(2):116-23.

27. Schepens M, Dossche K, Morshuis W, Heijmen R, van Dongen E, Ter Beek H, Kelder H, Boezeman. Introduction of adjuncts and their influence on changing results in 402 consecutive thoracoabdominal aortic aneurysm repairs.Eur J Cardiothorac Surg. 2004 May;25(5):701-7.

28. Chiesa R, Melissano G, Civilini E, de Moura ML, Carozzo A, Zangrillo A. Ten years experience of thoracic and thoracoabdominal aortic aneurysm surgical repair: lessons learned.Ann Vasc Surg. 2004 Sep;18(5):514-20.

29. Coselli JS, Conklin LD, LeMaire SA. Thoracoab-

dominal aortic aneurysm repair: review and update of current strategies.Ann Thorac Surg. 2002 Nov;74(5):S1881-4.

30. Cina CS, Lagana A, Bruin G, Ricci C, Doobay B, Tittley J, Clase CM. Thoracoabdominal aortic aneurysm repair: a prospective cohort study of 121 cases.Ann Vasc Surg. 2002 Sep;16(5):631-8. Epub 2002 Aug 19.

31. Sanchez L. Total transposition of the visceral arteries for thoracoabdominal aneurysms. In: Thoracic Aorta Endografting, A Multidisciplinary approach, Amor M, Bergeron P, Castriota F, Cremonesi A, Mathias K and Raithel D eds, p.177-180.

32. Bell P. Extra anatomical and Combined methods for treating thoracoabdominal aneurysms. In: Thoracic Aorta Endografting, A Multidisciplinary approach, Amor M, Bergeron P, Castriota F, Cremonesi A, Mathias K and Raithel D.eds, p.181-185.

33. Achouh PE, Madsen K, Miller CC 3rd, Estrera AL, Azizzadeh A, Dhareshwar J, Porat E, Safi HJ. Gastrointestinal complications after descending thoracic and thoracoabdominal aortic repairs: a 14-year experience.J Vasc Surg. 2006 Sep;44(3):442-6.

34. Pawlowski E, Pettit J, Harrison L, Cina CS. Endovascular repair of perirenal and Group IV thoracoabdominal aortic aneurysms: a case study report.J Vasc Nurs. 2006 Sep;24(3):75-80; quiz 81.

35. Weigang E, Hartert M, Siegenthaler MP, Beckmann NA, Sircar R, Szabo G, Etz CD, Luehr M, von Samson P, Beyersdorf F. Perioperative management to improve neurologic outcome in thoracic or thoracoabdominal aortic stent-grafting.Ann Thorac Surg. 2006 Nov;82(5):1679-87.

36. Greenberg RK, West K, Pfaff K, Foster J, Skender D, Haulon S, Sereika J, Geiger L, Lyden SP, Clair D, Svensson L, Lytle B. Beyond the aortic bifurcation: branched endovascular grafts for thoracoabdominal and aortoiliac aneurysms.J Vasc Surg. 2006 May;43(5):879-86; discussion 886-7.

37. Kaviani A, Greenberg R. Current status of branched stent-graft technology in treatment of thoracoabdominal aneurysms.Semin Vasc Surg. 2006 Mar; 19(1):60-5.

38. Baril DT, Ellozy SH, Carroccio A, Marin ML. Branched endografts for treatment of complex aortic aneurysms.Surg Technol Int. 2005;14:245-52.

39. Anderson JL, Adam DJ, Berce M, Hartley DE. Repair of thoracoabdominal aortic aneurysms with fenestrated and branched endovascular stent grafts.J Vasc Surg. 2005 Oct;42(4):600-7.

40. Suzuki K, Kazui T, Ohno T, Sugiki K, Doi H, Ohkawa Y. Re-reconstruction of visceral arteries with thoracoabdominal aortic replacement using a branched graft.Jpn J Thorac Cardiovasc Surg. 2005 Apr;53(4):217-9.

41. Chuter TA. Branched stent-grafts for endovascular repair of aortic and iliac aneurysms.Tech Vasc Interv Radiol. 2005 Mar;8(1):56-60.

42. Eide TO, Romundstad P, Saether OD, Myhre HO, Aadahl P. A strategy for treatment of type III and IV thoracoabdominal aortic aneurysm.Ann Vasc Surg. 2004 Jul;18(4):408-13.

43. Cowan JA Jr, Dimick JB, Henke PK, Huber TS, Stanley JC, Upchurch GR Jr. Surgical treatment of intact thoracoabdominal aortic aneurysms in the United States: hospital and surgeon volume-related outcomes.J Vasc Surg. 2003 Jun;37(6): 1169-74.

44. Miller CC 3rd, Porat EE, Estrera AL, Vinnerkvist AN, Huynh TT, Safi HJ. Analysis of short-term multivariate competing risks data following thoracic and thoracoabdominal aortic repair.Eur J Cardiothorac Surg. 2003 Jun;23(6):1023-7; discussion 1027.

45. Cambria RP, Clouse WD, Davison JK, Dunn PF, Corey M, Dorer D. Thoracoabdominal aneurysm repair: results with 337 operations performed over a 15-year interval.Ann Surg. 2002 Oct;236(4):471-9; discussion 479.

46. Svensson LG, Crawford ES, Hess KR, Coselli JS, Safi H. Experience with 1509 patients undergoing thoracoabdominal aortic operations.J Vasc Surg 1993;17(2):357-368.

47. Gawenda M, Aleksic M, Heckenkamp J, et al. Hybrid-procedures for the treatment of thoracoabdominal aortic aneurysms and dissections.Eur J Endovasc Surg 33, 71-77(2007).

48. Testi G, Freyrie A, Gargiulo M, et al. Endovascular and hybrid treatment of reccurent thoracoabdominal aneurysms in an HIV-positive patient. Eur J Endovasc Surg 33, 78-80(2007).

49. Rao Vallabhaneni, Harris PL. Lessons learnt from the EUROSTAR registry on endovascular repair of abdominal aortic aneurysm repair: Endovascular Grafting: state of the art. Eur. j. radiol. 2001, vol. 39, n1, pp.34-41(20 ref).

Magnet assisted contralateral stump cannulation using a repositionable aortic endograft

Nikolaos Melas, Nikolaos Saratzis, Athanasios Saratzis, Dimitrios Kiskinis

INTRODUCTION – THE NEED FOR BIFURCATED ENDOGRAFTS

Parodi et al in 1991 first implanted a physician-fabricated **aortoaortic tube endograft** comprised of a balloon-expandable stent and a Dacron graft.[1] Three of the first five procedures eventually failed because the graft was only fixated proximally. Blood-reflux around the distal end of the Dacron graft, which was not attached to the aorta, led to persistent sack perfusion. The graft design was modified to include a second distal Palmaz stent to accomplish fixating of the Dacron graft in the terminal aorta, so success was achieved in excluding the AAA from the arterial circulation. Soon afterwards **aortouniiliac grafts** (AUI) were used in conjunction with femoro-femoral crossover grafts, but tube configuration remained a mainstay of endovascular AAA treatment for the first years due to the advantage of being more straightforward in its deployment, with a limited potential for graft twisting or kinking.[2] Parodi and colleagues deployed 51 aortoaortic tube endografts (in a total of 109 patients) and reported no increase in early endograft failure or any adverse events at that time.[2] During the following years, other investigators, reported that tube grafts may not provide effective long-term exclusion of AAAs.[3] Secondary type I distal endoleaks, despite an apparent adequate length of the distal neck, were reported in sporadic cohorts.[3,4,5,6,7] In addition, growth of the inferior aneurysm neck and recontouring that appeared to be unrelated to endoleaks was also reported and correlated to morphological alterations of the abdominal aorta after EVAR.[8] So, the need for a bifurcated endograft fixated distally to the common iliac arteries was more than obvious in order to overcome the defects of "tube" and "AUI" endoprostheses. From 1993 to 1997 many articles were published showing the initial results of custom made bifurcated endoprostheses in Australia, USA and Europe.[9-18] As the technique evolved, experience was gained and gradually many commercial-industrial modular **bifurcated endografts** were released in the market. EVAR soon become popular proving equal or even superior results versus open AAA repair.[19-25] At the same time, complications, pitfalls, defects and special considerations regarding this new technique became apparent (endoleak, migration, material fatigue, sack enlargement, leg dislocation or thrombosis, reinterventions etc.).

CONTRALATERAL STUMP CANNULATION

The vascular community soon reached consensus and agreed that modular bifurcated endografts should be first choice implants in AAA. These grafts consist of a uniform main body-ipsilateral leg attached distally to the ipsilateral common iliac artery and a separate contralateral leg attached distally to the contralateral common iliac artery. In certain configurations the graft consists of three segments: main body; ipsilateral leg and contralateral leg. Bifurcated endografts proved superior results over time, but in either configuration (two or three parts) the main defect is contralateral stump cannulation. Once the main body-ipsilateral leg is deployed, the contralateral stump should be catheterized from the contralateral iliac axis with a wire. The contralateral leg is then advanced over this wire inside the contralateral stump up to the docking zone. The problem is that this procedure may occasionally prove difficult and time consuming implicating many catheters, especially in AAAs with a wide lumen, or in the event of angulated common iliac arteries. Several techniques have been proposed to confirm that the contralateral wire will be correctly inserted through the contralateral stump and not into the aneurismal sack:

1. **Pigtail test**: Once the contralateral wire is thought to have been inserted through the stump, a pigtail catheter is advanced over the wire at the level of the proximal body attachment zone (proximal neck). The wire is then withdrawn a few cm backwards. If the pigtail can be rotated easily, the catheter is located inside the main body and not between the graft and the neck.

2. **Angiography test**: The procedure is similar to the aforementioned. Instead of simply rotating the pigtail the wire is removed and an angiography is obtained. If the pigtail is in the main body the dye is first seen inside the graft. In the event of malpositioning, the dye is seen scattered between the graft and the neck.

3. **Dual wire confirmation**: Before deploying the main body-ipsilateral leg, a simple guide wire is advanced from the contralateral iliac artery over the renal arteries. Once the main body-ipsilateral leg is deployed, a second wire is advanced to catheterize the contralateral stump. When the second wire is thought to be located inside the main body, an arrow sheath is advanced over both contralateral wires and against the stump. The first wire is outside and the second inside the main body; therefore the sheath cannot be further advanced but simply pushes the stump upwards.

4. **90 degrees biplane sequential fluoroscopy**: Once the contralateral wire is thought to have been inserted inside the sump, it is advanced proximally over the renal arteries. A pigtail catheter is advanced over the wire at the point of the proximal neck. The wire is removed and the pigtail is slowly filed with dye. The imaging device is then rotated 90 degrees. If the catheter is outside the main body it can easily be seen between the graft and the aortic neck.

Unfortunately, more than one test should be performed in some cases. Therefore, the procedure can be time, fluoroscopy and contrast media consuming. Moreover, there are cases were the catheterization is impossible implicating crossover maneuvers from the ipsilateral leg to the contralateral stump or brachial artery access. Rarely, conversion to aortouniiliac configuration has been described.

OVERCOMING THE STUMP CATHETERIZATION DEFECTS

Vascutek (Vascutek USA Inc., Ann Arbor, MI, USA) recently released the Anaconda AAA Stent Graft System. The specific device has been developed for the treatment of infrarenal aortic aneurysms and is a modular system constructed of polyester fabric material and self-expanding nitinol ring-stents. It features a repositionable, woven polyester body, which is sealed in the infrarenal neck by two nitinol ring-stents, and is anchored in position by four pairs of nitinol hooks. The two separate legs of the device are supported by individual nitinol ring-stents. They are separately deployed into position sequentially. The contralateral stump is catheterized with the use of two guidewires which are equipped with a magnetic tip. The first wire is attached on the main body from the ipsilateral main body introducing system to the contralateral stump. The second wire is inserted from the contralateral iliac, advanced opposite to the previous magnetic tip and with simple manoeuvres the two magnetic tips attach and can be pushed proximally so that the contralateral wire enters the contralateral stump.

The specific abdominal aortic endograft has recently been approved by the European Union (CE Mark) for all appropriate applications but is still being evaluated in order to achieve FDA approval; therefore the experience and long term results that has been gained so far remains limited.

DESCRIPTION AND CHARACTERISTICS OF THE DEVICE

The specific endo-graft consists of three separate segments which form a modular bifurcated endoprosthesis: one main bifurcated body, deployed at the level of the abdominal aorta and two (2) independent peripheral segments, the so called "iliac legs" (Figure 1). The leg which is inserted from the contralateral iliac is called contrallateral leg and the one that is intro-

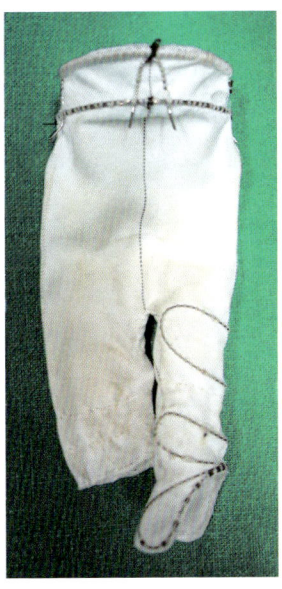
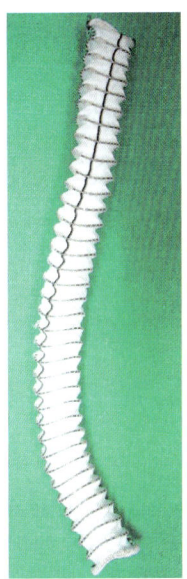
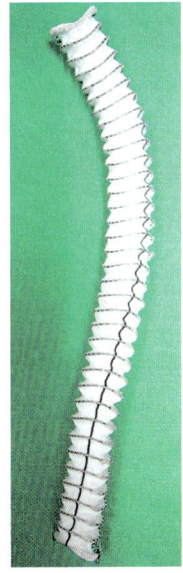

FIGURE 1: Anaconda (Vascutek, USA Inc., Ann Arbor, MI, USA) AAA Stent Graft System is a modular bifurcated endoprosthesis consisting of one main bifurcated body, deployed at the level of the abdominal aorta and two (2) independent peripheral segments, the so called "iliac legs".

duced from the ipsilateral iliac is called ipsilateral leg.

The endoprosthesis is constructed of ultrathin woven polyester fabric and a nitinol skeleton which consists of separate ring stents. Each ring stent consists of several nitinol wires put together in a spiral manner, which reduces the danger for ring stent rapture due to pulse tension. The main body of the device is equipped with two separate ring stents fixed at a distance of 8 mm from each other, while the iliac legs are consisted of 18 to 36 separate ring stents, depending on the length of the graft that is being deployed (Figure 1). Several markers located at various segments of the endoprosthesis assist proper positioning, orientation and deployment of the device (Figure 2).

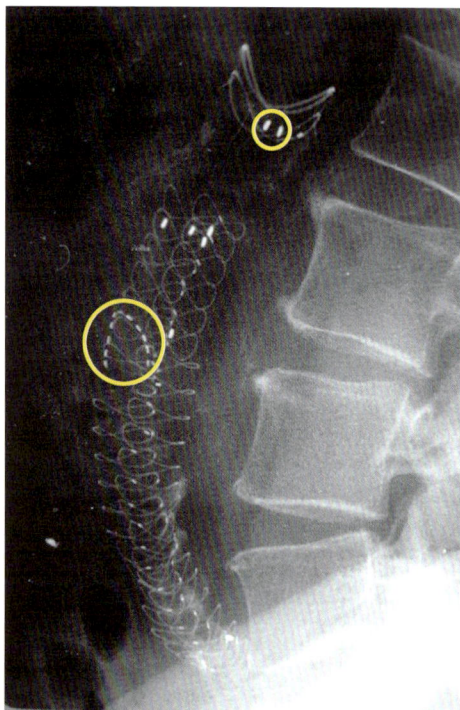

FIGURE 2: Several markers located at various segments of the endoprosthesis assist proper positioning, orientation and deployment of the device

FIXATION AND SEALING

No supra-renal fixation stent is present. The affixation of the prosthesis is achieved by:

1. The two independent ring stents of the main body. A certain amount of oversizing (10-15%) is critical to ensure proper fixation and sealing proximally (Figure 3).
2. A total of four pairs of stainless steel hooks, which are located between the two ring stents of the main body. The specific hooks are partially inserted into the aortic wall after the device has been fully deployed at the level of the proximal neck. Their main goal is anchoring against distal migration (Figure 3).

The iliac legs are inserted sequentially into position (docking zones) on the main body with 25 mm of overlapping. A specific amount of oversizing (10-15%) is crucial here as well to achieve proper sealing and fixation in the docking zones and in the distal iliac landing zones as well (Figure 1).

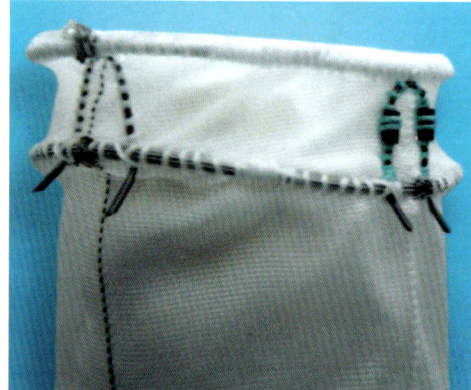

FIGURE 3: The two independent ring stents of the main body. A total of four pairs of stainless steel hooks are located between the two ring stents. The specific hooks are partially inserted into the aortic wall after the device has been fully deployed at the level of the proximal neck. Their main goal is anchoring against distal migration.

DELIVERY SYSTEM

The main body delivery system of the device (120 cm in length) consists of the following components:

1. A flexible plastic sheath reinforced with an internal highly flexible metallic braided catheter shaft (65 cm in length) ending to a tapered flexible top tip, which enchances the trackability of the device through tortuous iliac arteries. The endograft is located inside the specific sheath (Figure 4). The outer diameter of the sheath is between 20.4-22.5 Fr and the inner diameter is 18-20 Fr, depending on the diameter of the prosthesis that has been selected.

2. The control handles located at the distal end of the sheath, which enable the operator to control the positioning and deployment of the prosthesis (Figure 4). In specific, the "sheath slider" enables the deployment of the main body. The "delivery handle" retracts the top tip. The "control collar" enables the operator to compress the main body re-adjust the position of the graft (rotate or advance - retract) and redeploy it for accurate positioning (Figure 5). Moreover, the "control collar" can be used for "canting" the two main stents of the body for better positioning in angulated necks (Figure 6). The two "release-wire rings" hold the endo-prosthesis in place and enable the operator to cant and re-deploy the graft in order to achieve optimum positioning.

3. The sheath is equipped with 2 "ports".

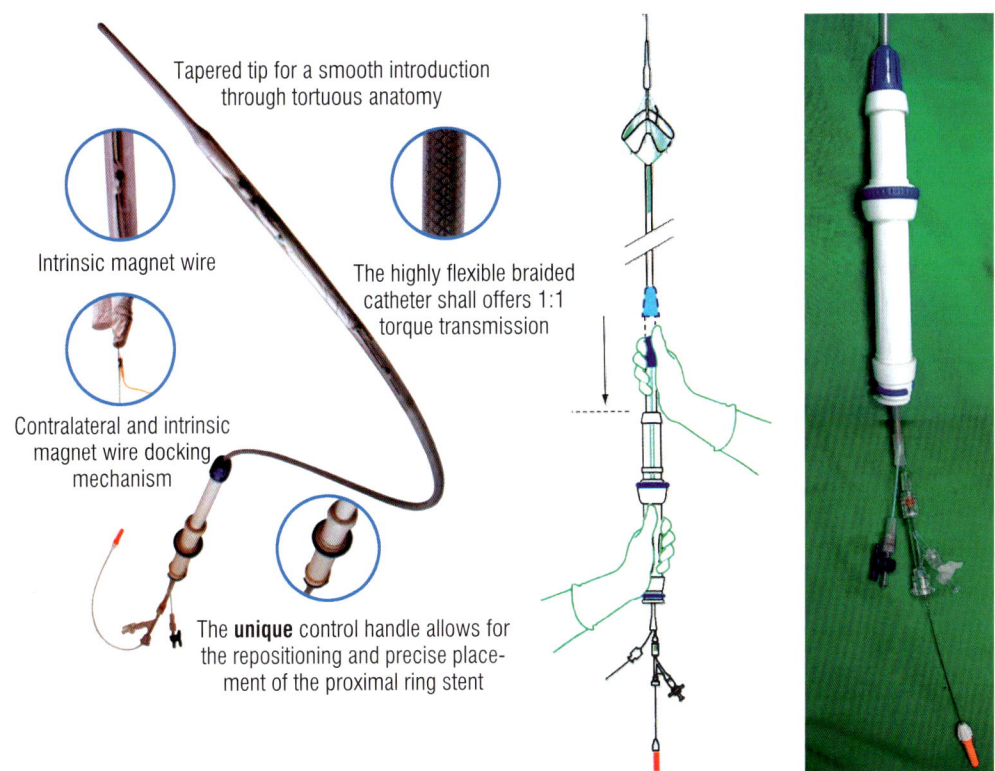

Tapered tip for a smooth introduction through tortuous anatomy

Intrinsic magnet wire

The highly flexible braided catheter shall offers 1:1 torque transmission

Contralateral and intrinsic magnet wire docking mechanism

The **unique** control handle allows for the repositioning and precise placement of the proximal ring stent

FIGURE 4: Delivery system and control handles of the device. The intrinsic magnet wire is the one with the orange rotator.

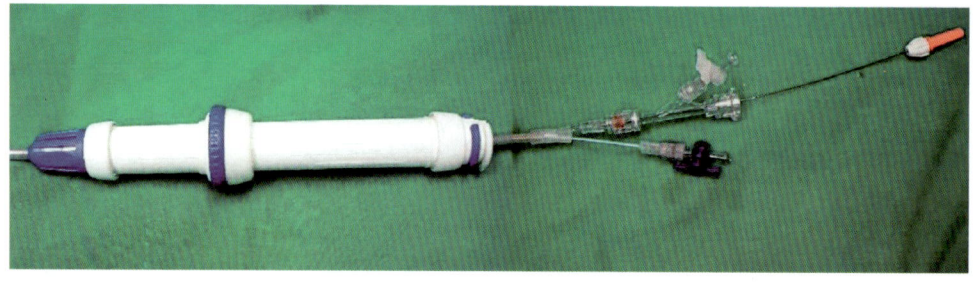

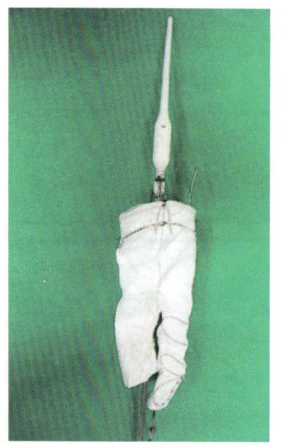 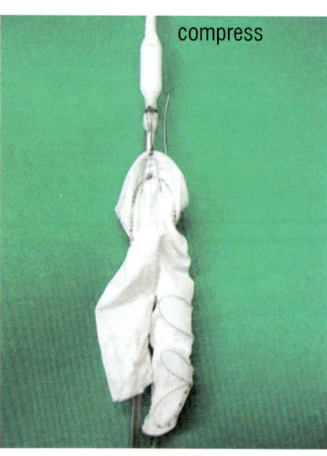 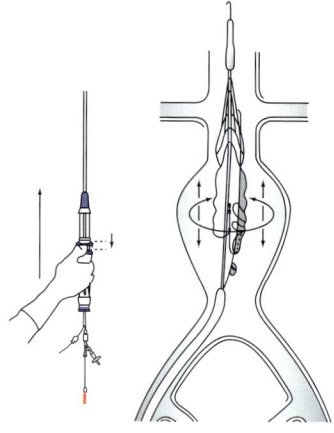

compress

FIGURE 5: The "control collar" enables the operator to compress the main body re-adjust the position of the graft (rotate or advance-retract) and redeploy it for accurate positioning.

The first is the main guide-wire port, equipped with a haemostatic valve. The second is the magnetic wire port, equipped with a haemostatic valve and with side flushing port enabling angiography through the device. The magnet wire passes from the main body sheath, outside the main body graft but inside the contralateral stump and bears a magnet which assists the catheterization of the contra-lateral leg. This characteristic is unique to the specific endo-prosthesis (Figure 4 and 7).

The configuration of the delivering system of the two separate iliac legs is very much similar. The overall length of the system is 113 cm and the length of the delivering sheath is 55 cm. However,

no magnetic wire or "control collar" is present.

CHOICE OF THE APPROPRIATE SIZE

The proximal diameter of the main body is chosen based on the diameter of the proximal aneurismal neck adding a total of 10-15 % oversizing to ensure optimum fixation and sealing. The same amount of oversizing is applied to both iliac legs. Special attention is mandatory to ensure that the iliac legs match the main body in size, so that the docking zones and the overlapping parts are all coherent. Beware that not all iliac leg diameters match all main body diameters. The iliac legs are tubular in shape (the proximal and distal

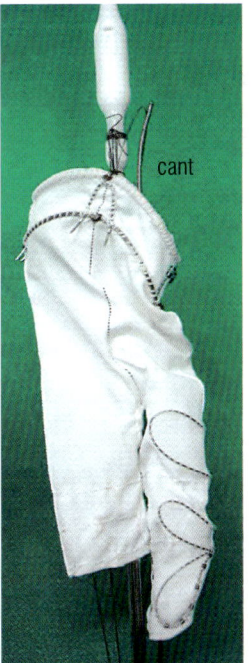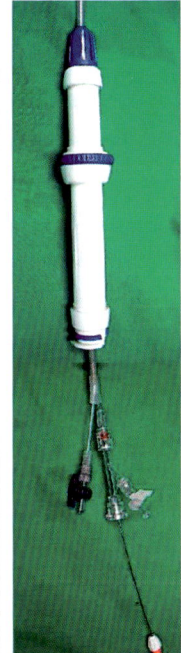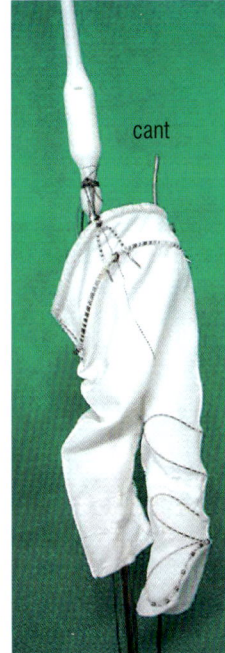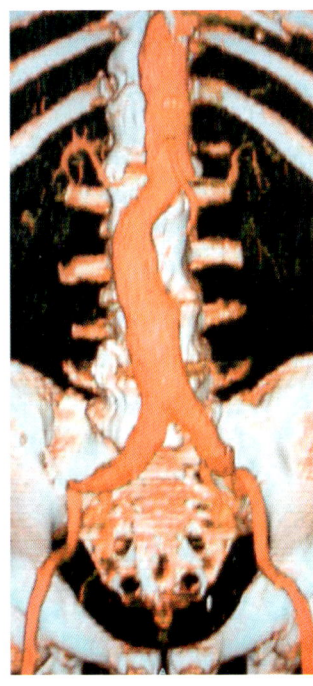

FIGURE 6: The "control collar" can be used for "canting" the two main stents of the body for better positioning in angulated necks.

diameter match) but recently bell bottom shaped legs are available.

PROCEDURE

All manipulations should be carried out in a fully equipped operating room under fluoroscopic control, using a mobile C-arm and a radiolucent table. Standard patient monitoring should be available, including ECG and arterial pressure. Preparation and flushing of endovascular devices and endoprostheses should be carried out in the usual fashion. Both common femoral arteries are surgically exposed. Heparin is administered intravenusly. The ipsilateral common femoral artery is punctured using a Seldinger needle. A.035" standard guidewire is introduced into the vessel and advanced proximally - beyond the orifice of the two renal arteries. A 7 Fr short sheath is

inserted into the vessel. An angiography catheter is introduced over the wire and beyond the renal arteries. The first wire is exchanged for a non-magnetic ultra stiff guide-wire and the angiography catheter is removed. A.035" standard guidewire is sequentially inserted into the contralateral common femoral artery and advanced proximally beyond the renal arteries. A 7Fr Arrow (Arrow International, Inc., Reading, PA, USA) sheath (length: 45 cm) is introduced over the wire and advanced forward - up to the level of the two renal arteries. An initial angiography is performed through the Arrow sheath in order to visualize renal arteries, the aortic bifurcation and the configuration of the iliac axis. The short sheath (ipsilateral femoral artery) is removed and the delivery system of the bifurcate body is advanced over the stiff guidewire. The radiopaque markers of the top ring stent are positioned below the orifice of the lower re-

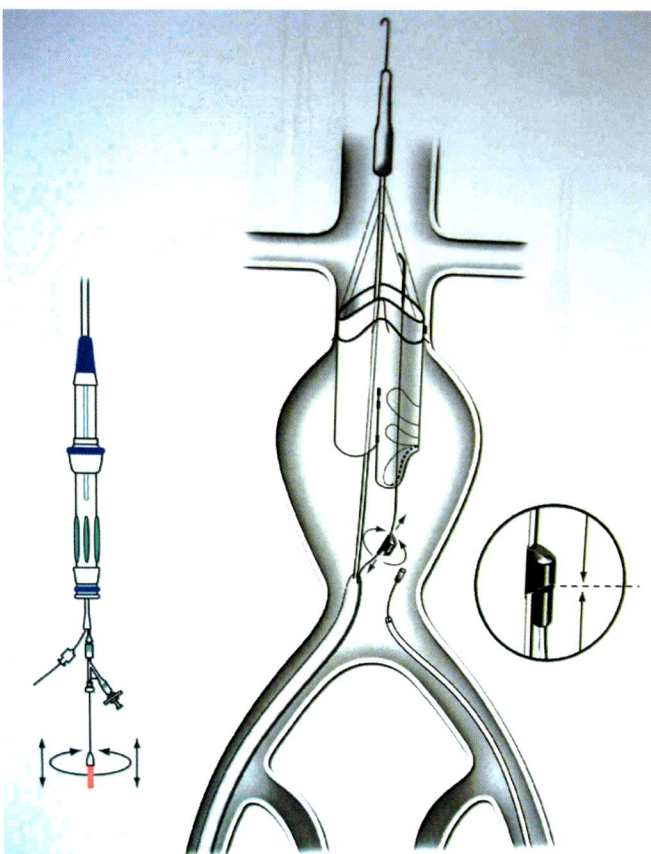

FIGURE 7: The intrinsic magnet wire of the main body and the contralateral magnet guidewire are both manipulated in such a manner that allows the attachment of the two separate magnets.

nal artery. The contralateral stump of the graft should be positioned towards the contralateral iliac artery (the contralateral radiopaque marker and the magnetic tip of the body should be turned over towards the contralateral iliac axis). When proximal positioning and orientation has been confirmed, the outer sheath of the delivery system is withdrawn by pulling the sheath slider backwards. The main body is fully deployed but is still tied to the delivery system by the two releasing-wires that control the top stents. An angiography performed through the Arrow sheath confirms correct positioning. The top ring stents of the graft can be repositioned in relation to the renal arteries using the delivery system control collar. To achieve this, the collar is retract-

ed backwards, causing the main body and top ring stents to compress and the anchors to be removed from the aortic wall, thus enabling the operator to re-adjust the position of the graft (either rotate or advance-retract it). If an angulated proximal neck is detected, the top ring stents can be canted left or right in relation to the longitudinal axis of the aorta by retracting the control collar and then rotating it clockwise or anti-clockwise, allowing the graft to conform to the anatomical configuration of the aneurysm neck. Once correct positioning of the main body is confirmed, contralateral leg cannulation is attempted. In order to cannulate the contralateral stump of the bifurcate body, a.035" magnetic (standard or flexible) guidewire is inserted into the Arrow sheath (Figure 7). The intrinsic magnet wire of the main body and the contralateral magnet guidewire are both manipulated in such a manner that allows the attachment of the two separate magnets. The two magnetic guidewires are then simultaneously advanced - until the magnets can be visualized in a supra-renal position. The contralateral magnet guidewire is fixed and the intrinsic wire is advanced another 2 cm. The intrinsic wire is then withdrawn and the contralateral magnet guidewire is advanced further proximally. The Arrow sheath is advanced up to the orifice of the two renal arteries and an angiography is performed to confirm the patency of the renal arteries and the contralateral internal iliac artery. The Arrow sheath is sequentially removed and the contralateral iliac leg delivery system is advanced over the contralateral guidewire. Once the proximal radiopaque marker of the leg has been positioned into the docking zone, the contralateral iliac endoprothesis is deployed by retracting the sheath slider backwards. The release wire ring is retracted and the leg is fully detached from the introducing system. Confirmation of the patency of the ipsilateral internal iliac artery can be achieved by angiography from the side port of the contralateral leg delivery system just before the retraction of the top tip. If an extension graft is necessary, it can be deployed in the same manner.

At this stage, the main body is still attached to its delivery system (release wires), allowing it to be slightly repositioned, if necessary, as described above. The main body is fully detached from the introducing system after retracting the release wires. No further repositioning or canting is now possible. The top tip is then retracted and an angiography performed through the side port confirms the position of the ipsilateral internal iliac artery. The main body delivery system is removed and the ipsilateral leg is inserted, advanced and deployed in the same manner as the contralateral leg. Completion angiography can be performed be inserting the Arrow sheath through the contralateral axis.

INSTITUTIONAL EXPERIENCE

Fifty-one (51) patients were treated with the Anaconda (Vascutek USA Inc., Ann Arbor, MI, USA) stent-graft during a period of 21 months for an infra-renal abdominal aortic aneurysm in our Department, located in a tertiary hospital. There were 48 men (94,11%) and 3 women (5,9%) with a mean age of 71 ±8 years (range: 62-89 years). Six (6) patients were considered at high-risk for surgical intervention [defined as ASA (American Society of Anesthesiology) grade 3]. The mean duration of the follow-up was 16 months (range: 1-21 months). Four (4) patients were lost to follow-up (4/51-7,84%).

Preoperative assessment

Preoperative assessment included spiral contrast enhanced computed tomography (CT) scans acquired at 3 or 5 mm intervals with 2 –or 3– dimensional reconstruction in all cases. 12 patients underwent digital subtraction angiography (DSA) prior to EVAR. Neck diameter ranged from 22 to 30mm with a mean value of 26 mm, while neck length ranged from a minimum of 14 mm to a maximum of 35 mm (mean: 18.5 mm). Mean neck angulation (proximal neck) was 30 degrees (range: 5-60 degrees).

Procedure

All procedures were carried out in an operating theatre with a radiolucent table under fluoroscopic guidance. Epidural or spinal anesthesia was used in all patients. Exposure of the femoral arteries was performed with a vertical groin incision. Aspirin and clopidogrel were initiated from the day of the operation.

Procedural results

The stent-graft was successfully deployed in all patients (technical success rate: 100%). In one (1) case the graft was compressed and repositioned due to renal artery occlusion. The renal arteries were eventually patent on completion angiography. In six (6) cases (6/51-11,71%) the graft was compressed and repositioned proximally, towards the lower renal artery due to a proximal endoleak. The leaks were subsequently sealed on completion angiography in 5 out of 6 patients. One proximal cuff [EndoFit (LeMaitre Vascular, Burlington, MA, USA); size: 30 x 5 with a suprarenal stent] was deployed in the case were the proximal leak insisted and once graft-repositioning was no longer feasible. Modular iliac extensions were used in 10 patients (10/51-19,6%). Blood transfusion was required in 8 cases (mean: 1,5 unit; range: 1-2 units).

Early follow-up (<30 days)

No peri-operative aortic rupture or death occurred. Local wound complications including seroma, hematoma and infection occurred in 3 cases (5,88%). One patient developed a pulmonary infection while hospitalized and was treated conventionally (1,96%). Ten (10) patients developed post-implant syndrome (19,06%) and remained hospitalized until the condition had resolved. One patient (1,96%) developed postoperative renal impairment during hospitalization, which subsided while he remained hospitalized. The major-complications rate during early follow-up was 5,88% (3/51 patients). Mean hospitalization was 3 ±2,3 days. ICU hospitalization was not required in any case.

Late Follow-Up (>30 days)

Death
One patient developed an aorto-duodenal fistula on the 8th post-operative month

and was subsequently admitted to our institution with hematemesis. Prompt surgical intervention was decided. At laparotomy, the endo-graft was excised and the aorta was ligated. An axillo-femoral by pass was performed to restore blood flow. The patient eventually died of MODS (multiple organ deficiency syndrome) on the 3rd post-operative day. Another patient died of an acute myocardial infarction on the 6th post-op month. Total mortality rate was (2/51 - 3,92%).

Endoleaks and major complications

One **iliac limb thrombosis** was detected on the 3rd post-op month (1,96%). The complication was attributed to the anatomical configuration of the terminal aorta (14 mm in diameter) which resulted in low blood-flow towards the limb. A femoro-femoral cross-over bypass was performed (using an 8 mm PTFE graft) to overcome intermittent claudication.

Graft migration occurred in one case (1,96%), diagnosed on the 6th post-op month. The proximal ring stents migrated distally (30 mm) and the aneurismal sack was re-perfused causing aneurysm expansion (type I endoleak). A proximal (EndoFit) cuff had been deployed intra-operatively in the specific patient, as described previously. Both the cuff and the Anaconda prosthesis had migrated distally. The complication was attributed to neck deficiency (bulge), which had been initially underestimated. Re-intervention was performed attempting to deploy an EndoFit (Le Maitre Vascular, Burlington, MA, USA) proximal abdominal cuff, but the main body of the initial prosthesis was compressed and rotated, restricting EVAR. The patient was converted to open-repair and has survived uncomplicated.

Endoleak was observed in a total of 5 cases (9,80%) during follow-up. Four (4) retrograde side-branch leaks (type II endoleak; 4/51 patients-7,84%) were detected and remained under surveillance (the aneurismal sack had remained stable in diameter and the patients were free of any vascular complications). A type 1 endoleak (1,96%) was observed in one case - as described previously (graft migration).

Aneurysm sac enlargement was detected only in the case of the patient who presented with a proximal endoleak and graft migration (1,96%).

The **re-intervention rate** during the late follow-up was 3,92% (2/51 patients). Major complications (as defined previously) were detected in 8 patients during the late follow-up (15,68%). No events of rupture were noted throughout the follow-up.

CONCLUSION

Having described the characteristics of the Anacoda (Vascutek USA Inc., Ann Arbor, MI, USA) endograft and the implantation procedure, it is clear that this graft features certain advantages:

1. **Repositionable main body** (unique characteristic of this device). Offers the advantage for accurate positioning almost until the end of the procedure. There is no need for an extra proximal cuff in case an intraoperative proximal endoleak is detected due to improper deployment.
2. **Magnet assisted contralateral stump cannulation** (unique characteristic of this device). Overcomes the limitation of difficult cannulation in large AAAs or in the event of angulated iliac arteries and minimizes the operative time and contrast medium needs.
3. **Dual top ring stent**.
4. **Separate multiple ring stents in the iliac legs**. Enables dealing with angulated iliacs against leg thrombosis.
5. **Highly sophisticated low profile flexible reinforced delivery system**. Offers adequate control during every stage of

the procedure and good trackability through tortuous iliac arteries.
6. **Canting ability of the dual top ring stents** (unique characteristic of this device). Enables the graft to conform to angulated proximal necks.

On the other hand special attention should be drawn to the following aspects:
1. The endograft is contraindicated to short (<15 mm) or wide (>30 mm) proximal neck
2. Rotation of the device while repositioning should be carried out very meticulously to avoid graft twisting because between the first dual ring stents and the main body bifurcation there is no metallic skeleton. This is more important in highly angulated necks were friction against the angle of the neck while rotating could twist the graft.

A single center report on the preliminary results of the device has already been published, showing good peri-operative results in the treatment of infrarenal AAAs with a neck length not less than 15 mm.[26] The midterm results from our cohort are promising. We believe that the Anaconda endograft features unique advantages for specific AAAs. Greater series from more centres and longer follow up is crucial to justify the long term durability of the specific endoprosthesis.

REFERENCES

1. Parodi JC, Palmaz JC, Barone HD. Transfemoral intraluminal graft implantation for abdominal aortic aneurysms. Ann Vasc Surg 1991;5:491-9.
2. Parodi JC, Barone A, Piraino R, Schonholz. Endovascular treatment of abdominal aortic aneurysms: lessons learned. J Endovasc Surg 1997;4:102-10.
3. Nasim A, Thompson MM, Sayers RD, et al. Is endulominal abdominal aortic aneurysm repair using an aortoaortic (tube) device a durable procedure? Ann Vasc Surg. 1998;12:522-8.

4. Schurink GW, Aarts NJ, van Bocket JH. Endoleak after stent-graft treatment of abdominal aortic aneurysms: a meta-analysis of clinical studies. Br J Surg 1999;86:581-7.

5. Raithel D. Results of endovascular Abdominal Aortic Aneurysm Repair (EVAR) Zentralbl Chir. 2002;127:660-3.

6. Hinchliffe R.J., Hopkinson B.R. Endovascular repair of abdominal aortic aneurysm: current status J.R.Coll.Surg.Edinb. 2002;47:523-527.

7. Bernhard VM, Mitchell RS, Matsumura JS, et al. Ruptured abdominal aortic aneurysm after endovascular repair. J Vasc Surg. 2002;35:1155-62.

8. Broeders IA, Blandensteijn JD, Gvakharia A, et al. The efficacy of transfemoral endovascular aneurysm management: a study on size changes of the abdominal aorta during mid-term follow-up. Eur J Vasc Endovasc Surg 1997;14:84-90.

9. Chuter TA, Green RM, Ouriel K, Fiore WM, DeWeese JA. Transfemoral endovascular aortic graft placement. J Vasc Surg. 1993;18:185-95; discussion 195-7.

10. Moore WS, Vescera CL. Repair of abdominal aortic aneurysm by transfemoral endovascular graft placement. Ann Surg. 1994;220:331-9; discussion 339-41.

11. Chuter TA, Donayre C, Wendt G. Bifurcated stent-grafts for endovascular repair of abdominal aortic aneurysm. Preliminary case reports. Surg Endosc. 1994;8:800-2.

12. Sayers RD, Thompson MM, Bell PR. Regarding "Transfemoral endovascular aortic graft placement". J Vasc Surg. 1994;19:758. No abstract available.

13. May J, White GH, Yu W, Waugh RC, McGahan T, Stephen MS, Harris JP. Endoluminal grafting of abdominal aortic aneurysms: causes of failure and their prevention. J Endovasc Surg. 1994;1: 44-52.

14. White GH, Yu W, May J, Stephen MS, Waugh RC. A new nonstented balloon-expandable graft for straight or bifurcated endoluminal bypass. J Endovasc Surg. 1994;1:16-24.

15. Chuter TA, Wendt G, Hopkinson BR, Scott RA, Risberg B, Walker PJ, White G. Transfemoral insertion of a bifurcated endovascular graft for aortic aneurysm repair: the first 22 patients. Cardiovasc Surg. 1995;3:121-8.

16. Quinones-Baldrich WJ, Deaton DH, Mitchell RS, Berry G, Piplani A, Quiachon D, Edwards WH, Moore WS. Preliminary experience with the Endovascular Technologies bifurcated endovascular aortic prosthesis in a calf model. J Vasc Surg. 1995;22:370-9.

17. White GH, Yu W, May J, Waugh R, Chaufour X, Harris JP, Stephen MS. Three-year experience with the White-Yu Endovascular GAD Graft for transluminal repair of aortic and iliac aneurysms. J Endovasc Surg. 1997;4:124-36.

18. Lawrence-Brown M, Sieunarine K, Hartley D, van Schie G, Goodman MA, Prendergast FJ. The Perth HLB bifurcated endoluminal graft: a review of the experience and intermediate results. Cardiovasc Surg. 1998;6:220-5.

19. UK Evar trial 1: Comparison of endovascular aneurysm repair with open repair in patients with AAA (Evar trial 1), 30-day operative mortality results: randomised controlled trial. The Lancet 2004;364:843-48.

20. FA. Lederle et al. Abdominal Aortic Aneurysm - Open versus Endovascular Repair. New England Journal of Medicine. 2004;351:1677-1679.

21. Mortality results for randomized controlled trial of early elective surgery or ultrasonographic surveillance for small AAA. The UK Small Aneurysm Trial Participants. Lancet 1998;352:1649-55.

22. Johnston KW. Nonruptured AAA: Six-year follow-up results from the multicenter prospective Canadian aneurysm study. Canadian Society for Vascular Surgery Aneurysm Study Group. JVS 1994;20: 163-70.

23. Schermerhorn ML, Finlayson SR, Fillinger MF et al. Life expectancy after endovascular versus open repair of AAA: Results of a decision analysis model on the bases of data from EUROSTAR. JVS 2002;36:1112-20.

24. Heller JA, Weinberg A, Arons A, et al. Two decades of AAA repair: have we made any progress? JVS 2000;32;1091-1100.

25. Lottman PE, Laheij RJ, Cuypers PW, et al. Health related quality of life outcomes following elective open or endovascular AAA repair: A randomized controlled trial. JEVT 2004;11:323-329.

26. Freyrie A, Gargiulo M, Rossi C, Losinno F, Testi G, Mauro R, Faggioli G, Stella A. Preliminary Results of Anaconda trade mark Aortic Endografts: A Single Center Study.Eur J Vasc Endovasc Surg. 2007.

Double tube endografts for treatment of abdominal aortic aneurysms

Section 1
Early application of double tube graft techniques

Geoffrey White, Keith Baxter, Weiyun Yu

INTRODUCTION

Tube grafts are preferred over bifurcated grafts for conventional open repair of abdominal aortic aneurysms (AAA) for a variety of reasons, including reduced morbidity and mortality associated with the operative procedure, and improved long term patency of the grafts.[1,2] In the early stages of development of endovascular graft techniques, tube grafts were also seen as the preferred option[3,4] for similar reasons, including ease of use, reduced morbidity and the perception that long term patency of a bifurcated endovascular device may be compromised by the requirement to implant the iliac limbs within the relatively narrow iliac arteries. It became clear, however, that only a small proportion of patients with AAA had anatomic features suitable for durable implant and sealing of a tube graft device, particularly with reference to the absence of a true distal attachment zone. With time, modular bifurcated grafts became and remain the preferred option for almost all cases, and tube graft devices are now available only as extension pieces for the majority of commercial devices.

Recently, there has been a move to re-consider the application of tube grafts for endovascular repair of selected aortic conditions, especially when deployed in overlapping or "trombone" fashion.

Role of tube grafts in the early history of endovascular repair

Parodi's initial clinical experiences with endovascular AAA graft repair procedures involved the use of polyester tube grafts held in position by large Palmaz stents.[5,6] Early cases featured stent attachment only at the proximal end within the infrarenal neck of the AAA. It was quickly appreciated that a freely-hanging graft allowed persistent blood reflux distally into the AAA sac, and thus it was necessary to include stent attachment at the distal aspect as well –this led to the distal segment of abdominal aorta being referred to as the "distal neck". In a sense this was an extrapolation of the surgical situation whereby open tube grafts are sutured in to a distal cuff of aortic wall surrounding the orifice of the iliac arteries. The early commercial device known as the EndoVascular Technologies graft (EVT) worked on this principle, with both the proximal and the distal attachment of a tube graft being accomplished by a self-expanding row of hooks which were pushed into the aortic wall by balloon-expansion technique.[7] Most AAAs, however, do not have a true distal neck, and early anatomic and morphologic studies showed that only approximately 5% of AAA that were large enough to require treatment had anatomy suitable for tube graft implant.[8-10]

Ongoing experience showed that endovascular tube grafts had a higher incidence of late failure than bifurcated grafts, due to late expansion of the distal aortic segment ("neck zone") causing development of type I endoleak and upward migration of the graft device.[11,12] In an analysis of the relationship of procedure outcome to graft configuration, we showed that early aortoaortic tube grafts had a significantly increased rate of mid-term failure due to the development of late endoleaks, and recommended a reassessment of the criteria for selecting the tube configuration, but we believed that tube grafts should not be abandoned altogether.[12]

The "trombone technique": overlapped tube grafts as a modular device

The first reported use of overlapping modular straight tube grafts to repair AAAs endoluminally concerned non-commercial devices deployed by balloon-expansion techniques.[8,13-15] The term "trombone technique" was coined to describe the variable, sliding overlap of two tube grafts, or the iliac limbs of a modular bifurcated device[13] (Figure 1).[13,14] This technique was preferred over simple deployment of a single tube graft, and is acknowledged as allowing the determination of precise device lengths using off-the-shelf devices.[16] In these procedures, two straight tube grafts were overlapped to exclude an infra-renal aneurysm, deploying the proximal graft immediately below the renal arteries and overlapping the second graft in such a

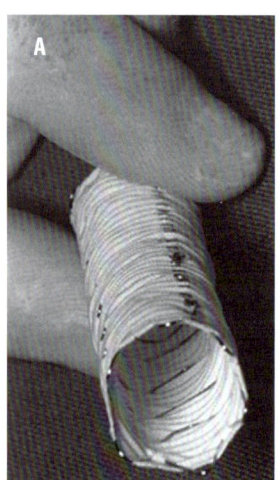
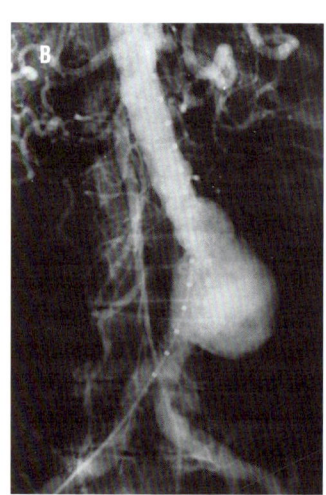
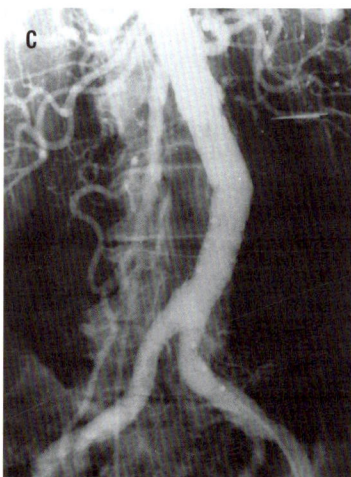

FIGURE 1: Early use of overlapped endovascular tube grafts for saccular AAA repair. **A.** The White-Yu Endovascular GAD Graft demonstrating the structure of the overlapped straight tube components. **B.** Preoperative angiogram of a 5.6 cm diameter AAA, with predominant saccular morphology. **C** Postoperative angiogram showing aneurysmal flow excluded by 2 overlapping tube grafts. Note the flexibility conveyed by overlap technique.

manner that the distal end was precisely at the desired distal attachment zone, just above the orifice of the iliac arteries (Figure 2). In an early report, the success rate for a series of 39 patients with AAA treated in a similar fashion was greater than 80%, and a primary endoleak rate of less than 15% was achieved.[8] A multi-center trial of overlapped tube graft application was undertaken in the USA (Figure 3).

At a later interval, when commercial AAA endovascular tube grafts were no longer readily available, this technique was re-explored by York and colleagues in 2002 who reported on the use of short aortic tube extension grafts to repair saccular infrarenal AAAs in 5 patients.[17] In this more recent series, short aortic extension cuffs were stacked together with 1.5 to 2 cm of overlap to exclude flow into the aneurysms. 3 patients needed only 2 extenders, while 2 patients required 3 extension cuffs. The most proximal graft was positioned 1.5 above the origin of the saccular aneurysm. Reported results were favourable with most patients demonstrating a reduction in aneurysm diameter, and no patients exhibited signs of endoleak or graft migration. The advantage of this technique was the ability to treat saccular AAAs with endografts that could be easily adapted to patient's differing anatomies (ie aortic length); this would spare having to customize unibody devices for each patient. Drawbacks of this approach include the potential for graft migration (due to short proximal and distal landing distances), and type III endoleak through the cuff overlapping zones. Though these two issues were not appreciated in the short term follow-up of patients in this series, one would be concerned that migration or endoleak may become apparent over time.

Single or double tube grafts? UniBody or modular?

The relative features of single or modular

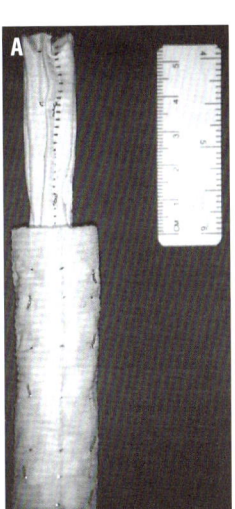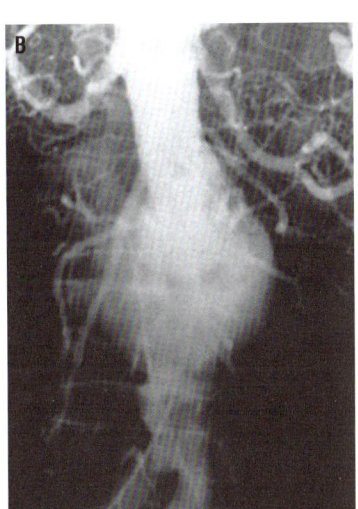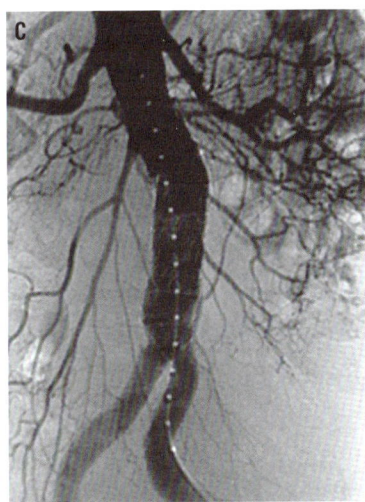

FIGURE 2: Case example of application of overlapped tube grafts for fusiform AAA repair. **A.** Example of the custom-made grafts and the technique of overlap by balloon-deployment method. **B.** Preoperative angiogram showing anatomy suitable for overlapped tube-graft repair (apparent distal neck or attachment zone). **C.** Post-deployment angiogram. Two devices have been implanted, covering the aortic lumen from just below the renal arteries to the aortic bifurcation.

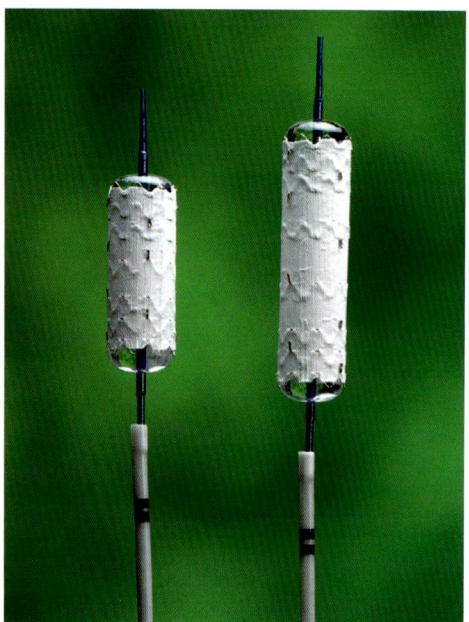

FIGURE 3: Photograph of the Baxter balloon-expandable endograft system, designed for overlap tube deployment and trialed in a multi-center FDA study from 1996. Two alternative lengths of graft are shown, mounted on the square-ended balloons designed for safer deployment.

device designs are summarized in Table 1. Placing a single tube graft in the aorta has the advantage of avoiding the potential for type III endoleak between stacked or overlapping graft components. Furthermore, a single component would be easier and quicker to deploy. There are, however, several drawbacks to treating aortic pathologies with just one stent-graft. In order to bridge a length of aorta reaching from the just below the renal arteries to the aortic bifurcation, a customized length of graft would have to be manufactured. This would add significant cost and delay a patient's treatment while just a device was being constructed. A double tube technique is advantageous in that the two components have the potential of telescoping into one another, thus providing added flexibility for more tortuous vessels (see Figure 2).

Indications for infrarenal aortic tube endografts

Certain aortic pathologies may be better suited for repair using a tube as opposed to a bifurcated configuration of the endoluminal graft. It is well documented that fusiform infrarenal AAAs are best treated with bifurcated modular devices, particularly those with no distal neck region.[11,12] However, other aortic diseases may be more suitable for treatment by tube graft application (see Table 2). Saccular AAA's can be repaired without significant graft-related complications using tube grafting,[8,17,18] and this may be the best appli-

TABLE 1

COMPARISON OF SINGLE-PIECE AND MODULAR ENDOVASCULAR GRAFTS

Single piece	Modular (multi-piece)
Complex graft construction and delivery system	Simple graft components and delivery system
Graft dimensions determined at time of manufacture	Customized graft component selection may be available at time of procedure
Single piece construction may reduce potential for fabric leak or graft failure	Potential for leakage, disconnection or stenosis at graft over-lap zone
Difficult to deliver fully stented (may require addition stents implanted into graft limbs)	Can be delivered as a fully supported stent-graft

TABLE 2
CONDITIONS POTENTIALLY SUITABLE FOR TUBE GRAFT REPAIR

Thoracic, iliac, and peripheral aneurysms
Saccular AAA
Anastomotic aneurysms
Aorto-enteric fistula
Aortic dissection
Penetrating aortic ulceration
"Shaggy aorta"
Ruptured calcified plaque
Infected AAA's

cation (see Figure 1). Other relative indications include many types of anastomotic aneurysms, and perhaps focal infective lesions. For example, Berchtold et al described using a tube stent-graft to treat a patient with a symptomatic AAA related to Salmonella septicaemia.[19] Repair of anastomotic aneurysms following open aortic surgery using tube stent-grafts is well documented.[20-22] Other potential uses for tube aortic stent-grafting in the infrarenalaorta include the repair of penetrating aortic ulceration, aorto-enteric fistula,[23] "shaggy aorta",[24] aortic dissection, and ruptured calcified aortic plaque.

Recent re-evaluation of double - tube overlapped grafts

To avoid the potential complications associated with stacking 2 or 3 short cuff extension components, a double tube stent-graft design has recently been revisited.[18] With this technique, two long stent-grafts with an overlapping distance of 6 to 8 cm are used to line the aorta from the lowest renal artery to the aortic bifurcation. Recent experience with the double-tube overlap is presented by Umschied and co-authors in the second section of this chapter.

Section 2

Contemporary application of double tube technique

Thomas Umscheid, Joerg Tessarek, Volker Ruppert, Wolf J. Stelter, Giovanni Torsello

INTRODUCTION

Early custom-made endovascular grafts were tubular structures due to lack of bifurcated technology.[5,6] The initial commercially available grafts were also tube graft designs, but they proved to have poor long term results[11,25,26] and thus they almost vanished from the market. In the Eurostar registry only 2% of all endografts are tubular.[27]

On the other hand bifurcated grafts make the procedure more complicated and have specific complications as well, particularly limb occlusion. During our 15 years practice with EVAR we learnt that there is a subset of patients who may benefit from tube graft devices and a double tube concept was developed.[18, 27]

RE-EXPLORATION OF THE DOUBLE TUBE CONCEPT

Treatment of the infrarenal aorta with a tube graft relies on proximal and distal neck fixation. If a bifurcated graft is used the distal anchoring points are in the iliacs rather than the distal aorta. If a tube graft is used one has to take away as much of the force from the proximal and distal fixation as possible. By putting two tubes in a "trombone technique" in the aorta, the two components, provided there is a long overlap, can move against each other. There is graft length to conform to the anatomy of the aorta and the aneurysm. The pull out forces at both ends are reduced

(Figures 4-5). Advantages of this approach, compared to simple stacking of short-cuff extensions, are numerous: longer proximal and distal landing zones help to resist graft migration and type I endoleak, greater stent overlapping distance diminishes the opportunity for type III endoleak, and differences between the proximal and distal aortic landing zone diameter can be accommodated by using different sized devices and placing the larger into the smaller stent-graft. (Tables 3-4)

IMPLANTATION TECHNIQUE

This section summarises the aspects of double-tube technique that we have found are important. For each procedure, two tube grafts are used in overlapped fashion. Both components are delivered through the same groin. On the contralateral side, percutaneous access is required only for angiography during the procedure. Adequate proximal and distal landing zones in the aorta are mandatory for the double tube technique; we believe that 10mm proximal and distal implant zones are the minimum acceptable. These zones may be shorter than those proposed for bifurcated grafts, since the movement of two grafts against each other reduces the forces at the landing zones. The distal part should be placed as low as possible (close to the aortic bifurcation) to utilize the maximum amount of the neck for sealing. The same should be done with the proximal component. To assist in placing

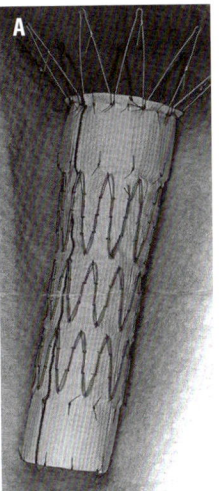 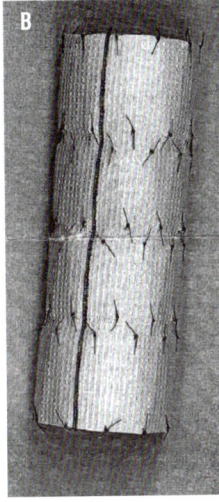

FIGURE 4: **A.** and **B.** double tube proximal part with suprarenal fixation, distal part without additional hooks or barbs.

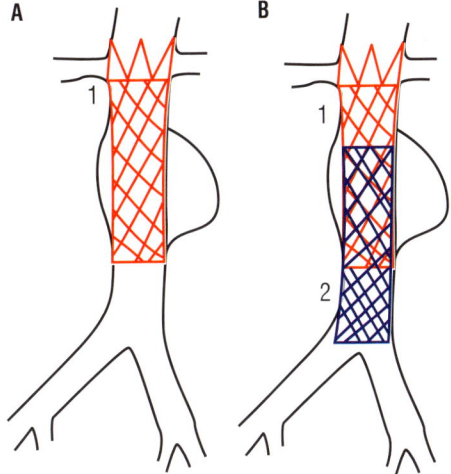

FIGURE 5: Proximal tube is placed first, distal second, extending to aortic bifurcation as close as possible.

the distal graft as close as possible to the bifurcation, it is useful to advance a guidewire across the bifurcation as shown in Figure 6.

Both grafts may be of the same diameter, different diameter or tapered. Depending on the diameter of the aorta the distal part can be smaller, but should then be implanted first, or be tapered (Figure 6). Logically it seems preferable to routinely place the distal component first (Figure 7) since this creates an imbricated feature of the graft. Sometimes however this is prevented by graft dimensions. As

long as there is no diameter mismatch and there is a long overlapping zone no adverse events have been observed to date when using the "top first method".

RESULTS

Our experience with tube graft techniques has been presented in two articles published during 2007.[18,27] Perioperative mortality was 0% in the overall series of 45 patients. Four endoleaks were observed. Aneurysm shinkage was significant in all

TABLE 3

ADVANTAGES OF DOUBLE GRAFT TECHNIQUE

* easy deployment sequence
* quicker procedure
* no limb occlusion concerns
* only one large access
* bifurcated graft later possible
* open repair easier, if required later

TABLE 4

DISADVANTAGES OF DOUBLE TUBE TECHNIQUE

* lack of commercially available grafts
* limited number of patients with suitable anatomy
* potential for dislocation of the distal part during implantation
* occlusion of iliac artery possible

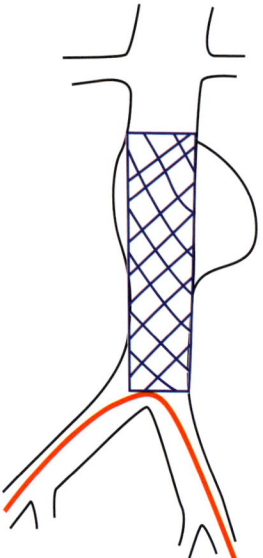

FIGURE 6: Wire crossover from contralateral groin marks bifurcation. Exact positioning of the distal tube possible. If the graft does not conform properly, dilation in kissing balloon technique is recommended.

patients. Comparison to the EUROSTAR data revealed a shorter intervention time and a lower rate of type II endoleak, but

no statistically significant advantage in perioperative mortality rate.[27] Today about 10% of our patients are treated with tube grafts, 90% of them with double tubes (Figures 8-9).

DISCUSSION

We believe that tube endovascular grafts, especially when used in overlapped double tube fashion, can still be a useful tool for a subset of patients requiring repair of AAA (see Table 2). A current problem is the lack of commercially available tube grafts. They are offered as custom made devices by several companies, but only two offer them off-the-shelf. Alternatively, in patients with narrow aorta, off-the-shelf limb extensions can be used, if they are long enough (60 to 80 mm at least). For bigger diameters, thoracic grafts can sometimes be used. We believe that the use of infrarenal extender cuffs, as proposed by several authors,[17] is not a generally acceptable alternative, because it the overlap between these components is too

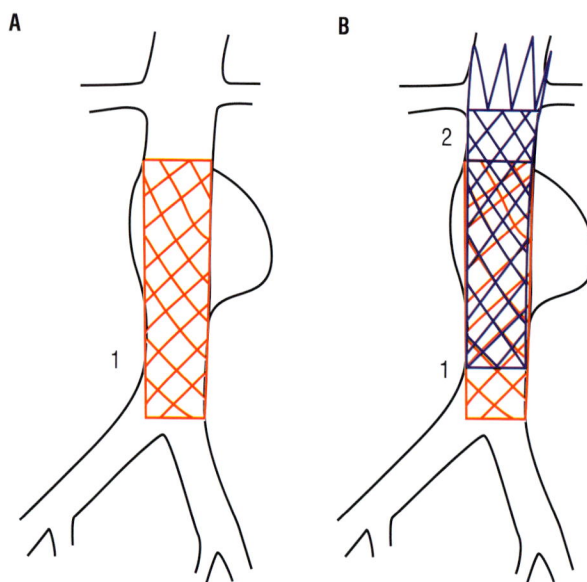

FIGURE 7: Distal tube placed first. Theoretically a higher incidence of dislocation of the distal part is possible.

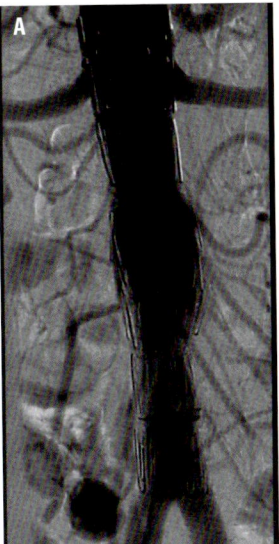
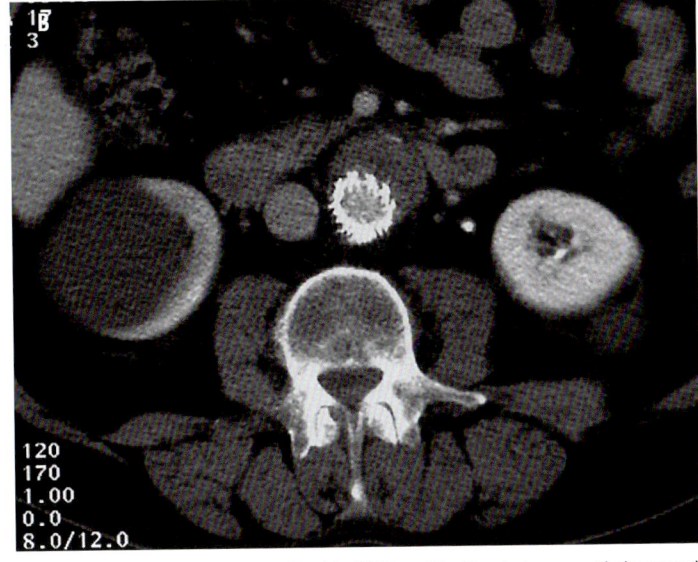

FIGURE 8: A. Completion angiogram after double tube implantation (Zenith, CMD graft) . Exact placement below renal arteries and above aortic bifurcation. **B.** CT-scan of the same patient with a saccular aneurysm

short; we feel that an overlap of at least 50 mm is mandatory. The available extender cuffs can not provide this, because their length is between 36 and 50 mm only.

Patients with saccular aneuryms are ideal candidates for tube grafts. These patients often have calcified access vessels. The opportunity to use only one femoral artery for access is therefore an advantage in such patients.

FIGURE 9: A. Pre interventional angiogram of a more fusifom infrarenal aneurysm with a distal neck. **B.** Angiogram after double tube implantation (Zenith CMD graft).

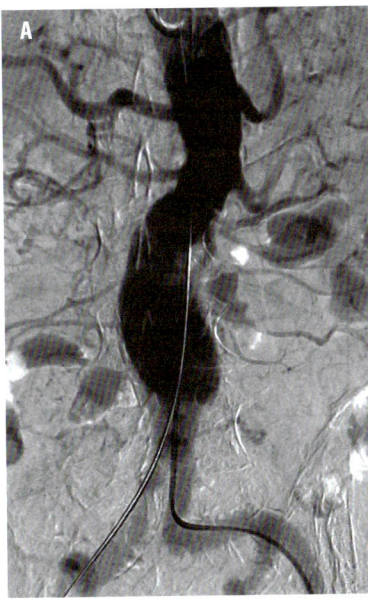
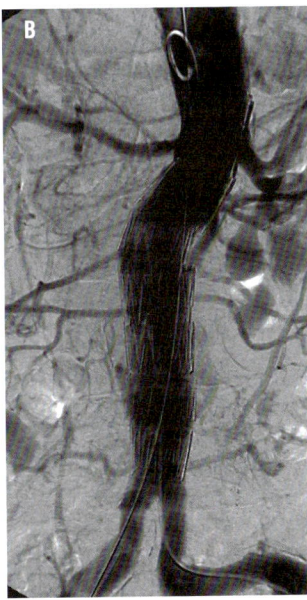

The outcome of overlapped tube grafts does not rely on proximal and distal fixation alone, but also on the flexibility of the overlap zone.[28] Implantation technique is easier than for a bifurcated graft and implantation time is shorter. It is mandatory to have a long overlap and to choose each graft as long as possible. Because of the ability to deploy either the proximal or distal part first, different proximal and distal diameters can be compensated for. In our experience, aortic necks or implant zones as short as 10 mm are possible. In patients with narrow distal necks, use of tube graft avoids the problem of limb compression which often occurs when a bifurcated graft is used in such anatomy. Bifurcated grafts need a distal diameter of 24 mm or more to allow both limbs unrestricted space in which to expand.

The double graft overlapping concept is of use during bifurcated graft procedures as well. We have used it in the proximal trunk section of composite grafts in more than 600 cases to date (Figure 10). The bifurcated distal component can sit

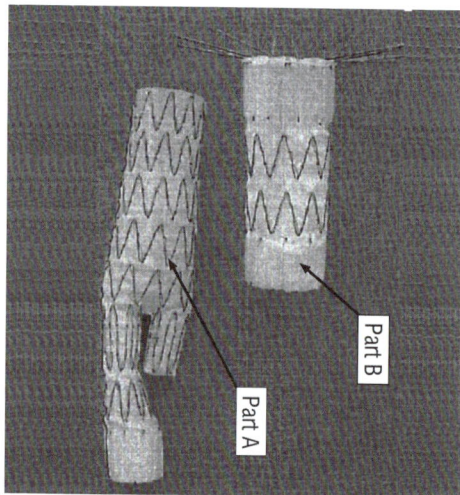

FIGURE 10: Devices used in the double "tube" concept for bifurcated grafts (picture of one of the first Cook Zenith composite grafts developed for implantation in patients in 1998).

on the natural aortic bifurcation (or close to it) to provide stability, and the proximal tube part can be placed as close as possible to the renal arteries separately. This is especially useful for fenestrated graft procedures, where an independent rotation of the proximal part is necessary for exact placement.

REFERENCES

1. Wilson SE, White G, Williams RA. Straight segmental versus bifurcation grafts for repair of abdominal aortic aneurysm. Cardiovasc Surg 1993;-1:23-6.
2. Hassen-Khodja R, Feugier P, Favre JP, Nevelsteen A, Ferreira J. Outcome of common iliac arteries after straight tube-graft placement during elective repair of infrarenal abdominal aortic aneurysms. J Vasc Surg 2006;44:943-8.
3. Lazarus HM Endovascular grafting for the treatment of abdominal aortic aneurysms. Surg Clin North Am 1992;72:959-68.
4. Andrews SM, Cuming R, Macsweeney ST, Barrett NK, Greenhalgh RM, Nott DM. Assessment of feasibility for endovascular tube correction of aortic aneurysms.Br J Surg 1995; 82:917-9.
5. Parodi JC, Palmaz JC, Barone HD. Transfemoral intraluminal graft implantation for abdominal aortic aneurysms. Ann Vasc Surg 1991;5:491-499.
6. Laborde JC, Parodi JC, Clem MF, Tio FO, Barone HD, Rivera FJ, Encarnacion CE, Palmaz JC Radiology 1992;184:185-90.
7. Moore WS, Rutherford R. Transfemoral endovascular repair of abdominal aortic aneurysm: Results of the North American EVT phase 1 trial. J Vasc Surg 1996; 23:543-553.
8. White GH, Yu W, May J, Waugh RC, Stephen MS, Harris JP. Three year experience with the White-Yu GAD graft for transluminal repair of aortic and iliac aneurysms. J Endovasc Surg 1997; 4:124-136.
9. Nasim A, Thompson MM, Sayers RD, Boyle JR, Maltezos C, Fishwick G, et al. Is endoluminal abdominal aortic aneurysm repair using an aortoaortic (tube) device a durable procedure? Ann Vasc Surg 1998;12:522-8.
10. Allen RC, White RA, Zarins CK, Fogarty TJ. What

are the characteristics of the ideal endovascular graft for abdominal aortic aneurysm exclusion? J Endovasc Surg 1997;4:195-202.

11. Faries PL, Briggs VL, Rhee JY, Burks JA Jr, Gravereaux EC, Carroccio A, Morrissey NJ, Teodorescu V, Hollier LH, Marin ML. Failure of endovascular aortoaortic tube grafts: a plea for preferential use of bifurcated grafts. J Vasc Surg. 2002 May;35(5):868-73.

12. May J, White GH, Yu W, Waugh RC, Stephen MS, Arulchelvam M, Harris JP. Importance of graft configuration in outcome of endoluminal aortic aneurysm repair: A 5-year analysis by the life table method. Eur J Vasc Endovasc Surg 1998;15:406-411.

13. White GH, Yu W, May J, Waugh RC, Stephen MS, Harris JP. A new non-stented balloon-expandable graft forstraight or bifurcated endoluminal bypass. J Endovasc Surg 1994; 1:16-24.

14. Yu W, White GH, May J, Stephen MS. Endoluminal repair of abdominal aortic aneurysms using the trombone technique. Asian J Surg 1996; 19:37-40.

15. May J, White GH, Yu W, Waugh RC, Stephen MS, Sieunarine K,Chaufour X, Harris JP.. Endoluminal repair of abdominal aortic aneurysms: Strengths and weaknesses of various prostheses observed in a 4.5 year experience. J Endovasc Surg 1997;4: 147-51.

16. Marin ML, Hollier LH, Avrahami R, Parsons R. Varying strategies for endovascular repair of abdominal and iliac artery aneurysms. Surg Clinics North America 1998.

17. York JW, Sternbergh III, C, Lepore MR, Yoselevitz M, Money SR. Endovascular exclusion of saccular AAAs using "stacked" AneuRx aortic cuffs. J Endovasc Ther 2002;9:295-98.

18. Ruppert V, Kerstin E, Burklein D, Treitl M, Steckmeier B, Stetler W, Umscheid T. Double tube stent-grafts for infrarenal aortic aneurysm: a new concept. J Endovasc Ther 2007;13:144-149.

19. Berchtold C, Eibl C, Seelig MH, Jakob P, Schon-leben K. Endovascular treatment and complete regression of an infected abdominal aortic aneurysm. J Endovasc Ther 2002;9:543-8.

20. van Herwaarden JA, Waasdorp EJ, Bendermacher BLW, van den Berg JC, Teijink JAW, Moll FL. Endovascular repair of paraanastomotic aneurysms after previous open aortic prosthetic reconstruction. Ann Vasc Surg 2004;18:280-6.

21. Zhou W, Bush RL, Bhama JK, Lin PH, Safaya R, Lumsden AB. Repair of anastomotic abdominal aortic pseudoaneurysm utilizing sequential AneuRx aortic cuffs in an overlapping configuration. Ann Vasc Surg 2006;20:17-22.

22. Piffaretti G, Tozzi M, Lomazzi C, Rivolta N, Caronno R, Castelli P. Endovascular treatment for para-anastomotic abdominal aortic and iliac aneurysms following aortic surgery. J Cardiovasc Surg 2007;48:711-7.

23. Danneels MIL, Verhagen HJM, Teijink JAW, Cuypers Ph, Nevelsteen A, Vermassen FEG. Endovascular repair for aorto-enteric fistula: A bridge too far or a bridge to surgery? Eur J Vasc Endovasc Surg 2006;32:27-33.

24. Hollier LH, Kazmier FJ, Oschner J, et al. "Shaggy" aorta syndrome with atheromatous embolization to visceral vessels.Ann Vasc Surg 1991;5:439-444.

25. Raithel D. Results of endovascular Abdominal Aortic Aneurysm Repair (EVAR). Zentralbl Chir 2002;127(8):660-3.

26. Brewster DC, Geller SC, Kaufmann JA, et al. Initial Experience with Endovascular Aneurysm Repair: Comparision of early results with outcome of open Repair. J Vasc Surg 1998;27(6): 992-1003

27. Ruppert V, Leurs LJ, Hobo R, Buth J, Rieger J, Umscheid T; EUROSTAR Collaborators: Tube Stent-grafts for Infrarenal Aortic Aneurysm: A matched-Paired Analysis Based on EUROSTAR Data. Cardiovasc Intervent Radiol 2007;30(4):611-618

28. Umscheid Th, Stelter WJ. Time-Related Alterations in Shape, Postion and Structure of Self-Expanding Modular Aortic Stent-Grafts: A 4-year Single-Center Follow-up. J Endovasc Surg 1999;6:17-32

Emergency endovascular AAA rupture repair: EVAR vs open surgery

Frank J. Veith, Mehta Manish, Nicholas J. Gargiulo III

This work was supported in part by grants from the William J. von Liebig Foundation.

When ruptured abdominal aortic aneurysms (AAAs) rupture and are not treated, they invariably lead to the patient's death. In addition, ruptured abdominal aortic aneurysms (RAAAs) have high mortality (35-70%) and morbidity rates when treated by standard open surgical methods.[1-5] These high perioperative mortality and morbidity rates have not been substantially reduced despite the introduction of many improvements in open operative technique or perioperative care.[1-6] The introduction of endovascular approaches to treat AAAs in the early 1990s seemed like an opportunity to alter substantially treatment outcomes when ruptured occurred.[7,8] The present chapter details how these endovascular approaches, which include endovascular stented grafts, can be applied to the treatment of RAAAs, and what advantages these new catheter based approaches to treatment offer.

OBSTACLES TO USE OF ENDOVASCULAR GRAFTS IN THE RUPTURED ANEURYSM SETTING

The less invasive nature of endovascular treatment of RAAAs offers many potential advantages. However, one obstacle in the early days of endovascular AAA treatment was the selection of the appropriate graft for each patient which required complex measurements of aneurysmal and adjacent arterial lengths and diameters. These measurements are usually based on high quality contrast CT scans and arteriography which take time to perform and which may not be available in the RAAA setting. Moreover, it may not be possible to have available a stock of grafts suitable for most patients. A second obstacle to the use of endovascular grafts was that standard surgical practice mandated early proximal aortic control, and it was thought that this could be achieved most rapidly and most effectively by laparotomy with placement of a supraceliac or infrarenal aortic clamp.[9]

SUITABLE ENDOGRAFTS FOR ENDOVASCULAR REPAIR IN THE RAAA SETTING

To overcome the first obstacle, we have had available since 1993 a derivative of the original Parodi endograft[10] to treat aortic and aortoiliac aneurysms. This Vascular In-

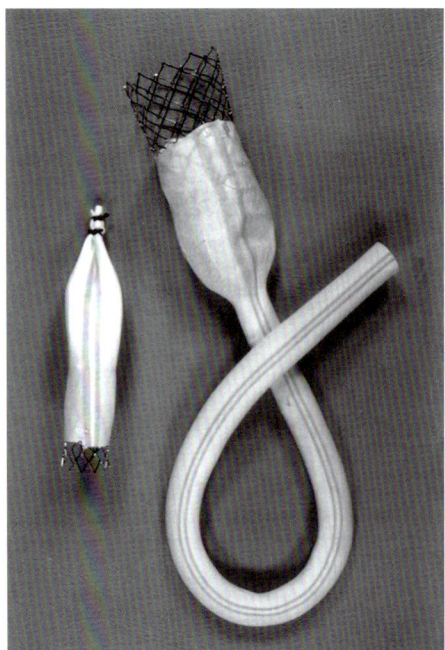

FIGURE 1: Vascular Innovation (VI) graft. A large Palmaz stent is attached to the PTFE graft. A surgeon-made occluder device is shown on the left. However, there are many other commercially made occluders available, and any of these can be used to block the opposite common iliac artery.

novation (VI) graft,* which is used in an aortofemoral configuration, is comprised of a large proximal Palmaz balloon expandable stent affixed to a long tulip shaped PTFE graft (Figure 1).[11] This graft is "a one size fits most" since the proximal diameter can vary between 20 and 27 mm depending on the inflation pressure applied to the deployment balloon, and the excess graft length can be cut off and tailored appropriately before the distal graft is sutured to the graft introduction site within the common femoral artery (Figure 2).

Having this graft sterilized and available has had the potential for eliminating the need for preoperative measurement and fabricating or procuring a suitable graft for use in the urgent RAAA setting. Moreover, as the commercially made modular endografts became available, components of these grafts could be stocked in the operating room and could be used to treat RAAAs.

EARLY EXPERIENCE WITH ENDOVASCULAR TREATMENT OF RUPTURED AAAS

Because we had available a surgeon-made VI graft, on April 21, 1994, we had a patient with a ruptured abdominal aorta and all the clinical sequellae thereof, i.e., severe abdominal pain, hypotension and a large pulsatile abdominal mass. Because the patient had had a total cystectomy and ileal bladder, and because he had severe symptomatic coronary artery disease with an ejection fraction of 20%, he was deemed unsuitable for an open repair of his ruptured aortic aneurysm. We were able to perform an endovascular graft repair of his RAAA along with placement of a right common iliac artery occluder and a femorofemoral bypass (Figure 3).[7] The patient did well following this procedure until he died from cardiac disease three years later. To our knowledge this was the first endovascular graft repair of a ruptured aortic aneurysm, although another early case was reported by Yusuf, Hopkinson et al.[8]

Following our experience with our first successful case we performed similar operations on another 11 patients with ruptured aortoiliac aneurysms.[11] All these patients had major contraindications to open operation with serious medical comorbidities (e.g., coincident major myocardial infarction, chronic obstructive pulmonary

---

* This graft was originally made by us from available materials but is now to be commercialized as the Vascular Innovation (VI) Graft, Vascular Innovation, Inc., Perrysburg, OH 43551.

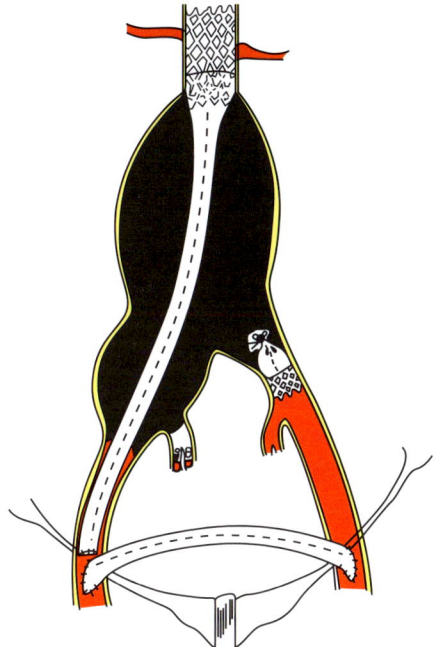

FIGURE 2: Schematic drawing illustrating how the VI graft is used This graft is fixed within the proximal neck with a large Palmaz stent (p). The cranial end of the graft is denoted by a metallic marker (m) attached to the graft. The bare portion of the stent is deployed across the orifice of the renal arteries so that the graft is implanted immediately below the renal arteries (r). An endoluminal anastomosis (e) is performed at the distal end of the endograft. The occluder device (o) is deployed in the contralateral common iliac artery to preserve at least one internal iliac artery (i). c, embolization coil; f, femorofemoral bypass; s, sutures to occlude the end of the occluder.

disease (COPD) requiring home oxygen therapy) or surgical problems producing a hostile abdomen (e.g., abdominal infection or massive recurrent incisional hernias). All 12 of these first patients had been stable enough to undergo preoperative CT scanning to confirm the aneurysmal rupture. In all 12 of these original patients, the ruptured aneurysm was successfully excluded by the endovascular graft. Moreover, only two of the patients died within 2 months of the procedure, a 17% operative mortality.

HYPOTHESIS REGARDING ENDOVASCULAR TREATMENT OF RUPTURED AAAS AND CURRENT

Management plan

This low operative mortality prompted us to speculate that all RAAAs should be treated endovascularly. Such an approach might lead to better outcomes than were currently being achieved with open repair. In 1995, we therefore adopted the following treatment plan.[12] All patients with a presumed diagnosis of a RAAA were taken immediately to the operating room. A diagnosis of RAAA was presumed if two or more elements of the diagnostic triad were present; namely syncope, abdominal or back pain, and a known or palpable AAA.[9] In the operating room, with preparation for fluoroscopy of the patient from the neck to the knees, via a femoral or brachial puncture under local anesthesia a wire was placed in the supraceliac aorta. Using this guidewire a catheter was placed to visualize the abdominal aorta and iliac arteries angiographically. This angiogram, which was best performed with a power injector, allowed a determination of whether or not an endovascular graft repair of the RAAA was possible on the basis of aortic neck and iliac artery anatomy. If not, a standard repair was carried out.

CONTROL OF BLEEDING AND BLOOD PRESSURE: RESTRICTED RESUSCITATION, HYPOTENSIVE HEMOSTASIS AND PROXIMAL BALLOON CONTROL

As already noted, it is widely believed that with RAAAs, it is necessary to perform immediate laparotomy to permit clamp control of the aorta proximal to the aneurysm. With major arterial bleeding in other circumstances, however, restricted fluid re-

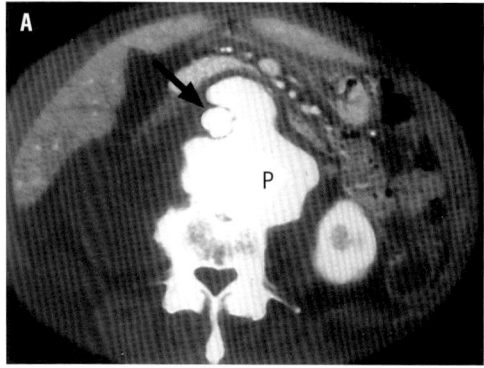

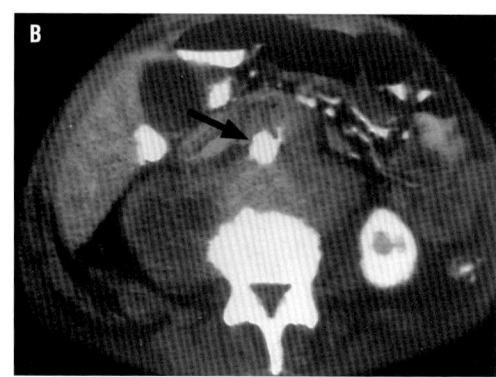

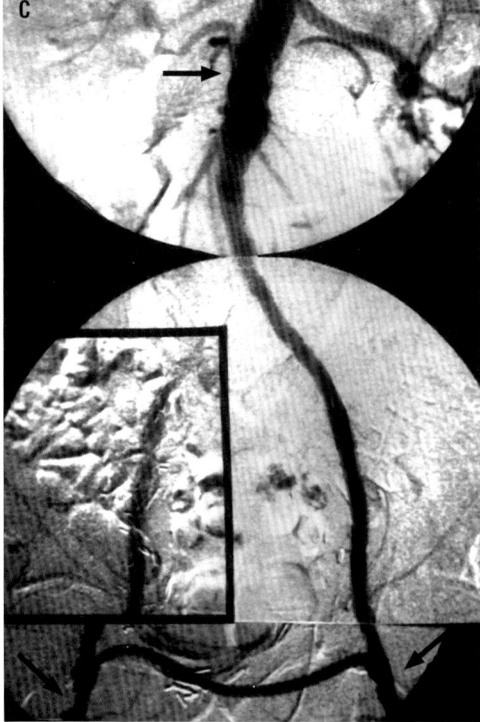

FIGURE 3: Transfemoral repair of a rupture of a distal aortic aneurysm (**A**) A spiral CT scan demonstrates extravasation of contrast material from the aorta (*arrow*) into a large, partially clot-filled pseudoaneurysm (P). (**B**) A spiral CT scan performed after transfemoral insertion of an endovascular graft demonstrates that the pseudoaneurysm is excluded and vascular continuity within the lumen of the aorta (*arrow*) is preserved. (**C**) A postoperative transfemoral arteriogram at 1 week demonstrates vascular continuity between the aorta (*open arrow*) and the common femoral arteries (*arrows*). The inset shows flow up the external iliac artery to the right hypogastric artery. An occluder has been placed in the right common iliac artery. (Reproduced with permission.[7])

suscitation and withholding blood transfusions have been shown to decrease blood loss and improve outcomes.[13-16] One editorial in 1991 also advocated restriction of fluid resuscitation in the preoperative management of RAAAs.[17] We also believe that restriction of fluid resuscitation and blood transfusion in the RAAA setting is not only desirable but mandatory. If the blood pressure is in the 50-70 mmHg range, it should

be left there. If the patient is moving and talking, no fluids should be given. This should continue when the patient is first in the operating room being prepared for treatment and having a guidewire and catheter placed in the suprarenal aorta under local anesthesia via either a femoral or brachial puncture.

Patients with RAAAs frequently deteriorate with induction of anesthesia. If that occurs and the blood pressure falls below 50 mmHg or is unobtainable, administration of fluid and blood become necessary. We believe such deterioration warrants proximal balloon control and have used this technique selectively in our current management plan for ruptured aneurysms.

Proximal Balloon Control

If and when patients deteriorate before, during or after induction of anesthesia, a larger size (14-16 Fr) hemostatic sheath is inserted over the previously placed guidewire via either the femoral or brachial artery With the wire in place a 27, 33 or 40 mm compliant (latex) balloon is inserted through the sheath and inflated with dilute contrast under fluoroscopic control (Figure 4) in either the supraceliac or pararenal aorta (depending on the length of the infrarenal neck). If the femoral route is chosen for the balloon placement, the sheath must be kept in place in the aorta to support the balloon and to facilitate its removal after graft placement. With the balloon inflated, the remainder of the procedure is conducted as rapidly as possible to minimize the duration of visceral and renal ischemia. If the infrarenal neck is too short, too flared or too angulated for an endovascular repair, open aortic control, preferably below the renal arteries, is obtained and a standard AAA repair performed. If a bifurcated endograft is inserted, an infrarenal balloon should be placed within the graft to replace the more proximal balloon as soon as possible. Then the endograft procedure is completed in a deliberate fashion.

EXPERIENCE WITH ENDOVASCULAR TREATMENT OF RUPTURED AAAs

To date, we have treated 48 patients with ruptured aortoiliac aneurysms using endovascular techniques. Included are the 12 original patients already described and another 34 patients treated according to our current management plan. Of these

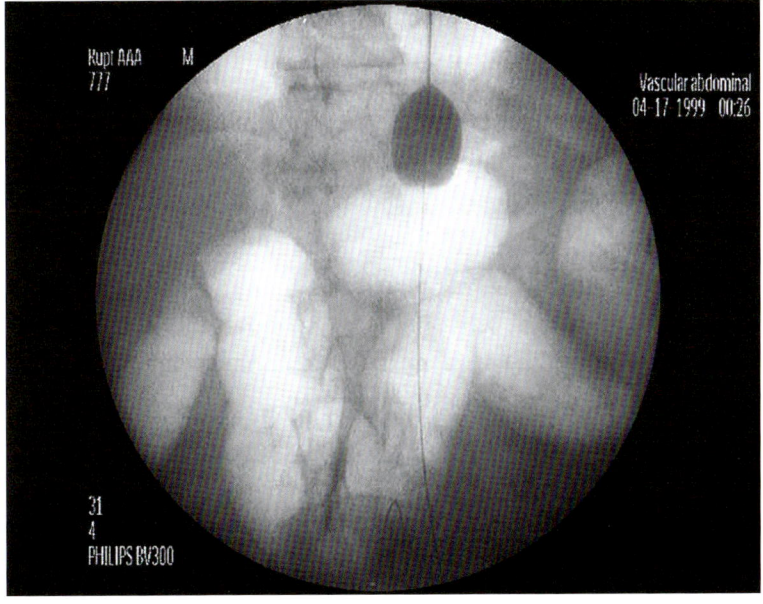

FIGURE 4: Fluoroscopic view of a proximal occlusion balloon introduced through the brachial artery.

48 patients, 8 were deemed unsuitable for endovascular treatment because of their aortic neck or iliac anatomy. These 8 underwent open repair, only 3 required inflation of the proximal balloon. All survived for more than two months after operation.

Of the remaining 40 patients who received an endovascular graft, 31 had the graft inserted without the need for proximal balloon control. Only 9 of the 48 required balloon control. Twenty-five of these patients were treated with a VI graft, and 15 received an industry made graft (AneuRx, Zenith, Excluder). In all 38 patients, the graft was deployed successfully and completely excluded the ruptured aneurysm. There were no significant endoleaks and all surviving patients became and remained asymptomatic. Five of the 40 patients died during the 30 days after their procedure, but all had serious medical comorbidities (coincident major myocardial infarctions and/or oxygen dependent COPD). Thus, in this entire series of 48 ruptured AAAs, there was a procedural mortality of only 10%.

Two patients receiving endovascular grafts required evacuation of a large retroperitoneal hematoma for abdominal compartment syndrome. In one of these patients the decompression was required immediately after graft placement; in the other it was required 7 days later. Two groin wound infections required drainage but healed without graft involvement.

COLLECTED WORLD EXPERIENCE WITH ENDOVASCULAR GRAFT TREATMENT OF RAAAS

Over the last 3 years, a collaborative group, the EVAR for Ruptured Aneurysm Investigators, have been pooling their results with the use of endovascular graft repair of RAAAs. The data collection is still in progress. However, to date many centers have submitted their results which will be published as a multiauthored report. Of 571 RAAA patients collected to date and treated with endografts, 463 have survived more than 30 days, giving an encouragingly low procedural mortality rate of 19%. Although patients were selected for endovascular treatment by a variety of criteria, some of the patients had free intraperitoneal rupture and many were severely hypotensive. In addition, many were prohibitive risks for a standard open repair (Figure 5). The low mortality for endograft repair coupled with the inclusion of many high risk RAAA patients strongly suggests that endovascular graft repair, when feasible, will improve treatment outcomes for RAAAs.

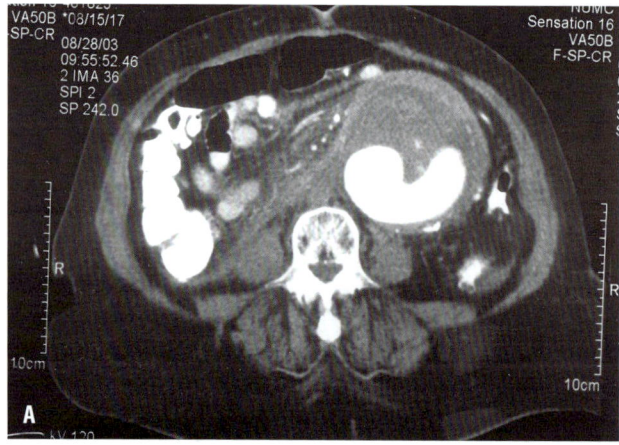

FIGURE 5: Eighty-six year old Jehovah's Witness with a 10 cm RAAA.
A. Contrast CT showing RAAA.

FIGURE 5: B. Contrast CT showing an unfavorable short angulated neck. Open repair was advised but patient refused blood transfusion. The hematocrit fell to 17% and the systolic arterial blood pressure to 60 mmHG. Open repair was thought to carry a prohibitive risk.

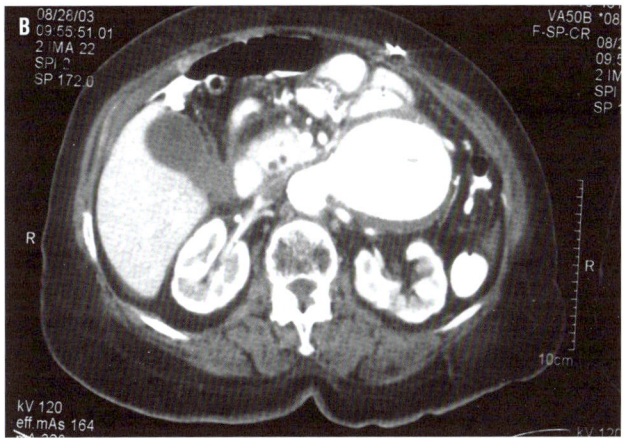

Advantages of endovascular treatment of ruptured AAAs

Among the advantages of endovascular repair of ruptured aneurysms are the ability to obtain proximal control without general anesthesia, the ability to deploy the graft from a remote access site, reduced blood loss, and minimizing hypothermia by eliminating laparotomy.

Proximal control without general anesthesia

Patients with ruptured AAAs may be severely hypotensive. However, many patients may have their blood pressure stabilized at a nonlethal level. This is due to sympathetically mediated vasoconstriction in response to hypotension. It is not uncommon for this vasoconstriction to be re-

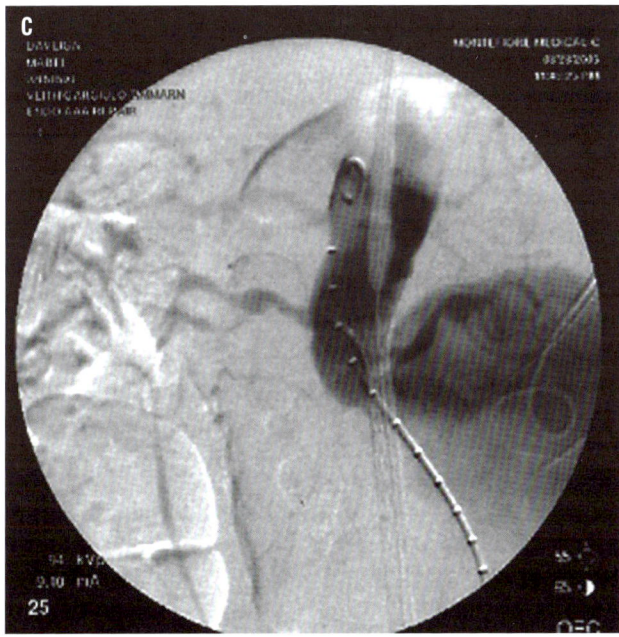

FIGURE 5: C. Endovascular repair was performed despite the angulated short neck. Note left renal artery appearing to arise from the aneurysm. The endograft is in place but not yet deployed.

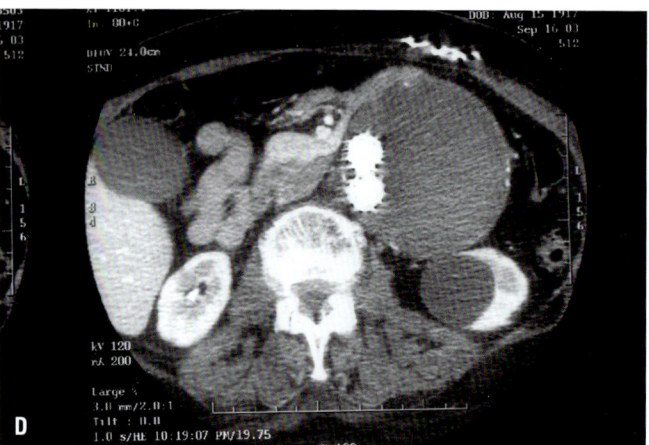

FIGURE 5: D. Contrast CT scan 6 weeks after the procedure. The aneurysm sac is excluded from the circulation.

leased during the induction of general anesthesia, which results in a sudden drop in blood pressure. Therefore, a relatively stable patient may become severely hypotensive, mandating urgent application of a proximal aortic clamp. However, a guidewire can be inserted in the upper abdominal or lower thoracic aorta through a percutaneous puncture under local anesthesia, while maintaining the vasoconstriction. Once the guidewire is inserted in the aorta, the patient can then safely undergo induction of general anesthesia because proximal control can be rapidly and relatively safely obtained by an occlusion balloon placed over the previously inserted guidewire.

Deployment of graft from a remote access Site

Endovascular grafts can be inserted and deployed through a remote access site, thereby obviating the need for laparotomy and, more importantly, eliminating the technical difficulties that are encountered when performing a standard repair in the rupture setting. With the associated bleeding, the anatomy of the retroperitoneal structures is often distorted and obscured

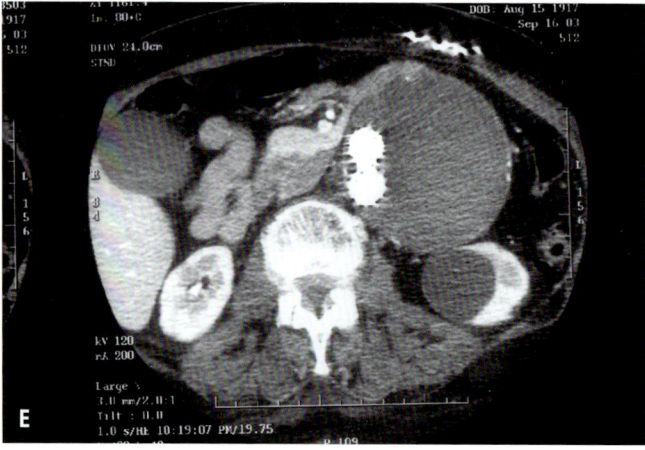

FIGURE 5: E. Contrast CT scan 6 weeks after the procedure. The aneurysm is excluded. The left renal artery is perfused. The patient remains well over 2 years later.

by a large hematoma, which may lead to technical difficulties as well as inadvertent injury of the inferior vena cava, the left renal vein or its genital branches, the duodenum, or other surrounding structures. These iatrogenic injuries have been the cause of significant operative morbidity and mortality following standard surgery for RAAAs. In contrast, endograft repair is performed within the arterial tree, which is unaffected by extravasated blood or previous operative scarring. Thus, the technical difficulty encountered when treating a RAAA with an endograft is similar to that for elective cases. Moreover, this approach completely eliminates the risk of inadvertent injury to surrounding structures.

Reduced blood loss

In our experience, endovascular repair for RAAAs was accomplished with a relatively small amount of additional blood loss (800 ml) compared with that which occurs during open RAAA repair. This advantage is more important in patients with RAAAs because these patients have already lost a significant amount of blood following rupture, and coagulopathy or disseminated intravascular coagulation secondary to further blood loss can be serious and often lethal complications. There are several reasons why blood loss was limited, including the maintenance of the tamponade effect within the retroperitoneum. In addition, back-bleeding from the iliac and lumbar arteries and bleeding from the anastomotic suture lines and from iatrogenic venous injuries are eliminated.

Minimizing hypothermia

Hypothermia secondary to poor perfusion and laparotomy can exacerbate coagulopathy, which is one of the causes of mortality following open surgical repair. Endovascular graft repair can minimize the extent of hypothermia by avoiding laparotomy.

DISCUSSION

The relatively low mortality rates in RAAA patients treated endovascularly are encouraging, particularly because many were high-risk patients who were poor surgical candidates.[12,18-21] These results show that endograft repair of RAAAs is feasible and effective in selected cases. However, before the universal use of these techniques is adopted, many questions must be answered. Should endovascular repair be attempted in all RAAA patients or just those who are relatively stable? In what proportion of RAAA patients should an endograft repair be used? Should a CT scan be obtained before RAAA patients are taken to the operating room or endovascular suite? In which patients should a proximal balloon be placed? How should this be done? Is a randomized prospective comparison with open repair necessary or justified? Should an aortounilateral graft be used or a modular bifurcated graft? What kind of anesthesia should be employed? What resources are required for an institution to undertake endograft repairs of RAAAs? Until these questions are answered, we will not know the optimal approach to endovascular repair of RAAAs. Nevertheless, we believe that endovascular grafts represent a potentially better way to treat this entity since previous open surgical methods have had such a persistently high morbidity and mortality. We currently believe that these endovascular grafts can and should be used in over 50-60% of patients who present with a RAAA. Indeed some of the sickest, most urgent hypotensive patients may benefit the most from endograft treatment rather than subjecting them to an emergent open repair under suboptimal conditions. Moreover, we believe that the use of fluoroscopic techniques to facilitate the placement of proximal occlusion balloons, an old idea,[22-25] will make this endovascular adjunct a practical and valuable one, even if an endovascular graft procedure is not possible and an open repair is required. And finally, we believe that hypotensive hemostasis or restricted fluid resuscitation will prove valuable in the RAAA setting and will become the standard of care for this entity leading to improved treatment outcomes for this lethal condition.

REFERENCES

1. Johansen K, Kohler TR, Nicholls SC, Zierler RE, Clowes AW, Kazmers A. Ruptured abdominal aortic aneurysm: The Harbor view experience. J Vasc Surg 1991;13:240-247.
2. Gloviczki P, Pairolero PC, Mucha P. Ruptured abdominal aortic aneurysms: Repair should not be denied. J Vasc Surg 1992;15:851-859.
3. Marty-Ane CH, Alric P, Picot MC, Picard E, Colson P, Mary H Ruptured abdominal aortic aneurysm: Influence of intraoperative management on surgical outcome. J Vasc Surg 1995;22:780-786.
4. Darling RC, Cordero JA, Chang BB. Advances in the surgical repair of ruptured abdominal aortic aneurysms. Cardiovasc Surg 1996;4:720-723.
5. Dardik A, Burleyson GP, Bowman, Gordon TA, Williams GM, Webb TH, Perler BA. Surgical repair of ruptured abdominal aortic aneurysms in the state of Maryland: Factors influencing outcome among 527 recent cases. J Vasc Surg 1998;28: 413-423.
6. Noel AA, Gloviczki P, Cherry KJ Jr, Bower TC, Panneton JM, Mozes GI, Harmsen WS, Jenkins JD, Hallet JW, Jr. Ruptured abdominal aortic aneurysms: The excessive mortality rate of conventional repair. J Vasc Surg 2001;34:41-46.
7. Marin ML, Veith FJ, Cynamon J, Sanchez LA, Lyon R, Levine BA, Bakal CW, Suggs WD, Wengerter KW, Rivers SP, et al. Initial experience with transluminally placed endovascular grafts for the treatment of complex vascular lesions. Ann Surg 1995;222:1-17.
8. Yusuf SW, Whitaker SC, Chuter TA, Wenham PW, Hopkinson BR. Emergency endovascular repair of leaking aortic aneurysms. Lancet 1994;344:1645.
9. Veith FJ. Emergency abdominal aortic aneurysm surgery. Compr Ther 1992;18:25-29.
10. Parodi JC, Palmaz JC, Barone HD. Transfemoral intraluminal graft implantation for abdominal aortic aneurysms. Ann Vasc Surg 1991;5:491-499.
11. Ohki T, Veith FJ, Sanchez LA, Cynamon J, Lipsitz EC, Wain RA, Morgan JA, Zhen L, Suggs WD, Lyon RT. Endovascular graft repair of ruptured aorto-iliac aneurysms. J Am Coll Surg 1999;189:102-123.
12. Veith FJ, Ohki T. Endovascular approaches to ruptured infrarenal aorto-iliac aneurysms. J Cardiovasc Surg 2002;43:369-378.
13. Andresen AFR. Results of treatment of massive gastric hemorrhage. Am J Digest Dis 1939;6: 641-650.
14. Andresen AFR. Management of gastric hemorrhage. NY State J Med 1948;48:603-611.
15. Shaftan GW, Chiu CJ, Dennis C, Harris B. Fundamentals of physiologic control of arterial hemorrhage. Surg 1968;58:851-856.
16. Bickell WH, Wall MJ Jr, Pepe PE, Martin RR, Ginger VF, Allen MK, Mattox KL. Immediate versus delayed fluid resuscitation for hypotensive patients with penetrating torso injuries. N Engl J Med 1994;331:1105-1109.
17. Crawford ES. Ruptured abdominal aortic aneurysm: an editorial. J Vasc Surg 1991;13:348-350.
18. Yusuf SW, Whitaker SC, Chuter TAM, Ivancev K, Baker DM, Gregson RH, Tennant WG, Wenham PW, Hopkinson BR Early results of endovascular aortic aneurysm surgery with aortouniiliac graft, contralateral iliac occlusion, and femorofemoral bypass. J Vasc Surg 1997;25:165-172.
19. Yusuf SW, Hopkinson BR. Is it feasible to treat contained aortic aneurysm rupture by stent-graft combination? In Greenhalgh RM (ED), Indications in Vascular and Endovascular Surgery, pp 153-165, London, W B Saunders, 1998.
20. Greenberg RK, Srivastava SD, Ouriel K, Waldman D, Ivancev K, Illig KA, Shortell C, Green RM. An endoluminal method of hemorrhage control and repair of ruptured abdominal aortic aneurysms. J Endovasc Ther 2000;7:1-7.
21. Lachat ML, Pfammatter T, Witzke HJ, Bettex D, Kunzli A, Wolfensberger, U, Turina MI. Endovascular repair with bifurcated stent-grafts under local anaesthesia to improve outcome of ruptured aortoiliac aneurysms. Eur J Vasc Endovasc Surg 2002;23:528-536.
22. Hughes LCCW. Use of an intra-aortic balloon

catheter tamponade for controlling intraabdominal hemorrhage in man. Surgery 1954;36:65-68.

23. Hesse FG, Kletschka HD. Rupture of abdominal aortic aneurysm: control of hemorrhage by intra-luminal balloon tamponade. Ann Surg 1962;155: 320-322.

24. Anastacio CN, Ochsner EC. Use of Fogarty cathe-ter tamponade for ruptured abdominal aortic an-eurysms. Am J Roentgenol 1977;128:31-33.

25. Hyde GL, Sullivan DM. Fogarty catheter tampon-ade of ruptured abdominal aortic aneurysms. Surg Gynecol Obstet 1982;154:197-199.

Instant home made fenestrations for emergency EVAR in AAAs without an adequate sealing zone

Robert J. Hinchliffe, Nuno V. Dias, Martin Malina, Krassi Ivancev

INTRODUCTION

Endovascular stent-graft technology has evolved in to a technique, which has reduced the morbidity and mortality of aneurysm repair in selected patients.[1,2] The applicability of the endovascular technique is limited to those patients with suitable aneurysm morphology. Unsuitable proximal neck morphology, particularly short neck length is the most common reason patients are turned down for EVAR. In one study 44 of 154 (29%) patients studied with AAA had unacceptably short necks.[3]

Patients with adverse anatomy have traditionally received open surgery. However, the presence of adverse anatomy also increases the risks of open surgery.[4] In one recent study the mortality from open juxta-renal AAA repair (with supra-renal clamp) tended to be higher (6.1% versus 3%, p = 0.058) compared with a group of matched controls undergoing standard infra-renal AAA repair. There were more frequent pulmonary (p = 0.021) complications and re-operations (p = 0.019) in those patients with juxta-renal aneurysms.[5] As a result many patients are turned down for operative repair because they are not fit enough to withstand the rigours of open surgery.

Fenestrated stent-graft technology was developed in order to increase the morphological applicability of EVAR and offer an alternative to open repair. The technique was developed in 1996 and has subsequently been refined into a system (based on the Zenith stent-graft, William A. Cook Ltd, Brisbane, Australia) which is now commercially available.[6,7]

Fenestrated stent-grafts are individually customised and require some weeks to manufacture. Consequently they are not suitable for patients presenting emergently with acute symptomatic or ruptured AAA. Unfortunately, studies of patients with AAA reveal that many present acutely. In one study from the U.K. 26% of patients presented as an emergency.[8]

However, these patients may just be the group who would benefit the most from fenestrated stent-graft technology. A significant proportion of patients presenting with acute symptomatic or ruptured aneurysms are considered too frail to undergo open surgery.[8] Patients with large symptomatic aneurysms are more likely to have adverse anatomical features of the proximal neck.[9] Furthermore, the mortality from open repair of symptomatic AAA is significantly higher than in patients who are operated on electively. In one recent literature review, the mortality rate was 16%.[10]

DEVELOPMENT AND CURRENT RESULTS OF FENESTRATED STENT-GRAFTS

The technique of fenestrated stent-grafting has evolved with increasing experience. Major refinements include the use of a modular system to assist independent alignment of the stent-graft in the aortic neck and bifurcation. Diameter reducing restraining ties limit initial stent-graft expansion to permit alignment of the stent-graft prior to catheterization of target vessels. Reinforced fenestrations facilitate catheterization and prevent late vessel occlusion.

Most data on fenestrated stent-grafts has been published between 2005 and 2006. Sun and co-workers have performed a systematic review of the literature 1999-2006.[11] Short-term results are encouraging. Peri-operative target vessel patency rate was 97% (95% CI 92%-100%) and 90% (85%-95%) during follow-up. No conversions to open surgery were required. Peri-operative mortality was 1.1% (0.4-2.7) and the endoleak rate after 30 days was 9.4% (2.6-16.3). Long-term data is limited with only four studies reporting more than 12 months mean follow-up.

INDICATIONS, REQUIREMENTS AND EVOLUTION OF THE HOME-MADE FENESTRATED STENT-GRAFTS

Many of the early infra-renal aortic aneurysm stent-graft systems were surgeon manufactured.[12] Experience with the original first generation stent-graft systems demonstrated that it was possible to manufacture and customise the stent-graft systems "on the operating table" with low rates of graft related failure.[13,14] Over time

industry manufactured infra-renal stent-grafts improved significantly. Consequently, surgeon manufactured and customised devices became unnecessary.

The concept of a home-made fenestrated stent-graft was born out of the need to treat patients presenting acutely with symptomatic aneurysms, who were not candidates for open repair and where proximal neck morphology precluded standard EVAR.

At present, we employ the technique in patients presenting with acute symptomatic aneurysms. Morphologically they must be unsuitable for standard infra-renal EVAR. The morphological inclusion criteria we use are identical to those used in patients treated electively with fenestrated stent-grafts. All are medically high risk for standard open repair or have a hostile abdomen.

The technique we use for stent-graft fenestration is based on the fenestrated Zenith stent-graft. The technique has been modified and refined following the first report.[15]

The procedure of home-made stent-graft fenestration manufacture and implantation is technically challenging. Operating surgeons must be experienced in elective standard infra-renal and fenestrated EVAR and have access to good quality high resolution spiral CT for pre-operative planning. A good working knowledge of the Zenith stent-graft and its delivery system is required. They must be experienced in planning elective fenestrated stent-graft procedures. Excellent intra-operative imaging is required. Operators must be familiar with a variety of wires and catheters and be experienced in the catheterisation of renal and visceral vessels.

PRE-OPERATIVE ASSESSMENT

i) Aneurysm morphology

Aneurysm morphology should be assessed using high resolution multislice helical computed tomographic angiography. Calibration angiography is unnecessary. In Malmo we use an Aquarius workstation (TeraRecon, San Mateo, CA, USA) to reconstruct the aneurysm morphology from axial CT and calculate the required stent-graft size (Figure 1).

The main morphological indication for fenestrated stent-grafts is the presence of a short proximal aneurysm neck. Patients with an aneurysm neck length greater than 15 mm should receive a standard infra-renal aortic stent-graft. In cases where neck lengths decrease to 10 mm a standard infra-renal device can be used with a high probability of success, assuming there are no other adverse features. Those with neck lengths less than 10 mm are unlikely to seal with a standard infra-renal graft and require fenestrated stent-grafts.

A detailed assessment of all morphological aspects is required. The diameter at the level of the renal arteries and the length of the aneurysm neck is calculated. Distances are measured between the ostia of the coeliac axis, the superior mesenteric and renal arteries. The distance between fenestrations should be measured from the centre of the ostium whereas those target vessels receiving scallops should be measured from the most caudal point of the ostium. The location and relationship of the renal and visceral ostia are recorded in a clock-dial configuration.

There are a number of morphological factors that significantly increase the chances of failure with current fenestrated stent-graft technology. The aorta should measure no greater than 31 mm diameter at the level of the target vessels (normally

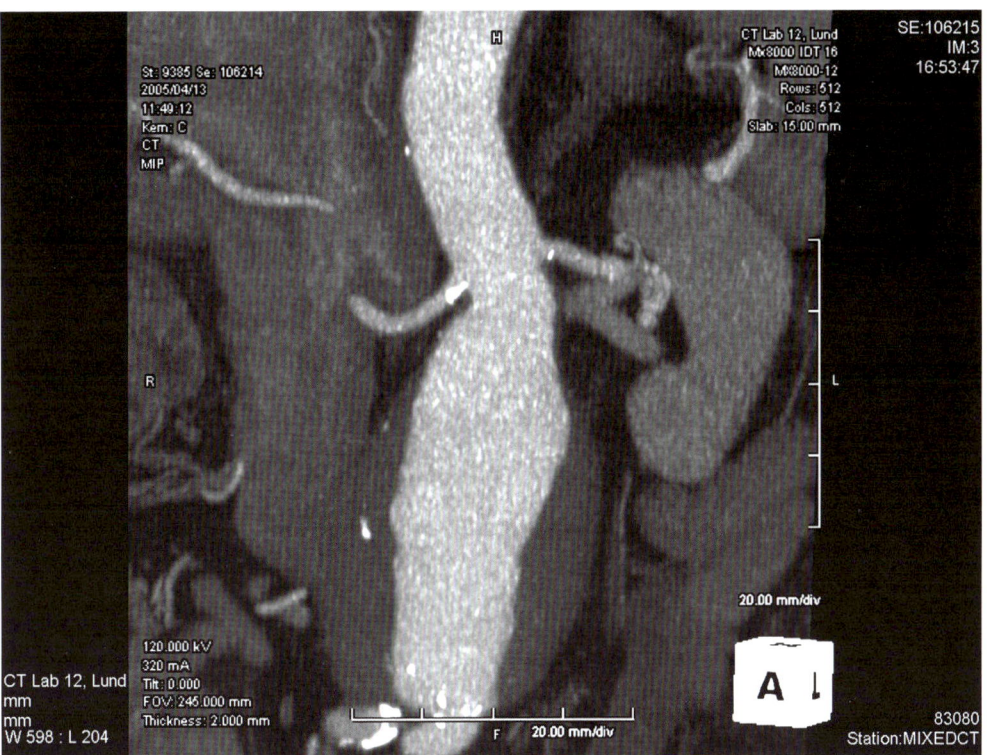

FIGURE 1: MIP reconstruction of juxta-renal AAA subsequently treated with home-made fenestrated stent-graft.

the renal arteries). Stent-grafts should be oversized by 10-20% in the aortic neck. An aortic diameter greater than 31 mm usually requires open repair or branched stent-graft technology.

In the Western Australia experience the factors associated with loss (occlusion) of target vessels were unstented fenestrations/vessels; greater than 60 degrees of angulation of the aneurysm neck; multiple fenestrations and target vessels of 4 mm diameter or less.[14]

Angulation of the aortic neck makes it difficult to size the stent-graft. There may be significant discrepancy between distances measured from orthogonal (mid flow-line) and axial views. Furthermore, it is not always possible to reliably predict the lie of the stent-graft in vivo. The angulation of the neck also increases the technical demands of fenestration/target vessel catheterisation.

Increasing the number of fenestrations increases the difficulty in terms of planning and deployment.

Multiple renal vessels, especially where less than 4 mm diameter (accessory) or stenosed are associated with catheterisation failure or subsequent occlusion.

Thrombus in the aneurysm neck is not necessarily, in itself, a contraindication to fenestrated EVAR (whether industry or surgeon made) but is associated with an increased risk of embolisation.

ii) Clinical

The position of open repair as the gold standard treatment for juxta-renal AAA is being challenged. Although, one may argue that fenestrated EVAR is justified in all patients with juxta-renal and symptomatic aneurysms. These patients have significantly worse outcome than those receiving standard open elective infra-renal aneurysm surgery.

However, until more data is available, patients should probably be selected for customised stent-graft fenestration on the grounds that they are medically at prohibitively high risk from open repair. The decision on which technique to offer patients may depend, in part, on local expertise and experience.

STENT-GRAFT PREPARATION

Stent-graft preparation is performed in a sterile environment in the operating theatre. If time permits it is best to prepare the stent-graft the night before the operation (assuming appropriate facilities are available for stent-graft and delivery system sterlisiation).

A Zenith stent-graft bifurcated main body (Cook Europe, Bjaereskov, Denmark) is selected according to the proximal neck diameter and renal artery-aortic bifurcation length. The first one or two covered stents are deployed (on the bench) by withdrawing the sheath of the main delivery system. The supra-renal stent is restrained within the top cap. The safety trigger wire is removed only from the top cap using artery forceps to permit deployment of the uncovered supra-renal stent. The inner cannula which is attached to the top cap is then advanced to deploy the supra-renal stent.

Fluoroscopy of the stent-graft is performed ex-vivo to identify and assess the orientation of the stent-graft markers, particularly the lateral markers identifying the contralateral iliac stump. These markers will be helpful later to aid orientation at the aortic bifurcation and to ensure the stent-graft is not twisted when re-loaded. The markers of welding of each stent are also helpful in the orientation and checking for possible rotation on reloading (Figure 2).

One of the drawbacks of the emergency fenestration system is that it does not permit independent alignment of the fenestrations in the aortic neck and the con-

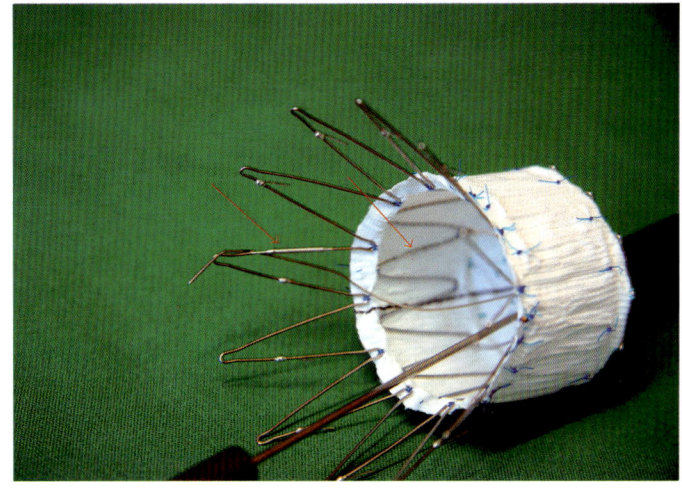

FIGURE 2: Welding on each stent strut acts as a useful marker to confirm correct alignment (*arrow*).

tralateral stump at the aortic bifurcation. The composite design of the commercially manufactured system allows independent alignment. The composite design has the potential drawback of modular disconnection between the two large components (proximal fenestrated tubular and distal bifurcated). However, some authors have suggested that the composite design may reduce the forces on the proximal fenestrated tubular component by placing them on the distal bifurcated segment instead.[16]

The stent-graft is fenestrated according to the measurements required. An indelible marker pen is used to mark the Dacron (Figure 3). Careful measurement is required to mark the longitudinal and axial distances. Low-power ophthalmic cautery (Medtronic Xomed, Jackonsville, FL) is used to create fenestrations or scallops in the Dacron (Figure 4). Dacron is flammable and care should be taken to avoid uncontrolled burning of the fabric (have a syringe containing saline available).

A variety of fenestrations or scallops can be made, all based on the standard

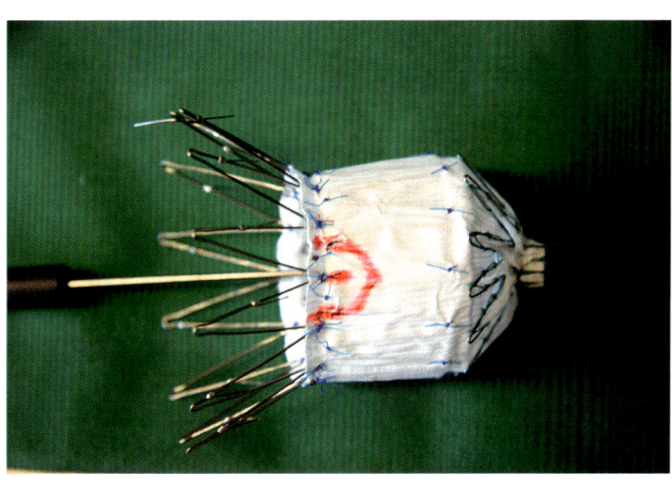

FIGURE 3: Indelibe pen to mark position of scallop/fenestrations. Note position of supra-renal stent strut. The strut was moved by bending adjacent struts and re-sutured to the Dacron. This permits free and easy endovascular access to the scallop.

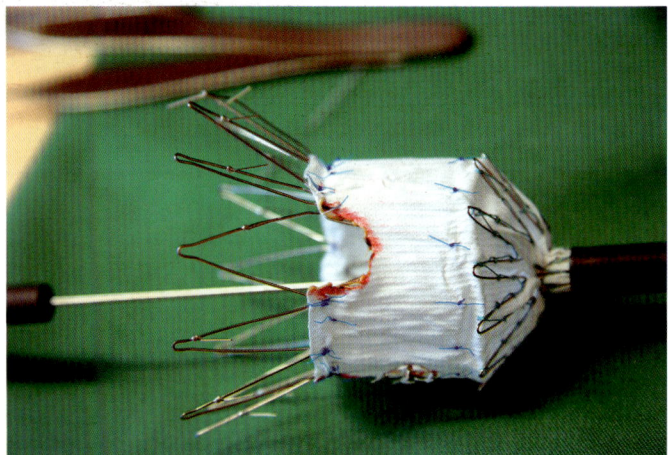

FIGURE 4: Scallop created with low power diathermy. The supra-renal stent strut has been moved and re-sutured to the Dacron.

Zenith fenestrated stent-graft. It is wise to adhere to the principles and sizes of standard stent-graft fenestrations and not to create other sizes.[17] In brief, small fenestrations have a diameter of 6-8 mm and are located at a minimum of 15 mm distal to the top of the fabric. The small fenestrations are placed between stent struts to allow unimpeded access to the target vessel. If a stent strut crosses the intended site of fenestration it is possible to move the strut (Figure 5). This is done by bending adjacent struts closer together or wider apart as necessary to clear the fenestration. Small fenestrations are designed to be stented to resist longitudinal and rotational migration and maintain alignment between the stent-graft and target vessel. Scallop fenestrations are hemi-oval, 6-10 mm in height and 8-12 mm in diameter and are located on the proximal portion of the graft. Large fenestrations cannot be stented due to the presence of stent struts traversing the fenestration. They are designed to be much larger than the target vessel.

Small fenestrations are generally used for the renal arteries and scallops for the SMA or sometimes the coeliac axis. Large

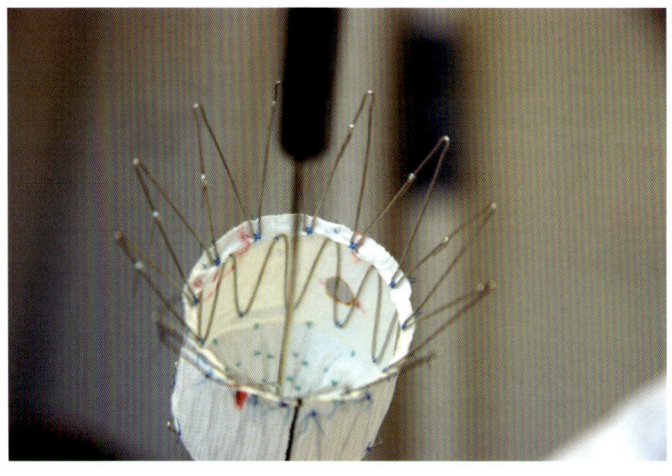

FIGURE 5: Renal fenestration. Note stent strut traversing fenestration. The strut was moved to the side of the fenestration by bending adjacent struts.

fenestrations are rarely used, but can be used to accommodate the visceral vessels.

The fenestrations are identified with radiopaque (gold) marker beads (Accellent, Wilmington, MA, USA). The gold markers are sutured close to, but not on the edge of the fabric using a CV-6 monofilament non-absorbable suture (PTFE, Gore, Flagstaff, AZ, USA) (Figure 6). Alternatively, if gold markers are not available, the four markers from the graft on the proximal edge of the Zenith graft may be removed and re-sutured to identify one of the fenestrations. The circular fenestrations are marked with four beads, one in each quadrant, whilst scallops are marked with three. It is actually and advantage to remove the markers from the proximal Zenith graft. They do not identify any useful point during fenestrated EVAR and are a potential source of confusion. If gold markers are not available it is possible to use a guidewire as a marker. First, remove the core from a 0.014" guidewire. Remove the outer wire and suture it to the circumference of the fenestration or scallop with CV-6 suture to act as a marker. Fluoroscopy of the stent-graft *ex-vivo* confirms the position and identification of the markers. The stent-graft must be placed accurately *in vivo*.

Once the fenestrations have been created the stent-graft can be re-loaded in to the delivery system. The supra-renal stent is re-captured in the top cap by using a cotton (umbilical) tape surrounding the struts and pulled together. The stent is pulled carefully back in to the top cap and the metal inner cannula replaced in its original position. The safety trigger wire is then repositioned in the top cap.

The covered stents are now withdrawn in to the delivery system. Each stent is sequentially and concentrically collapsed using umbilical tapes. Care should be taken not to compress adjacent stents into one another.

When re-loading the covered stents, it is vital to ensure correct alignment. It is possible to twist the stent-graft. It is crucial to check alignment of the multiple markers at the joints of the Z stents (leading down to the contralateral iliac limb stump) with fluoroscopy before the stent-graft is inserted in to the patient. Failure to do so may result in incorrect fenestration or contralateral stump alignment.

THE PROCEDURE

The procedure should be performed in an

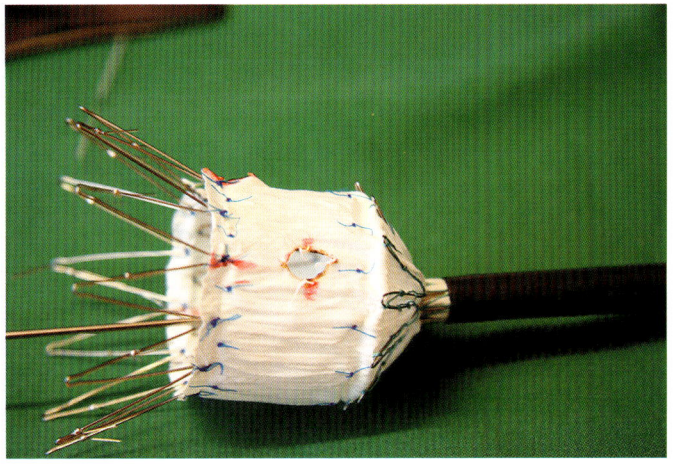

FIGURE 6: Gold markers sutured in four quadrants adjacent to fenestration.

operating theatre or interventional suite with high resolution imaging. The type of anaesthesia should remain at local discretion. We prefer general anaesthesia due to the length of the procedure and the frequent number of breath holds required with repeat angiography.

We perform the procedure percutaneously using the pre-close technique which has been described elsewhere.[18] The patient is systemically heparinised (100 units/kg). Activated clotting times are maintained at greater than 300 secs with additional doses of heparin. A 4 Fr universal flush catheter is introduced percutaneously from the contra-lateral (opposite to the side used for introduction of the main delivery system) common femoral artery and placed in the visceral aorta to perform intraoperative angiography. The main delivery system is advanced in to the aorta over an extra stiff guidewire (Lunderquivst, Cook Europe, Bjaereskov, Denmark) to the level of the renal arteries. A 20Fr sheath (Check-Flo, Cook Europe, Bjaereskov, Denmark) is inserted through the contralateral common femoral artery to allow the introduction of multiple sheaths and catheters. Angiogra-

phy is performed through the 4 Fr universal flush catheter to ensure the stent-graft is in the correct position. The outer sheath of the delivery system is withdrawn until the contra-lateral iliac stump (short leg) is deployed. Small degrees of rotational and longitudinal movements are possible to align the stent-graft fenestrations with their target vessels (Figure 7).

Access to the lumen of the main body of the graft is through cannulation of the short contralateral leg in the standard fashion. The target vessels (renal arteries in most cases) are catheterised using a C2 cobra (Cordis) or another suitable catheter and a 0.035" glidewire (Terumo Corporation, Tokyo, Japan). The glidewire is exchanged for an Amplatz wire and guiding catheters are used to introduce the stent-grafts in to the renal arteries.

If there is contact between the stent-graft and the target vessel ostium then a simple balloon expandable stent can be used. In most cases we use balloon expandable stent-grafts to minimise the chances of leak between the aortic stent-graft and the fenestration.

The JoStent (Abbott Vascular Devices,

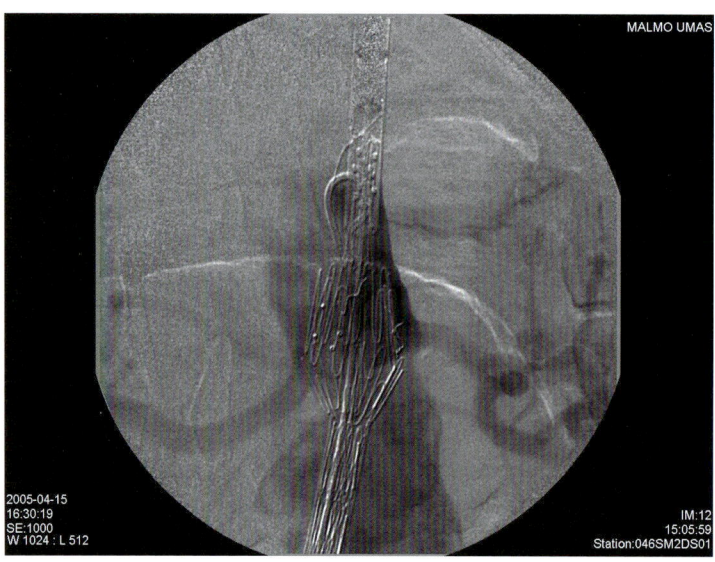

FIGURE 7: Introduction of fenestrated stent-graft and alignment of fenestrations with renal arteries and scallops with SMA.

Redwood City, Calif, USA) flares well but is not pre-mounted. The Atrium (Atrium Medical Corp, Hudson, NH, USA) is pre-mounted but tends to rebound more than the JoStent and flare less well. The size of the stents is usually in the region of 7-9 mm in diameter and 15-30 mm in length.

The balloon expandable stents are deployed. The aortic portion of the stent is flared with a 10 mm angioplasty balloon. Balloon expandable stents with larger cell sizes flare better than those with small cell designs. A semi-compliant latex balloon (Coda, Cook Europe, Bjaereskov, Denmark) is then inflated to ensure seal between the renal stent-graft and the main body of the aortic stent-graft.

The uncovered supra-renal stent is then deployed. The top cap trigger wire is removed and the top cap pushed off to release the stent. The distal trigger wire is removed to fully release the main body of the stent-graft. The ipsilateral and contra-lateral iliac limbs are inserted and deployed down to both common iliac artery bifurcations. Care should be taken when inserting the iliac limbs not to disturb the renal stent-grafts. Balloon moulding of the stent-graft is performed in the seal zones using the Coda balloon.

A completion angiogram is performed and if the aneurysm is satisfactorily excluded, the heparin is reversed with protamine sulphate, the delivery systems are removed and the groins closed with pre-close sutures (Figure 8 and Figure 9).

EARLY CLINICAL RESULTS

In Malmo, 18 patients (14 male) have been treated with home-made fenestrated stent-grafts October 2000-May 2006. Nine of these patients were either symptomatic (n = 8) or ruptured (n = 1). Median age of patients was 72 (inter-quartile range 68-78) years. The ASA distribution was grade II (n = 4); III (n = 9); IV (n = 5).

The median aneurysm diameter of treated patients was 65 (IQR 59-76) mm. A total of 37 target vessels were accommodated with either scallops or fenestrations (median of two per patient).

Five target vessels out of a total of 37 were lost intra-operatively. Two patients suffered bilateral renal artery occlusion.

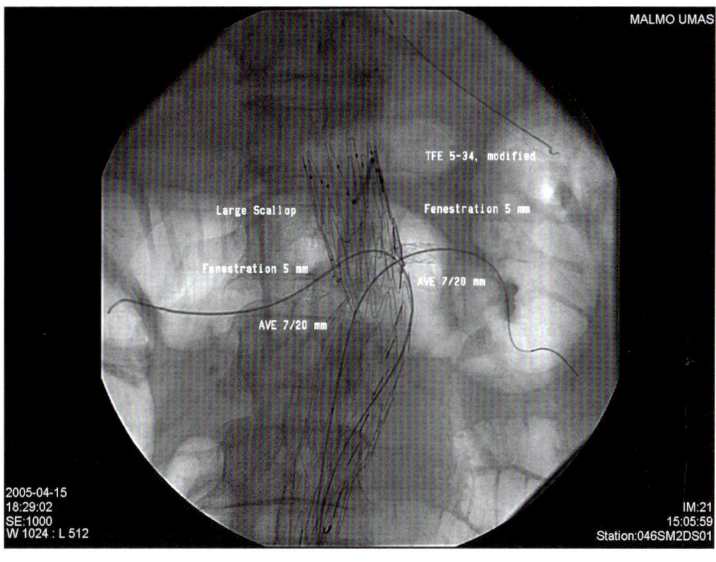

FIGURE 8: Fully deployed stent-graft (native).

MALMO UMAS **FIGURE 9:** Completion angiography.

One of these underwent immediate conversion to open repair. The other patient with bilateral renal artery occlusion had a ruptured AAA and was not converted to open repair. He survived two months post-operatively on dialysis. He died from uraemia and multiple organ failure.

A total of two patients died peri-operatively. One of these patients had a symptomatic AAA.

During a median follow-up of 24 (3-46) months there was one aneurysm related death (as described above). One patient developed renal artery stenosis which was treated successfully with a balloon expandable stent. Three patients developed type 2 endoleaks. One of these patients also developed a distal type 1 endoleak. Two of these three patients had expanding aneurysm sacs and underwent endovascular correction.

This model does not incorporate diameter reducing restraint ties. These are present on the industry made stent-graft. The feature limits the initial expansion of the stent-graft and facilitates longitudinal and rotational movement prior to target vessel catheterisation. Movement of the stent-graft can be difficult in vivo without partial constraint, especially in patients with tortuous vessels. Manipulation of a fully expanded stent-graft also increases the risk of embolisation. We have created a diameter reducing restraint tie using a 0.018" guidewire passed along the length of the delivery system and 2/0 prolene suture loops. This has been used successfully on the bench and in one patient. However, we have abandoned the technique because it is very time consuming and technically difficult. The stent-graft requires complete deployment from the delivery system. We have found there is a significant risk of twisting of the device on re-loading. We do not believe the potential advantages outweigh these significant difficulties.

FUTURE PROSPECTS/ REQUIREMENTS

Fenestrated stent-grafts are technically challenging and are lengthy procedures. Excessive endovascular manipulation potentially contributes to the morbidity and mortality of the procedure.

One potential method to reduce this problem is to pre-load wires through the fenestrations. In this way only the target vessel (and not the fenestration) require catheterisation. Employing this technique would significantly reduce catheterisation times.

Improved fenestrated technology is required to accommodate more than one patient's aneurysm morphology. Having a small number of fenestrated grafts available on the shelf to fit a large number of patients would allow endovascular specialists to treat more patients with acute aneurysms.

CONCLUSIONS

A significant proportion of patients with AAA present as an emergency and have adverse morphological features, particularly of the length of the proximal neck. Large symptomatic or ruptured AAA are more likely to have adverse features of the proximal neck. Both these features substantially increase the risks associated with open repair. They cannot be managed with standard infra-renal aortic stent-grafts.

Fenestrated stent-graft technology has evolved to offer a realistic alternative to open repair. However, custom manufacture by industry limits the availability of the fenestrated stent-grafts to elective surgery.

The surgeon performed custom fenestration technique described here is an alternative to open repair. The technique requires considerable endovascular experience, excellent imaging and a good working knowledge of the Zenith endovascular stent-graft system. The technique should be reserved for patients who are clinically and morphologically suitable for standard fenestrated stent-graft repair where time does not permit commercial manufacture.

Early experiences with the technique are encouraging. A number of issues need to be addressed regarding the relability, liability and durability of the customised stent-grafts.

INVENTORY

A number of items are required in addition to those used for standard infra-renal and fenestrated endovascular aneurysm repair.
- Rule/tape measure.
- Clock dial template.
- Waterproof marking pen.
- Low-power ophthalmic cautery (Medtronic Xomed, Jackonsville, FL).
- Umbilical (cotton) tapes.
- Artery forceps (Halstead).
- Standard forceps/needle holders.
- Wire cutters/benders.
- Gold marker beads (Accellent, Wilmington, MA).
- CV-6 sutures (PTFE, Gore, Flagstaff, AZ, USA).

KEY POINTS IN PATIENT SELECTION, MANUFACTURE AND DEPLOYMENT OF HOME-MADE FENESTRATED EVAR

- Excellent pre-operative CT imaging and reconstruction.
- Morphological criteria as for standard fenestrated EVAR.
- Angulated necks and small target vessels increase technical difficulty.
- Carefully measure distances on the Dacron fabric.
- Dacron is flammable (care during creation of fenestrations/scallops).
- Remove the proximal gold markers from the stent-graft to avoid confusion with the fenestrations/scallop during fluoroscopy.
- Avoid twisting the stent-graft on re-loading.
- Check stent-graft under fluoroscopy ex-vivo before insertion.
- Excellent intra-operative imaging with road-map/fluoro-fade facilities.

- No diameter reducing ties are available so ensure good alignment before withdrawing the sheath.

REFERENCES

1. Blankensteijn JD, de Jong SE, Prinssen M, van der Ham AC, Buth J, van Sterkenburg SM, Verhagen HJ, Buskens E, Grobbee DE; Dutch Randomized Endovascular Aneurysm Management (DREAM) Trial Group. Two-year outcomes after conventional or endovascular repair of abdominal aortic aneurysms. N Engl J Med. 2005;352:2398-405.

2. EVAR trial participants. Endovascular aneurysm repair versus open repair in patients with abdominal aortic aneurysm (EVAR trial 1): randomised controlled trial. Lancet. 2005;365:2179-86

3. Armon MP, Yusuf SW, Latief K, Whitaker SC, Gregson RH, Wenham PW, Hopkinson BR. Anatomical suitability of abdominal aortic aneurysms for endovascular repair. Br J Surg. 1997;84:178-80.

4. Dias NV, Ivancev K, Malina M, Resch T, Lindblad B, Sonesson B. Does the wide application of endovascular AAA repair affect the results of open surgery? Eur J Vasc Endovasc Surg. 2003;26:188-94.

5. Ockert S, Schumacher H, Bockler D, Malcherek K, Hansmann J, Allenberg J. Comparative early and midterm results of open juxtarenal and infrarenal aneurysm repair. Langenbecks Arch Surg. 2007 Jan 23; [Epub ahead of print]

6. Park JH, Chung JW, Choo IW, Kim SJ, Lee JY, Han MC. Fenestrated stent-grafts for preserving visceral arterial branches in the treatment of abdominal aortic aneurysms: preliminary experience. J Vasc Interv Radiol. 1996;7:819-23

7. Faruqi RM, Chuter TA, Reilly LM, Sawhney R, Wall S, Canto C, Messina LM. Endovascular repair of abdominal aortic aneurysm using a pararenal fenestrated stent-graft. J Endovasc Surg. 1999;6:354-8.

8. Magee TR, Galland RB, Collin J, McPherson GA, Orr MM, Ratliff DA, Rutter P, McWhinnie DL. A prospective survey of patients presenting with abdominal aortic aneurysm. Eur J Vasc Endovasc Surg. 1997;13:403-6.

9. Hinchliffe RJ, Alric P, Rose D, Owen V, Davidson IR, Armon MP, Hopkinson BR. Comparison of morphologic features of intact and ruptured aneurysms of infrarenal abdominal aorta. J Vasc Surg. 2003;38:88-92.

10. Leo E, Biancari F, Kechagias A, Ylonen K, Rainio P, Romsi P, Juvonen T. Outcome after emergency repair of symptomatic, unruptured abdominal aortic aneurysm: results in 42 patients and review of the literature. Scand Cardiovasc J. 2005;39:91-5.

11. Sun Z, Mwipatayi BP, Semmens JB, Lawrence-Brown MM. Short to midterm outcomes of fenestrated endovascular grafts in the treatment of abdominal aortic aneurysms: a systematic review. J Endovasc Ther. 2006;13:747-53.

12. Alric P, Hinchliffe RJ, Wenham PW, Whitaker SC, Chuter TA, Hopkinson BR. Lessons learned from the long-term follow-up of a first-generation aortic stent graft. J Vasc Surg. 2003;37:367-73.

13. Yusuf SW, Whitaker SC, Chuter TA, Ivancev K, Baker DM, Gregson RH, Tennant WG, Wenham PW, Hopkinson BR. Early results of endovascular aortic aneurysm surgery with aortouniiliac graft, contralateral iliac occlusion, and femorofemoral bypass. J Vasc Surg. 1997;25:165-72.

14. Ivancev K, Malina M, Lindblad B, Chuter TA, Brunkwall J, Lindh M, Nyman U, Risberg B. Abdominal aortic aneurysms: experience with the Ivancev-Malmo endovascular system for aortomonoiliac stent-grafts. J Endovasc Surg. 1997;4: 242-51.

15. Uflacker R, Robison JD, Schonholz C, Ivancev K. Clinical experience with a customized fenestrated endograft for juxtarenal abdominal aortic aneurysm repair. J Vasc Interv Radiol. 2006;17:1935-42.

16. Semmens JB, Lawrence-Brown MM, Hartley DE, Allen YB, Green R, Nadkarni S. Outcomes of fenestrated endografts in the treatment of abdominal aortic aneurysm in Western Australia (1997-2004). J Endovasc Ther. 2006;13:320-9.

17. Greenberg RK, Haulon S, O'Neill S, Lyden S, Ouriel K. Primary endovascular repair of juxtarenal aneurysms with fenestrated endovascular grafting. Eur J Vasc Endovasc Surg. 2004;27: 484-91.

18. Borner G, Ivancev K, Sonesson B, Lindblad B, Griffin D, Malina M. Percutaneous AAA repair: is it safe? J Endovasc Ther. 2004;11:621-6.

Chimney grafts. A promising but still unproven technology

Martin Malina, Tomas Ohrlander, Björn Sonesson

BACKGROUND

The applicability of endovascular stent grafts is often limited by the presence of vital aortic side branches originating from the potential landing site for a conventional stent graft. Fenestrated stent grafts have been developed for this group of patients but require customized devices for each patient. This makes the fenestrated stent graft unsuitable for urgent cases. Furthermore, tortuous vessel morphology may jeopardize safe deployment of a fenestrated stent graft. Several investigators have, therefore, investigated the applicability of a novel technology commonly referred to as the chimney graft (CG) or snorkelling graft. The chimney graft consists of a covered stent that is placed parallel to the proximal portion of the aortic stent graft in order to ensure blood supply to an over-stented aortic side branch (Figure 1). The CG technology has been successfully applied to one or both renal arteries, the SMA and all the branches of the aortic arch.

TECHNICAL ASPECTS

The side branch that originates from the potential landing site of an aortic stent graft is cannulated. The renal arteries, the SMA, the brachiocephalic trunk and the left subclavian artery are cannulated from a brachial puncture while the left common carotid artery is cannulated from a carotid cut down. A covered stent is parked in appropriate position within the side branch. The side branch is then over-stented with a standard aortic stent graft. After the aortic stent graft has been deployed, the side branch is reconstituted by expanding the covered stent. It is important to allow the covered stent to protrude proximally beyond the proximal end of the aortic stent graft. Simultaneous inflation of compliant balloons both within the aortic stent graft and the CG allows moulding of the aortic stent graft around the CG in order to minimize the so called gutters running alongside the covered stent. This may minimize the risk for a proximal type I endoleak.

Both self expanding and balloon expandable covered stents may be used for CG. The balloon expandable stent has the advantage of greater radial force but it may kink and seems too rigid in some settings.

INDICATIONS

We have applied the CG technology successfully in urgent repair of juxta renal aortic aneurysms and also for those lesions of the thoracic aorta that reach

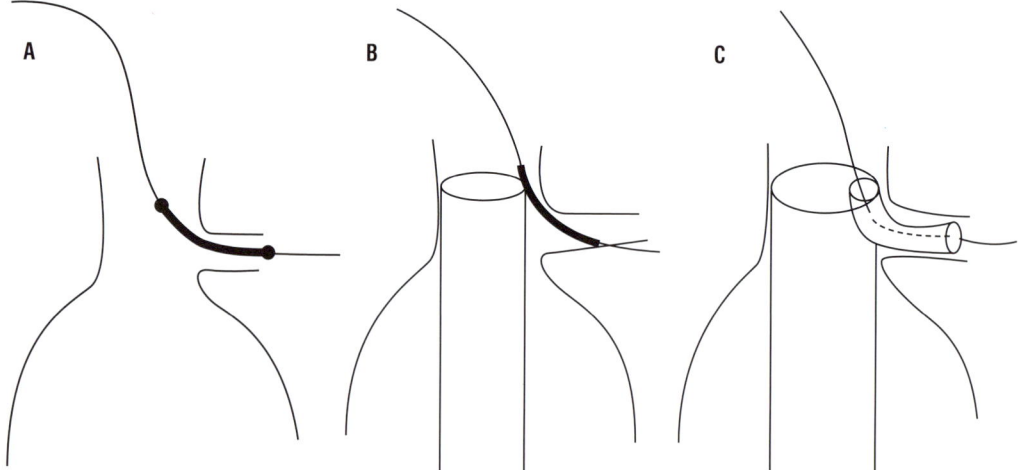

FIGURE 1: Placing a CG: **A.** A vital aortic side branch originating from the aneurysmal neck is catheterized and a covered stent is parked in position. **B.** A standard aortic stent graft is deployed across the side branch. **C.** The side branch is reconstituted by expanding the covered stent.

close to the branches of the aortic arch (Figure 2).

The implantation technique is somewhat modified when the CG is applied to salvage a vital aortic side branch that has been accidentally over-stented during EVAR. This has been particularly helpful for the over-stented SMA and left common carotid artery. The over-stented SMA cannot be cannulated from the aorta and in this setting, regrade cannulation of the SMA via laparotomy has been performed.

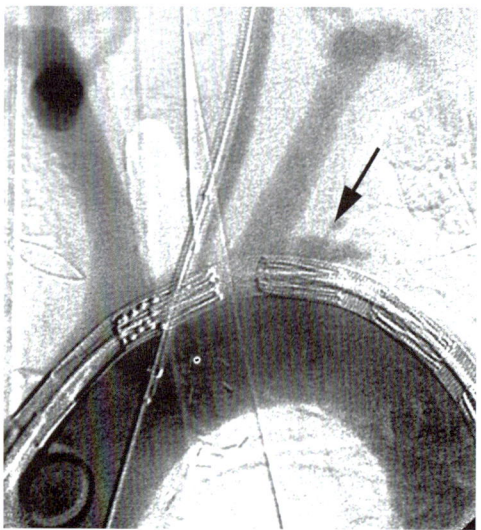
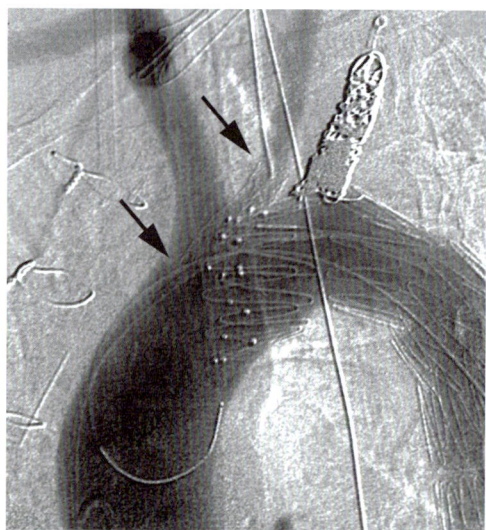

FIGURE 2: A. Road traffic accident with aortic rupture at the level of the left common carotid and subclavian arteries (*arrow*). **B.** The rupture was successfully sealed with a standard thoracic stent graft and a carotid CG (*between arrows*) combined with coil embolisation of the left subclavian artery.

In a series of 12 patients with one or multiple CGs there has only been one proximal type-I endoleak associated with the CG. The endoleak occurred in a patient with a CG in the brachiocephalic trunk. This was the largest diameter CG used by us. Consequently, the gutters alongside the chimney graft were large and probably contributed to the fact that the proximal seal was inadequate. The leak was successfully sealed with coils. No proximal type I endoleak has occurred in the remaining cases. It should, however, be emphasized that the overall experience remains limited with a short follow-up and the durability of this type of repair remains to be proven.

Summary

The CG technique is promising for a challenging group of patients, namely the ones that have an urgent large aneurysm without an adequate neck for fixation of a standard stent graft and without enough time to manufacture a customized fenestrated device. This group of patients is also challenging for open repair and remains associated with significant morbidity and mortality. The chimney graft technique allows instant endovascular exclusion of such lesions with commercially available off-the-shelf devices. The chimney graft technique has also proven helpful for bail-out in situations when a vital aortic side branch has been accidentally covered during EVAR.

Reference

1. Greenberg R. K, Clair D, Srivastava S, et al: Should patients with challenging anatomy be offered endovascular aneurysm repair? J Vasc Surg. 2003 Nov; 38(5):990-6.
2. Criado FJ.: A percutaneous technique for preservation of arch branch patency during thoracic endovascular aortic repair (TEVAR): retrograde catheterization and stenting. J Endovasc Ther. 2007 Feb; 14(1):54-8.
3. Larzon T, Gruber G, Friberg O, et al: Experiences of Intentional Carotid Stenting in Endovascular Repair of Aortic Arch Aneurysms- Two Case Reports. Eur J Vasc Endovasc Surg. 2005;(30):147-151.
4. Hiramoto JS, Schneider DB, Reilly LM, et al: A Double Barrel Stent-Graft for Endovascular Repair of the Aortic Arch. J Endovas Therapy 2006;(13): 72-76.
5. Malina M, Sonesson B, Dias N, et al: How to fashion a home made fenestrated stent graft. An option for urgent aneurysms with an inadequate neck. Controversies and updates in Vascular surgery 2007: 143-48.

Complications following aortic endograft procedures, with particular reference to the post-implantation syndrome

Vasilios D. Tzilalis, Theodossios P. Perdikides,
Miltos K. Lazarides, Geoffrey H. White

INTRODUCTION

Endovascular treatment of abdominal aortic aneurysms (AAA) is now well- established as an indicated procedure in a large proportion of AAA cases, even though it may be a technically demanding procedure. In many centres, the endoluminal repair technique replaces conventional surgical repair for the majority of AAA in high risk patients. Endovascular procedures must be initiated by a preoperative assessment of the patient, followed by study of the CT imaging, selection of the proper graft, and endovascular repair. Meticulous clinical assessment of a vascular patient requires screening of cardiac, renal, and pulmonary function, as in open aortic surgery. Despite these assessments, various systemic complications still occur, and some of the most interesting are those that appear to be related to Systemic Inflammatory Response Syndrome (SIRS). The development of the current FDA-approved devices and research to develop new devices, as well as improved selection of the proper device for each patient, have diminished the incidence of technical complications

such as graft-related endoleak, type II endoleak, migration, kinking, occlusion and rupture. These technical complications and other medical complications are analysed in different chapters of this book. In this chapter, the role of the inflammatory process (and particularly its extreme form SIRS) is analysed and emphasized as a potential trigger for medical complications.

COMPLICATIONS AND THEIR MANAGEMENT

Complications have been classified as *remote or systemic* and local or vascular by the Ad Hoc Committee of the Joint Societies of Vascular Surgery and North American Chapter of the International Society for Cardiovascular Surgery for uniform reporting standards.[1,2] The remote/systemic complications after endoluminal AAA repair do not vary greatly from those following open aneurysm repair and are not covered further here. The *local/vascular* complications, however, are important, as many of them are specific to the endoluminal method of aneurysm repair. A general classification of these complications, based on their occurrence as either early or late events, is presented in Table 1.[3] The more important of these are considered in detail below.

INJURIES TO ACCESS ARTERIES

It is not surprising that the passage of comparatively large-bore access sheaths through tortuous and diseased femoral and iliac arteries may result in dissection or rupture. It is important to recognize that such problems may become apparent not only during the introduction of the various guidewires and catheters, but also following withdrawal of the delivery sheath. If iliac rupture occurs, the onset of bleeding will often be delayed by the tamponading effect of the sheath. Although later generation prostheses are capable of being introduced through iliac arteries with a considerable degree of tortuosity, the presence of heavy circumferential calcification considerably increases the risk of ruptur-

TABLE 1A

COMPLICATIONS FOLLOWING AORTIC ENDOGRAFTING: (A) EARLY AND (B) LATE, MEDICAL (M), TECHNICAL (T) AND SYSTEMIC (S)

(A) EARLY	
Trauma to access arteries	(T)
Trauma to aorta (stiff wires, catheters)	(T)
Microembolization	(T, M)
(Dislodgment of mural components or thrombus from the sac or the vessel wall)	
To: aortic arch orifices (manipulation of stiff wires): stroke	
visceral arteries: colonic ischemia, renal impairment	
lumbar / Adamkievitz: spinal cord ischemia (for AAA: rare as in open 0.25%)[19]	
peripheral arteries: trash foot	
Graft displacement or misplacement	(T)
Graft limb compression / stenosis / occlusion	(T)
Occlusion of major branch arteries	(T)
Hypogastric artery/arteries: buttock claudication/necrosis, colonic ischemia	
Inferior mesenteric (always): colonic ischemia	
Main or accessory renal arteries: renal insufficiency	
Endoleak	(T)
AAA rupture	(T)
Groin inscision complications (hematoma, lymphocele)	(T)
Coagulation trauma [84,85]	(M, S)
Post-Implantation syndrome	(M, S)
Myocardial infraction	(M, S)
Contrast allergy/nephropathy/ lactic acidosis (metformin)	(M, S)
Radiation Injury (long period of fluoroscopy attempting fenestrated grafts)	(M,S)
Hypertension[15] (thoracic endografting in young patients after thoracic aortic disruption)	(M,S)

TABLE 1B

COMPLICATIONS FOLLOWING AORTIC ENDOGRAFTING: (A) EARLY AND (B) LATE, MEDICAL (M), TECHNICAL (T) AND SYSTEMIC (S)

(B) LATE	
Graft migration	(T)
Endoleak	(T)
Endotension (thrombosis or lytic process into the sac, gelatinous condition, shear stess)	(M,T)
Late stenosis / kink / thrombosis of the graft or graft limb	(T)
Graft tear or failure / Material fatigue / stent or wire form breakage	(T)
AAA rupture	(T)
Graft Infection	(T, M, S)

ing the artery. When this complication is suspected, it is important to maintain guidewire access, so that immediate endovascular management can be achieved by deployment of iliac extension grafts. If necessary, bleeding can be controlled by inflation of an angioplasty balloon more proximal in the iliac system, while the extension graft is being prepared, or while open repair is done.

If it is not technically possible to correct an iliac dissection or rupture by endovascular means, we recommend placing a prosthetic surgical bypass graft from the common iliac artery to the common femoral artery via an extraperitoneal approach. This allows simultaneous revascularization of the affected limb and ensures access to the common iliac artery for delivery of the endovascular device into the aneurysm.

Suprarenal arteries are also vulnerable to injury when the brachial route is used to complement access of the AAA. The seemingly harmless passage of a guide wire from the brachial artery down the descending thoracic aorta may result in substantial intraperitoneal bleeding if it passes inadvertently and unnoticed into the superior mesenteric artery and ruptures one of the terminal branches of this artery.

EMBOLIZATION

Manipulation of endovascular devices within the sac of an AAA has resulted in widespread microembolization and death from renal failure.[4] Every effort should be made to reduce the catheter introduction process to one pass in which the prosthesis is delivered to the level of the renal arteries. The movement of all component parts of the catheter from this point should be in the direction of withdrawal, not advancement, to minimize the risk of thrombus dislodgment.

Embolic stroke can occur due to guidewire movements within the aortic arch. To avoid this complication, the position of the top end of the various guidewires should be monitored by fluoroscopic imaging, and kept out of the arch. The straighter descending aorta is a safer place for the guidewire, but debris may still be displaced causing renal, splenic or bowel infarcts.

Distal embolization resulting in leg ischemia is also a recognized complication. There may be a greater risk of significant limb embolization when endografts are deployed into diseased aortic necks which have regions of eccentric mural thrombus or irregular atheroma. When the endoluminal method is used in patients with these features, it is recommended to clamp both common femoral arteries to capture any released emboli which may otherwise travel to the leg arteries.

ENDOLEAK

Angiography is always performed at the completion of device deployment, to confirm wide patency of the graft and to exclude endoleak, incomplete sealing or exclusion of the aneurysm sac by the endograft.[5-9] Digital subtraction cine-angiography is done antegradely at the level of the renal arteries, and also by retrograde injection at the distal ends of the iliac limbs, looking for any sign of peri-graft leakage. Type II endoleaks due to retrograde flow into the AAA sac from patent lumbar arteries do not require active treatment; most of these will close spontaneously over the next 1-3 months.[8] Type I and type III endoleaks, however, should be treated immediately by either balloon dilatation of the involved graft component, endograft extension pieces or supportive stent, or by combinations of these techniques.[8-10] Every attempt should be made to close such endoleaks before the patient leaves the operating room, since the AAA remains at risk of rupture until sealed.

If endoleaks cannot be successfully sealed at the time of the procedure, we do not recommend proceeding to open repair at the same time, since the patient has already undergone a prolonged operation, often with high contrast load and other factors that increase peri-operative morbidity and mortality rates.

GRAFT LIMB STENOSIS OR THROMBOSIS

Narrowing of the iliac limb grafts may occur due to external compression, kinking within angulated iliac segments or graft twist. Such narrowing predisposes to early or late occlusion. Early generation endografts with unsupported fabric were prone to thrombosis of the limbs of the graft due to kinking and twisting within the native iliac arteries. Even with later prostheses, in which the fabric is supported by a metallic frame, the problem persists. Postprocedure on table angiography in one plane is no guarantee that kinking has not occurred. When graft limb stenosis is suspected, pressure measurements should be obtained by connecting a pressure line to the femoral sheath on that side, with comparison of the pressure to the radial line parameters. A pressure differential of more than 10-20 mm Hg should prompt management by adjunctive balloon dilatation, with or without stent implantation. Plain x-ray studies in anteroposterior and lateral planes in the immediate postoperative period are recommended to identify a problem in the metal frame before thrombosis occurs and while correction may be carried out by endovascular rather than open means.

Successful endoluminal repair often results in reduction in the size of the aneurysm sac in both length and transverse diameter. This may lead to kinking of the previously straight limbs of an endoluminal graft, with progression to thrombosis. Such kinking may also encourage or result in dislocation of the limbs of endograft from the native iliac arteries or the contralateral limb from the contralateral stump of the endograft. Fortunately, kinks in the iliac arteries and within the aneurysm sac are amenable to endovascular correction, thus avoiding open operation.

CONVERSION TO OPEN REPAIR

Acute conversion to open repair may be required if aortic rupture occurs during the implantation procedure.[11] In this situation, blood loss may be reduced by inflation of an occlusion balloon at or above the level of the renal arteries. In some situations, continuation with the endovascular technique may be a reasonable method to achieve sealing. As described above, immediate conversion to open repair is not recommended for management of endoleak. This is best done as a separate procedure with the patient and operating team fully prepared.

POST IMPLANTATION SYNDROME

Post implantion syndrome is characterized by back pain, fever, leukocytosis and CRP elevation in the absence of any evidence of infection.[12] It follows implantation directly, generally lasts for 2-3 days but sometimes up to 7 days, and is usually associated with thrombosis within the aneurysm sac. The cause is unknown, and the incidence may be as high as 50%. Despite some early reports of an associated coagulopathy, the course of post implant syndrome is generally considered to be benign; indeed, some hold it to be a favorable sign signifying thrombosis of the aneurysm sac and successful endoluminal repair. Treatment is not often required, and for severe cases should be supportive, including anti-pyretic and/or anti-inflammatory medications. Further features of the post-implantation syndrome are discussed in more detail below.

INCIDENCE OF COMPLICATIONS

The major complications are death and conversion to open repair. There is evidence that the incidence of these and other serious complications is declining, but many of these still necessitate further interventions, usually by radiological means. A recent report from the EURO-STAR registry, covering 6787 patients in Europe that received a variety of endograft designs, indicated an annual incidence rate of conversion to open repair in 3% of the patients, with a range that varied from 5.4% for an early graft to 0.6% for a more modern design with the best performance.[13] Mortality occurred in 7% of the cases overall and the annual incidence rate for rupture was 0.5%. Improved results with more recent devices were also shown in a report based on research conducted by the Minnesota Evidence-Based Practice Center under the Agency for Healthcare Research and Quality: this study reported frequencies of 1.5% for 30-day mortality and 2% for Abdominal Aortic Aneurysm (AAA)-related mortality.[14] The overall incidence for AAA-related death was 3%, with an early (within 30-days) rupture rate of 0.2% and a delayed rupture rate of 0.5%. Finally, primary conversion to open repair was 2.2%, while the delayed conversion was 1.8%.

PHYSIOLOGICAL FACTORS MAY INFLUENCE THE INCIDENCE OF COMPLICATIONS

Some of the less understood factors that may influence complications include several natural physiological and systemic responses. For example, endograft implants in young thoracic aortas after blunt thoracic trauma can trigger mechanisms that result in severe hypertension.[15] Relatively rigid endografts affect the elastic properties of a young aorta through a mechanism that remains unknown. Recently, Volodos noted the adverse effect of arterial hypertension on the outcome of endovascular grafting of aortic aneurysms.[16] Another influence appears to be related to the body's inflammatory response mechanisms: A Post-Implantation syndrome (PI syndrome) is now well recognised, but its mechanisms remain unclear. Elucidation of the mechanisms leading to these complications and establishment of prevention and treatment strategies in the future will lower peri-procedure morbidity rates.

Regarding the effects of ASA classification, in a population of 167 patients undergoing EVAR, postoperative complication and 30-day morality rates did not significantly differ among the different ASA classifications.[17] Patients at high surgical risk (ASA class IV) benefit from AAA repair, except for patients with aneurysms less than 6 cm in diameter with risk of death at one year due to co-morbidities that are higher than the risk of rupture.[18] Spinal cord ischemia is equally rare following open aortic surgery or EVAR (1/400 and 0.21% respectively), which is evidenced in the EUROSTAR database.[19] Microembolism is the probable cause[19] and can be prevented or treated by maintenance of intra-operative pressure, systemic heparinization, and preservation of the pelvic circulation,[20] including surgical internal iliac artery revascularization (Figure 1). Drainage of the spinal cord may offer decompression and improve the artery flow reservoir.[21]

THE SYSTEMIC INFLAMMATORY RESPONSE SYNDROME

Systemic Inflammatory Response Syndrome (SIRS) represents a pathophysiological cascade that can occur after any major surgery. For vascular surgeons, it is particularly a concern with respect to either elective or emergency abdominal aortic aneurysm repair.[22] A "normal" initial inflammatory response is essential for the continued survival of the patient, but excessive activation of inflammatory cascades leads to SIRS. The line between a normal "physiologic" response and abnormal triggering of a cytokine burst should be drawn and correlated with clinical outcome, not only in vascular surgery, but in all major interventional specialties, including anesthesiology and interventional radiology.[23-33]

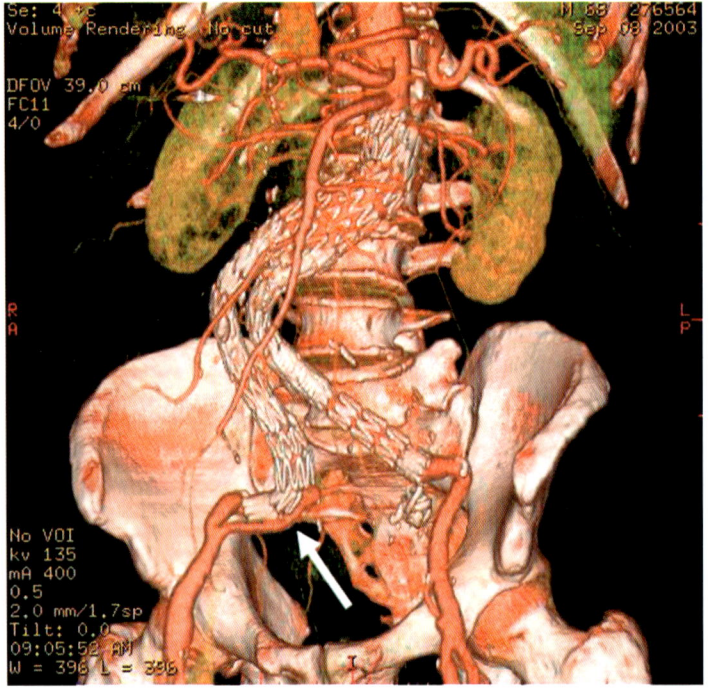

FIGURE 1: EVAR in a case of aneurysmal disease: of infrarenal aorta, both common iliac arteries and left internal iliac artery (that was preoperatively embolized). Since both internal iliac arteries had to be occluded, this patient unfortunately developed paraparesis postoperatively, that was resolved after a right external to internal iliac bypass (*white arrow*) was performed.

SIRS is known to occur after elective vascular surgery. There is evidence that the SIRS response is reduced by the application of endovascular techniques, although a few studies have suggested the opposite[34] or have proposed a different mechanism for inflammation.[35,36] Most of the studies support the idea that endografting correlates with a reduced inflammatory response, when compared to open surgery.[37-51] On the other hand, SIRS is undoubtedly a major threat to the outcome of repaired ruptured abdominal aortic aneurysms (AAA).[22] The endovascular alternative approach for ruptured AAA in critically ill patients will be indicated at experienced well equipped centers and will further decrease the frequency of SIRS development. SIRS incidence in conventional vascular surgery repair of elective, urgent, and ruptured AAA is 89%, 92% and 100%, respectively, as shown in a very recent study of 100 consecutive AAA.[22] There is strong evidence from the literature that the endovascular approach to the cardiovascular system limits postoperative systemic immune and inflammatory responses. This leads to a more favorable procedure with fewer complications and improved morbidity and mortality. In nine studies that compared the endovascular approach to open repair, the clinical parameters of PI syndrome, temperature, C-reactive protein (CRP), and leukocytes (WBC), were generally lower in the endovascular group, with differences that reached statistical significance in five articles (Table 2). In these studies, data taken from cytokine projects showed that the endoluminal approach was less aggressive. This has been reported in many previous studies of the inflammatory response after endoluminal AAA repair (eAAA).

EFFECTS OF ACUTE AORTIC CONDITIONS

The presence of an "Unstable Aneurysm",

sometimes also described as Acute Aortic Syndrome,[52] followed by specific, easy to obtain markers may allow for prompt recognition of insidious changes in the aneurysm sac and lead to timely algorithmic management. Factors such as AAA size, the amount of thrombus within the AAA sac, the presence of subacute dissection, or a penetrating ulcer in a severely diseased aorta may all be important. Difficulties may arise from the fact that aortic aneurysms are almost always "surrounded" by other sites of inflammation, such as carotid, femoral, or coronary artery plaques. C-reactive protein, Interleukin-6, fibrin D-dimer, and coagulation factors have been studied in coronary heart disease,[53] and are referenced in the definition of an unstable carotid plaque[54] and in endovascular procedures below the knee.[55] The secretion level of these markers also seems to correlate with the size of an aneurysm or its thrombus; for example it has been shown that the bigger an aneurysm or the amount of thrombus within it (dimensions expressed as surface area in different studies), is the more IL-6 is secreted into the circulation.[56] We formed a similar conclusion following a prospective study of PI syndrome following EVAR: the group with a larger amount of newly formed thrombus in the AAA sac after EVAR (surface area) frequently had evidence of inflammatory responses.[57]

THE POST-IMPLANTATION SYNDROME AFTER EVAR

The Post-Implantion (PI) syndrome is the clinical and biochemical expression of an inflammatory response that is commonly observed following endovascular aortic aneurysm repair.[40,46-48] It is characterized by fever, elevated C-reactive protein, and leukocytosis in the absence of an infectious agent.[46,47] After its first description, it was further characterised in a retrospective

Concomitant References of Cytokine Studies and Post-Implantation Syndrome (PI) or Any of Its 3 Characteristics as a Complication After Endovascular Intervention

Reference	Number of patients treated endoluminally/open				Clinical Markers			Inflammatory Markers			
	AAA	Peripheral	PI	SIRS	Temperature	CRP	WBC	TNF-a	IL-6	IL-8	Other
1997 Norgen, Swartbol[36]	7 endo 11 open			1 (14%)	Lower * day 1 Lower 2-5 days			+ -	Lower * P<0.005 +++		C1q, C3, C4 lower in endo group CD11b,c, lower * in open group
1997 Hayoz et al[42]		11	4 (36%)					-	+		Fibrinogen, C3,C4, ASAT, ALAT, IL-1β, CD4, CD8
1998 Syk et al[43]	23 endo 14 open				(Not significant)					89 pg/ml 249 pg/ml	Sigmoid colon pH
2000 Galle et al[41]	7 endo 5 open				Lower (P<.05)	Lower (P<.01)	Lower (P<.01)	higher Not signif	parallel parallel	higher Not signif	Monocl. Antibodies, sol. Adh Molecules, vWF, C3-4.
2000 Odegard et al[44]	10 endo 10 open				Mean 38.3°C Mean 38.3°C	max 123 mg/L P<0.01 max 196 mg/L	++ +	* P<0.001 max	max 2.4 ng/ml 3.7 ng/ml	134 pg/ml P<0.01 379 pg/ml	Complement, Platelets, fibrinogen, MPO
2000 Elmarasy et al[45]	9 endo 10 open				Mild + Mild + higher * between 4-12h			+ higher * 4-16h	+ higher * 3-23h		PCO2 gap sigmoid co mucosa

Reference	Number of patients treated endoluminally/open				Clinical Markers				Inflammatory Markers		
	AAA	Peripheral	PI	SIRS	Temparature	CRP	WBC	TNF-a	IL-6	IL-8	Other
2001 Parodi et al[37]	14 endo					333+/-102 **lower *** P<.005				+	IL-1RA fell quicker
	10 open					923+/-116 mg/L				+	Lower TGFb-1
2002 Sweeney et al[39]	8 endo			1 (12.5%)							IL-2, IL-10, CD25, CD69,CD62L Endo reduces T-cell activation
	12 open			4 (33%)							
2003 Decker et al[38]	8 endo 16 open						**Lower *** (P<.005)				IFN-γ, IL-4, HLA-DR, CD23
2006 Englberger[84]		15 endo					not signif different	Signif 1st day (P<0.05)			Fibrin monomers * and TAT complex* levels were higher in the EVAR group (P<.0001) FPA and d-dimmers not significantly different
		15 open									

* Significantly different

study that attempted to interpret its etiology.[48] Post-Implantation syndrome is accepted to be an immunological response to the implantation of an endovascular device and the manipulation of catheters and wires in large diseased vessels that receive iodine contrast in a patient that is also exposed to radiation. All of these aspects may have an influence on this inflammatory process. A major fundamental difference of endovascular surgery for aneurysms relative to conventional surgery is that the aneurysm sac and its components remain in the patient and are hopefully excluded from systemic circulation. The "hand grenade" has been secured, but formation of a new thrombus and changes within the old thrombus can trigger biological phenomena, such as PI syndrome.

According to the current definition of PI syndrome, temperature is elevated above 38°C, WBC is greater than 12.000 cells/L, and the CRP level is elevated. The absolute level of CRP elevation remains to be determined in a future study, but, in the case of PI, it is up to tenfold higher than the preoperative value. Temperature and WBC, as described above, are only two of several criteria required for the

identification of SIRS.[49] Fulfillment of at least two of these criteria defines SIRS. So, PI as it was defined by Blum et al,[46] could be regarded as a modified form of SIRS, or can be more precisely defined as SIRS following endovascular procedures or eSIRS (Figure 2).

In none of the prior reports, nor in our own clinical experience, did the occurrence of either PI syndrome embody the other more serious characteristics of SIRS, such as hypothermia, tachycardia, changes in $PaCO_2$, or respiratory rhythm alterations and leukopenia. The incidence of PI syndrome varies between 3-70.3% in various reports depending on the vessels involved, the number of patients studied, and the criteria used for definition of the PI. In the largest series of 1554 endovascular procedures for AAA, sepsis or prolonged fever was described in only 52 patients (Table 3), but, as in other similar studies, the focus remained on the major device-related complications and gave scant attention to these "minor" complications. The frequency of PI in thoracic endovascular procedures ranges from 36 to 75%, while in iliac and peripheral arteries, this value is about 55% and 4.5-36%, re-

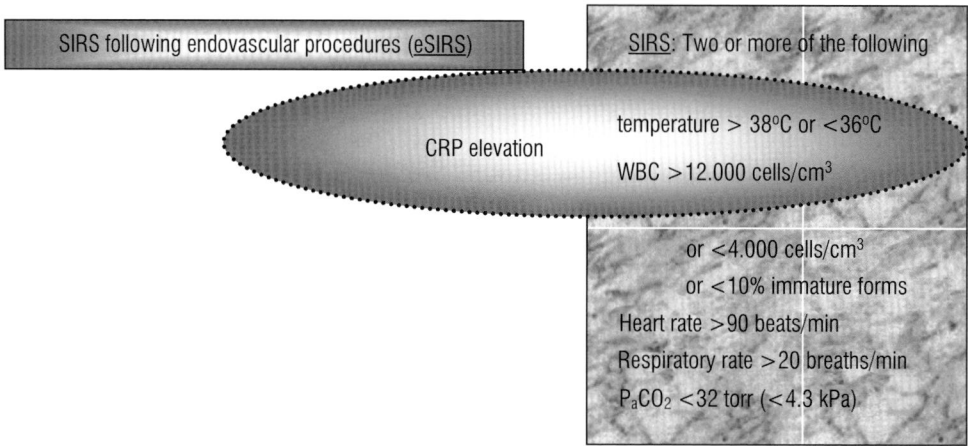

FIGURE 2: Definition of Systemic Inflammatory Response Syndrome (SIRS) and Post Implantation syndrome or SIRS following endovascular procedures (eSIRS).

TABLE 3 References of Post-Implantation Syndrome (PI) or Any of Its 3 Characteristics as a Complication After Endovascular Intervention in AAA, Thoracic Aorta, Iliac or Peripheral Arteries

Reference	Number of patients treated endoluminally						Number of patients (%)				
	Lab Study	AAA	Thoracic	Iliac	Peripheral lesions	PI	SIRS	Fever mild >38°	CRP	WBC	Sepsis
1987 Weibull et al[50]					127 (134 lesions)			6 (4.5%) mild fever, shivering			
1996 Moore et al[51]		46						3 (21%)			
1997 Blum et al[46]		154				87 (56%)		87 (56%)	87 (56%) 40-341 mg/L	87 (56%) 9800-29500/dl	
1997 Norgen, Swartbol[36]	Yes	7					1 (14%)	Sign. lower * day 1 but higher 2-5 days			
1997 Hayoz et al[42]	Yes				11	4 (36%)			+ 77.5 +/- 15 mg/L	– 7.2 +/- 0.9	
1997 Mialhe et al[58]		79						45 (57%)			
1998 Syk et al[43]	Yes	23						Not differ significantly to 14 open repair			
1998 Coppi et al[59]		60						60 (100%) 25 (42%)			
1998 Maynar et al[60]		11						8 (73%)			
1999 Gorich et al[61]		49				25 (45%)			25 (45%)	>10000/µL	

(continued)

TABLE 3 — References of Post-Implantation Syndrome (PI) or Any of Its 3 Characteristics as a Complication After Endovascular Intervention in AAA, Thoracic Aorta, Iliac or Peripheral Arteries (continued)

Reference	Number of patients treated endoluminally						Number of patients (%)				
	Lab Study	AAA	Thoracic	Iliac	Peripheral lesions	PI	SIRS	Fever mild >38°	CRP	WBC	Sepsis
1999 Nienaber et al[62]			12			9 (75%)		+ (max 148mg/L)	+	Mild + (11+ /-9 x 10^6/cm^3)	
1999 Velazquez et al[48]		12						2 (17%)	8 (67%)	7 (58%) >11000/dl	
1999 Ruchat et al[63]		5				3 (60%)					
2000 Buth et al[64]		1554						52 (3%) **sepsis, prolonged fever**			1
2000 Galle et al[41]	Yes	7						Temperature lower 7 Endo to 5 open **(P <.05)**	Lower compared to 5 open **(P <.01)**	Lower compared to 5 open **(P <.01)**	
2000 Scheinert et al[65]				20				11(55%) **mean 38.6°C**	13(65%) **mean 116 mg/L**	10 (50%) **14.6 x 10 9**	
2000 Guo et al[66]		6	4	1				5 (45.5%) prolonged fever			
2000 Henry et al[67]					48	4 (8%)					
2000 Odegard et al[44]	Yes	10						38.2-38.4°C	Max 123 mg/L	+	

Reference	Number of Patients treated endoluminally					Number of patients (%)					
	Lab Study	AAA	Thoracic	Iliac	Peripheral lesions	PI	SIRS	Fever mild >38°	CRP	WBC	Sepsis
2000 Elmarasy et al[45]	Yes	10						Mild +			
2001 Wolpert et al[68]				18				10 (56%) >101°F		+ 12.8 x 109/L (8.5-22.9)	
2001 Kato et al[33]			15			+					
2001 Won et al[69]			23			10 (43%)		+	+	+	
2001 Parodi et al[37]	Yes	14						3 (21%)	333+/-102 mg/L lower *than 10 open	7 (50%)	
2002 Sweeney et al[39]	YES	8					1 (12.5%)				
2002 Shim et al[70]			14			9 (64%)					1
2002 Espinoza et al[71]		134					8 (6%)	70.3% (37.6-38.9°C)			
2003 Decker et al[38]	Yes	8								Lower * compared to 16 open (P <.005)	
2003 Schoder et al[72]			28					10 (36%)	24 (92%)	10 (37%)	

*Lab study: Study that included cytokine project . * Significantly different*

spectively (Table 3). Not only does PI follow endovascular treatment of AAA, it occurs in all interventional specialties.[12]

ROLE OF C-REACTIVE PROTEIN IN THE POST-IMPLANTATION SYNDROME

One measurable factor and criterion for the determination of PI is C-reactive protein (CRP). This is an acute phase protein that has the potential to influence one or more inflammatory stages and has many pathophysiologic roles in the inflammatory process.[73] Measurement of the CRP level is a reliable, practical biological test, and is a consistent, specific marker of the acute inflammatory reaction. Most normal subjects have plasma CRP concentrations of 2 mg/L or less, but some individuals have concentrations as high as 10 mg/L. Slightly elevated concentrations of CRP, within the range of normal subjects, have been found to predict subsequent coronary events, often years later, in patients with angina and in healthy individuals.[74,75] The level of CRP correlates with endovascular disease and may serve to identify otherwise asymptomatic patients at cardiovascular risk sufficient to warrant aggressive therapy.[76] The CRP level increases rapidly, as early as 6 hours after an inflammatory trigger, reaches its peak in 1-2 days, and returns to baseline after 4 to 10 days.[73] This economical biological warning sign is the "vanguard and the rearguard" of even the subtlest disease as it assists in the observation of a patient's correlative situation, the intensity of inflammation, and the efficacy of treatment. Among 29 studies that describe, either accurately or incompletely, PI syndrome in endoluminal interventions (Table 2), only 10 refer to CRP. In these series, the percentage of participation varies from 56-92%, with CRP levels ranging from 40 to 435 mg/L.

CRP, as has been demonstrated in many studies, can serve as an indicator in the diagnosis of PI or eSIRS in patients following endovascular procedures.

ROLE OF CYTOKINES

Cytokines play a crucial role in the inflammatory response and PI. Cytokines are components of a large, complex signaling network that can broadly be classified as growth factors, chemotactic factors or chemokines (IL-4, IL-8), modulators of lymphocyte function (IL-2, IL-4), and modulators of the inflammatory response (IL-1β, TNF-α, IL-6). The internal balance is maintained by recently discovered naturally occurring soluble receptors for TNF-α (sTNFr1, sTNFr2), the competitive antagonist for IL-1 (IL-1ra), and the anti-inflammatory cytokines IL-10, IL-4, IL-13.[77-79] Despite their incontestable role in PI, their clinical significance is outshined by the fact that cytokine investigation is expensive and infrequently performed in clinical settings. Rather, analysis of cytokine levels occurs more in experimental and research settings. Difficulties in obtaining blood samples, variable sampling patterns, incalculable factors that can affect the results and different laboratory methods make the study of cytokines a complex procedure. In a recent study from Greece, fever was more common in a group of patients who received polyester endovascular grafts than in those that received PTFE graft. Interestingly, IL-8 was higher in the first group,[80] a finding which suggests a stronger host reaction to the specific synthetic prosthesis.[81] Other studies that have assessed inflammatory markers are shown in Table 2. IL-6 has been proven to be released from the aneurysmal thrombus;[82] this finding has been very recently endorsed.[56] Additionally, aneurysm surface area and mean plasma IL-6 levels are correlated.[56] PI syndrome and aneurysm surface area were also correlated in an anecdotal prospective sub-study of an RPAH study presented in Melbourne in 2003.[57] Furthermore, future combined studies that assess IL-6, thrombus volume, the coagulation cascade, and clinical parameters such as fever patterns, CRP, and leucocytes and their types, will answer many of our "eSIRS-PI syndrome" questions.

Obtaining clinically useful and cost-effective conclusions regarding eSIRS is related to the golden aim of assessing cost-effective, specific markers in a timely manner that fits with the patient's short hospital stay.

COAGULATION AND MAJOR ENDOVASCULAR PROCEDURES: ROLE OF ANTI-THROMBIN III

Other clinical and experimental investigations have focused on the role of coagulation in aortic endovascular procedures. Data from the early 2000's suggest that there is a low risk for consumption coagulopathy after endografting for the thoracic aorta.[83]

Recent data from various studies suggest the possibility of an increased procoagulant state in patients undergoing EVAR.[84,85] Englberger et al showed that there is increased perioperative production of coagulation markers, including fibrinopeptide A (FPA), fibrin monomers, thrombin/antithrombin complex (TAT) and D-dimers. Interestingly, the levels of fibrin monomers and TAT complex were higher in the EVAR group compared to the OAR group[84] (Table 2). The theory expressed above, that the endovascularly excluded aneurysm with new/old thrombotic material serves as a "dynamically potential inflammatory grenade", needs to be addressed. Van Nes et al[85] showed that the patients undergoing EVAR repair who developed growth of the aneurysm sac postoperatively (presence of endoleak type II or endotension) had increased levels of FDP and D-dimers in the aneurysm sac fluid, which suggests the occurrence of hyperfibrinolysis. The fact that peri-procedural use of antithrombin can decrease hypercoagulation and inflammatory activation during conventional abdominal aortic surgery strengthens the hyperfibrinolysis hypothesis.[86] Elective use of AT III when there is evidence of consumption, coagulopathy, may decrease the frequency of these adverse events.

The above data suggest that there may be a correlation between PI and disturbances in the coagulation equilibrium. However, this correlation remains to be proven.

CONCLUSIONS

The main issue regarding PI syndrome that concerns endovascular surgeons, cardiologists and interventional radiologists is its pathophysiology. Is it a reaction of the vessel wall[87] to the synthetic graft, which serves as a sign of a peri-vessel reaction; or is the PI the result of aseptic inflammation caused by the preexisting or newly formatted thrombus between the graft and the aneurysm sac? The latter hypothesis seems to be more likely since there is evidence that the inflammatory reaction is proportional to the amount of thrombus inside the lumen of AAA and its release of IL-6.[82,88] Increased platelet activity during aneurysm thrombosis is another attractive factor that contributes to the role of the thrombus in PI syndrome.[89] The hypothesis that cytokine release and burst from the fresh thrombus, which is formed in the sandwich of the endoluminal graft and the diseased vessel wall, may be the key to interpreting PI.

PI is a definitive physiologic response to the implantation of an endovascular graft. However, PI needs to be redefined in order to describe more specifically the postoperative clinical and biochemical responses after endostenting or endografting. As demonstrated in figure 1, the commonly observed parameters, temperature >38°C, leucocytes >12.000 cells/L, and increased CRP, can be defined as SIRS following endovascular procedures or eSIRS. PI syndrome may also describe the broad intermediate condition after endovascular procedures, while eSIRS is a more specific term that simultaneously and accurately applies to all three factors (temperature, leucocytes and CRP) with certain abnormal values.

Is it an academic dilemma to treat eSIRS/PI syndrome, or does it really affect the patients less than some vascular surgeons suggest? The economic hindrance for treating PI syndrome/eSIRS, apart from the special tests required for diagnosis, is the prolongation of hospital stay,[90,65] and the tests done to exclude other reasons for fever. Following elucidation of its cause and after reviewing feedback from our patients, we will predict the requirements for therapy and address the concerns mentioned here. Finally, the interpretation of its pathophysiology will facilitate differentiation of the septic cases that mimic eSIRS/PI syndrome. Veith stated in 1997 that "the causes remain obscure" for the inflammatory reactions to endografts; since then there has been enormous progress, but there is still a way to go.[91]

REFERENCES

1. Chaikof EL, Blankensteijn JD, Harris PL, White GH, Zarins CK, Bernhard VM, Matsumura JS, May J, Veith FJ, Fillinger MF, Rutherford RB, Kent KC; Ad Hoc Committee for Standardized Reporting Practices in Vascular Surgery of The Society for Vascular Surgery/American Association for Vascular Surgery. Reporting standards for endovascular aortic aneurysm repair. J Vasc Surg. 2002 May;35(5):1048-60.
2. Ahn SS, Rutherford RB, Johnston KW, et al: Reporting standards for infrarenal endovascular abdominal aortic aneurysm repair. J Vasc Surg 25:405-410, 1997.
3. White GH, May J. Basic Techniques of endovascular Aneurysm Repair-Complications. Ch. 52, 971-976 in Vascular Surgery edited by Robert Rutherford. Sixth Edition
4. Parodi JC: Endovascular repair of abdominal aortic aneurysms and other arterial lesions. J Vasc Surg 21:549-555, 1995
5. White GH, Yu W, May J, et al: Endoleak as a complication of endoluminal grafting of abdominal aortic aneurysms: Classification, incidence, diagnosis, and management. J Endovasc Surg 4:152-168, 1997.
6. White GH, May J, Waugh RC, Yu W: Type I and type II endoleak: A more useful classification for reporting results of endoluminal repair of AAA (Letter). J Endovasc Surg 5:189-191, 1998.
7. White GH, May J, Waugh RC, Chaufour X, Yu W. Type III and type IV endoleak: toward a complete definition of blood flow in the sac after endoluminal AAA repair. J Endovasc Surg. 1998 Nov;5(4):305-9.
8. Faries PL, Cadot H, Agarwal G, Kent KC, Hollier LH, Marin ML Management of endoleak after endovascular aneurysm repair: cuffs, coils, and conversion. J Vasc Surg. 2003 Jun;37(6):1155-61.
9. Chuter TA, Faruqi RM, Sawhney R, Reilly LM, Kerlan RB, Canto CJ, Lukaszewicz GC, Laberge JM, Wilson MW, Gordon RL, Wall SD, Rapp J, Messina LM. Endoleak after endovascular repair of abdominal aortic aneurysm. J Vasc Surg. 2001 Jul;34(1):98-105.
10. Marin ML, Veith FJ, Cynamon J, et al: Initial experience with transluminally placed endovascular grafts for the treatment of complex vascular lesions. Ann Surg 222:449-469, 1995
11. May J, White GH, Yu W, et al: Endovascular grafting for abdominal aortic aneurysms: Changing incidence and indications for conversion to open operation. Cardiovasc Surg 6:194-197, 1998
12. Storck M, Scharrer-Palmer R, Kapfer X, et al. Does a Postimplantation Syndrome Following Endovascular Treatment of Aortic Aneurysms Exist? Vasc Surg 2001;35:23-29.
13. van Marrewijk CJ, Leurs LJ, Valladhaneni SR, et al, on behalf of EUROSTAR collaborators. Risk-Adjusted Outcome Analysis of Endovascular Abdominal Aortic Aneurysm Repair in a Large Popu-

lation: How Do Stent-Grafts Compare? J Endovasc Ther 2005;12:417-429

14. Wilt TJ, Lederle FA, Macdonald R, Jonk YC, Rector TS, Kane RL. Comparison of endovascular and open surgical repairs for abdominal aortic aneurysm. Evid Rep Technol Assess (Full Rep). 2006 Aug;(144):1-113. Review.

15. Tzilalis VD, May J, White GH, Stephen MS, Harris JP. Severe hypertension following implantation of endovascular grafts into the thoracic aorta of young patients. J Endovasc Ther. 2005 Feb;12(1):142-3.

16. Volodos SN. An adverse effect of arterial hypertension on the outcomes of endovascular grafting of aortic aneurysms. Angiol Sosud Khir. 2006;12(3): 7-12.

17. Conners MS 3rd, Tonnessen BH, Sternbergh WC 3rd, Carter G, Yoselevitz M, Money SR. Does ASA classification impact success rates of endovascular aneurysm repairs? Ann Vasc Surg. 2002 Sep;16(5):550-5. Epub 2002 Sep 4.

18. Sbarigia E, Speziale F, Ducasse E, Giannoni MF, Ruggiero M, Palmieri A, Fiorani P. What is the best management for abdominal aortic aneurysm in patients at high surgical risk? A single-center review. Int Angiol. 2005 Mar;24(1):70-4.

19. Berg P, Kaufmann D, van Marrewijk CJ, Buth J. Spinal cord ischaemia after stent-graft treatment for infra-renal abdominal aortic aneurysms. Analysis of the Eurostar database. Eur J Vasc Endovasc Surg. 2001 Oct;22(4):342-7

20. Clavert P, Chakfe N, Edah-Tally S, Beaufigeau M, Hassani O, Thaveau F, Kahn JL, Kretz JG. Paraplegia secondary to surgery of the abdominal aorta. J Mal Vasc. 1999 Jun;24(3):229-32

21. Huynh TT, Miller CC 3rd, Safi HJ. Delayed onset of neurologic deficit: significance and management. Semin Vasc Surg. 2000 Dec;13(4):340-4.

22. Bown MJ, Nicholson ML, Bell PRF, Sayers RD. The Systemic inflammatory response syndrome, organ failure, and mortality after abdominal aortic aneurysm repair. J Vasc Surg 2003;37:600-6.

23. Cremer J, Martin M, Redl H, et al. Systemic Inflammatory Response Syndrome After Cardiac Operations. Ann Thorac Surg 1996;61:1714-20.

24. Taylor KM. SIRS - The Systemic Inflammatory Response Syndrome After Cardiac Operations. Ann Thorac Surg 1996;61:1607-8.

25. Royston D, Kovesi T, Marczin N. The unwanted response to cardiac surgery: Time for a reappraisal? J Thorac Cardiovasc Surg 2003;125:32-5.

26. Ortolano GA, Aldea GS, Lilly K, et al. A review of leukofiltration in cardiac surgery: the time course of reperfusion injury may facilitate study design of anti-inflammatory effects. Perfusion 2002; 17 Suppl:53-62

27. Markewitz A, Lante W, Franke A, Marohl K, Kuhlmann WD, Weinhold C. Alterarions of cell-mediated immunity following cardiac operations: clinical implications and open questions. Shock 2001; 16 Suppl 1: 10-5.

28. Schaller B. Craniocerebral trauma--new pathophysiological and therapeutic viewpoints. Swiss Surg 2002;8:145-58.

29. Burgi U, Stocker R. Intensive care concepts after traumatic spinal cord injury. Schweiz Med Wochenschr 2000;130:811-5

30. Folgar C, Lindsey RW. C-Reactive protein in orthopedics. Orthopeadics. 1998;21:687-691.

31. Deitch EA, Goodman ER. Prevention of multiple organ failure. Surg Clin North Am 1999;79:1471-88.

32. Payen D, Faivre V, Lukaszewicz AC, Losser MR. Assessment of immunological status in the critically ill. Minerva Anestesiol 2000;66:351-7.

33. Kato N, Hirano T, Shimono T, et al. Treatment of chronic aortic dissection by transluminal endovascular stent-graft placement: preliminary results. J Vasc Interv Radiol 2001;12:835-40.

34. Morikage N, Esato K, Zenpo N, Fujioka K, Takenaka H. Is endovascular treatment of abdominal aortic aneurysms less invasive regarding the biological responses? Surg Today 2000;30:142-6.

35. Swartbol P, Norgren L, Albrechtsson U, et al. Biological responses differ considerably between endovascular and conventional aortic aneurysm surgery. Eur J Vasc Endovasc Surg 1996;12:18-25.

36. Norgren L, Swartbol P. Biological responses to endovascular treatment of abdominal aortic aneurysms. Review. J Endovasc Surg 1997; 4:169-73.

37. Parodi JC, Ferreira LM, Fornari MC, Berardi VE, Diez RA. Neutrophil Respiratory Burst Activity and Pro- and Anti-inflammatory Cytokines in AAA Surgery: Conventional versus Endoluminal Treatment. J Endovasc Ther 2001;8:114-124.

38. Decker D, Springer W, Decker P, et al. Changes in TH1/TH2 Immunity after Endovascular and Conventional Infrarenal Aortic Aneurysm Repair:

lst Relevance for Clinical Practice. Eur J Vasc Endovasc Surg 2003;25: 254-261.

39. Sweeney KJ, Evoy D, Sultan S, et al. Endovascular Approach to Abdominal Aortic Aneurysms Limits the Postoperative Systemic Immune Response. Eur J Vasc Endovasc Surg 2002;23:303-308.

40. Swartbol P, Truedsson L, Norgren L. The Inflammatory Response and its Consequence for the Clinical Outcome Following Aortic Aneurysm Repair. Review Article. Eur J Vasc Endovasc Surg 2001;21:393-400.

41. Galle C, De Maertelaer V, Motte S, et al. Early inflammatory response after elective abdominal aortic aneurysm repair: A comparison between endovascular procedure and conventional surgery. J Vasc Surg 2000;32:234-46.

42. Hayoz D, Do Do-Dai, Mahler F, Triller J, Spertini F. Acute Inflammatory Reaction Associated With Endoluminal Bypass Grafts. J Endovasc Surg 1997;4:354-360.

43. Syk I, Brunkwall J, Ivancev K, et al. Postoperative fever, bowel ischaemia and cytokine response to abdominal aortic aneurysm-a comparison between endovascular and open surgery. Eur J Vasc Endovasc Surg 1998;15:398-405.

44. Odegard A, Lundbom I, Muhre HO, et al. The Inflammatory Response Following Treatment of Abdominal Aortic Aneurysms: a Comparison Between Open Surgery and Endovascular Repair. Eur J Vasc Endovasc Surg 2000 ;19:536-544.

45. Elmarasy NM, Soong SV, Walker SR, et al. Sigmoid Ischemia and the Inflammatory Response Following Endovascular Abdominal Aortic Aneurysm Repair. J Endovasc Ther 2000;7:21-30.

46. Blum U, Gotz V, Lammer J, et al. Endoluminal Stent-Grafts for Infrarenal Abdominal Aortic Aneurysms. N Engl J Med 1997;336:13-20.

47. Kahn RA, Moskowitz DM. Endovascular aortic repair. J Cardiothorac Vasc Anesth 2000 Apr;16(2): 218-33.Review.

48. Velazquez OC, Carpenter JP, Baum RA, et al. Perigraft Air, Fever, and Leukocytosis after Endovascular Repair of Abdominal Aortic Aneurysms. Am J Surg 1999;178:185-189.

49. Nystrom Per-Olof. The systemic inflammatory response syndrome: definitions and aetiology. J Antimicrob Chemoth 1998;41:Suppl.A,1-7.

50. Weibull H, Bergqvist D, Jonsson K, Karlsson S,

TakolanderR. Complications after transluminal angioplasty in the iliac, femoral, and popliteal arteries. J Vasc Surg 1987;5:681-6.

51. Moore WS, Rutherford RB, for the EVT Investigators. Transfemoral endovascular repair of abdominal aortic aneurysm: Results of the North American EVT phase 1 trial. J Vasc Surg 1996;23:543-53.

52. Ahmad F, Cheshire N, Hamady M. Acute aortic syndrome: pathology and therapeutic strategies. Postgrad Med J. 2006 May;82(967):305-12.

53. Luigi M. Biasucci. CDC/AHA Workshop on Markers of Inflammation and Cardiovascular Disease Application to Clinical and Public Health Practice Clinical Use of Inflammatory Markers in Patients With Cardiovascular Diseases. A Background Paper. Circulation. 2004 Dec 21;110(25):e560-7.

54. Alvarez Garcia B, Ruiz C, Chacon P, Sabin JA, Matas M. High-sensitivity C-reactive protein in high-grade carotid stenosis: risk marker for unstable carotid plaque. J Vasc Surg. 2003 Nov; 38(5):1018-24.

55. Schillinger M, Exner M, Mlekusch W, et al. Endovascular revascularization below the knee: 6-month results and predictive value of C-reactive protein level. Radiology. 2003 May;227(2):419-25. Epub 2003 Mar 20.

56. Dawson J, Cockerill GW, Choke E, Belli AM, Loftus I, Thompson MM. Aortic aneurysms secrete interleukin-6 into the circulation. J Vasc Surg. 2007 Feb;45(2):350-6.

57. Tzilalis V, Dubenec SR, Choy ET, Pasenau JEH,et al. A prospective study of systemic inflammatory syndrome in patients following endoluminal aortic aneurysm repair. Archived Presentation in ANZSVS 2003 www.anzsvs.org.au/abstract.asp?PresentationNo=67

58. Mialhe C, Amicabile C, Becquemin JP. Endovascular treatment of infrarenal abdominal aneurysms by the Stentor system: preliminary results of 79 cases. Stentor Retrospective Study Group. J Vasc Surg 1997;26:199-209.

59. Coppi G, Pacchioni R, Moratto R, et al. Experience with the Stentor Endograft at Four Italian Centers. J Endovasc Surg 1998;5:206-215.

60. Maynar M, de Blas M, Reyes R, et al. Endovascular treatment of abdominal aorta aneurysms using bifurcated endoprosthesis. Rev Clin Esp 1998; 198(4):200-6.

61. Gorich J, Rilinger N, Soldner J, et al. Endovascular repair of aortic aneurysms: treatment of complications. J Endovasc Surg 1999;6:136-46.

62. Nienaber CA, Fattori R, Lund G, et al. Nonsurgical reconstruction of thoracic aortic dissection by stent-graft placement. N Engl J Med 1999;340:1539-45.

63. Ruchat P, Capasso P, Hayoz D, Genton A, Schnyder P, von Segesser LK. Endovascular treatment of abdominal aortic aneurysm. Preliminary experiences with the Talent endoprosthesis. Swiss Surg 1998;Suppl 2:4-7.

64. Buth J, Laheij RJF on behalf of the EUROSTAR Collaborators. Early complications and endoleaks after endovascular abdominal aortic aneurysm repair: Report of a multicenter study. J Vasc Surg 2000;31:134-36.

65. Scheinert D, Ludwig J, Steinkamp HJ, Schroder M, Balzer JO, Biamino G. Treatment of Catheter-Induced Iliac Artery Injuries With Self-Expanding Endografts. J Endovasc Ther 2000;7:213-220.

66. Guo W, Zhang G, Liang F, et al. Endoluminal stent-graft repair of aortic aneurysms. Zhonghua Wai Ke Za Zhi 2000;38:179-81.

67. Henry M, Amor M, Henry I, et al. Percutaneous endovascular treatment of peripheral aneurysms. J Cardiovasc Surg (Torino) 2000;41:871-83.

68. Wolpert LM, Dittrich KP, Hallisey MJ, et al. Hypogastric artery embolization in endovascular abdominal aortic aneurysm repair. J Vasc Surg 2001;33:1193-8.

69. Won JY, Lee DY, Shim WH, et al. Elective endovascular treatment of descending thoracic aortic aneurysms and chronic dissections with stent-grafts. J Vasc Interv Radiol 2001;12:575-82.

70. Shim WH, Koo BK, Yoon YS, et al. Treatment of Thoracic Aortic Dissection with stent Grafts. J Endovasc Ther 2002;9:817-821.

71. Espinoza G, Marchiori E, Silva LF, De Araujo AP, Riguetti C, Perez Baquero RA. Initial Results of Edovascular Repair of Abdominal Aortic Aneurysms with a Self-expanding Stent-Graft. J Vasc Interv Radiol 2002 13:1115-23.

72. Schoder M, Cartes-Zumelzu F, Grabenwoger M, et al. Elective Endovascular Stent-Graft Repair of Atherosclerotic Thoracic Aortic Aneurysms: Clinical Results and Midterm Follow-Up. AJR 2003;180:709-715.

73. Gabay C, Kushner I. Mechanisms of Disease: Acute-Phase Proteins and Other Systemic Responses to Inflammation. Review Article. N Engl J Med 1999;340:448-454.

74. Haverkate F, Thompson SG, Pyke SDM, Gallimore JR, Pepys MB. Production of C-reactive protein and risk of coronary events in stable and unstable angina. Lancet 1997;349:462-6.

75. Ridker PM, Cushman M, Stampfer MJ, Tracy RP, Hennekens CH. Inflammation, aspirin, and the risk of cardiovascular disease in apparently healthy men. N Engl J Med 1997;336:973-9.

76. Zimmerman MA, Selzman CH, Cothren C, Sorensen AC, Raeburn CD, Harken AH. Diagnostic Implications of C-Reactive Protein. Review Article. Arch Surg 2003;138:220-224.

77. Lin E, Calvano SE, Lowry SF. Inflammatory cytokines and cell response in surgery. Surgery 2000;127:117-126.

78. Gilliand HE, Armstrong MA, Carabine U, McMurray TJ. The choise of anesthetic maintenance technique influences the anti-inflammatory cytokine response to abdominal surgery. Anesth Analg 1997;85:1394-1398.

79. Dinarello CA. Proinflammatory cytokines. Chest 2000;118:503-508.

80. Gerasimidis T, Sfyroeras G, Trellopoulos G, et al. Impact of endograft material on the inflammatory response after elective endovascular abdominal aortic aneurysm repair. Angiology. 2005 Nov-Dec;56(6):743-53.

81. Shindo S, Ogata K, Kubota K, et al. Vascular prosthetic implantation is associated with prolonged inflammation following aortic aneurysm surgery. J Artif Organs. 2003;6(3):173-8.

82. Swartbol P, Truedsson L, Norgren L. Adverse reactions during endovascular treatment of aortic aneurysms may be triggered by interleukin 6 release from the thrombotic content. J Vasc Surg 1998;28:664-8.

83. Shimazaki T, Ishimaru S, Kawaguchi S, Yokoi Y, Watanabe Y. Blood coagulation and fibrinolytic response after endovascular stent grafting of thoracic aorta. J Vasc Surg. 2003 Jun;37(6):1213-8.

84. Englberger L, Savolainen H, Jandus P, et al. Activated coagulation during open and endovascular abdominal aortic aneurysm repair. J Vasc Surg. 2006 Jun;43(6):1124-9.

85. van Nes JG, Hendriks JM, Tseng LN, van Dijk LC, van Sambeek MR. Endoscopic aneurysm sac fenestration as a treatment option for growing aneurysms due to type II endoleak or endotension.J Endovasc Ther. 2005 Aug;12(4):430-4.

86. Nishiyama T. Antithrombin can modulate coagulation, cytokine production, and expression of adhesion molecules in abdominal aortic aneurysm repair surgery. Anesth Analg. 2006 Apr;102(4): 1007-11.

87. Gordon FAA, Stewart-Lee AL, Anggard EE. Arterial response to mechanical injury: balloon catheter de-endothelialization. Review Article. Atherosclerosis 1992;92:89-104.

88. Juvonen J, Surcel HM, Satta J, et al. Elevated circulating levels of inflammatory cytokines in patients with abdominal aortic aneurysm. Arterioscler Thromb Vasc Biol 1997;17:2843-2847.

89. Boyle JR, Goodall S, Thompson JP, Bell PRF, Thompson MM. Endovascular AAA Repair Attenuates the Inflammatory and Renal Responses Associated with Conventional Surgery. J Endovasc Ther 2000;7:359-371.

90. Chaikof EL, Blankensteijn JD, Harris PL, et al. Reporting standards for endovascular aortic aneurysm repair. J Vasc Surg 2002;35:1048-1060.

91. Veith FJ. Inflammatory Reactions to Endografts: The Causes Remain Obscure. Commentary. J Edovasc Surg 1997;4:361.

Advances in management of endoleaks type I, II, III

James May, Geoffrey H. White, Kathryn Busch, John P. Harris

BACKROUND

The endoluminal method of aneurysm repair has proven to be a much less invasive method than the conventional open operation. Blood loss at operation, the need for postoperative intensive care, and length of hospital stay are significantly less with the endoluminal technique.[1]

Failure to isolate the aneurysm from the general circulation, however, remains a cause for concern. Such failure is likely to result in further expansion of the aneurysm sac with the potential for rupture.

TERMINOLOGY

Failure to isolate the aneurysm from the circulation may be detected by angiography, CT, or duplex ultrasound imaging. This phenomenon had been described in the early literature on endoluminal aneurysm repair as a "leak". This term, however, was confusing because it has been common practice to use the word "leak" to refer to extravasation of blood outside the aorta associated with aneurysm rupture. We proposed that a more specific term for failure to exclude the aneurysm from the circulation would be "endoleak."[2]

This term would be unique to endoluminal grafts because the leak of blood remains within the confines of the vessel but external to the endoluminal graft. We suggested the following definition of endoleak:

Endoleak is a condition associated with endoluminal vascular grafts, defined by the persistence of blood flow outside the lumen of the endoluminal graft but within an aneurysm sac or adjacent vascular segment being treated by the graft. Endoleak is due to incomplete sealing or exclusion of the aneurysm sac or vessel segment as evidenced by imaging studies such as contrast-enhanced CT, ultrasonography, or angiography.[3]

We further proposed that a clear distinction should be made between endoleak related to the graft device itself and endoleak associated with flow from collateral arterial branches.[4] We proposed that these be identified as being type I or type II endoleak, respectively.

Type I endoleak occurs when a persistent channel of blood flow develops because of an inadequate or ineffective seal at the graft ends.

Type II endoleak occurs when there is persistent collateral blood flow into the aneurysm sac flowing retrogradely from patent lumbar arteries, the inferior mesenteric artery, the intercostals arteries (in thoracic aneurysm), or other collateral vessels. In this situation there is usually a complete seal around the graft attachment zones so that the complication is not related directly to the graft itself.

We subsequently proposed that the term type III endoleak be introduced for leakage through a defect in the graft fabric or between segments of a modular endograft.[5] In the same paper, we suggested that blood flow through an intact but porous fabric, should be termed type IV endoleak.

CLASSIFICATION OF ENDOLEAKS

The Ad Hoc committee on reporting standards for endovascular aortic aneurysm repair has recommended a classification of endoleak by site of origin[6] (Table 1 is a

modification of this classification and Figure 1 is a diagrammatic representation of the various types of endoleak).

RELATED CONDITIONS

Microleaks

Matsumura et al reported a failure mode after endovascular AAA repair not previously recognized.[7] They termed this a "transgraft microleak" which resulted from a fabric defect at the site of suture holes leading to a persistent type III endoleak for up to 2½ years after operation. The authors have emphasized that they are not describing previously unrecognized endoleaks but rather endoleaks that had been seen on standard contrast computed tomography (CT) without the exact site of origin being identified. The authors describe a number of special manouvres that allow the site of

TABLE 1	CLASSIFICATION OF ENDOLEAKS, MODIFIED FROM THE JOURNAL OF VASCULAR SURGERY[6]

Classification of endoleak

Type Cause of perigraft flow

I a) Inadequate seal at proximal end of endograft
    b) Inadequate seal at distal end of endograft
    c) Inadequate seal at iliac occluder plug

II Flow from visceral vessel (lumbar, IMA, accessory renal, hypogastric) without attachment site connection

III a) Flow from module disconnection
     b) Flow from fabric disruption

IV Flow from porous fabric (<30 days after graft placement

V Flow visualised but source unidentified

Modified from Journal of Vascular Surgery.[6]

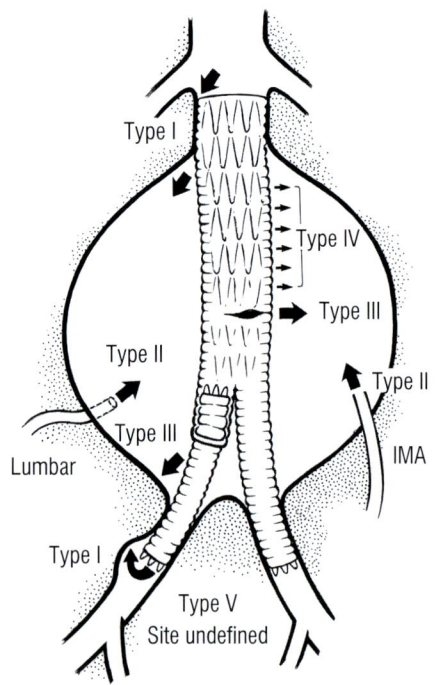

FIGURE 1: Diagram depicting sites of graft related and collateral circulation related endoleaks.

these small type III endoleaks to be identified. These included "directed" angiography with balloon occlusion of the iliac limbs and careful colour flow duplex ultrasound scanning by skilled sonographers.

Endotension

Endotension has been defined as aneurysm enlargement after endovascular repair in the absence of a detectable endoleak. Explanations for persistent or recurrent pressurization of aneurysm sac include blood flow in the sac that is below the sensitivity limits for detection with current imaging technology[5,8,9] or pressure transmission through thrombus[10,11] or the endograft fabric. The aneurysm may be pulsatile on physical examination and intra-sac pressure measurement may be in the near systemic range

DIAGNOSIS OF ENDOLEAKS

The imaging for diagnosis of endoleak may be considered during the operative period and in the postoperative period.

Intraoperative diagnosis of endoleak

When primary endoleak occurs it will often be detected during the operative procedure by completion angiography. At other times, primary endoleak may not be diagnosed until the early postoperative studies, such as CT scan or color duplex ultrasound scan, are performed.

All cases of endoleak detected within the perioperative period should be classified as primary endoleak. The cause of these early cases will usually be related to problems in the case selection, design/sizing of a particular graft or technical problems encountered during the graft implantation. Although an endovascular graft may appear to be sealed at the time of completion angiography and

then develop an endoleak at the time of perioperative imaging, it seems more likely that this is in fact and primary endoleak that went undetected initially.

Intraoperative angiography

Angiograms are usually done at intervals during the implantation procedure and at its completion. Endoleak is diagnosed by the presence of contrast media outside of the graft lumen, filling completely or partially the lumen of the aneurysm sac. In patients with a large amount of laminated thrombus within the aneurysm, the residual lumen may be reduced to such an extent that contrast outside the graft lumen may be missed. Completion angiography should be performed using a power injector in a precise manner at several sites along the graft length. A pigtail catheter with multiple holes in the tail is preferred to deliver a large quantity of contrast at the one level. Angiography may also be performed via the side ports of introducing sheaths in the common femoral arteries bilaterally. This serves to check for perigraft reflux around the iliac limbs of the endograft, that has not been detected on previous films. Cine-loop angiography (set at 2-4 frames per second) with the capability for digital subtraction and frame-by-frame replay is essential.

Some graft fabrics being used in endografts are porous and completion angiography may demonstrate contrast outside the endograft lumen. This may present a diagnostic dilemma. Contrast in the sac due to the porosity usually appears late during the digital subtraction angiogram (DSA) and is usually generalized along the length of the graft. By contrast type I endoleaks appear early and are localized.

Postoperative diagnosis of endoleak

The modalities for postoperative imaging of endoleak, may be surrogate or direct.

Surrogate modalities

Since the vast majority of endografts have a radio-opaque metallic frame, a plain abdominal x-ray is a useful investigation. It may demonstrate faulty fixation more clearly and earlier than contrast CT and preceed the detection of endoleak.[12] The accuracy of detecting migration can be improved by following a protocol of performing A-P, lateral and oblique views at the level of the umbilicus.

Studies have confirmed that the presence of endoleak is usually associated with an increase in the size of the aneurysm sac.[13,14] Measurement of AAA diameter by B mode ultrasound can therefore be used as a surrogate method of detecting endoleak. CT may also be used for a similar purpose with the option of monitoring an increase in volume of the sac in addition to the diameter of the sac.

Direct modalities for imaging endoleaks

The direct methods of imaging for endoleak comprise colour duplex ultrasound, contrast enhanced CT and angiograpy. Contrast enhanced CT has been accepted as the gold standard for detecting the presence of an endoleak. Once an endoleak has been detected, however, carefully planned arteriography is more useful in characterizing the origin and nature of the endoleak. Colour duplex ultrasound has the advantage of imaging type II endoleaks in real time as distinct from contrast CT and arteriography, both of which have to rely on accurate timing to image the contrast arriving in the sac via collateral circulation.

Colour duplex ultrasound

From the beginning of the endoluminal method of treating abdominal aortic aneurysm, computed tomography (CT) scanning has been considered the optimal diagnostic method to monitor patients after endoluminal repair. More recently color duplex ultrasound (CDU) has emerged as an important alternative imaging modality.[15] CDU with the advantages of low cost and risk can accurately monitor aneurysm size, detect endoleak and provide dynamic and hemodynamic information not available with other testing methods. The technique is however operator dependent, can be time consuming and certain aspects of device failure, notably wire fracture, cannot be detected.[16]

Duplex ultrasound evaluation of aortic endografts

Technique

- The patient should fast overnight to minimize intestinal gas and schedule the study for a morning appointment. The examination will take approximately one hour.
- Obtain operative information prior to the examination on what type of endograft has been used as there are different types and some designs feature bare stents that extend above the renal arteries.
- Use a high-resolution color duplex ultrasound system with pulsed Doppler transducers ranging in frequency from 2.25 MHz to 5.0 MHz allowing adequate depth penetration.
- Perform the examination with the patient in the supine position with the head slightly elevated. For the obese patient and the patient with excessive bowel gas, the examiner may have to position the patient in various positions using other windows to visualise the endograft.
- Commence the study using B-mode imaging in the transverse plane. Identify the aorta at the level of the superior mesenteric artery. Look for the reflective metal struts of the aortic stent graft, which in some grafts can be visualised above the level of the renal arteries. The proximal extent of the graft (material) is seen as a

hyperechoic signal along the aortic lumen and can be visualised just below the level of the renal arteries. This is the superior attachment site. If the stent graft is uni-iliac or a bifurcated graft, then the inferior attachment site(s) would be the native common or external iliac artery.

- In the transverse plane, take maximum diameter measurements of the aneurysm sac. Over time there should be a decrease in the size of the residual sac. Any increase in size suggests flow to the sac and therefore a continued risk of rupture.

- Confirm patency of the renal arteries with spectral Doppler and measure the distance of the superior attachment in relation to the renal level for possible graft migration. Then scan from the superior attachment to the inferior attachment site(s) in both transverse and sagittal planes in B-mode. The addition of Harmonic Imaging improves image quality and contrast resolution and will aid in diagnostic accuracy.

- Using color and spectral Doppler assess the stent graft looking for any perigraft flow, graft stenosis, thrombosis or kinking recording flow velocities throughout the body of the graft and graft limb(s). Optimize color settings so that color completely fills the graft lumen avoiding excessive artifact. The examiner should be confident in differentiating between a true endoleak and color artifact. The addition of Power Doppler may be useful in detecting perigraft leak. Assess patency of the native iliac and femoral arteries beyond the endograft and perform spectral Doppler analysis.

- It is important to be aware of potential sites of perigraft leak. A true leak will have reproducible arterial waveforms with **different** spectral Doppler characteristics compared to flow within the aortic endograft. Try to determine the source of leak and direction of flow.

Color duplex ultrasound imaging is an accurate modality to detect early and late endoleak and device complications after endoluminal aortic surgery. The test is emerging as the diagnostic test of first choice for surveillance, allowing CT scanning and aortography to be used more selectively to plan secondary intervention. Further investigation is required to confirm the accuracy of this test and the optimal intervals for surveillance programs.

ADVANCES IN MANAGEMENT OF ENDOLEAKS

Type I and type II endoleaks

We have recently become aware of the intermittent nature of some endoleaks. A 65 year old male patient was shown on colour duplex ultrasound & CT to have a type I distal iliac endoleak. He was admitted for an aortogram and subsequent secondary extension graft to the culprit iliac limb. Following bed rest in hospital, however, despite careful and detailed angiography no leak could be detected. Subsequent outpatient investigation by color duplex ultrasound and contrast CT demonstrated the type I endoleak at the original site. Since successfully managing this patient by deployment of an extension endograft, we have become aware of type III endoleaks, whose presence may be demonstrated only in the right or left lateral decubitus positions. Such a case is demonstrated in Figure 2.

Our attention was first drawn to the concept of intermittent and posture dependent endoleaks by a case managed by one of the authors (GHW). In 1998, a 76 year old male patient underwent endovascular repair of a 5 cm AAA using an AneuRx prosthesis. There were no complications, but the aneurysm sac gradually and consistently increased in diameter to 6.6 cm. This enlargement was accompa-

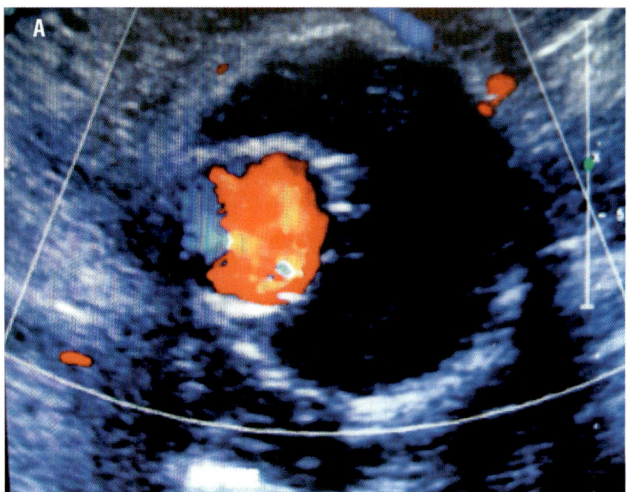

FIGURE 2: Colour duplex ultrasound demonstrating **A**. No type III endoleak while the patient is lying supine.

nied by a change in the shape of the sac and the appearance of streaks of echolucency in the thrombus within it.

In 2002, in the absence of any evidence of endoleak, a Cook aortic cuff was deployed on the suspicion of pressure transmission through thrombus between the proximal portion of the body of the endograft and the native aorta. The aneurysm ruptured in 2003 and conversion to open repair was required. When the endograft was explanted and re-pres-

surised with blood, a type III fabric defect was noted, but only in certain positions. The flow of blood through the endoleak could by controlled and stopped by flexion and extension of the endograft (Figure 3).

Changes to colour duplex ultrasound protocol

Since becoming aware of intermittent and posture dependent endoleaks, we have

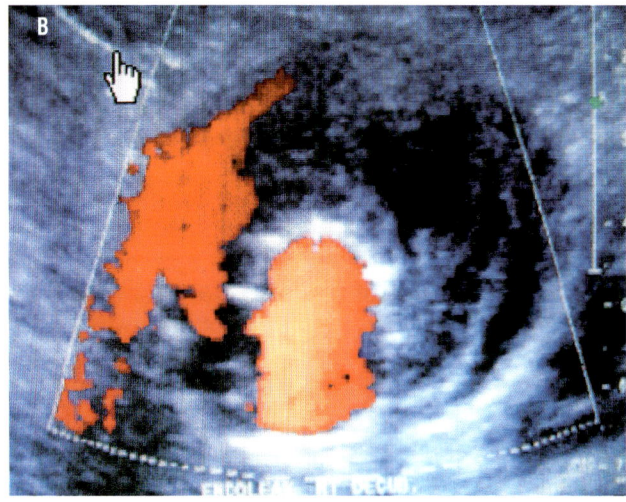

FIGURE 2: **B**. Type III endoleak while the paitent is lying in the right lateral decubitis position.

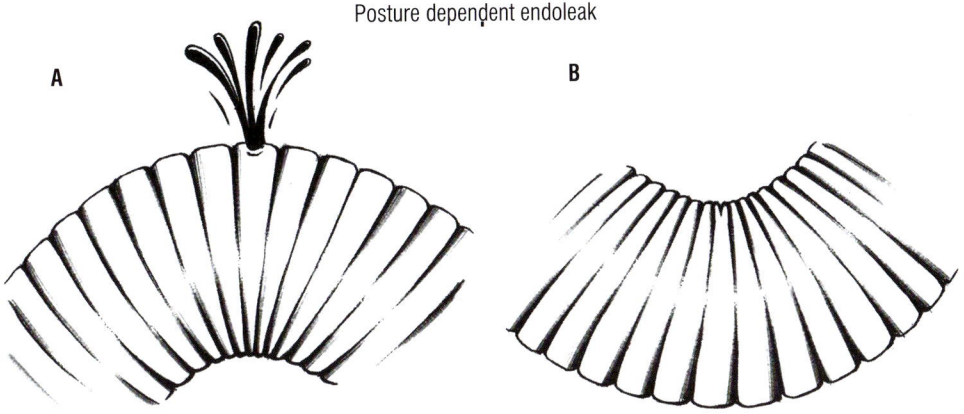

Posture dependent endoleak

A

B

FIGURE 3: Diagram demonstrating how a type III endoleak may change from **A**. Being closed when the endograft is in the flexed position to. **B**. Being open when the endograft is in the extended position.

changed our ultrasound protocol for examining patients with endotension.[17,18] These changes included:

1. Changing the patient's position from supine to left and right lateral decubitus.
2. Optimising colour gain settings
3. Use of harmonic imaging

Changes in technique of treating type I and type III endoleaks

Type I endoleaks are largely treated by proximal extension cuffs and distal extension grafts to the limbs. Advances on these established methods have included coil and glue embolization techniques and fenestrated cuff technology where the proximal neck has undergone, degeneration resulting in type I endoleak.

Type III endoleaks have traditionally been treated by deployment of a secondary endograft at the site of a localised fabric defect or modular disconnection. If the fabric defect is more generalised, techniques are now available to generalise re-line the original endograft. The Cook company has developed two devices (Renu) (Figure 4) for this purpose.

TYPE II ENDOLEAKS

From the outset of endovascular aneurysm repair, type II endoleaks have been assumed to be an anavoidable consequence of the endovascular method of repair and independent of the kind of endograft used. More recently, there have been some suggestions that the incidence of type II endoleaks may be graft dependent. A definitive paper by Sheehan and his colleagues,[19] however, encompassing 1909 elective endovascular AAA repair with six types of endogrft in five university institutions, revealed that no graft had a long-term statistically significant difference in the rate of type II endoleak formation.

Changes in indications and techniques for treating type II endoleaks

Traditionally type II endoleaks have been regarded as benign, unless they result in progressive expansion of the AAA sac. Recent reports, however, have questioned this approach.[20,21] The Massachusetts General Hospital group reported on two cohorts of patients, 131 with complete and

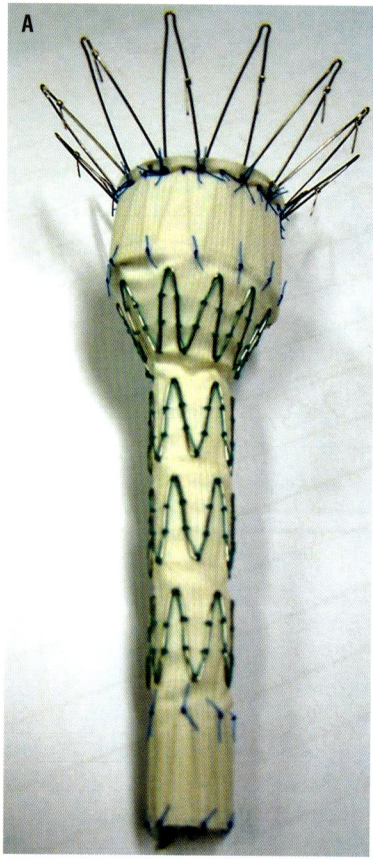

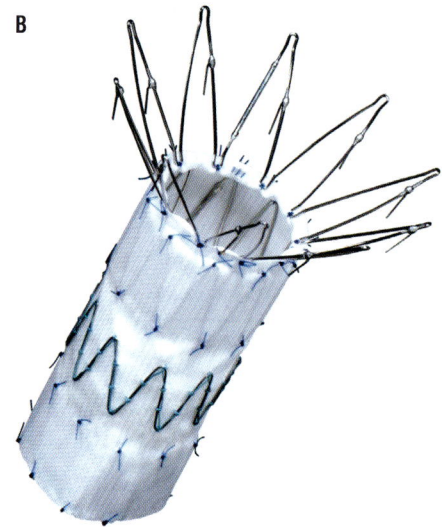

FIGURE 4: Photographs of the Renu endografts developed by Cook Inc specifically for repair of primary endografts which have undergone degeneration and/or migration. **A.** Converter. **B.** Body extension.

permanent resolution of early type II endoleak in less than 6 months and 33 whose endoleak persisted beyond 6 months.[21] The group concluded that persistent type 2 endoleak is associated with an increased incidence of adverse outcomes, including aneurysm sac growth, the need for conversion to open repair, reintervention rate, and rupture. These data suggest that patients with persistent type 2 endoleak (>6 months) should be considered for more frequent follow-up or a more aggressive approach to reintervention.

Treatment of type II endoleaks has also undergone a change from percutaneous endoluminal embolization of lumbar and inferior mesenteric leaks via the ascending lumbar and superior mesenteric/marginal

colonic arteries respectively, to puncture of the AAA sac.[22] Sac puncture is followed by sacography to identify the nidus of the type II endoleak and its communications to inferior mesenteric and/ or lumbar arteries. All the components of the type II endoleak are thus able to be treated by coil and/or glue embolization. Baum and his colleagues[22] have recommended trans-lumbar direct needle puncture to access the sac. More recently, Mansueto and his colleagues[23] have made a good case for transcatheter, transcaval embolization. Compared with translumbar embolization, the technique has the advantage that the entire procedure is performed in the angiography suite in the supine position, under fluoroscopic control. Of the 12 patients with expanding AAA in the study, the tran-scaval approach was able to be used in 11. A favourable outcome with reduction in sac diameter was achieved in 10 of the 11 patients at 1 year follow-up.

REFERENCES

1. May J, White GH, Yu W. et al: Concurrent comparison of endoluminal versus open repair in the treatment of abdominal aortic aneurysms: Analysis of 303 patients by life table method. J Vasc Surg 1998;27:213-222.
2. White GH, Yu W, May J. "Endoleak": A proposed new terminology to describe incomplete aneurysm exclusion by an endoluminal graft (letter). J Endovasc Surg 1996;3:124-125.
3. White GH, Yu W, May J, et al. Endoleak as a complication of endoluminal grafting of abdominal aortic aneurysms: Classification, incidence, diagnosis, and management. J Endovasc Surg 1997;4:152-168.
4. White GH, May J, Waugh RC, et al. Type I and type II endoleak: A more useful classification for reporting results of endoluminal repair of AAA (letter). J Endovac Surg, 1998;5:189-191.
5. White GH, May J, Petrasek P, Waugh RC, Yu W. Type III and type IV endoleak: toward a complete definition of blood flow in the sac after endoluminal repair of AAA. J Endovasc Surg 1998;5:305-9.
6. Chaikof EL, Blankensteijn JD, Harris PL, White GH, Zarins CK, Bernhard VM, Matsumura JS, May J, Veigh FJ, Fillinger MF, Rutherford RB, Kent KC for the Ad Hoc Committee for Standardized Reporting Practices in Vascular Surgery of The Society for Vascular Surgery/American Association for Vascular Surgery. Reporting Standards for Endovascular Aortic Aneurysm Repair. Journal of Vascular Surgery 2002;35:1048-1060.
7. Matsumura JS, Ryu RK, Ourier K. Identification and implications of transgraft microleaks after endovascular repair of aortic aneurysms. J Vasc Surg 2001;34:190-7.
8. White GH, May J, Petrasek P, Waugh R, Stephen M, Harris J. Endotension: an explanation for continued AAA growth after successful endoluminal repair. J Endovasc Surg 1999;6:308-15.
9. Schurink GW, Aarts NJ, Wilde J, van Baalen JM, Chuter TA, Schultze Kool LJ, et al. Endoleakage after stent-graft treatment of abdominal aneurysms: implications on pressure and imaging: an in-vitro study. J Vasc Surg 1998;28:234-41.
10. Faries PL, Sanchez LA, Marin ML, Parsons RE, Lyon RT, Oliveri S, et al. An experimental model for the acute and chronic evaluation of intra-aneurysmal pressure. J Endovasc Surg 1997;4:290-7.
11. Schurink GW, van Baalen JM, Visser MJ, van Bockel JH. Thrombus within an aortic aneurysm does not reduce pressure on the aneurismal wall. J Vasc Surg 2000;31:501-6.
12. May J, White GH, Yu W. Sieunarine K. Importance of plain x-ray in endoluminal aortic graft surveillance. Eur J Vasc Endovasc Surg 1997;13:202-206.
13. May J, White GH, Yu W, Waugh RC, Stephen MS, Harris JP. A prospective study of changes in morphology and dimensions of abdominal aortic aneurysm following endoluminal repair: preliminary report. J Endovasc Surg 1995;2(4):343-347.
14. May J, White GH, Yu W, Waugh RC, Stephen MS, Harris JP. A prospective study of anatomico-pathological changes in abdominal aortic aneurysms following endoluminal repair: is the aneurysmal process reversed? Eur J Vasc Endovasc Surg 1996;12:11-17.
15. Thurnher S & Cejna M. Imaging of aortic stent-grafts and endoleaks. Radiologic Clinics of North America 40:799-833, 2002.
16. Carter KA, Gayle RG, DeMasi RJ, Marcinczyk MJ, Gregory RT. The incidence and natural history of type I and II endoleak: a 5-year follow-up assessment with color duplex ultrasound scan. J Vasc Surg 35:595-597, 2003.
17. May J, White GH, Busch K, Makeham V, Harris JP. Intermittent and posture-dependent endoleaks: An increasingly recognized cause of endotension following EVAR. J Endovasc Ther, 2007;14(Suppl 1):1-18.
18. Busch KJ, Kidd J, White GH.Harris J, Kelly A. What are the duplex ultrasound signs that characterise an unstable abdominal aortic aneurysm sac after endograft implantation ? J Vascular Ultrasound 2007; 31:143-146.
19. Sheehan MK, Ouriel K; Greenberg R; McCann R; Murphy M, Fillinger M, Wyers M, Carpenter J, Fairman R, Makaroun MS. Are type II endoleaks

after endovascular aneurysm repair endograft dependent?

20. Gelfand DV, White GH, Wilson SE. Clinical significance of type II endoleak after endovascular repair of abdominal aortic aneurysm. Ann Vasc Surg 2006;20(1):69-74.

21. Jones JE, Atkins MD, Brewster DC, Chung TK, Kwolek CJ, Lamuraglia GH, Hodgman TM, Cambria RP. Persistent type 2 endoelak after endovascular repair of abdominal aortic aneurysm is associated with adverse late outcomes [In Process Citation] J Vasc Surg 2007;46(1): 1-8.

22. Baum RA, Carpenter JP, Golden MA et al. Treatment of type 2 endoleaks after endovascular repair of abdominal aortic aneurysms: comparison of transarterial and transluminal techniques. J Vasc Surg. 2002;35:23-29.

23. Mansueto G, Cenzi D, Scuro A, Gottin L, Griso A, Gumbs AA, Mucelli RP. Treatment of type II endoleak with a transcatheter transcaval approach: results at one-year follow-up. J Vasc Surg 2007;45:1120-7.

Secondary interventions following EVAR – Managing complications

Peter Ziegler, Efthimios D. Avgerinos, Konstantinos Lagios,
Anastasios Chronopoulos, Theodossios P. Perdikides

For the last 15 years endovascular treatment has been progressing towards the optimal and least invasive management of abdominal aortic aneurysms. During the early years commercial devices encountered various problems leading to various complications. Devices, following various modifications, have gradually improved and nowadays EVAR has gained widespread acceptance. However, complications still exist and considerable rates of secondary interventions are the "achilles heel" of EVAR and a major point of controversy against open repair. Recently, the Eurostar reported an 8.7% (at a mean follow up of 12 months) rate of secondary interventions, while the EVAR-1 and DREAM trials reported significantly higher rates compared to open repair.[1,2,3]

By studying and understanding the cause and nature of EVAR complications, the preoperative planning can be more focused and the rates of secondary interventions can be diminished. Understanding EVAR complications could potentially improve decision making for a secondary intervention (which and when) and its outcome.

Whoever is offering EVAR to his patient should keep in mind that treatment does not end by deploying the graft. EVAR users should feel responsible for the long term treatment success which includes follow-up and treatment of late complications.

The majority of complications following EVAR can be managed by interventional techniques; sometimes a minor surgical procedure is necessary to solve the problem and less frequently a major operation is inevitable. Some of them (e.g. leaks) are very difficult to uncover. In case of recurrent problems it depends mostly on the patient's condition, as to whether the "final solution" of conversion to open repair (with total or partial graft removal) will be the best option.

EVAR complications could be categorized according to various parameters (e.g cause related, or treatment oriented). The following classification of EVAR complications in three groups seems to facilitate categorization and treatment orientation.

1. Vessel (renal or internal iliac artery), graft limb or side-branch (for fenestrated and branched grafts) stenosis or occlusion (thrombosis).
2. Endoleaks.
3. Graft migration.

Vessel (Penal or Internal Iliac Artery), Graft Limb or Side-Branch (for Fenestrated and Branched Grafts) Stenosis or Occlusion (Thrombosis)

a. Renal artery stenosis or occlusion

Upwards slipping of a graft, which was initially placed very close to the renal ostium can lead to renal artery stenosis or occlusion. Depending on the grade of stenosis or occlusion, an unexplained hypertension or sudden renal impairement should alert the physician for such a complication

Proposed intervention

A pull-down manoeuvre of the graft mainbody with a cross-over wire from one groin to the other could liberate the renal ostia. Securing of the renal arteries with

stents, would potentially prevent the recurrence of the complication (Figure 1).

b. Internal iliac artery stenosis or occlusion

Occlusion or stenosis of the hypogastric ostium occurs when the graft limb is chosen too long or placed too far distally. Downward migration of graft limb might happen when the common iliac artery is severely kinked and the distal end of the limb slips downwards. Depending on the status of the contralateral internal iliac artery variable symptoms may occur, ranging from no symptoms to colonic ischemia. However, the most frequent symptom is buttock claudication.

Proposed intervention

The only option, besides removing the limb is to try to push back the distal graft end using an inflated balloon over a stiff

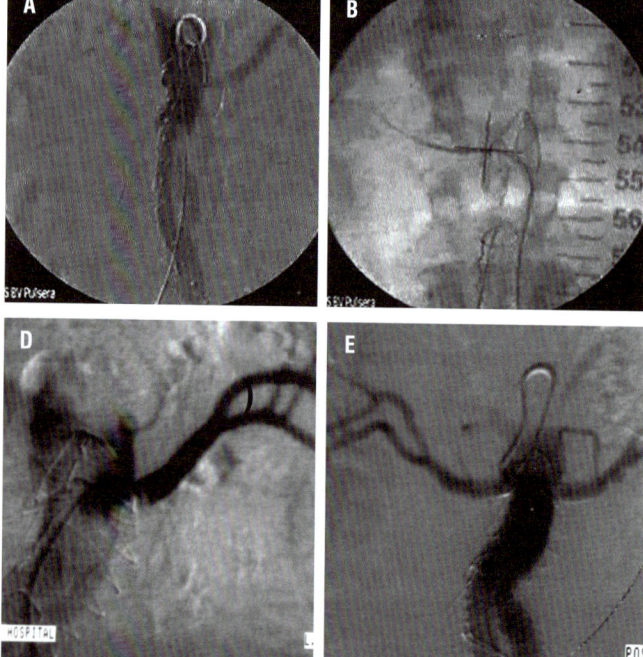
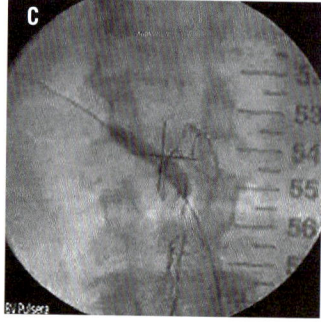

FIGURE 1: Final angiography reveals right renal artery occlusion and severe left renal artery stenosis. An attempt to pull down the graft failed. **A, B, C.** A Simmons catheter was used to cannulate the right renal artery behind the graft and ballon angioplasty and stenting followed. **D, E.** Next day, a stent was placed in the left renal artery and final angiography shows patent both renal vessels.

wire or the edge of a large sheath. Usually only a couple of millimetres can be gained by this manoeuvre.

c. Graft limb stenosis or occlusion

Graft limb occlusions following EVAR have been reported to occur with an incidence up to 15%.[4-6] Late graft limb stenosis/ thrombosis may be due to

- angulated, kinked and stenosed iliac arteries,
- limb kinking following gradual aneurysm shrinkage,[7]
- twisting of the limb during deployment,[8]
- excessive oversizing of the endograft leading to infolding of the graft material within the lumen[8] or due to
- insufficiently flexible graft limbs.

Such a complication usually occurs within the first year and can be suspected in a patient complaining for recent onset of claudication or by a weak femoral pulse in the groin. Sometimes and in the longer term occlusions, it can occur silently because of good collateralisation through the hypogastric arteries.

Proposed intervention
A limb stenosis can be managed by deploying a short length balloon expandable stent ("Palmaz-type"), inserted by the "back-loading technique", e.g using a sheath to pass the stenotic graft limb portion with the balloon-mounted stent.

An occlusion can be managed by initially performing a retrograde recanalization of the occluded limb with a stiff Terumo wire followed by replacement with an ultra-stiff wire (e.g. "back-up Meier"). In older (>4-6 weeks) occlusions the hard consistency of the thrombus and the presence of kinking might require significant force to pass the wire. To center the wire and to gain better push ability it is often helpful to place a large non-compliant balloon at the distal entrance of the limb (Figure 2). After successfully passing the occlusion ballooning of the thrombotic material with a 12 mm angioplasty balloon and deployment of an adequate Palmaz stent will restore the flow (Figure 2). "Ballooning" is generally the preferred intervention, since "Fogarty Manoeuvring" to extract thrombus frequently leads to occlusion of the internal iliac artery. In case an old occlusion fails to be recanalized, cross-over bypass is the final solution.

d. Side-branch stenosis or occlusion in fenestrated grafts

Late loss of side branches in fenestrated grafts can be attributed to angulated, kinked and stenosed target vessels lead-

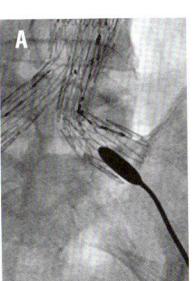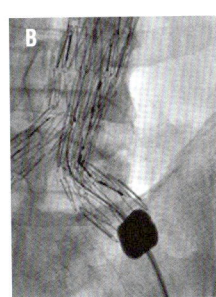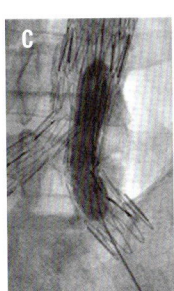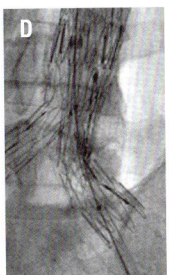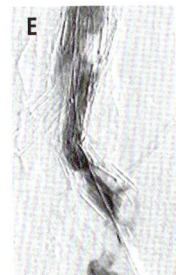

FIGURE 2: Management of limb occlusion, **A**. Attempt to recanalize the limb using an olive dilator through a sheath, **B**. Retrograde recanalization of the occluded limb with a stiff wire centered and supported by an inflated balloon, **C**. Stent deployment, **D**. Final angiography with patent internal iliac artery.

ing to stent deformation and subsequent thrombosis.[9] Neointimal hyperplasia could also be an attributing factor.[10] Migration of the graft's aortic component could also deform the stent and lead to stenosis or occlusion.

Vessel losses in fenestrated grafts can also happen in non-stented target vessels in cases of graft migration.

The symptoms depend on the severity of stenosis or occlusion, the vessel affected and the collateral networks. Our team has experienced superior mesenteric artery occlusion that was initially presented with diarrhoeas that gradually subsided. Following angiography, no further intervention was scheduled, since the collateral network from the open celiac tripod was enough to perfuse the intestines (Figure 3).

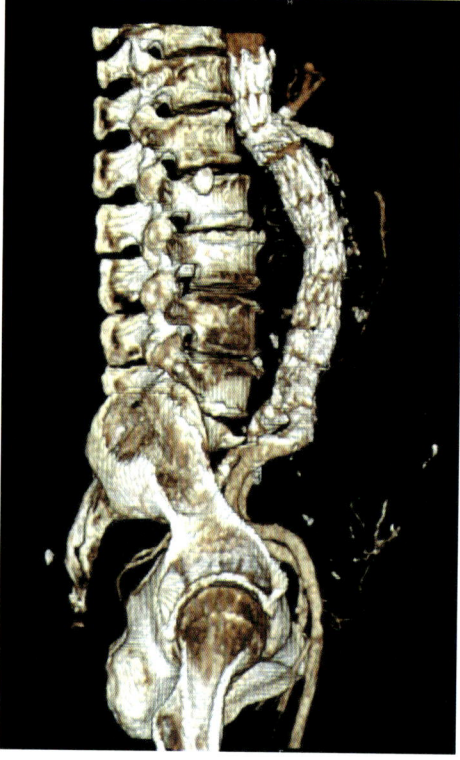

FIGURE 3: Occluded SMA branch. No intervention was necessary since the collateral network from the open celiac tripod was enough to perfuse the intestines.

Proposed intervention
Repeat angioplasty and stenting whenever needed and if possible (Figure 4).

ENDOLEAKS AND GRAFT MIGRATION

a. Type I endoleak

Proximal type I leaks may be due to main body under sizing or inadequate fixation (angled, short, wide or conical necks) of the stent graft (usually primary leak) or due to late dilatation of the infra renal neck (secondary leak), both leading to graft migration.[11-14]

Distal type I leaks may be also due to limb under sizing, inadequate fixation (aneurysmatic or tortuous iliacs) of the limb or due to late dilatation of the common iliac artery.

Since primary leaks are always managed intraoperatively, a secondary intervention usually concerns a secondary one. Sometimes though, it may be a primary one that had not been detected at the time of the operation. Type I leaks should be treated the soonest possible as the risk of aneurysm rupture is multiplied.

Proposed intervention
Treatment options for proximal type I leaks depend on the neck's anatomy and on the graft's position. If the covered part of the graft is more than 5 mm below the lower renal ostium, a cuff (2 mm larger than the original proximal graft diameter) should be deployed and, if required, further secured by a "Palmaz Maxi" stent (self-mounted on a 25 mm PTA balloon, back-loading technique). Recently, modern devices (e.g Zenith® Renu™ AAA Ancillary Graft) are available to seal these type of leaks and improve proximal fixation. These devices are available in configurations offering either a main body proximal extension with a suprarenal bare stent, either an one-piece

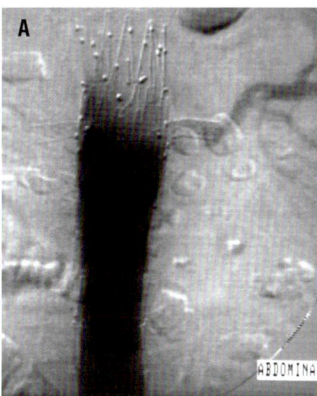
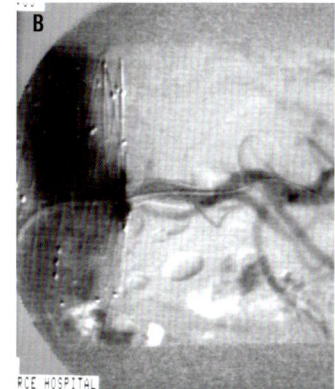
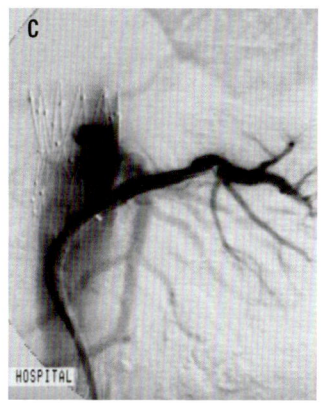

FIGURE 4: One year post-EVAR (fenestrated endograft with two renal side branches) the patient manifests acute renal deterioration, following hospitalization for bladder tumor. **A.** Angiography reveals total occlusion of his right renal and severe stenosis of his left renal artery. **B.** The left renal is catheterized, ballooned and re-stented. **C.** Final angiography shows a patent left renal artery.

converter that finally converts the graft to aortouniiliac, depending on the old graft's configuration (Figure 5).

If the graft is already placed in optimal position, stenting with "Palmaz Maxi" will help only when a calcified tortuous neck prevents the proximal part of the graft to fully expand. Otherwise, the only alternative to open conversion is "neck banding", which however requires an open transabdominal access and can be technically very demanding.

For distal type I leaks, if the distance between the limb and the internal iliac artery is long enough an iliac extension graft of larger diameter can seal the leak without interrupting the hypogastric circulation. If this not possible, alternative options are:

1. Overstenting of the internal ilac artery with an iliac extension graft up to the external iliac artery (preliminary elimination of the internal iliac "back-flow" by coiling is not always necessary).
2. Iliac extension graft to the external iliac

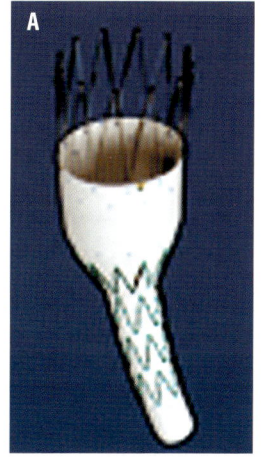
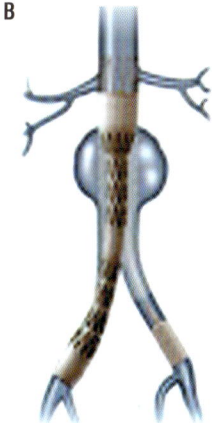

FIGURE 5: Zenith® Renu™ AAA Ancillary Graft for type I leak sealing. The one-piece converter converts the graft to aortouniiliac.

artery and re-implantation-transposition of the internal iliac artery (only in anatomically suitable patients, demanding surgical procedure)

3. Banding of the common iliac artery over the insufficient graft limb, by an oblique lateral flank incision (retroperitoneal access).

4. Secondary implantation of an iliac bifurcation device. This is an alternative for cases of aneurysmal common iliac artery and patent, non-stenosed, internal iliac offspring and remains a demanding interventional procedure.[15]

Our team has also encountered a distal type I leak from the distal end of the side branch of an iliac bifurcation device. Ballooning sealed the leak (Figure 6).

b. Type II endoleak

Type II endoleaks, arising from branches of the aorta (inferior mesenteric or vertebral arteries for infrarenal AAA) occur frequently and may appear either early (within a year) either late (within 3 years or more).[8]

In many cases, the presence of a type II endoleak may not be of great consequence because most of these follow a more indolent course and resolve spontaneously without a need to subject the patient to any additional interventions.

During the early experience of EVAR, the significance and natural history of endoleaks was not well understood, thus most patients had an intervention for treatment of their endoleak. Current knowledge and experience dictates that type II endoleaks, do not justify conversion, unless there is evidence of significant expansion of the aneurysm sac. As a result, many surgeons have taken a less aggressive stance in treating these endoleaks; however, exact treatment patterns and timing of intervention may vary from surgeon to surgeon.

Proposed intervention

Coil embolization seems to be the preferred method. However, selective embolization with coils placed at the origin of the IMA may not be a sufficient treatment for type II endoleaks because some collateral branches may lead to reperfusion of the aneurysm. Combining injections of thrombogenic materials directly into the sac may improve the long term ourcomes and the reduce the risk of relapse. Selective catheterization of the arch of Riolan and of the IMA permits embolization of the aneurysm sac. Embolization of the lumbar arteries is also feasible in certain cases (Figure 7). The direct transTlumbar puncture of the aneurysm sac under fluoroscopic or CT guidance can be attempted as an alternative treatment

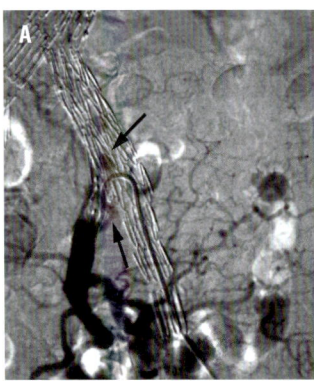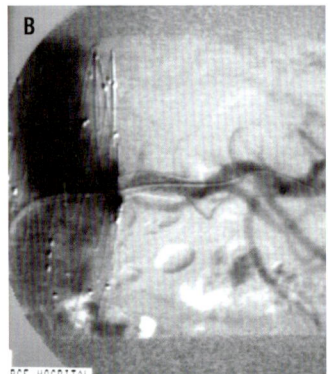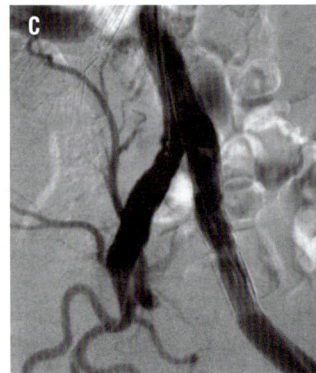

FIGURE 6: Type I endoleak from the distal end of the side branch of an iliac bifurcation device. Balloon inflation into the side branch and internal iliac artery seals the leak.

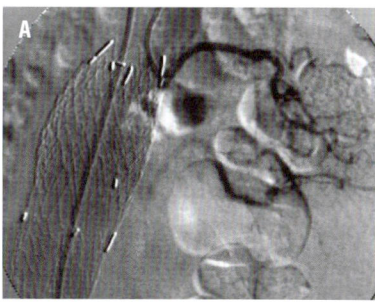
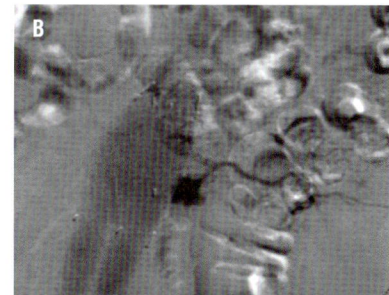
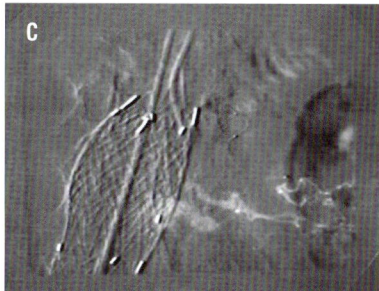
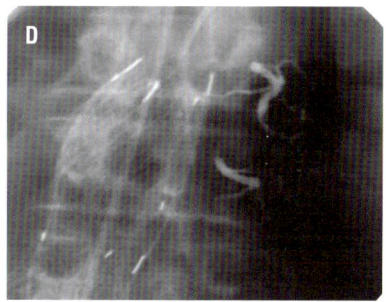

FIGURE 7: Type II endoleak from lumbar arteries. Through a Simmons catheter a microcatheter (Rebar MTI) is advanced in the lumbar collateral circulation and a liquid embolic agent (ONYX MTI) is infused to occlude both lumbars.

modality. Surgical or laparoscopic clipping of the arteries involved or open exposure of the aneurysm sac remain the last solution.

c. Type III endoleak

Type III endoleaks occur when there is a structural failure of the endovascular device and may be due to device disruptions, due to suture holes or due to disconnection of the modular graft's components (main body –limb or proximal tube– distal bifurcated body for composite grafts). Disconnection, under the forces of strong blood stream pulsations, can be attributed to insufficient between-components fixation and the most usual cause seems to be insufficient overlapping. Immediate management is necessary.

Proposed intervention
Deployment of a bridging graft (2 mm larger than the original proximal graft diameter) would most of the times resolve the leak.

d. Type IV endoleak

Type IV endoleaks are attributed to graft matereial failure (porosity) or to overtime small graft lesions that both lead blood egression through the pores or the lesions in the fabric. These are mostly seen in early generation grafts usually many years after implantation (solid thrombus) and are difficult to detect. Angiography does not help to detect these lesions.

Proposed intervention
In case of growing aneurysm open exposure and conversion is the safest option to reveal the suspected reason of graft failure. Alternatively an aortouniiliac "conversion graft" with a contralateral iliac occlusion and a femoro-femoral bypass can be used.

GRAFT MIGRATION

Graft migration is the most insidious complication of endovascular repair. Migration can be downward, but also upward and lateral or anterior.[16] Migration is usually the result of insufficient proximal or distal fixation: device (suprarenal stirixis or not, hooks, barbs, over or undersizing etc), anatomy (wide, angled or conical necks) and physician related (experienced or not). Whichever is the reason of migration the final result would be a vessel stenosis or occlusion, or a type I or III endoleak. The proposed interventions have already been described above.

Conclusions

The need for secondary interventions has tended to decline in recent years, attributed partly in improved devices and partly in experience growth. However EVAR experience has not yet matured for many vascular interventionalists and complications continue to evolve. It is however apparent that most complications can by managed endovascularrly. Most of the secondary interventions can be carried out percutaneously, usually via transfemoral procedures. Accurate parameters that define the need for secondary interventions to treat endoleaks have not yet been fully established. Expansion of the aneurysm sac is, however, an accepted indication for reintervention.[1]

References

1. Hobo R, Buth J. Secondary interventions following endovascular abdominal aortic aneurysm repair using current endografts. A EUROSTAR report. J Vasc Surg 2006;43:896-902.
2. EVAR trial participants. Endovascular aneurysm repair versus open repair in patients with abdominal aortic aneurysm (EVAR trial 1): randomised controlled trial. Lancet 2005; 365: 2179-86.
3. DREAM Trial Group. Two-Year Outcomes after Conventional or Endovascular Repair of Abdominal Aortic Aneurysms. N Engl J Med 352;2398-405.
4. Conners MS, Sternbergh WC, Carter G, et al. Secondary procedures after endovascular aortic aneurysm repair. J Vasc Surg 2002;36: 992-6.

5. Carpenter JP, Anderson WN, Brewster DC, et al. Multicenter pivotal trial results of the lifepath system for endovascular aortic aneurysm repair. J Vasc Surg 2004;39:34-43.
6. Krajcer Z, Gilbert JH, Dougherty K, et al. Successful treatment of aortic endograft thrombosis with rheolytic thrombectomy. J Endovasc Ther 2002;9:756-64.
7. Buth J, Lheij RJF. Early complications and endoleaks after endovascular abdominal aortic aneurysm repair; report of a multicenter study. J Vasc Surg 2000; 31:134-146.
8. Lalka S, Dalsing M, Cikrit D, Sawchuk A, Shafique S, Nachreiner R, Pandurangi K. Secondary interventions after endovascular abdominal aortic aneurysm repair. Am J Surg 2005; 190: 787-794.
9. Semmens JB, Lawrence-Brown M, Hartley DE, et al. Outcomes of Fenestrated Endografts in the Treatment of Abdominal Aortic Aneurysm in Western Australia (1997-2004) J Endovasc Ther 2006;13:320-329.
10. Halak M, Goodman MA, Baker SR. The Fate of Target Visceral Vessels After Fenestrated Endovascular Aortic Repair-General Considerations and Mid-term Results Eur J Vasc Endovasc Surg 2006; 32:124-128.
11. Zarins CK, White RA, Fogarty TJ. Aneurysm rupture after endovascular repair using the AneurRx stent graft. J Vasc Surg 2000; 31:960-970.
12. Politz JK, Newman VS, Stewart MT. Late abdominal aortic aneurysm rupture after AneurRx repair: a report of three cases.J Vasc Surg 2000; 31:599-606.
13. Saghal A, Veith FJ, Lipitz E, et al. Diameter changes in isolated iliac artery aneurysms 1 to 6 years after endovascular graft repair. J Vasc Surg 2000; 33:289-295.
14. Chuter TA, Risberg B, Hopkinson BR, et al. Clinical experience with a bifurcated endovascular graft for abdominal aortic aneurysm repair. J Vasc Surg 1996; 24:152-168.
15. Ziegler P, Avgerinos ED, Umscheid T, Perdikides T, Erz K, Stelter WJ. Branched iliac bifurcation: 6 years experience with endovascular preservation of internal iliac artery flow. J Vasc Surg 2007; 46:204-10.
16. Umscheid T, Stelter WJ. Time-related alterations in shape, position and structure of self expanding, modular aortic stent grafts: a 4-year single-center follow up. J Endovasc Surg 1999;6:17-32.

Percutaneous endovascular AAA repair

Aysel Can, Giovanni Torsello

INTRODUCTION

Endovascular repair of an abdominal aortic aneurysm (AAA) has proven to decrease operative morbidity and postoperative patient discomfort. The implantation of stent grafts requires the use of large-bore sheaths (16 F-24 F) usually needing surgical exposure of the common femoral artery (CFA). The bilateral groin dissection is associated with local complications such as wound infection, lymphocele and hematoma usually requiring re-exploration.[1] In addition, postoperative scar tissue makes future access to the femoral arteries more difficult and increases the frequence of complications. With the objective of further decreasing the invasiveness of the procedure, the preclosing technique using Prostar XL (Perclose, Redwood City, CA) has been developed for complete percutaneous endovascular aneurysm repair. Prostar XL is a suture based closure device and has been used for more than 8 years at our institution in many patients after a wide variety of percutaneous interventions. This device was first effectually evaluated in patients undergoing peripheral and coronary angiography or intervention. The use of this device was then extended for the endovascular treatment of AAA. Until today, many studies have been published analyzing the advantages and disadvantages of this device as well as the procedure related complications.[2-8]

DEVICE DESCRIPTION

The Perclose device (Prostar XL) is made up of two components. The first component is a sheath containing four lance-like needles which are connected at their tips to two suture loops. The second component of the device includes a deployment ring and a barrel. This is positioned above the artery to guide the needle trajectory through the subcutaneous tissue once the sutures have been pulled through the arterial wall from inside out. The 6 F device (Techstar, Perclose) delivers two needles and one suture through the arterial wall, whereas the 8 F and 10 F devices (Prostar XL, Perclose) deliver four needles and two sutures. Usually, the two-needle (single suture) device is employed to close arterial puncture sites after diagnostic or interventional catheterization procedures performed through 5 F and 6 F introducer sheaths. The four-needle device (two sutures) is used to achieve hemostasis after interventional procedures performed through 7 F to 10 F introducer sheaths.[9,10] For endovascular exclusion of abdominal aortic aneurysms larger sheaths are used requiring the application of a pre-close technique. For this purpose a 10F device is deployed at the start of the procedure, ensuring that the needles penetrate the arterial wall before the arteriotomy is enlarged by the use of sheaths up to 24 F.[3,4,6,11] The use of this device requires slight enlargement of the skin incision and subcutaneous track dilation at the puncture site. The sutures are fastened at the end of the procedure after removing of the sheath. Hemostasis is achieved by sliding a self-locking surgical knot to the artery. The positioning of the knot can be adjusted by using a knot pusher.

PRE-CLOSE TECHNIQUE

Arterial access is achieved with an 18-gauge needle by introducing an 8 F sheath into the common femoral artery. The puncture should be performed at level of the in-guinal ligament to avoid placement of the introducers in the superficial femoral or profunda artery. The sheath is then exchanged over a 0.035 inch nonhydrophilic guide wire for a 10 F Prostar XL (Figure 1). In order to facilitate device introduction and making correct device positioning possible, the subcutaneous tissue should be prepared by simply rotating the device barrel (Figure 2) after slightly extending the cutaneous incision using a scalpel. In some cases an extended atraumatic preparation of the subcutaneous tissue is needed, accomplished by using a mosquito clamp in order to advance smoothly the device. A pulsatile back bleeding from a marker lumen (Figures 3 and 4) indicates when the device has reached its correct position through the arterial wall. After 90° anti-clockwise rotation of the ring shaped handle the lance-like needles can be deployed by pulling back the ring (Figure 4). The arterial wall is now captured by the sutures and the needles are removed with a needle holder (Figure 5). After cutting the suture at the tip of the nitinol needles, the device is

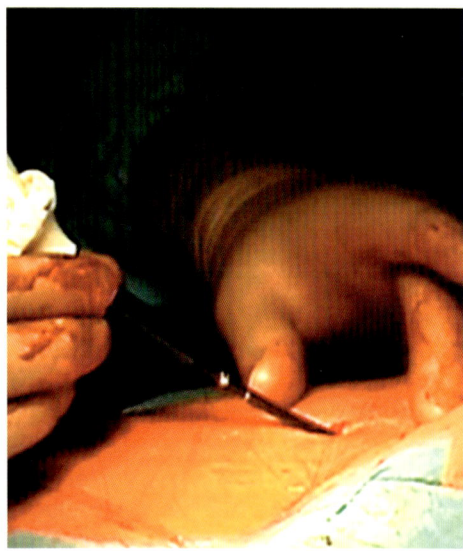

FIGURE 1: Placement of the Prostar XL, the guide wire is already removed.

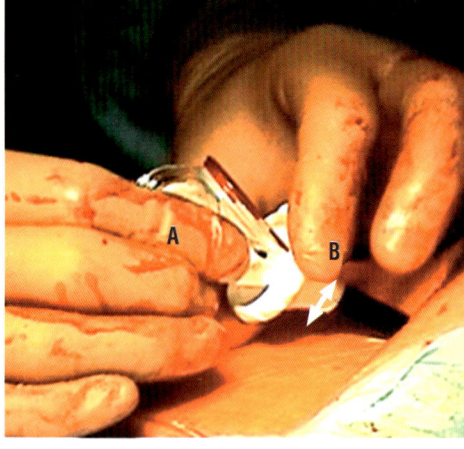

FIGURE 2: To achieve a pulsatile back bleeding from the marker lumen the device has to be compressed slightly (**A**) and the barrel (**B**) needs to be rotated (arrow in the picture) after atraumatic preparation of the subcutaneous tissue.

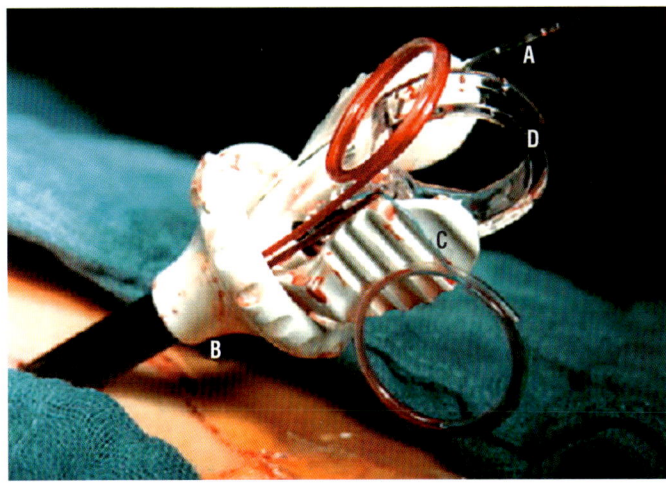

FIGURE 3: The Prostar XL device with the marker lumen (**A**) and the device barrel (**B**). After compression of the device (**C**) the ring shaped handle (**D**) has to be rotated 90° anti-clockwise. Then it can be pulled as far as it will go.

partially withdrawn from the vessel. The sutures are then hold by a mosquito clamp until the end of the endovascular procedure. Next, the device is exchanged for a large introducer sheath (12 F or 14 F) via a guide wire for dilation of the vessel at the access site. After completion of the endovascular procedure the sutures are tied using the fisherman knot technique (Figure 6). The introducer sheath is removed under manual compression of the groin and the prepared knots are advanced to the vessel wall (Figure 7). Hemostasis is achieved by sliding the self-locking knot and by holding the knot with the knot pusher for a while (Figure 8). It is helpful to soak the sutures generously with heparin saline solution and to ensure that they run freely before advancing the knot. Finally, the skin incision is approximated by a single stitch knot or sterile strips and covered by a sterile dressing. Additionally, a low pressure bandage is applied for 4-6 hours.

PATIENT SELECTION

The feasibility, safety and efficacy of percutaneous repair of aortic aneurysms depend on the adequate selection of patients and appropriate puncture and suture technique.

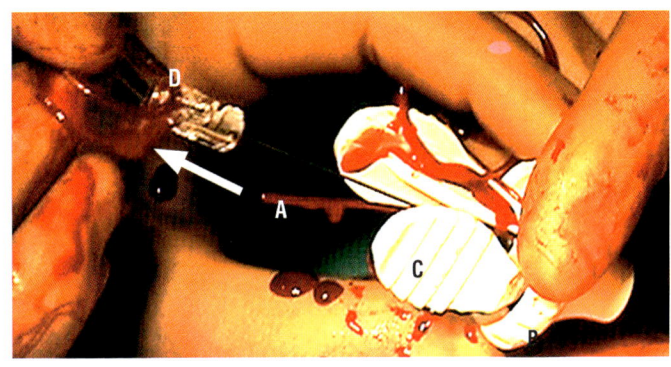

FIGURE 4: A pulsatile back bleeding (**A**) indicates correct position of the device through the vessel wall. By pulling back the ring shaped handle (**D**) the needles can be deployed.

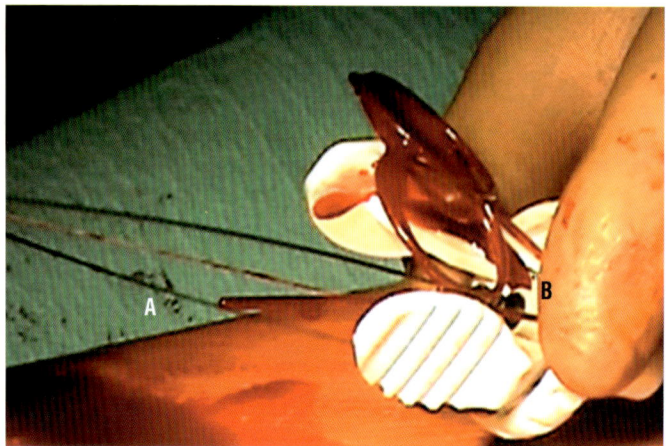

FIGURE 5: With a needle holder the needles (**A, B**) can be removed.

Obesity is one major risk factor affecting the success of the percutaneous technique. The puncture is technically demanding. Nevertheless, the treatment of obese patients by a percutaneous technique can reduce the rate of wound infections and should be seen as the first approach option. One more important risk factor is calcification of the common femoral artery. The presence of calcifications of the anterior vessel wall at the puncture site is a contraindication for the percutaneous approach. The nitinol needles are not able to capture the vessel wall and can deflect into the subcutaneous tissue.

A further significant risk factor is the presence of an inguinal arterial prosthesis or aneurysm of the femoral artery. We do not recommend using the perclose device in these patients either.

The use of the PVS device in patients with PAOD was considered a disadvantage for a long time because of the higher rate of severe calcifications of the com-

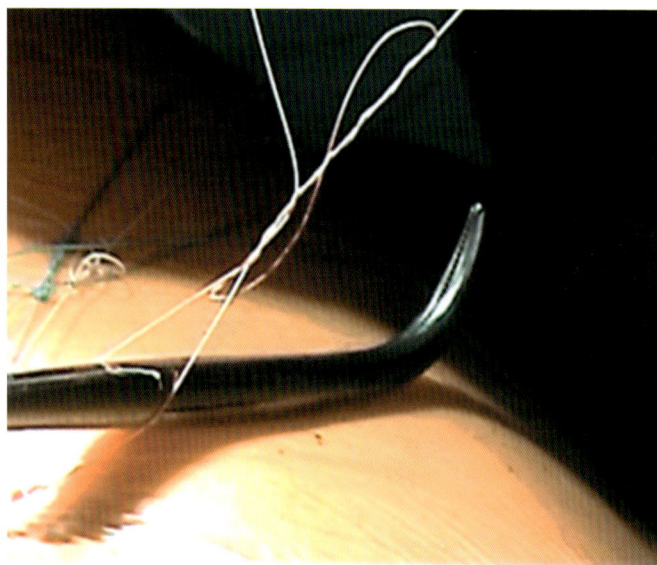

FIGURE 6: After completion of the endovascular procedure the sutures are tied using the fisherman knot technique.

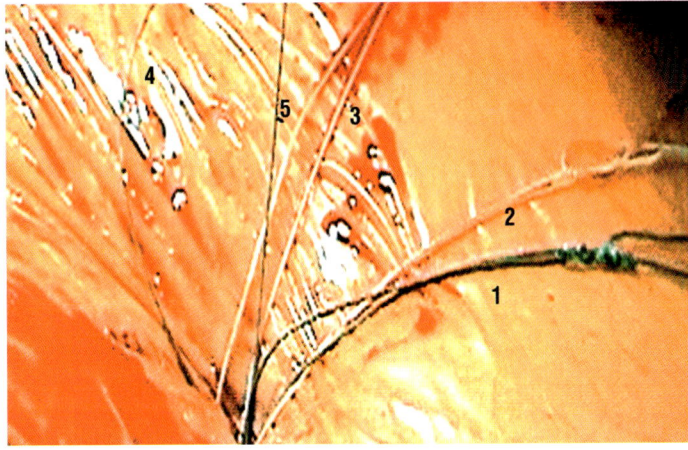

FIGURE 7: The prepared knots **(1-4)**, are advanced to the vessel wall by pulling them slightly in direction of the femoral artery and simultaneous removing of the guide wire **(5)**.

mon femoral artery in this particular group of patients. However, Starnes et al showed that percutaneous closures were successfully achieved also in arteries with anterior calcification.[12]

A closure device failure can also occur in patients with a small vessel diameter (<6 mm) or when the femoral bifurcation is on a higher level than usual. Therefore, a duplex ultrasound of the groin should be performed to assess the feasibility of the percutaneous technique. In these cases the risk of an arterial wall rupture is increased as well.

COMPLICATIONS AND TROUBLE SHOOTING

The percutaneous technique is an important step forward for less invasive treatment of aortic aneurysms. However, satisfactory hemostasis after use of large introducer sheaths depends on a careful pa-

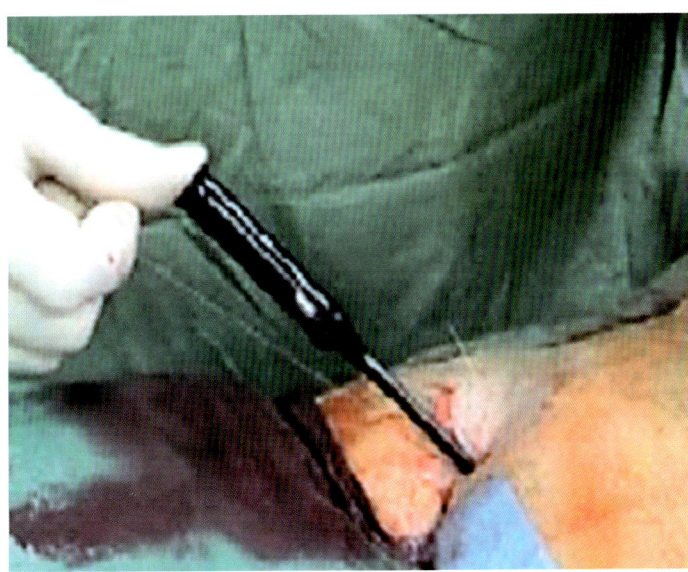

FIGURE 8: A knot pusher can be used for further advancement of the knot.

tient selection, an appropriate suture technique and trouble shooting. Based on the stage of the procedure we distinguish several sources of complications.

Device introduction

If the femoral puncture has been made too low, the introduction of large introducers through the superficial femoral or profunda artery would tear the vessel wall. Therefore, it is important to identify the common femoral artery by taking into account the preoperative imaging (Duplex scan, CT or angiography) or by performing an angiography during the procedure. We recommend a puncture at level of the inguinal ligament.

In the presence of tortuosity of the iliac arteries or of the aneurysm neck, the forced advancement of Prostar XL can be dangerous, leading to peripheral embolism or rupture of the arterial wall. In such cases we do not exceptionally remove the guidewire before the tip of the Prostar XL has passed the tortuosity even after the wire entry port has passed under the skin.

Needle deployment

Another complication occurs when the nitinol needles cannot be retrieved. This complication is extremely rare and can simply be treated by reinserting the wire and using another Prostar XL device.

In case of scarring of the groin or calcification of the anterior vessel wall, the flexible nitinol needles can deflect while retracting the handle. If possible, the handle should be pushed back into the hub and after the guidewire has been reinserted, the Prostar XL device can be removed. If this manoeuvre is not possible, removal of the deflected needle must be performed after enlargement of the skin incision. A digital exploration should be avoided. Under fluoro control the needle should be identified and removed using a clamp or needle holder.

Getting flow through the marker lumen

If no pulsatile flow through the marker lumen is achievable, the needles cannot grasp the arterial wall. In this case, it is not advisable to retract the handle. Especially, in obese patients it is mandatory to create a sufficient subcutaneous tunnel between the skin and the vessel wall. In case of unsufficient back flow we recommend to flush the port with heparin saline solution and to slightly rotate the device to exclude mechanical obstruction of the marker lumen.

Knot slipping

Disruption of the vessel wall during slipping of the fisherman knot can be avoided by preventing twisting of the sutures and testing the free run before performing the knot, we recommend to irrigate the multifilament sutures and remove accurately fibrin and debris from the suture surface.

It is also helpful to pull gently the long end of the suture in the right direction while slipping the knot and using the knot pusher for advancing the knot to the vessel wall.

When feeling resistance while advancing the knot, the reason should be carefully evaluated.

Final bleeding control

The guidewire should be removed first after successful bleeding control has been achieved. If this is not sufficient, the knot should be moved against the vessel wall with the knot pusher for a while compressing manually the artery above the puncture site. High blood pressure should be normalized. If the above mentioned measures are not effective, a PTFE felt pledget can be sewn using the sutures of Prostar XL. This technique, well known from conventional cardiovascular surgery, is useful to avoid surgical exploration of the femoral vessel.

POSTOPERATIVE PATIENT CARE

After successful hemostasis is achieved, an appropriate sterile pressure dressing is applied to the puncture site. Patients can be permitted to get up 2-4 hours after suture when no or minimal subcutaneous oozing is present. The femoral access site and pulses should be monitored and duplex ultrasound should be performed before hospital discharge. Any suspected bleeding complication or incomplete hemostasis can be treated with adjunctive compression and prolonged application of pressure bandage. False aneurysms require surgical treatment.

DISCUSSION

The percutaneous endovascular aneurysm repair provides a less invasive access to the aorta in contrast to the surgical cutdown of the femoral arteries. The percutaneous closure technique enables the physician to perform the complete endovascular procedure in local or regional anesthesia. Especially, the treatment of ruptured aortic aneurysms benefits from this alternative.

Success rates of percutaneous endograft implantation without conversion to an open groin incision described in several clinical studies ranges between 46.2 % to 93 %.[1-7]

It is hypothesized that results of percutaneous closure of 16 F access sites are better than those of larger access sites (22-25 F).[4,7,8]

Therefore, most teams use tandem devices for sheaths over 18 F with different recommendations for rotation of the second device.[2] In our experience the use of two Prostar 10 F devices has no advantage. Too many threads can cause catching on other sutures, disrupting the vessel wall during fastening of the knot.[6] Nevertheless, we believe that the success

rate depends on the learning curve of the physician.

Pseudoaneurysm, arteriovenous fistula as well as arterial occlusion or stenosis are possible complications of this technique. In a recent prospective study Watelet et al described one pseudoaneurysm and three bleedings in four out of 29 cases which healed spontaneously.[8] No late complication was detected after a mean follow-up of 17.5 months. The incidence of infection after placement of percutaneous suture-mediated devices is low. Watelet et al reported no infection.[8] As consequences of this complication may be disastrous, prevention is best provided by pre-procedural antibiotics, together with a sterile technique and environment. We further recommend a Duplex scan of the groin before and 3 months after discharge to maintain adequate follow-up.

When comparing both procedures, femoral cutdown and percutaneous technique, regarding the total costs there is no significant difference.[6] There is only another distribution of fixed and instrumentation costs. The surgical cutdown approach necessitates a longer mean operation time and longer postoperative hospital stay associated with accordant hospital costs.

REFERENCES

1. Borner G, Ivancev K, Sonesson B, Lindblad B, Griffin D, Malina M. Percutaneous AAA repair: Is it safe? J Endovasc Ther. 2004;11:621-626.
2. Howell M, Villareal R, Krajcer Z. Percutaneous access and closure of femoral artery access site associated with endoluminal repair of abdominal aortic aneurysm. J Endovasc Ther. 2001;8:68-74.
3. Howell M, Doughtery K, Strickmann N, Krajcer Z. Percutaneous repair of abdominal aortic aneurysms using the AneuRx stent graft and the percutaneous vascular surgery device. Cathet Cardiovasc Intervent. 2002;55:281-287.
4. Rachel ES, Bergamini TM, Kinney EV, Jung MT, Kaebnik HW, Mitchell RA. Percutaneous endovas-

cular abdominal aortic aneurysm repair. Ann Vasc Surg. 2002;16:43-49.

5. Teh LG, Sieunarine K, van Schie G, Goodman MA, Lawrence-Brown M, Prendergast FJ et al. Use of the percutaneous vascular surgery device for closure of femoral access sites during endovascular aneurysm repair: lessons from our experience. Eur J Vasc Endovasc Surg. 2001;22:418-423.

6. Torsello GB, Kasprzak B, Klenk E et al. Endovascular Suture versus cutdown for endovascular aneurysm repair: A prospective randomized pilot study. J Vasc Surg. 2003;38:78-82.

7. Traul DK, Clair DG, Gray B, O'Hara PJ, Ouriel K. Percutaneous endovascular repair of infrarenal abdominal aortic aneurysms: a feasibility study. J Vasc Surg. 2000;32:770-776.

8. Watelet J, Gallot JC, Thomas P, Douvrin F and Plissonier D. Percutaneous Repair of Aortic Aneurysms: A Prospective Study of Suture-Mediated Closure Devices. Eur J Vasc Endovasc Surg. 2006;32:261-265.

9. Baim D, Pinkerton C, Vetter J. Acute results of the STAND II percutaneous vascular surgical device trial. (Abstr.). Circulation. 1997;96:(Suppl I)1-442.

10. Gerckens U, Caatelaens N, Muller R. Percutaneous suture of femoral artery access sites after diagnostic heart catheterization and or coronary intervention. Safety and effectiveness of a new arterial suture technique. Herz. 1998;23:27-34.

11. Haas PC, Krajcer Z, Diethrich EB. Closure of large percutaneous access sites using Prostar XL percutaneous vascular surgery device. J Endovasc Surg. 1999;6:168-170.

12. Starnes BW, O'Donnell SD, Gillespie DL, Goff JM, Rosa P, Parker MV, Chang A. Percutaneous arterial closure in peripheral vascular disease: A prospective randomized evaluation of the Perclose device. J Vasc Surg. 2003:38;263-71.

13. Singh N, Adams E, Neville R, Deaton DH. Percutaneous Endovascular AAA Repair. Endovascular Today. April 2005;39-44.

Chapter 29

325

29. IS REMOTE INTRASAC PRESSURE MEASUREMENT A RELIABLE ALTERNATIVE SURVEILLANCE MODALITY?

Is remote intrasac pressure measurement a reliable alternative surveillance modality?

Pegge Halandras, Ross Milner

INTRODUCTION

Endovascular aortic aneurysm repair (EVAR) has become a widely utilized alternative to open abdominal aortic aneurysm repair since its introduction by Juan Parodi in 1991.[1] Initially, this technique was applied to patients that had significant comorbidities making the risks of open surgery prohibitive. Since its inception fifteen years ago, use of EVAR has dramatically increased with as many as 40% of all elective infrarenal abdominal aortic aneurysms (AAA) in Medicare patients repaired with endografts in 2003.[2] The number of patients treated by EVAR continues to increase as more devices become FDA-approved. Currently, there is a scarcity of long-term data regarding EVAR and lifelong endograft surveillance is essential. Surveillance techniques are aimed at detecting device migration, endoleaks, evaluation of residual aneurysm sac size and predicting the need for reintervention. The importance of surveillance is demonstrated by reports of a 10% per year reintervention rate with long-term analysis of EVAR patients.[3]

SURVEILLANCE

Current standard of care

Standard surveillance techniques and schedules consist of obtaining what is currently considered the gold standard study, computed tomography angiography (CTA). CTA's are usually obtained at one month, six months and 12 months after the implant, and then annually thereafter. CTA is frequently augmented with additional studies such as plain abdominal radiographs to detect device orientation and structural abnormalities. Duplex ultrasonography can also be used to detect endoleaks and changes in residual aneurysm sac dimensions. If no device abnormalities or changes in the excluded aneurysm sac are detected, surveillance is usually continued on an annual basis. Limitations of the current methods of surveillance are directly related to obtaining frequent CT scans. This modality exposes patients to radiation and nephrotoxic contrast. In addition, surveillance protocols add significant expense to EVAR with one study reporting an average follow-up cost per year after EVAR of roughly $1000.[4] Alternative surveillance methods that limit nephrotoxicity have been proposed and include following aneurysm sacs with non-contrast CT scans and endoleak evaluation with magnetic resonance angiography (MRA). Recently, the addition of continuous contrast infusion during contrast-enhanced ultrasound studies was reported to demonstrate increased detection of endoleaks when compared to CTA.[5] Although hampered by operator dependency, this may prove to be a cost-efficient alternative to CTA in the future. The above described limitations (Table 1) have lead to interest in alternative imaging protocols or novel techniques for endograft surveillance.

Advances in surveillance techniques

One notable new surveillance technique that promises a noninvasive, convenient, and sensitive mechanism for predicting EVAR failure is remote pressure sensing. The technology of remote pressure sensing devices involves implantation of wireless sensors into the excluded aneurysm sac at the time of aortic endograft placement. The main function of these sensors is to obtain intrasac measurements of the systolic and diastolic pressures.

The utility for surveillance by remote pressure sensor devices is supported by the observation that successful EVAR results in complete exclusion of the aneurysm sac and the reduction of aneurysm sac pressurization. In theory, by protecting the aneurysm sac from exposure to systemic pressure, the risks of dilation and rupture of the aneurysm sac will be eliminated. Several investigators have studied the relationship between excluded aneurysm sac pressures and the degree of success of EVAR. These studies have required invasive techniques and involve comparing systemic pressures to intrasac pressures obtained by sensors placed by translumbar puncture. In patients with documented excluded AAA's, intrasac pressures were dramatically lower than intra-aortic pressures and minimal pulsatile variations were recorded.[6] In patients with known endoleaks, access to the preserved aortic sacs was obtained by cannulation of patent inferior mesenteric arteries through superior mesenteric arteries, direct cannulation around attachment sites, or translumbar sac punctures in the perioperative period. In contrast, these measurements were consistent with elevated and pulsatile sac pressures.[7] These findings support the use of remote pressure sensors as a means of detecting exclusion of a residual aneurysm sac and a means of noninvasive surveillance of abdominal endografts.

REMOTE PRESSURE SENSORS

Two devices are currently being used and evaluated. The design and investigation of each device will now be discussed.

Impressure sensor

The first device is the Impressure Sensor (Remon Medical Technologies, Caesarea, Israel). This device consists of a transducer that is 3 mm x 9 mm x 1.5 mm in size (Figure 1). In initial clinical studies, the de-

TABLE 1 PROBLEMS WITH CURRENT MONITORING TECHNIQUES
Safety
Radiation exposure
Renal toxicity
Inaccurate
Inconvenient
Expensive
Patient compliance

327

29. IS REMOTE INTRASAC PRESSURE MEASUREMENT A RELIABLE ALTERNATIVE SURVEILLANCE MODALITY?

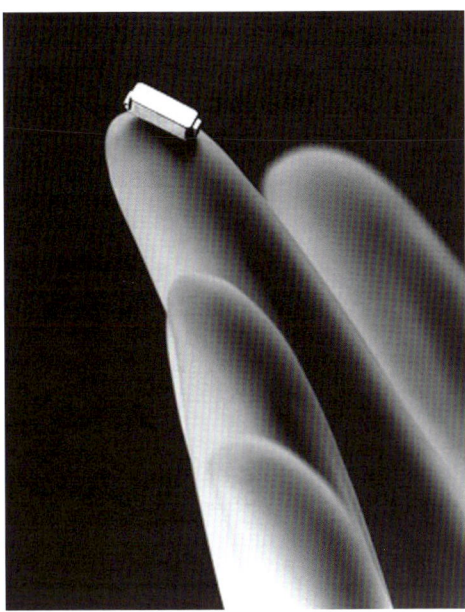

FIGURE 1: Impressure sensor by Remon Medical Technologies. The sensor measures 3 mm x 9 mm x 1.5 mm in size.

vice has been sutured to the endograft prior to insertion (Figure 2). The technology involves activation of a capacitor by conversion of ultrasound energy from a hand-held external ultrasound probe to electrical energy. This activated capacitor then provides energy for the transducer to obtain ambient pressure measurements. This data is then converted from an electrical signal to an ultrasound signal that is relayed to the external ultrasound probe. The converted measurement is then displayed on a monitor.

The Initial evaluation of the Impressure Sensor was conducted in a porcine model. In this study, abdominal aortic aneurysms were surgically created and excluded. Sensor devices were then implanted within the excluded aneurysm sac. Sensor pressure measurements were obtained in a noninvasive transcutaneous method with an ultrasound probe and compared to invasive catheter pressure measurements taken from the aorta

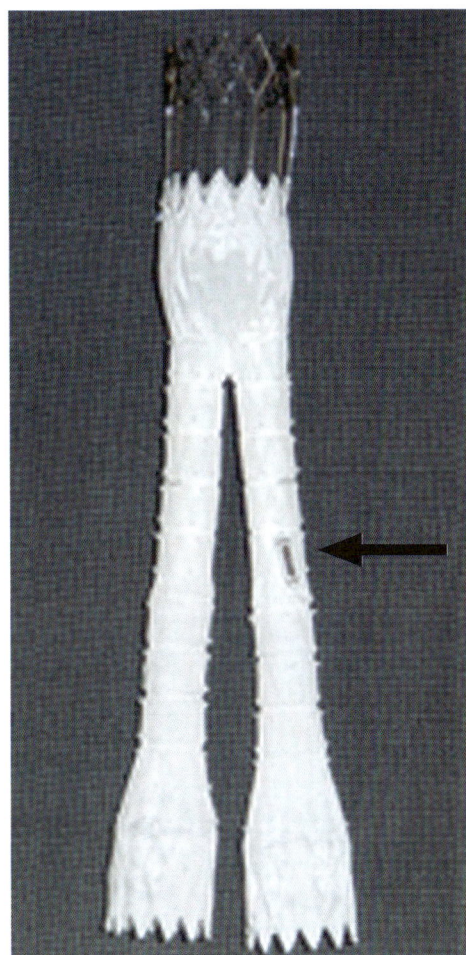

FIGURE 2: Impressure sensor sutured to the left-sided limb of an aortic endograft. The sensor is highlighted by the black arrow.

and excluded aneurysm sac. Type II and III endoleaks were created and the sensor pressures were shown to correlate with the associated elevated catheter pressure readings.[8]

Ellozy et al performed the first prospective study in humans in which fourteen patients undergoing EVAR had Impressure Sensors sewn to endografts prior to their deployment. These patients were followed for a mean of 2.6 months. Of those patients followed, only one device became nonfunctional in this time period. At one month, one patient with a type I endoleak demonstrated an elevated sac pressure that decreased appropriately with correction of the type I endoleak at three month follow-up evaluation. Four of the six patients without endoleaks demonstrated significant decreases in sac pressures during this time period. The remaining two patients without endoleaks had persistently elevated sac pressures of an indeterminate nature. One suggestion is that this elevation can be attributed to the phenomenon of endotension. Of the three patients with documented type II endoleaks, sac pressure was also noted to gradually diminish but not as dramatically as the sac pressures in those patients without endoleaks.[9] Additional investigation by this group has confirmed that those aneurysms that continue to shrink in size following EVAR also demonstrate more dramatic decreases in intrasac pressures.[10]

EndoSure sensor

The second device is the CardioMems Endosure Wireless AAA Pressure Sensor (CardioMems, Inc., Atlanta, GA). This device consists of an inductive-capacitive resonant circuit with a variable capacitor (Figure 3). The device is placed in the aneurysm sac through its own delivery sheath and the circuit is charged by radio-frequency energy transmitted by an external antenna (Figure 4 and 5). The resonant frequency of the activated circuit is altered by the pressure detected in the aneurysm sac and the sensor transmits a resonant frequency signal back to the antenna. This signal is subsequently converted to a pressure measurement by the Endosure software and displayed on an external monitor. The EndoSure Wireless Pressure Sensor has received FDA clearance for acute exclusion of an aneurysm sac during endograft repair. Clinical trials are planned to gain clearance for long-term surveillance

Data collected in the Acute Pressure Measurement to Confirm Aneurysm Sac Exclusion (APEX) trial has been instrumental in the FDA approval of implantation of the second type of device, the EndoSure Sensor. Currently, this approval

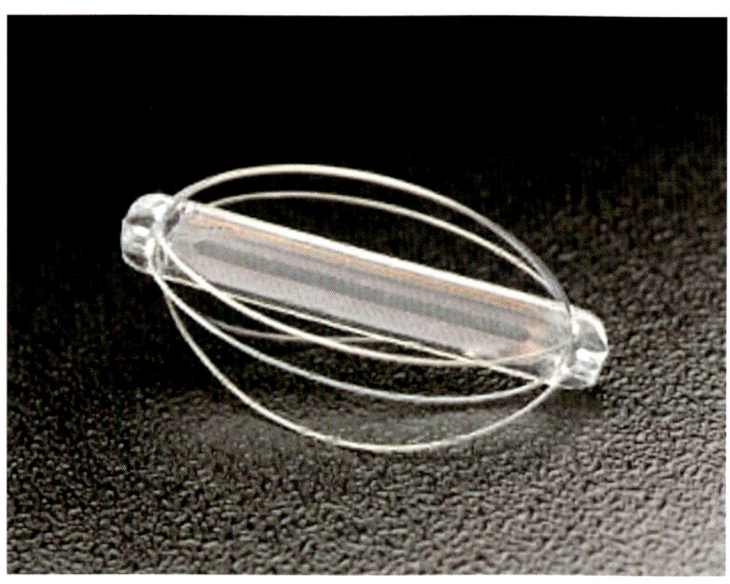

FIGURE 3: EndoSure Wireless AAA Pressure Sensor developed by CardioMems, Inc. This sensor has recently received FDA-clearance for marketing.

329

29. IS REMOTE INTRASAC PRESSURE MEASUREMENT A RELIABLE ALTERNATIVE SURVEILLANCE MODALITY?

FIGURE 4: EndoSure sensor within an excluded aneurysm sac after endovascular abdominal aortic aneurysm repair.

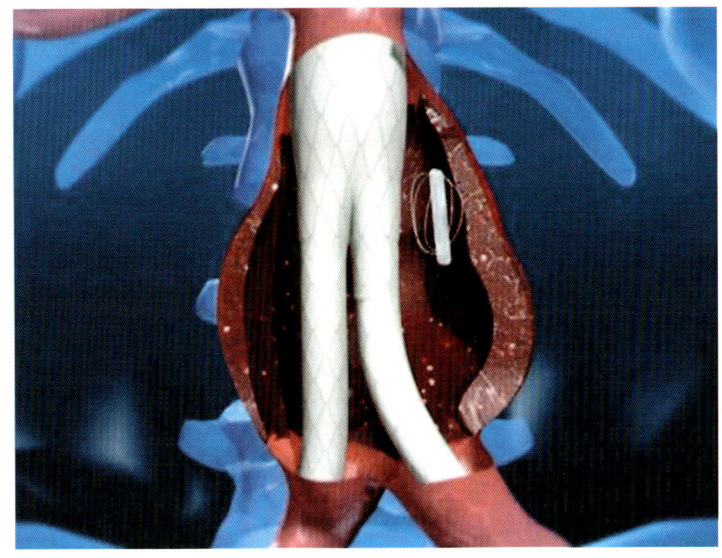

extends only to use of the device as a short-term surveillance modality.

This prospective study followed eighty-five patients from a total of twelve centers. Patients underwent EVAR with implantation of the sensor through the contralateral femoral artery into the aneurysm sac via a device specific delivery catheter. To verify the accuracy of initial sensor pressure measurements, an angiographic catheter was placed in the aneurysm sac and corresponding sac pulse pressure measurements were simultaneously recorded. To simulate a type I endoleak, pressure measurements were obtained after deployment of the main body of the endograft and prior to complete occlusion of the aneurysm with deployment of the con-

FIGURE 5: CT scan demonstrating the EndoSure sensor's independence from an aortic endograft. The two limbs of an endograft are clearly visualized within the large, residual aneurysm sac. The black arrow highlights the sensor residing in the mural thrombus of the abdominal aortic aneurysm in a separate location from the aortic endograft. The sensor is directly surrounded by its nitinol cage seen in Figure 3.

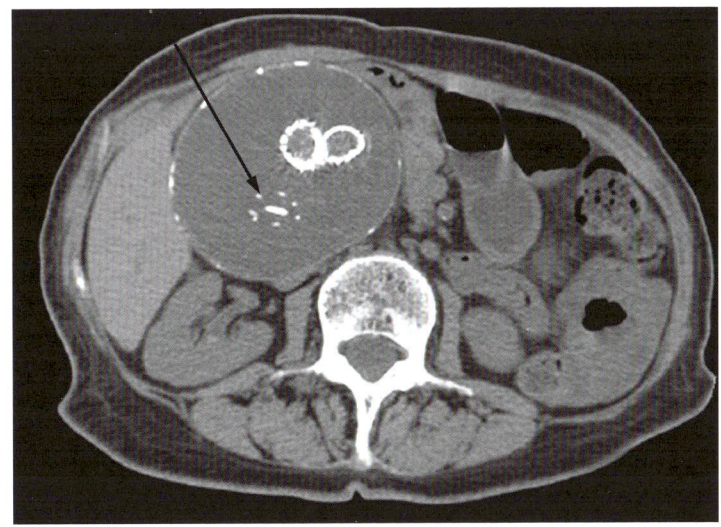

tralateral limb. Findings included a decrease in sac pressures with successful exclusions of the aneurysms and correlation between further declines in pressure measurements with aneurysm sac shrinkage over time (Figure 6). In addition, in cases with intraoperative type I and III endoleaks, pulse pressures were shown to decrease appropriately with resolution of the endoleaks.[11]

DETECTION OF ENDOLEAKS

The definition of successful EVAR can be defined as complete exclusion of an aneurysm sac from systemic circulation and pressure to prevent aneurysm rupture. Endoleaks represent the most frequent potential mechanism of failure of EVAR by providing persistent perfusion of an aneurysm sac. In fact, a persistent endoleak rate of 20% is frequently reported in the literature.[12] Currently, EVAR success is

most commonly determined by CTA demonstrating aneurysm sac shrinkage and the absence of contrast extravasation within an aneurysm sac. These parameters do not directly account for reduction of intra-aneurysm sac pressure and pulsatility which has been shown to correlate with successful exclusion of an aneurysm by endografting.[13] Therefore, the ability of remote pressure sensors to detect aneurysm sac pressures indicating early, persistent and late endoleaks supports the utility of this modality as a surveillance mechanism.

Type I and type III endoleaks

The large, multi-institutional EUROSTAR experience has provided a means to determine the natural history of various types of endoleaks. Specifically, this study determined that those patients with graft-related endoleaks (type I and type III) during a mean follow-up period of 15

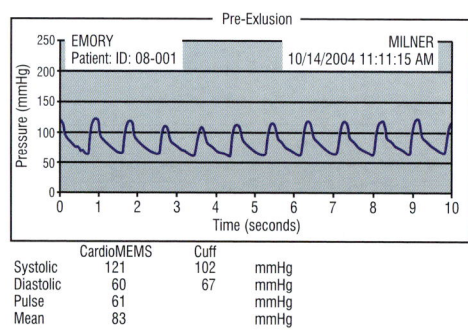

	CardioMEMS	Cuff	
Systolic	121	102	mmHg
Diastolic	60	67	mmHg
Pulse	61		mmHg
Mean	83		mmHg

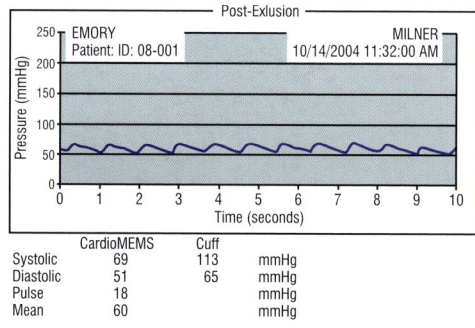

	CardioMEMS	Cuff	
Systolic	69	113	mmHg
Diastolic	51	65	mmHg
Pulse	18		mmHg
Mean	60		mmHg

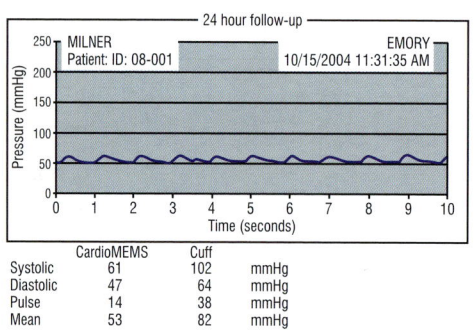

	CardioMEMS	Cuff	
Systolic	61	102	mmHg
Diastolic	47	64	mmHg
Pulse	14	38	mmHg
Mean	53	82	mmHg

FIGURE 6: Peri-operative pressure measurements in a patient treated at our institution as part of the APEX trial. The pre-exclusion pulse pressure is 61 mm Hg. The immediate post-exclusion pulse pressure is 18 mmHg. A reading was performed twenty-fours after the procedure and revealed a pulse pressure of 14 mmHg.

months had a greater risk of rupture and conversion to open repair than those patients without endoleaks or with type II endoleaks.[12] Therefore, the use of remote pressure sensors to identify pressure changes within aneurysm sacs in a chronic setting would help identify these at-risk patients. The feasibility of pressure sensing as a long-term surveillance modality is illustrated by the patient presented in Figure 7. This patient underwent EVAR with EndoSure sensor placement. Pressure readings taken one year postoperatively indicate an excluded aneurysm with both low aneurysm sac systolic and diastolic pressures and a low pulse pressure. At two years, the pressure sensor readings are increased as seen in Figure 8 and these findings correspond with an increase in sac size measured on surveillance CT. These changes ultimately correlate with a type III endoleak demonstrated by CTA (Figure 9). This endoleak was successfully treated with the placement of iliac extension cuffs and the pre- and post-intervention pressure readings are demonstrated in Figure 10a and

10b. In this setting, changes in pressure readings alone would have signaled a potential problem and eliminated the need for surveillance CT to measure aneurysm sac size.

One additional benefit of remote pressure sensing is that more frequent monitoring of aneurysm exclusion will be safe and practical. In the future, patients may be able to record their own aneurysm sac pressures via a personal wireless antenna and transmit this information to their physician on the internet for review. These measurements could be done more frequently, the risks of contrast and radiation exposure would be eliminated and an office visit would not be required. Most importantly, early detection of pressure changes would help identify endoleaks leading to rapid aneurysm expansion that would normally be missed with current intervals used for standard chronic surveillance.

Type II endoleaks

The significance of type II endoleaks re-

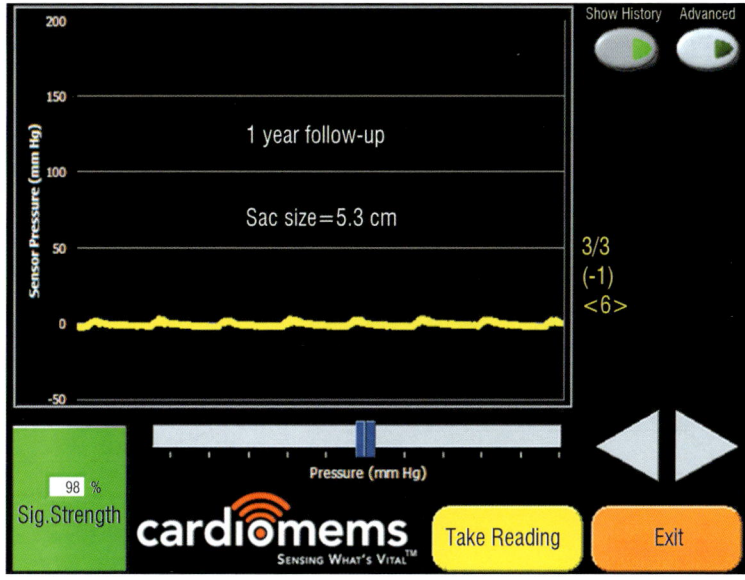

FIGURE 7: Surveillance at one year in an excluded aneurysm sac with a low pressure reading.

331

29. IS REMOTE INTRASAC PRESSURE MEASUREMENT A RELIABLE ALTERNATIVE SURVEILLANCE MODALITY?

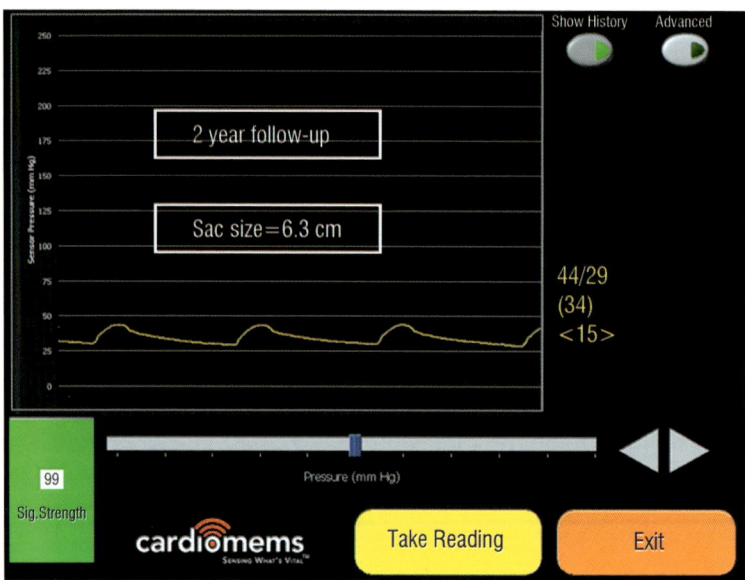

FIGURE 8: Surveillance at the two year timepoint in the same patient who has now developed a pulsatile pressure tracing with an elevated pressure within the aneurysm sac.

mains controversial. This debate centers mainly on the unpredictable natural history of type II endoleaks. Resolution of the majority of intraoperative type II endoleaks can be attributed to the thrombosis of aortic side branches and aneurysm sacs with the reversal of anticoagulation.[14] In contrast, it is the variable behavior of type II endoleaks that persist or develop in months or years after EVAR that contribute to the argument for mandatory long-term surveillance of patients. In a review of 2.617 patients included in 10 separate trials, the reported incidence of early endoleaks ranged from 6-17% and late endoleaks (6 months post-operatively) ranged from 1-8%. Although, aneurysm rupture associated with type II leaks has anecdotally been reported, this large review had no type II associated ruptures. Based on this review, recommended reintervention in the presence of type II endoleaks includes sac enlargement of >5 mm, symptomatic or pulsatile AAA sac, persistence of leak >12 months, or an aneurysmal sac pressure >20% of systolic pressure.[15] Therefore, with the exception of sac enlargement, pressure sensors offer a potential noninvasive method for monitoring trends in these parameters.

Currently, remote pressure sensors are unable to differentiate pressure elevations caused by endoleaks requiring more immediate reintervention such as

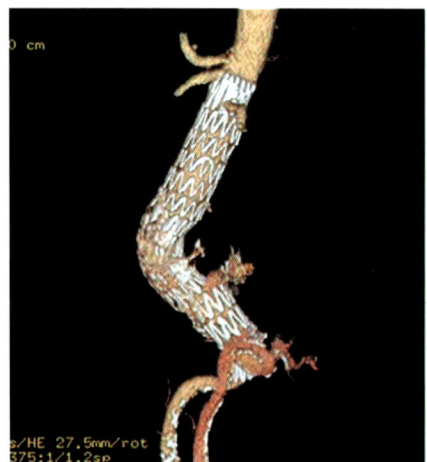

FIGURE 9: CTA of the same patient demonstrating a type III endoleak that has occurred at the junction of an iliac extension limb.

333

29. IS REMOTE INTRASAC PRESSURE MEASUREMENT A RELIABLE ALTERNATIVE SURVEILLANCE MODALITY?

FIGURE 10: Intra-operative surveillance during treatment of the type III endoleak. Panel **A** shows a pulsatile trace with an elevated pulse pressure that is markedly reduced in panel.

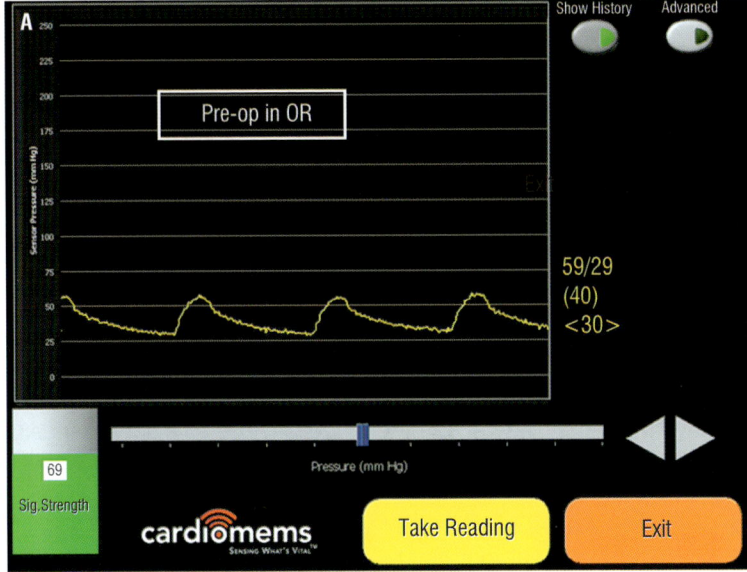

type I and III from those that may be followed more conservatively, namely type II. The ability to overcome this limitation will be one determinant in the development of pressure sensing technology as a primary chronic surveillance tool versus an enhancement to current surveillance methods.

LIMITATIONS OF REMOTE PRESSURE SENSORS

Preliminary studies evaluating remote pressure sensors have been promising but data regarding the value of this technology as a long-term surveillance tool is not currently available. Obviously with the

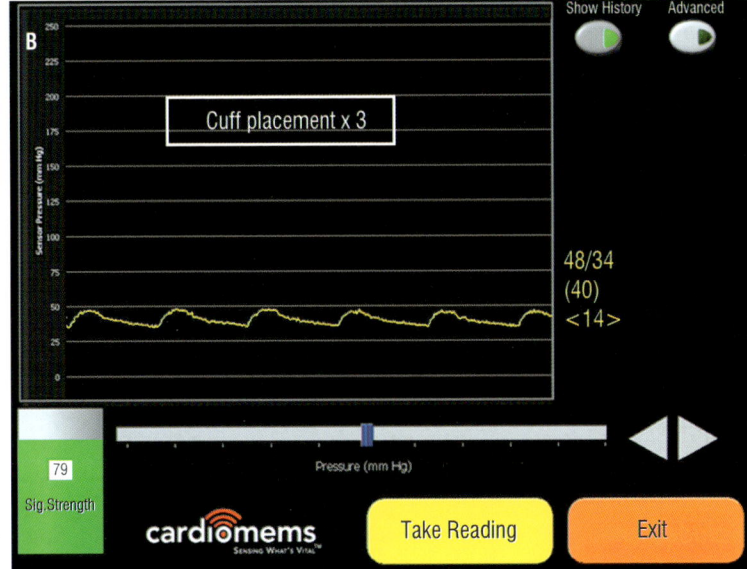

FIGURE 10: B after placement of extension cuffs.

limited data currently available, questions regarding the performance of pressure sensors over an extended time period, the possibility of device degradation or migration, or potential adverse reactions to implantation remain to be answered.

Another proposed limitation of pressure sensor technology is the ability of devices to accurately measure pressures while embedded in thrombus. Presumably, pressure measured within thrombus is not distributed uniformly and the characteristics of thrombus within an excluded aneurysm sac may vary according to location and age. Therefore, the currently available clinical studies in which only one device was implanted per patient during endograft deployment may not reflect this potential variability in pressure. This theory of aneurysm sac compartmentalization may also be a function of the relationship between endoleaks and pressure sensor positioning. Further investigation is needed to determine if pressure measurements obtained at sites remote from endoleaks accurately reflect changes in aneurysm sac pressures and predict the need for intervention.

Finally, the cost-effectiveness of this technology has yet to be defined. Currently, implantation of pressure sensors adds an additional expense to EVAR that is not covered by insurance companies due to its experimental nature. Its role for reducing surveillance expense by replacing more costly modalities remains to be determined.

CONCLUSIONS

Remote pressure sensing is a promising new surveillance technology that has currently been approved for initial monitoring of EVAR success. Current clinical studies have demonstrated the ability to detect excluded aneurysm sac pressures in the settings of successful endograft deploy-

ment, endoleaks and pressure changes associated with fluctuating aneurysm sac dimensions. Further studies are needed to determine if this technology will be successful in the earlier detection of endoleaks, graft migration and structural graft abnormalities. Currently, remote pressure sensing offers a surveillance technique that minimizes radiation and the risk of contrast nephropathy. Further investigation is needed to determine the efficacy of remote pressure sensors over an extended time period and to determine it role as a sole surveillance modality.

REFERENCES

1. Parodi JC, Palmaz JC, Barone HD. Transfemoral intraluminal graft implantation for abdominal aortic aneurysms. Ann Vasc Surg. 1991 Nov;5(6):491-9.
2. Dillavou ED, Muluk SC, Makaroun MS: Improving aneurysm-related outcomes: Nationwide benefits of endovascular repair. J Vasc Surg 2006;43:446-452.
3. Brewster DC, Jones JE, Chung TK, Lamuraglia GM, Kwolek CJ, Watkins MT, Hodgman TM, Cambria RP: Long-term outcomes after endovascular abdominal aortic aneurysm repair: The first decade. Ann Surg 2006;244:426-438.
4. Hayter CL, Bradshaw SR, Allen RJ, Guduguntla M, Hardman DTA: Follow-up costs increase the cost disparity between endovascular and open abdominal aortic aneurysm repair. J Vasc Surg 2005;42:912-918.
5. Henao EA, Hodge MD, Felkai DD, McCollum CH, Noon GP, Lin PH, Lumsden AB, Bush RL: Contrast-enhanced Duplex surveillance after endovascular abdominal aortic aneurysm repair: Improved efficacy using continuous infusion technique. J Vasc Surg 2006;43:259-264.
6. Sonesson B, Dias N, Malina M, Olofsson P, Griffin D, Lindblad B, Ivancev K: Intra-aneurysm pressure measurements in successfully excluded abdominal aortic aneurysm after endovascular repair. J Vasc Surg 2003;37:733-738.
7. Baum RA, Carpenter JP, Cope C, Golden MA, Velazquez OC, Neschis DG, Mitchell ME, Barker CF, Fairman RM: Aneurysm sac pressure meas-

urements after endovascular repair of abdominal aortic aneurysms. J Vasc Surg 2001;33:32-41.

8. Milner R, Verhagen HJ, Prinssen M, Blankensteijn JD: Noninvasive intrasac pressure measurement and the influence of type 2 and type 3 endoleaks in an animal model of abdominal aortic aneurysm. Vascular 2004;12:99-105.

9. Ellozy SH, Carroccio A, Lookstein RA, Minor ME, Sheahan CM, Juta J, Cha A, Valenzuela R, Addis MD, Jacobs TS, Teodorescu VJ, Marin ML: First experience in human beings with a permanently implantable intrasac pressure transducer for monitoring endovascular repair of abdominal aortic aneurysms. J Vasc Surg 2004;40:405-412.

10. Ellozy SH, Carroccio A, Lookstein RA, Jacobs TS, Addis MD, Teodorescu VJ, Marin ML: Abdominal aortic aneurysm sac shrinkage after endovascular aneurysm repair: Correlation with chronic sac pressure measurement. J Vasc Surg 2006;43:2-7.

11. Ohki T: Preliminary outcome of wireless pressure sensing for EVAR (the Apex Trial). Society for Vascular Surgery, Philadelphia, PA, June 18, 2005 presentation.

12. van Marrewijk C, Buth J, Harris PL, Norgren L, Nevelsteen A, Wyatt MG: Significance of endoleaks after endovascular repair of abdominal aortic aneurysms: The EUROSTAR experience. J Vasc Surg 2002;35:461-473.

13. Dias NV, Ivancev K, Malina M, Resch T, Lindblad B, Sonesson B: Intra-aneurysm sac pressure measurements after endovascular aneurysm repair: Differences between shrinking, unchanged, and expanding aneurysms with and without endoleaks. J Vasc Surg 2004;39:1229-1235.

14. Rhee SJ, Ohki T, Veith FJ, Kurvers H: Current status of management of type II endoleaks after endovascular repair of abdominal aortic aneurysms. Ann Vasc Surg 2003;17:335-344.

15. Gelfand DV, White GH, Wilson SE: Clinical significance of type II endoleak after endovascular repair of abdominal aortic aneurysm. Ann Vasc Surg 2006;20:69-74.

DREAM trial

AnNette F. Baas, Monique Prinssen, Eric Buskens,
Jan D. Blankensteijn

INTRODUCTION

Since the inception of endovascular AAA repair (EVAR) several large non-randomised studies comparing open repair (OR) and EVAR have been published. Two major biases with opposite effects limit the validity of these studies. EVAR was primarily designed for patients unfit to undergo laparotomy. As a consequence, a higher percentage of unfit patients has been treated with EVAR compared to OR in many of the non-randomised controlled studies, leading to less favourable results of EVAR. On the other hand, the very strict anatomical inclusion criteria used for EVAR may have biased outcome in favour of EVAR. To obtain the answer to the question which procedure is superior, randomised trials were initiated approximately 5 years ago.[1,2] In this chapter we discuss one of these trials in detail; the Dutch Randomised Endovascular Aneurysm Management (DREAM) trial.

PATIENT INCLUSION

The DREAM trial is a multi-center trial that included patients from 24 centers in the Netherlands and 4 centers in Belgium. Candidates had an AAA diameter of at least 50 mm, and were considered to be suitable for both EVAR and OR. EVAR suitability was primarily determined by anatomical criteria, while suitability for OR was decided by an internist or cardiologist. Emergency AAA surgeries were excluded from the trial, as were patients with inflammatory aneurysms, anatomical variations, connective-tissue disease, a history of organ-transplantation, or a life expectancy of less than 2 years.

351 patients were randomised, 178 were assigned to OR and 173 to EVAR. Six patients did not undergo AAA repair, and 6 patients crossed-over. There were 3 conversions from EVAR to OR, and 1 procedure was aborted. In total, OR was completed in 173 patients and EVAR in 171 patients. 323 patients (92%) underwent treatment as allocated.

SHORT-TERM RESULTS

Mortality and morbidity were analysed 30 days postoperative.[3] EVAR treated patients had significantly better surgical and peri-operative results in terms of duration of surgery, amount of blood loss, length of MCU or ICU stay, and duration of hospitalization. The operative mortality rate was 4.6% for OR against 1.2% for EVAR.

The risk ratio of 3.9 had a 95% confidence interval of 0.9-32.9 (P = 0.10). 10.9% of the OR treated patients had severe systemic complications, against 3.5% of the EVAR treated patients. The risk ration of 3.1 had a 95% confidence interval of 1.3-9.1 (P = 0.01).

The risk ratio of peri-operative mortality did not reach significance. But the results were almost identical to the results of the similar EVAR-1 trial that reported 30-day mortality rates of 1.7% for EVAR and 4.7% for OR.[4] Combining the mortality results of both trials yields a risk ratio of 3.1 with a 95% confidence interval of 1.7-6.2.

MID-TERM RESULTS

Complications, reinterventions and mortality were next analysed two years after randomisation.[5] The cumulative survival rates were 89.6% for OR and 89.7% for EVAR (P=0.86). The lives that were initially saved by EVAR were lost after the first postoperative year and from then on the survival rates were equal. Again, the EVAR-1 trial had equivalent results.[6] Mortality was divided in all-cause and aneurysm-related mortality. Aneurysm-related death was defined as death resulting from aneurysm rupture, graft infection, or thrombosis; any death occurring within 30 days after the procedure or a reintervention; or any death occurring more than 30 days after the procedure or reintervention, but during the same admission. The other causes of death were mainly due to cardiovascular disease, which is not surprising in an elderly, vascular comprised patient group as studied in the DREAM-trial. Aneurysm-related death after 2 years was 5.7% in OR treated patients and 2.1% in EVAR treated patients. It is important to note that the entire 3% difference is generated in the first 30 postoperative days, as any death (including coronary infarction and stroke) in that period is aneurysm-re-

lated by definition, and there were no documented postoperative AAA ruptures. Introducing the term "aneurysm-related" mortality enables the success of the surgery to exist beyond these 30 postoperative days, and to leave out death caused by so-called "competing-risks". In an elderly population like the DREAM trial death of competing risk may diminish the results of the indicated AAA treatment. But if death of frail patients is merely postponed and not prevented by EVAR, one should consider how representative the reflection of aneurysm-related mortality is. Clearly, the patient, his/her widow and family are not interested the cause of death, but most in preventing death.

In light of this, it is important to discuss that the overall survival curves appeared to converge in the second year after randomisation and that the data do not exclude the possibility of these curves to cross and produce an actual health-loss for EVAR beyond 2 to 3 years postoperatively. Although non-randomised, follow-up studies of patients after aneurysm repair have failed to show long-term benefit of OR over EVAR,[7,8] concerns remain as aneurysm-related mortality and reintervention-rates after EVAR have been reported to continue to increase.[9,10] Yet, the relevance of the prognosis of these patients beyond a few years after surgery could be questioned. In this severely compromised patient population, the reported 5-year mortality rates are 30% or higher.[7,8,11,12] Consequently, the first year benefits can be considered highly relevant even if not maintained in the period thereafter.

Reinterventions after EVAR occurred mainly in the first 9 postoperative months, and almost 3 times more than in OR treated patients (hazard ratio 2.9; 95% confidence interval 1.1-6.2, P = 0.03). From then on until 2 years postoperative, the reintervention rates of OR and EVAR treated patients were similar. A previous non-randomised study reported that the reintervention rates started to divergence after 2 years of follow-up.[8] Therefore, not only long-term results on mortality but also on reintervention rates are eagerly awaited for.

There were no major differences noted between OR and EVAR patients in the occurrence of complications.

QUALITY OF LIFE

An important aspect for determining which procedure is superior is quality of life (QoL). Although it is a complex and subjective phenomenon that is difficult to define, using standardized questionnaires it can be validly addressed. Moreover, the outcome of QoL studies weigh heavily in decision-making on introducing novel medication or techniques.

QoL was measured up until one year postoperative in 153 DREAM patients (141 male; 12 female) by using the Medical Outcome Study Short-form 36-item survey (SF-36) and the EuroQol 5 dimension questionnaire (EQ-5D).[13] QoL was reduced in both EVAR and OR treated patients, particularly in the first 3 weeks after surgery. Both groups recovered after 3 months, and returned to their pre-operative levels. Strikingly, after the first operative year the OR patients scored significantly better than the EVAR patients, suggesting that QoL after OR is superior to QoL after EVAR. Since an AAA is an asymptomatic condition it is expected to be difficult to improve QoL. However, it is recognized that after heavy surgery or severe illness people experience a relatively better QoL, most likely due to more appreciating life in general. As mentioned, the QoL results were based on the first postoperative year. Again, long-term outcomes are eagerly awaited. One can speculate that if anything would change it would most likely not by in favour of EVAR patients due to the frequent hospital visits and expected higher reintervention rates.

COST - EFFECTIVENESS

Another important aspect to consider is economics associated with the two procedures. In the DREAM trial, the direct costs for an OR patient were estimated to be 13.592 euros in the first postoperative year, versus 18.542 euros for an EVAR treated patient.[14] Detailed cost-effectiveness analysis in the DREAM trial patients clearly showed that EVAR cannot be considered as an efficient alternative for OR. This was concluded from a marginal short-term health gain against prohibitive costs of EVAR. The major cost drivers of the EVAR procedure were the expensive devices and life-long surveillance. Only if device costs would drop and durability of the device would increase EVAR can be considered cost-effective.

CONCLUSION

The results of the DREAM trial can be interpreted in different ways. On one hand, the better perioperative results after EVAR as compared to OR combined with a similar mid-term mortality risk can be used to claim superiority of EVAR over OR. On the other hand, one may argue that EVAR has no mid-term advantages, does not result in an improved QoL, is more expensive, has a higher reintervention rate, and is therefore inferior to OR.

Clearly, the randomised trials comparing OR and EVAR in AAA patients suitable for both have not provided a straightforward answer to the question which procedure is superior.

DISCUSSION

EVAR in patients fit to undergo OR provides some short-term benefits but without survival advantage beyond the first or second postoperative year. Many aspects, including quality of life and cost-effectiveness data, come into play when deciding which treatment option is best. From a patient perspective, however, none of these issues can compensate for a threefold increase in immediate (30-day) risk of dying from the proposed aneurysm repair procedure. Even the requirement of frequent and intensive follow-up in combination with a significant risk of reinterventions after EVAR causes few patients to choose the more dangerous OR procedure. Only if durability of the repair procedure is at stake in the not too distant future, some patients might prefer OR to EVAR. Long-term results from the DREAM trial are eagerly awaited.

REFERENCES

1. Prinssen M, Buskens E, and Blankensteijn JD: The Dutch Randomised Endovascular Aneurysm Management (DREAM) trial. Background, design and methods. J. Cardiovasc. Surg. (Torino) 2002;43:379-384.
2. Brown LC, Epstein D, Manca A, Beard JD, Powell JT, and Greenhalgh RM: The UK Endovascular Aneurysm Repair (EVAR) trials: design, methodology and progress. Eur. J. Vasc. Endovasc. Surg. 2004;27:372-381.
3. Prinssen M, Verhoeven EL, Buth J, Cuypers PW, van Sambeek MR, Balm R, Buskens E, Grobbee DE, and Blankensteijn JD: A randomized trial comparing conventional and endovascular repair of abdominal aortic aneurysms. N. Engl. J. Med. 2004;351:1607-1618.
4. Greenhalgh RM, Brown LC, Kwong GP, Powell JT, and Thompson SG: Comparison of endovascular aneurysm repair with open repair in patients with abdominal aortic aneurysm (EVAR trial 1), 30-day operative mortality results: randomised controlled trial. Lancet 2004;364:843-848.
5. Blankensteijn JD, de Jong SE, Prinssen M, van der Ham AC, Buth J, van Sterkenburg SM, Verha-
gen HJ, Buskens E, and Grobbee DE: Two-year outcomes after conventional or endovascular repair of abdominal aortic aneurysms. N. Engl. J. Med. 2005;352:2398-2405.
6. Endovascular aneurysm repair versus open repair in patients with abdominal aortic aneurysm (EVAR trial 1): randomised controlled trial. Lancet 2005;365:2179-2186.
7. Goueffic Y, Becquemin JP, Desgranges P, and Kobeiter H: Midterm survival after endovascular versus open repair of infrarenal aortic aneurysms. J. Endovasc. Ther. 2005;12:47-57.
8. Cao P, Verzini F, Parlani G, Romano L, De Rango P, Pagliuca V, and Iacono G: Clinical effect of abdominal aortic aneurysm endografting: 7-year concurrent comparison with open repair. J. Vasc. Surg. 2004;40:841-848.
9. Maher MM, McNamara AM, MacEneaney PM, Sheehan SJ, and Malone DE: Abdominal aortic aneurysms: elective endovascular repair versus conventional surgery-evaluation with evidence-based medicine techniques. Radiology 2003;228:647-658.
10. Zarins CK, Heikkinen MA, Lee ES, Alsac JM, and Arko FR: Short- and long-term outcome following endovascular aneurysm repair. How does it compare to open surgery? J. Cardiovasc. Surg. (Torino) 2004;45:321-333.
11. Long-term outcomes of immediate repair compared with surveillance of small abdominal aortic aneurysms. N. Engl. J. Med. 2002;346:1445-1452.
12. Biancari F, Ylonen K, Anttila V, Juvonen J, Romsi P, Satta J, and Juvonen T: Durability of open repair of infrarenal abdominal aortic aneurysm: a 15-year follow-up study. J. Vasc. Surg. 2002;35:87-93.
13. Prinssen M, Buskens E, and Blankensteijn JD: Quality of life endovascular and open AAA repair. Results of a randomised trial. Eur. J. Vasc. Endovasc. Surg. 2004;27:121-127.
14. Prinssen M, Buskens E, de Jong SE, Buth J, MacKaay AJ, van Sambeek MR, and Blankensteijn JD: DREAM Trial Participants: Cost-effectiveness of endovascular repair of abdominal aortic aneurysms. J. Vasc. Surg. 2007;46:883-890.

CAESAR Trial

Lydia Romano, Fabio Verzini, Gianbattista Parlani,
Federico Quaranta, Piergiorgio Cao

ABSTRACT

Objective: The CAESAR trial aims to assess the outcome of endovascular repair (EVAR) versus surveillance of small abdominal aortic aneurysms (AAA) measuring 4.1 to 5.4 cm in maximum diameter at Computerised Tomography (CT) scan.

Design: Patients between 50 and 80 years of age, with small AAA anatomically suitable for EVAR, are randomly allocated to early EVAR or surveillance. Primary outcome measure is patient survival. Secondary endpoints include aneurysm-related deaths (defined as any death caused directly or indirectly by rupture or endovascular/open aneurysm repair), AAA rupture, per-operative or late complications, conversion to open repair, complications associated with delayed treatment including loss of treatment options, growth rates, and quality of life. Target recruitment is 740 patients.

Progress: Inclusion started in September 2004. By the end of December 2006, 273 patients had been enrolled by 18 actively randomizing centers in Europe. Completion of recruitment is expected for September 2008, and publication of the results in mid 2009.

BACKGROUND

Population-based screening studies reveal that up to 9% of people over 65 years of age have unsuspected and asymptomatic abdominal aortic aneurysm (AAA), and it is estimated that ruptured AAA causes at least 15,000 deaths each year in the United States.[1]

Aneurysm size is the primary determinant of risk of aneurysm rupture and is an important predictor of long-term survival in patients with AAA.

There is long-standing evidence that elective surgical repair improves survival of patients with large AAA.[2,3] In contrast there is only limited evidence and much debate on the best management for patients with small AAA (4.1 to 5.4 cm).[3-9]

Treatment of AAA is appropriate when cumulative risk for rupture exceeds risk of repair. Two randomised controlled trials (UK Small aneurysm trial [UKSAT] and ADAM trial) found no advantage in overall survival for early open surgery compared to surveillance in patients with AAA 4.0-5.5 cm in diameter.[4,5]

In these trials, applying a strict follow-up protocol, AAA rupture in the surveillance group was low (about 1% per year) and there was no advantage for patients treated with early surgery. Many concerns remain unanswered.

- Those results were obtained by a combination of clinical follow-up, careful medical management, and strict ultrasound surveillance that are difficult to achieve in common practice outside RCTs.
- Some subgroups were at higher risk, such as women with a four-fold risk of rupture.
- Surveillance is almost in every case followed by AAA repair. In fact only 7% of surviving patients after 8 years from inclusion in the UK-SAT remained free from intervention.
- In-hospital mortality rates after delayed surgery were higher than those occurring with early surgery (7.2% vs. 5.8%, respectively).
- Long-term results of the UK trial indicated that 8-year mortality in the early surgery group was 7.2 percentage points lower than that in the surveillance group and since the autopsy rates were low, we could not exclude that this difference could be related to AAA.[10]

The only evidence from the results of both RCTs was that the critical issue for patients with small AAA is to define "when" and not "if" to treat and that patients with long life expetancy might benefit the most from early surgery.

If true benefit of open surgery remains unclear, with the advent of minimally invasive therapy, the option of early endovascular repair has gained widespread acceptance and application.[11]

Recently, two independent randomized trials, EVAR 1 (including subjects with AAA larger than 5.5 cm) and the DREAM Trial (AAA >5 cm) have reported a significant reduction in AAA-related deaths after EVAR compared to OR, starting from 4% immediate postoperative advantage that persisted during follow-up (aneurysm-related death estimates at 4 years: 4% vs 7%).[8,12-14]

Even more favorable results might be expected for endovascular repair of small AAA. In fact, analyses of clinical outcome after endovascular treatment of small versus large aortic aneurysms gave the impression that feasibility and durability of the endovascular procedure were improved.[15-17]

Zarins et al. recently published their results on 923 patients treated with EVAR, showing that preoperative aneurysm size is an important determinant in long-term outcome. Patients with small AAAs (<5.5 cm) are more favorable candidates for EVAR because they tend to be younger, with better surgical risk, and more favorable aortic neck anatomy. Five years after EVAR these patients were less likely to have died of an aneurysm-related event (1% vs 6%, p = .006) or to have had secondary intervention (25% vs 32%, p = .03), and presented a higher survival rate (69% vs 57%, p = .0002) than patients with large aneurysms after five year follow-up.[18]

Similary, Brewster et al, reviewing their 12-year experience with EVAR, reported a striking difference in late outcomes of small vs. large AAA, particularly in regard to perioperative mortality and late aneurysm-related death. Patients undergoing EVAR for large AAA were somewhat older (76.4 vs. 74.9 years) and had significantly increased comorbidities. Patients with large and small AAA were otherwise comparable with regard to other baseline parameters. No perioperative deaths occurred in 424 patients with AAA <55 mm (vs. 3.6% perioperative mortality in patients with large AAA) and aneurysm-related mortality was only 0.5% for patients with small AAA vs. 5.7% for large AAA.[19]

In the "real word" this uncertainty among optimal strategies for treatment of small AAA translates into a high rate of surgical treatment based on arbitrary indication and personal opinion. Data from large registries and multicenter experiences on AAA show that worldwide AAA repair (either endovascular or open) is performed on aneurysms with a diameter range from <4 cm to over 10 cm with variable results. Forty-five percent of the EUROSTAR patients and nearly 60% of the Cleveland patients treated with EVAR had aneurysms smaller than 5.5 cm.[15-16]

Also the ACC/AHA practice guidelines for the management of patients with AAA indicate a beneficial repair in patients with infrarenal or iuxatrenal AAAs 5-0 to 5.4 cm in diameter (class IIa recommendation, level of evidence: B).[20]

Endovascular repair may represent the treatment of choice for small AAAs, but there is a large area of uncertainty about the best treatment. Nevertheless, only a randomized study comparing observation and endovascular treatment of small AAAs will provide reliable answers on the eventual benefit of early treatment.

At this moment there are two ongoing randomized trials comparing early endovascular repair to surveillance in patients with small AAA. The first one is an American trial, the PIVOTAL study, headed by Kenneth Ouriel. It is designed to use the AneuRx (Medtronic Santa Rosa, CA) device in patients with AAAs between 4 cm and 5 cm in diameter. Sample size calculations suggest that approximately 1,700 patients will need to be enrolled. The primary end-point is rupture or aneurysm-related death, assessed at 3 years. The second one is a European trial, the CAESAR study.[21]

CAESAR Study Design

The **CAESAR** study (**C**omparison of **S**urveillance vs **A**ortic **E**ndografting for **S**mall **A**neurysm **R**epair study) is a randomized multicenter clinical trial designed to compare endovascular repair vs. surveillance and eventually delayed treatment in patients with small AAAs (measuring between 4.1 and 5.4 cm in maximum diameter defined by CT scan) suitable for EVAR.

The primary study endpoint is mortality from any cause. Secondary endpoints include: aneurysm-related deaths, AAA rupture, perioperative or late complications, conversion to open repair, complications associated with delayed treatment including loss of treatment options, growth rates, and quality of life.

A secondary cost analysis will be performed according to cost of the graft, operating time, length of hospital stay including intensive care admission, follow-up visits with imaging examination, need of reintervention, and blood transfusion.

Required sample size was estimated in 740 patients (370 patients per group) to detect a statistically significant difference(11%) in survival rates between the EVAR and the control group by log rank test, with 0.80 power and 0.05 two-sided type I error rate. The main outcome analyses will be conducted according to the intention-to-treat principle.

All standard-risk patients with AAA eligible for EVAR can be considered for participation in the CAESAR trial. Required entry criteria are shown in Table 1.

The CAESAR study includes experienced centers. Each participating center is required to comply with endovascular/open aortic repair and should have passed its learning curve in endovascular AAA repair prior to participation in the trial.

Centers must have obtained Human Ethics Committee approval from their institutions to conduct the randomized trial prior to enrolling patients in the study.

Pre-operative and follow-up CT scans obtained at each participating center will be read by experienced vascular specialists, and periodically validated by a core laboratory in the coordinating center, located in Perugia, Italy.

TABLE 1

ENTRY CRITERIA FOR CAESAR STUDY

Inclusion criteria

Patients 50-80 years of age

Non symptomatic infrarenal AAA of 4.1 to 5.4 cm in diameter measured by CT performed within 3 months before randomization

Adequate infrarenal aortic neck (length ≥15 mm diameter ≤30 mm) and other anatomical configurations suitable for EVAR

Patients have a life expectancy of at least 5 years

Signed informed consent

Exclusion criteria

Ruptured or symptomatic AAA

AAA maximum diameter ≥5.5 cm

Suprarenal or thoracic aorta aneurysm of more than 4.0 cm

Patient unsuitable for administration of contrast agent

Severe heart, lung, liver or renal disease (serum creatinine ≥3 mg/dl)

Need for adjunctive major surgical or vascular procedures within 1 month

High likelihood of non compliance with follow-up requirements

Randomization was designed with equal probability of assignment to either of the two groups by means of a computer-generated, random-number list. After eligibility is verified and the patient is considered suitable for the study, assignment is made using a computerized randomization table accessible on the web (http://www.caesarstudy.com). Because it is expected that many variables are specific for each participating center (i.e., team experience, case load, etc.), randomization is stratified by center. The allocated treatment is immediately available to the trial coordinator, surgeon, and patient.

The CAESAR study has been funded to use a single device in the trial: the Zenith® AAA Endovascular Graft (William Cook Europe, Bjaeverskov, Denmark). However the design of the study and the study itself are independently conducted. The use of a single graft model will also guarantee homogeneity of the results for all the EVAR patients included in the study. For patients randomized to early endovascular treatment, the repair has to be carried out within six weeks from randomization.

Before discharge, a color Duplex Ultrasound and abdominal plain X-ray (double projection) are carried out. Clinical and imaging follow-up are then performed at 30 days and every six months thereafter. Double projection plain abdominal X-rays are also used to follow patients after EVAR to assess stent integrity. CT scan with slice reconstruction at 5 mm or less is performed yearly.

All adverse events occurring after randomization, before or after treatment, (e.g., graft migration, disconnection, persisting endoleak, aneurysm growth, need for secondary procedures) are assessed, documented, treated if necessary, and recorded.

Patients assigned to the surveillance arm of the trial are evaluated every six months throughout the study. Follow-up assessment includes clinical, ultrasonography evaluations, and yearly CT scan. In patients under surveillance and with creatinine levels of 2 mg/100 ml or more, the use of contrast agent is not mandatory and left to the discretion of the investigator.

Ultrasonography is not used to define aneurysm baseline diameter but only to control aneurysm size and to assess achievement of threshold criteria that will need CT scan confirmation.

Surveillance visits continue until either the patient dies, the trial ends, or surgery is considered and performed. Surgery is considered only when the aneurysm grows to 5.5 cm, rapidly increases in diameter (>1 cm/year), or becomes symptomatic. Patients in the surveillance group who meet one or more threshold criteria to be converted to surgical repair will be evaluated to assess the persistence of anatomical suitability for EVAR.

Any patient in the surveillance group who requires repair during follow-up is followed until completion of the trial. Figure 1 shows the protocol for enrolled patients.

Quality of life is assessed in both groups at six-month intervals with Short-Form 36-items (SF-36) questionnaire administration.[13]

CURRENT STATUS

Recruitment began in September 2004 and by the end of December 2006 a total of 273 patients had been included in the CAESAR trial by 18 actively randomizing Centers throughout Europe.

Other Centers recently received Local Ethical Committee approval to actively randomize and the main Trial Office in Perugia is contacting several other centers willing to participate.

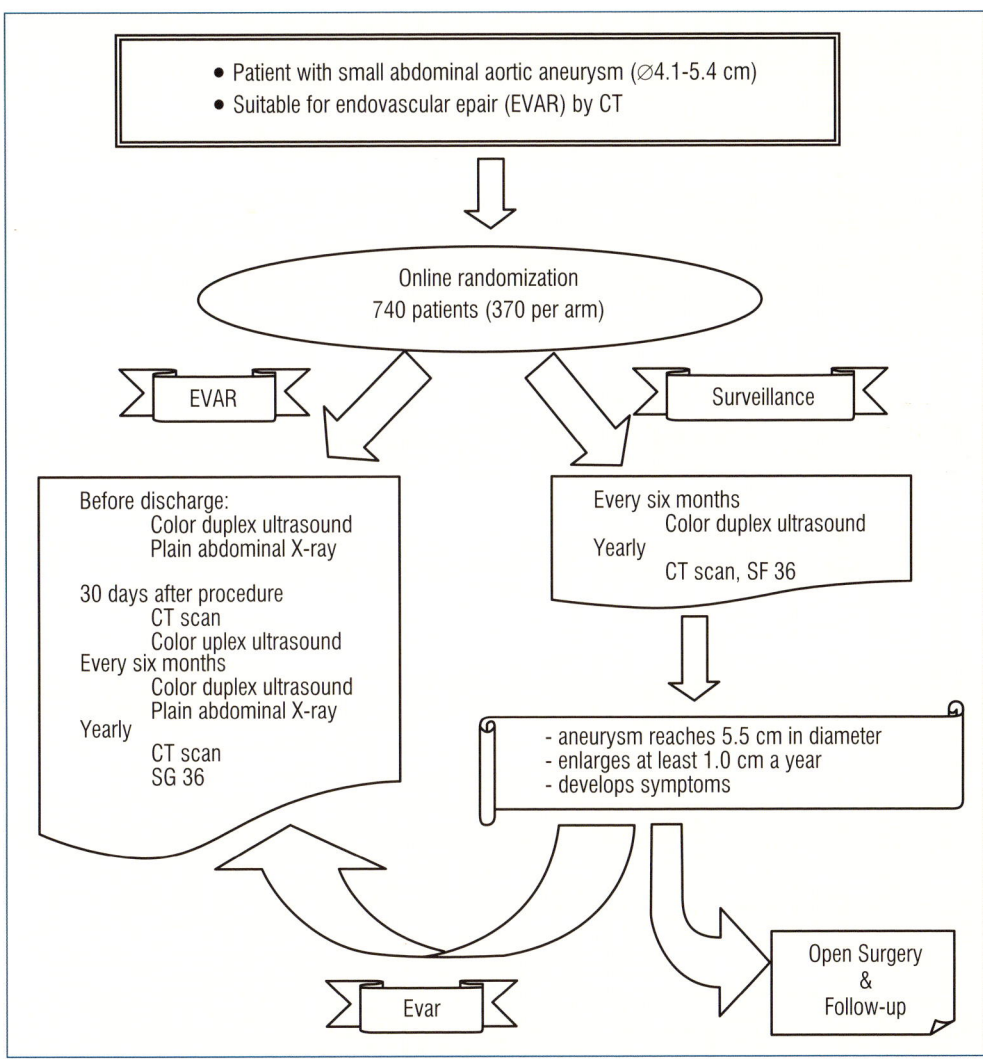

FIGURE 1: Flow chart for patients enrolled in CAESAR Trial.

The CAESAR Data Monitoring Committee has recommended that recruitment into the trial be completed within the end of August 2008. In order to accrue sufficient patient years of follow-up, a minimum of 1 year of follow-up is required per patient and on this timescale we might expect to publish the results of the trial in mid 2009. However, a final publication date has not been decided.

CONCLUSIONS

In the era of endovascular expansion, stent grafting for small AAA has been reported in several non-randomized trials with promising results.[8,9,11,15,16] Similarly, there are supporting data that surveillance and delayed treatment could be a safe choice for patients with small AAA. However, these results were based on open surgical treatment with a higher perioperative mortality rate than endografting.[8,12]

Endovascular treatment has been demonstrated to be associated with lower perioperative mortality than open surgery. However, EVAR has a number of complications that become apparent only during longer-term follow-up, such as late aortic rupture, endoleak, graf migration, and graft limb occlusion, requiring late reinterventions.

The high reintervention rate reported after endografting can make the cost effectiveness of this procedure unfavorable in patients with long life expectancy. Patients with small aneurysms usually have a greater anatomic suitability and the operation can be more durable lowering the need of reintervention.

At the moment the correct management of AAA measuring <5.5 is uncertain. Only a randomized trial will indicate the appropriate approach. The Caesar trial may help answer these controversial questions and will attempt to provide scientific evidence on the merits of endovascular repair of small AAAs.

APPENDIX I: PARTICIPANTS OF THE CAESAR STUDY *

Piergiorgio Cao, MD (Principal Investigator), FRCS, Dept. of Vascular and Endovascular Surgery, Universita degli Studi di Perugia, Ospedale S. Maria della Misericordia, Perugia, Italy; Carlo Pratesi, MD, Dept. of Vascular Surgery, Universita degli Studi di Firenze, Firenze, Italy; Stefano Michelagnoli, MD, U.O. Chirurgia Vascolare, Nuovo Ospedale S. Giovanni di Dio, Firenze, Italy; Enrico Vecchiati, MD, Dipartimento di Chirurgia Vascolare, Azienda Ospedaliera S.M. Nuova, Reggio Emilia, Italy; Roberto Troiani, MD, Unita di Chirurgia Vascolare, Azienda Ospedaliera di Carrara, Carrara, Italy; Francesco Mascoli, MD, Dipartimento di Chirurgia Vascolare, Ospedale S. Anna, Ferrara, Italy; Carlo Setacci, MD, U. O. Chirurgia Vascolare, Policlinico Le Scotte, Siena, Italy; Vicente Riambau, MD, Institute of Cardiovascular Diseases, Hospital Clinic, University of Barcelona, Barcelona, Spain; Giovanni Torsello, MD, Klinik fur Gefaesschirurgie, St. Franziskus Hospital, Muenster, Germany; Stephan Haulon, MD, Clinique de Chirurgie Cardiovasculaire, Hopital Cardiologique, Lille, France; Jacek Szmidt, MD, Naczyniowej I Transplantacyjnej Akademii Medycznej, Warsaw, Poland; Malgorzata Szostek, MD, Klinika Chirurgii Ogolnej i Chorob Klatki Piersiowej, Warsaw, Poland; Vaclav Prochazka, MD, Vitkovice Hospital, University Hospital Ostrava-Poruba, Ostrava, Czech Republic; Jaap Buth, MD, Dept. of Surgery, Catharina Hospital, Eindhoven, The Netherlands; Mike Jenkins, MD, Vascular Unit, St. Mary's Hospital, London, UK; Carlo Ruotolo, MD, U.O.C. Chirurgia Vascolare, Azienda Ospedaliera A. Cardarelli, Napoli, Italy, Domenico Tealdi, MD, Centro Cardiovascolare "E. Malan", Policlinico S. Donato, San Donato Milanese, Italy; Jan Brunkwall, MD, Department of Vascular Surgery, Koeln Universitaet, Koeln, Germany.

* listed in the timing of adhesion order.

REFERENCES

1. Alcorn HG, Wolfson SK Jr, Sutton-Tyrrel K, Kurrel LH. O'Learly. D. Risk factors for abdominal aortic aneurysms in older adults enrolled in the Cardiovascular Health Study. Arterioscler Thromb Vasc Biol 1996;16:963-970.

2. Nevitt MP, Ballard DJ, Hallett JW Jr.: Prognosis of abdominal aortic aneurysms: a population-based study. N Engl J Med 1989;321:1009-1014.

3. Glimaker H, Holmberg L, Elvin A, Nybacka O, Bjorck CG, Eriksson I: Natural history of patients with abdominal aortic aneurysm. Eur J Vasc Surg 1991;5:125-130.

4. The UK Small Aneurysm Trial participants: Mortality results for randomised controlled trial of early elective surgery or ultrasonographic surveillance for small abdominal aortic aneurysms. Lancet 1998;352:1656-1660.

5. Lederle FA, Wilson SE, Johnson GR, Reinke DB, Littooy FN, Acher CW, Ballard DJ, Messina LM, Gordon IL, Chute EP, et al.: Immediate repair compared with surveillance of small abdominal aortic aneurysms. N Engl J Med 2002;346:1437-1444.

6. Branchereau A: Small aortic aneurysm: is evidence evident? Eur J Vasc Endovasc Surg 2004; 27:363-365.

7. UK Small Aneurysm Trial Management Committee: Facts and not fiction: the small aneurysm trials do not justify early surgical intervention. Eur J Vasc Endovasc Surg 2004;28:227.

8. Prinssen M, Verhoeven ELG, Buth J, Cuypers PWM, van Sambeek MRHM, Balm R, Buskens E, Grobbee DE, Blankensteijn JD, for the DREAM Trial Group: A randomized trial comparing conventional and endovascular repair of abdominal aortic aneurysms. N Engl J Med 2004;351:1607-1618.

9. Lederle FA: Abdominal aortic aneurysm - Open versus endovascular repair. N Engl J Med 2004;351: 1677-1679.

10. The United Kingdom Small Aneurysm Trial Participants: Long-term outcomes of immediate repair compared with surveillance of small abdominal aortic aneurysms. N Engl J Med 2002;346:1445-1452.

11. Cao P, Verzini F, Parlani G, Romano L, De Rango P, Pagliuca V, Iacono G: Clinical effect of abdominal aortic aneurysm endografting: 7-year concurrent comparison with open repair. J Vasc Surg 2004;40:841-848.

12. Greenhalgh RM, Brown LC, Kwong GP, Powell JT, Thompson SG; EVAR trial participants: Comparison of endovascular aneurysm repair with open repair in patients with abdominal aortic aneurysm (EVAR trial 1), 30-day operative mortality results: randomised controlled trial. Lancet 2004; 364(9437):843-848.

13. EVAR trial participants: Endovascular aneurysm repair versus open repair in patients with abdominal aortic aneurysm (EVAR trial 1):randomised controlled trial. Lancet 2005;365:2179-2186.

14. Blankensteijn JD, De Jong SECA, Prinssen M, Van Der Ham AC, Buth J,Van Sterkenburg SMM, Verhagen HJM, Buskens E, Grobbee DE, for the Dutch Randomized Endovascular Aneurysm Management (DREAM) Trial Group: Two-year outcomes after conventional or endovascular repair of abdominal aortic aneurysm. N Engl J Med 2005;352:2398-2405

15. Ouriel K, Srivastava SD, Sarac TP, O'Hara PJ, Lyden SP, Greenberg RK, Clair DG, Sampram E, Butler B: Disparate outcome after endovascular treatment of small versus large abdominal aortic aneurysm. J Vasc Surg 2003;37:1206-1212.

16. Peppelenbosch N, Buth J, Harris PL, van Marrewijk C, Fransen G, EUROSTAR Collaborators: Diameter of abdominal aortic aneurysm and outcome of endovascular aneurysm repair: does size matter? A report from EUROSTAR. J Vasc Surg. 2004;39:288-297.

17. Chaikof EL, Blankensteijn JD, Harris PL, White GH, Zarins CK, Bernhard VM, Matsumura JS, May J, Veith FJ, Fillinger MF, et al.: Reporting standards for endovascular aortic aneurysm repair. J Vasc Surg 2002;35:1048-1059

18. Zarins CK, Crabtree T, Bloch DA, Arko FR, Ouriel K, White RA: Endovascular aneurysm repair at 5 years:does aneurysm diameter predict outcome? J Vasc Surg 2006;44:920-930.

19. Brewster DC, Jones JE, Chung TK, Lamuraglia

GM, Kwolek CJ, Watkins MT, Hodgman TM, Cambria RP: Long-term outcomes after endovascular abdominal aortic aneurysm repair: the first decade. Ann Surg 2006;244:426-438.

20. ACC/AHA 2005 Practice Guidelines for the management of patients with peripheral arterial disease (lower extremity,renal,mesenteric,and abdominal aortic).Circulation 2006;113:463-654.

21. CAESAR trial collaborators: Comparison of surveillance vs aortic endografting for small aneurysm repair (CAESAR) trial: study design and progress. Eur J Vasc Endovasc Surg 2005;30:245-251.

Training in vascular surgery.
The impact of endovascular procedures

Efthimios D. Avgerinos, Theodossios P. Perdikides, Marc A. Cairols, Christos D. Liapis

"Vascular surgery is the clinical and scientific discipline concerned with the diagnosis, treatment and prevention of diseases affecting arteries, veins and lymphatics ..."

INTRODUCTION

During the last 50 years vascular surgery has met an enormous evolution, paving the way for the development of modern vascular and endovascular surgery. Endovascular surgery has aroused during the last decade as a revolutionary, minimal invasive, weapon in the armamentarium of vascular surgeons. Through tiny incisions or transcutaneous procedures vessel access is maintained. Guide wires, catheters and sheaths find their way, intraluminnaly, to the vascular lesion and through real time x-ray guidance final treatment is applied.

Patients want specialist surgeons and not generalists. Certified proficient vascular surgeons achieve far better results, in all aspects of VS, than General or Cardiac or other occasional and sometimes amateurish, surgical professionals.[1,2]

Patients deserve the freedom to select less-proven but minimally invasive technology, with fewer immediate risks, even if conventional open surgery is more established and durable.[3]

Frank Veith told us just about a decade ago: "Become endocompetent or become extinct".[4]

Obviously, the changing face of vascular surgery demands a proportional modification of vascular training. This becomes particularly important and potentially complicated considering the two recent European directives that inevitably have altered the current status of vascular practice. The European working time directive 93 104 EC (48-hour week) has raised questions on the efficacy of training, while the "Recognition of Professional Qualifications" directive has raised questions on the actual ability of vascular professionals to practice in countries other than their own with diplomas and qualifications issued in their home country.

Vascular trainees, currently having less time to practice, need to be prepared for the forthcoming endovascular future, without though downgrading their open surgical skills. Modern vascular training becomes demanding and challenging and modern educational residency programmes need to be re-established towards both directions traditional open vascular surgery and cutting-edge endovascular-interventional surgery. It seems necessary to reduce some of the less relevant aspects of training and create a meaningful curriculum and move towards producing a hybrid surgeon with catheter skills.

EUROPEAN TRAINING MODEL

Vascular surgery is a recognized sub-specialty in Europe since the foundation of the Division of Vascular Surgery (initially incorporated in the European Board of Surgery) in 1993 and a recognized full specialty since its recognition by UEMS (Union Europeenne des Medicines Specialistes) as a separate section and board in 2004. However, regulations for the Certificate of Completion of Specialist Training in vascular surgery vary across Europe. Vascular surgery has, for many years, been a kind of subspecialty of General Surgery or Cardiac Surgery-depending on national or local situations. Some countries incorporate vascular surgery in the general surgery training and grant national certification in general surgery, while others allow the "common trunk" training in general surgery (2-5 years) followed by 2-4 years of training in vascular surgery to be certified in vascular surgery. For example, the duration of vascular surgical training varies from 5 years in Italy and Spain and 7 years in Greece to as long as 11 years in the UK. At present it is an independent monospecialty in nine out of 15 of the 'old' Member Countries of the European Union (EU) and presumably only in one of the 10 'new' ones.[5,6]

The body awarding the CCST also varies, governments, professional bodies and universities taking an almost equal share of responsibility across Europe.[7]

Perceiving Europe as an entity, there is a profound variability of exposure in general surgery, while vascular training varies among the nations of the European Union, both in quality and in quantity. Such variability has created a pressing need for accelerated harmonization of training and certification in Vascular Surgery. A structured training programme of knowledge and skills should be implemented in the form of a European curriculum and a minimum level of competence should be required in the specialty examinations.[8] The UEMS Section and Board of Vascular Surgery has been striving towards this end since 1996 and has made a tremendous contribution by developing and implementing the Annual European Board assessments in Vascular Surgery (EBSQ-VASC), referred to EBVS-exam since 2005.[9] The examination is now in its eleventh consecutive year. The minimum acceptable duration of surgical training for entry to the FEBVS assessments is 6 years. This must include a minimum total of 2 years in specialist vascular surgical units. The minimum acceptable total experience of specialist arterial reconstruction indicator procedures, open and endovascular, either as first assistant or as principal surgeon, is 200.[10] This includes at least 15 femoropopliteal bypasses, 15 abdominal aortic aneurysm repairs and 10 carotid endarterectomies performed as a principal surgeon assisted by trainer. Endovascular interventions were recently included in the indicator procedures, with a minimum number of 30 procedures required before a candidate can be admitted to the European vascular assessment. The candidate is then eligible to proceed to a viva voce examination covering clinical, scientific and logbook assessment as well as a technical skills exercise (Figure 1) to determine technical competence and correlation between log-book data and viva voce performance. Endovascular skills assessment will be part of the examination by year 2008, as the STRESS simulator is currently being tested and evaluated. Such a European examination could well be used as an exit examination in the interests of standardization and harmonization committed to guarantee free-

FIGURE 1: Technical skills exercise during the 7th Annual EBVS-exam, September 2002, Istanbul.

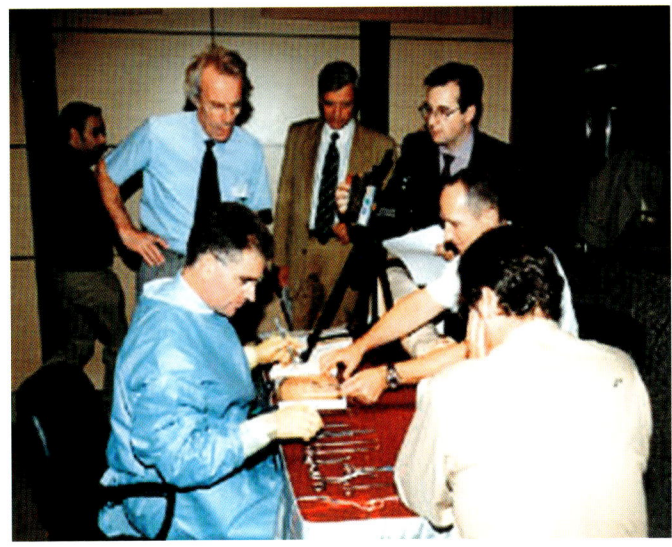

dom of movement and residence to all citizens of the European Union.[11]

USA Training Model

An American Board of Vascular Surgery (ABVS) was formed in 1996 to address the raising needs of vascular practice and to establish an independent American Board of Medical Specialties (ABMS) – approved ABVS. Despite its efforts to establish an independent board for vascular surgeons, conflicts with the American Board of Surgery have not yet allowed the full independency of the specialty. The ABVS had never official status as an examination or certifying body.

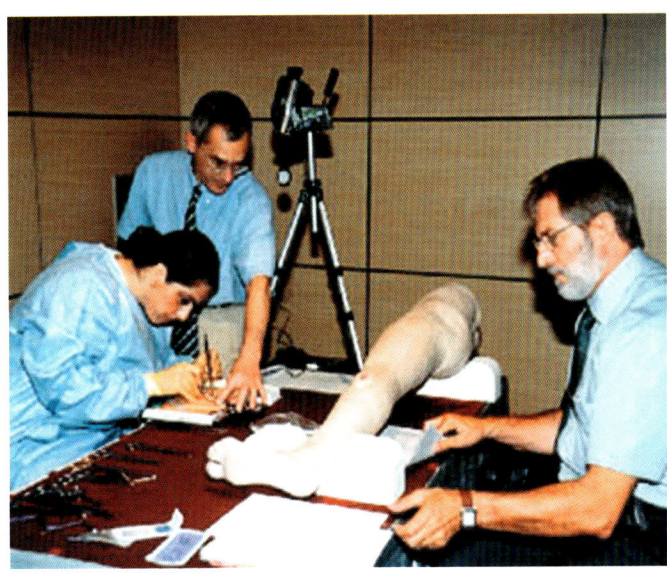

FIGURE 1: *(continued)*

Recently, the ABVS Board members voted for a name change from "The American Board of Vascular Surgery" to the "American Board of Vascular Specialists". The basis for this decision was considered because vascular surgeons perform services in many areas other than Vascular Surgery alone (endovascular Surgery, vascular medicine and imaging).[12]

The Directors of the ABVS are continuing to support exploratory talks on an examination that would cover vascular specialists. This four module examination would include open Vascular Surgery, endovascular surgery, elements of vascular medicine and imaging. If instituted, the first examinations would be open to applicants with knowledge in all four modules (vascular surgeons). In the future, and dependent on the Board's recommendations, this could be expanded to include other specialties. An offer has been made to the SVS Board for collaboration on the examinations content.[12]

For many years training and certification in Vascular Surgery required primary certification in General Surgery, a 7 year track ("5 + 2"). Following the 5 years of general surgery, graduates could follow a 2 year training in vascular surgery with eventual board certification in both specialties.

Since March 2005, the American Board of Surgery (ABS) has been approved from the American Board of Medical Specialties (ABMS) to offer a primary certificate in vascular surgery. Subsequently vascular surgeons in the US have the opportunity to become directly board-certified in vascular surgery without first becoming certified in general surgery. For the first time, medical students and residents who select vascular surgery as their specialty can undergo 3 years of general surgery and 3 years of vascular and endovascular surgery training without the need to obtain a general surgery board certificate.

Since February 2006 the Accreditation Council for Graduate Medical Education approved the Primary Certificate in Vascular Surgery. The primary certificate eliminates the requirement for pre-certification in General Surgery allowing more flexible and in-depth training paradigms. The available training pathways, apart from the "traditional" one, are either a six year track ("3 + 3") for residents who much in initial surgical training or a five year track ("3 + 2") for trainees who much during medical school. Following one of these two options board certification is granted only for vascular surgery.

By this reform opportunities to choose vascular surgery as a career choice are substantially increased, training periods are shortened and ultimately training in all new areas of vascular surgery is enhanced.

MODERN TRENDS TO INCORPORATE ENDOVASCULAR SKILLS IN VASCULAR SURGEON'S TRAINING

Revised curriculums

Vascular surgery has come of age and for a surgical specialty this means full development and integration of basic sciences, diagnostic tools, clinical refinement based on experience and evidence, medical engineering, new and sophisticated forms of treatment including Endovascular skills.[6]

There is currently a tremendous need to revise the traditional methods of training and certification in vascular surgery to produce competent vascular specialists in open surgery, catheter-maneuvering abilities and imaging experience.[13]

All over the world pilot programmes are established and some of these are discussed:

1. In USA some fellowship programmes are replacing the research training to endovascular training or incorporate an entire year of interventional radiology into vascular surgery training.[14] In San

Francisco, California, integration of vascular surgery and interventional radiology in one-year fellowships seems to work beneficial for both surgeons and radiologists.[15] Worth mentioning are also the 3-month endovascular mini-fellowships endorsed by the SVS Endovascular Program Evaluation and Endorsement Committee (EV-PEEC) offered by Vascular Centers such as Arizona Heart Institute, Baylor College, Cleveland Clinic Foundation etc to train graduates of vascular fellowship programs in endovascular treatment.

2. Accompanying the British residency training reform, the Vascular Society and the British Society of Interventional Radiology (BSIR) are scheduling a new joint programme that aims to enhance the cooperation between both disciplines and achieve a closer working relationship. The curriculum will be common for both specialties leading to better management of open or endovascular treatment. The proposed training programme will be divided into an initial co-operative two years post-foundation training (foundation = first two years of specialty training). Entrants should have either a radiological or surgical NTN. These two co-operative years will emphasize on imaging, interventional radiology, emergency and elective surgery. Following examination, that will lead to MRCS (Member of the Royal College of Surgeons) or FRCR (Fellow of the Royal College of Radiologists) the trainee (vascular surgeon or radiologist) follows 4 more years of core and advanced training in his specialty.

3. At the University of Milan, Italy, Giorgio Basi's team initiated a University certified Master in Endovascular Techniques (MET), open to vascular surgeons, interventional cardiologists and radiologists who have completed their CCST. It is an one-year training programme adjusted to the background and the needs of each trainee specialist. A vascular surgeon will spend 6 months in interventional radiology and 6 months in interventional cardiology and correspondingly the programme is revised for the cardiologist or the radiologist. The outcome brings out the "Endovascular Specialist". This new specialtist will have the competence to treat all vascular areas, including the coronaries.

Subsequently, all kinds of training and curriculum reform shorten the distance between surgeons and radiologists. Building bridges between these previously distinct specialties seems to be a sensible "political" and "scientific" decision. By these reforms, closer liaisons will be established and the combined knowledge and skills acquired will result in improved patient care and clinical outcomes. We are still in the start-point and there is a long way to go up to when uniform established training curriculums apply equally to all vascular specialists.

Vascular centers

The pressing need for vascular centers seems to be more important than ever. The expansion of vascular diseases along with the broadening of the vascular field in imaging and endovascular technology requires a setting for global vascular prevention, diagnosis and treatment. Integrated databases and research permit rapid accumulation of a large amount of data on new, cutting-edge endovascular therapy, an apparent advantage in today's rapidly changing technology

The experience with the Mayo Clinic Gonda Vascular Center, the Gonda Center at UCLA and the recent European efforts to set up multidisciplinary vascular centers throughout Europe suggest that multidisciplinary vascular centers can be beneficial for the patients and the stakeholders alike.[16]

Vascular centers can guarantee:

- Integrated training of endovascular specialists, integrated vascular conferences.
- Integrated clinical practice based on common credentialing and re-credentialing guidelines, and common quality control.
- Integrated research, common database.
- Integrated hospital service.

Endovascular simulators

Simulation can provide an excellent opportunity for training in procedures and management of potential complications. Although it does not replace clinical training, it does offer a means for mentored instruction in a more realistic way.

Currently available endovascular procedure simulators are useful educational tools to train the trainees. Incorporating skills training on computer-based learning modules and simulated cases can make a resident or fellow better prepared for "live" clinical cases. Studies from other surgical disciplines suggest that training in a skills laboratory reduces errors in actual practice.

Simulators modeling endovascular procedures are now commercially available (e.g AngioMentor, EndoVascular AccuTouch Simulator, Procedius VIST and SimSuite), while the preliminary publications[17,18] appear promising to facilitate a smooth transition from traditional vascular surgery to interventional technology.

REFERENCES

1. Pearce WH, Parker MA, Feinglass J, Ujiki M, Manheim LM. The importance of surgeon volume and training in outcomes for vascular surgical procedures. Eur J Vasc Endovasc Surg 1999;29:768-778.
2. Tu JV, Austin PC, Johnston KW. The influence of surgical specialty training on the outcome of elective abdominal aortic aneurysm surgery. J Vasc Surg 2001;33:447-452.
3. Gloviczki P. Vascular and endovascular surgeon: The vascular specialist for the 21st century and beyond. J Vasc Surg 2006;43(2):412-421.
4. Veith FJ. Presidential address Charles Darwin and vascular surgery. J Vasc Surg 1997;25:8-18.
5. Benedetti-Valentini F, Liapis CD. Vascular surgery: independence and identity as a monospecialty in Europe. Eur J Vasc Endovasc Surg. 2006 Jul;32(1):1-2.
6. Liapis CD, Paaske WP. Training in vascular surgery in Europe - the impact of endovascular therapy. Eur J Vasc Endovasc Surg 2002;23:1-2.
7. Buth J, Harris PL, Maurer PC, Nachbur B, van Urk H. Harmonization of vascular surgical training in Europe. A task for the European Board of Vascular Surgery (EBVS). Cardiovasc Surg 2000;8:98-103.
8. D Bergqvist. The European Board of Surgery Qualification in Vascular Surgery. In:Status of Vascular Surgery in Europe. Eds C Liapis, F Benedetti-Valentini, J Wolfe, M Horrocks, M Lepantalo.Elsevier International Congress Series 1272, p46-51, 2004.
9. C Liapis, B Nachbur. EBSQ-Vasc Examinations - Which Way to the Future? Eur J of Vasc and Endovasc Surg 2001;21(5):473-474.
10. Svetlikov AV, Nyheim T, Aksoy M. European Association of Vascular Surgeons in Training (EAVST). In Liapis D, Paaske W, eds. Status of Vascular Surgery in Europe. International Congress Series 1272, 2004, pp 76-94.
11. B Nachbur. The need for exit examinations for vascular surgeons in the various European countries. In: Status of Vascular Surgery in Europe. Eds C Liapis, F Benedetti-Valentini, J Wolfe, M Horrocks, M Lepantalo.Elsevier International Congress Series 1272, p72-75 2004.
12. Available in internet at URL:http://www.abvs.org.
13. Choi ET, Wyble CW, Rubin BG, Sanchez LA, Thomson RW, Flye MW, Sicard GA. Evolution of vascular fellowship training in the new era of endovascular techniques. J Vasc Surg 2001;33:S106-S110.
14. Cronenwett JL. Vascular surgery training in the United States, 1994 to 2003. J Vasc Surg 2004; 40:660-669.
15. Messina LM, Schneider DB, Chuter TAM, Reilly LM, Kerlan RK, LaBerge JM, Wilson MW, Ring EJ, Gordon RL. Integrated Fellowship in Vascular Sur-

gery and Intervention Radiology. A New Paradigm in Vascular Training. Ann Surg. 2002;236(4):408-415.

16. Duprez D, Allegra C, Bauersachs R, Belch J, Boccalon H, Hoffmann U, et al. Vascular centers in Europe. Results of a panel discussion at the 14th Meeting of the European Chapter of the International Union of Angiology (Cologne, Germany, May 25, 2001). Int Angiol 2002;21:96-98.

17. Dawson DL, Meyer J, Lee ES, Pevec WC. Training with simulation improves residents' endovascular procedure skills. J Vasc Surg 2007;45:149-54.

18. Chaer RA, DeRubertis BG, LinSC, Bush HL, Karwowski JK, Birk D, Morrissey NJ, Faries PL, McKinsey JF, Kent KC. Simulation improves resident performance in catheter-based intervention. Ann Surg 2006;244:343-352.

Nursing training in the new era of advanced endovascular techniques

Theofanis Fotis, Evangelos Konstantinou, Denise Giachetta-Ryan, Efthimios Avgerinos, Dimitrios Filippou, Theodosios P. Perdikides

INTRODUCTION

In the 21st century, there have been many new and exciting advances in medicine and surgery. The pace of these changes has been very rapid. The development of new technologies was accompanied by changes in the regulatory, economic aspects of medical care and in the planning and construction of minimally invasive operating suites. In the field of vascular surgery and particularly in aortic aneurysm repair, endovascular techniques, incorporating sophisticated endografts (e.g. fenestrated and branched) are becoming more widespread and are now available for diseases previously inoperable or requiring extensive surgery.[1,2] Designing and manpowering of modern vascular centers has created a need for reform in all aspects of vascular services, workforce and infrastructure, in order to provide comprehensive care, improve outcomes, coordinate care and standardize services as a center of excellence.

In accordance with all these developments, a change in the role of nursing has been necessary. Nursing has branched into a multidisciplinary service in which individuals or groups can perfect their areas of expertise. Perioperative Nursing in particular, encompasses the behavioral and technical components of professional nursing, in a flexible and diverse manner.[3] Perioperative nurses use their technical abilities to use surgical equipment and instruments while exercising sound judgment and problem-solving skills to ensure that each patient experiences a safe and effective surgical procedure.[4]

Vascular surgery is a complex technical area and theatre personnel need to be specially trained in the use of specialist instruments, prosthetics and techniques. The role of the vascular nurse within this model is instrumental in ensuring that these goals are met. Specialized, dedicated vascular nursing has to meet the challenge presented through progress and modern developments in vascular surgery.[5]

CURENT STATUS OF NURSING TRAINING

Currently endovascular techniques have revolutionized the elective treatment of abdominal aortic aneurysm (AAA). As such, traditional open treatment of AAA is currently scarce in institutions with endovascular equipment availability. Vascular surgeons and OR nurses are exposed in less open repair procedures than in the past.

The training of vascular surgeons is currently reevaluated; consequently, there is a great need for the development of a relevant training program for the nurses that will collaborate with endovascular surgeons in the modern endovascular setting.[8]

New graduates, while also experienced nurses who choose perioperative nursing need comprehensive training due to the specialized nature of the OR.[4] How will perioperative nurses be trained when nursing schools offer limited perioperative experience? Health care agencies must provide the necessary and proper training for perioperative nurses. Orientation programs are expensive, time-consuming, and use human resources. A high turnover of newly trained nurses wastes time and money.[4] It is very time-consuming to train inexperienced nurses to provide safety, quality and competent care in the OR. It can take as long as six months to train a novice nurse to practice independently in the perioperative arena. The costs of recruitment and retention are significant,[6] especially when we have to prepare a multiskilled nurse with skills in intraoperative procedure, emergency surgery, catheter and guide wire handlings.[7] The preparation of such a multiskilled nurse, a key member of the endosurgical team, should be the target of a vascular center performing basic and advanced (with fenestrated and branched grafts) endovascular procedures.

The framework and a detailed proposition of such program are discussed below.

THE TRAINING PROGRAM FRAMEWORK

The skill set required to perform such advanced interventions has not been included as significant component of general surgical education. Indeed, such skills have traditionally been the core compe-tencies for other specialties, namely interventional radiologists and cardiologists. The central importance of vascular surgeons integrating this skill set into their practice has been codified by the Association of Program Directors in Vascular Surgery.[9,10] Similarly nurses who participate in this kind of highly specialized surgical teams should obtain the same kind of knowledge in order to perform with high standards.

Today the traditional model of apprenticeship, based on "learning-by-doing", has been challenged, and clinical experience will have to be supplemented or replaced by workshops and simulators using virtual reality software in a non-clinical environment.[9,11] Simulations offer the possibility of reducing the learning curve and enabling the trainee to gain both cognitive and technical knowledge in a safe environment away from the patient. There is a number of simulation techniques available today, that can be used by educators, such as rating scales, checklists, bench models, motion analysis, endovascular simulators, and operating theatre environment simulators.[12-17]

SUGESSTED TRAINING PROGRAM

Learning objectives must be specific to the content and to the outcome behaviors expected in the clinical setting.[18] Objectives provide guidelines for the nature and purpose of the educational activity.[19] For that reason the development of a training manual for new workers that will contain these goals could be helpful.

The program must have at least 6 months duration at a surgical center of excellence in advanced endovascular techniques, with a large volume of cases, both EVAR and Open and it should be both in classroom and laboratory-OR settings.

The course will provide OR staff with

the information and training necessary to perform as an integral member of an endovascular support team. Didactic instruction, case review, and procedural observation will be conducted by the physicians and nurses of the faculty.

The subjects that could be taught will include vascular anatomy, radiation safety, radiographic equipment, operating room set-up, vascular access and positioning, endovascular equipment, complications and trouble shooting, procedure observation, and circulating-scrubbing for endovascular procedures.

The curriculum should be based on the standards of the Association of Perioperative Nurses (AORN). The 24 weeks of the educational program will be offered in 2 hour sessions of didactic lecture each week, focusing on concepts of perioperative nursing utilizing the nursing process. Topics that will be included encompass anesthesia, principles of sterilization, patient positioning, scrubbing, gowning, gloving, and aseptic technique.[20] The nurse will learn how to implement the plan of care during the intraoperative phase and will thoroughly discuss responsibilities for documentation and medico-legal requirements for perioperative nurses. The areas that will also emphasized during the class and in laboratory settings will include performing a surgical time out, verifying the correct surgical site, conducting surgical counts, processing specimens properly, retaining evidence, and ensuring security of patients who are of interest to law enforcement officials.[6]

Postoperative evaluation is also important to determine the effectiveness of the care provided, so the trainers will discuss the concept of "do no harm". The training will also focus on the care required for a patient with multiple traumas, urgent and emergent procedures, care of hemodynamically unstable patients, and participation in the care of a patient receiving moderate sedation.[6]

During the last 18 weeks the trainee will participate as an observer at the beginning, and then as a scrubbed nurse along with the trainer. The trainee will begin with small vascular peripheral procedures, followed by open repair of AAA. After that scrubbing for straight endovascular procedures with special focus on wire and catheter handling will follow. Finally, scrubbing for advanced endovascular procedures with fenestrated and branched grafts will complete the training program.

Especially for the radiation safety, nurse educators should take into account that legislation in most countries requires that individuals who take responsibilities for medical exposure must be properly trained in Radiation Protection. However, a training system and formal accreditation is still lacking in many countries. The International Commission on Radiological Protection (ICRP), states that interventional procedures are complex and demanding and tend to be operator dependent. It is particularly important that individuals performing the procedure are adequately trained both in clinical techniques and knowledge of radiation protection. Basic training and continuing training in radiation protection should be an integral part of OR nursing education for those practicing interventional procedures. This includes understanding the basic elements of X-ray imaging, the biological effects of radiation and the elements of patient and staff radiation safety.[21]

The training material could be provided as textbook which includes the conceptual framework, standards, and principles of perioperative practice, and it is a resource for information that learners can use for self-study. A textbook could provide perioperative nursing considerations with the nursing process as a framework. A book which includes general and specialty surgical interventions with detailed steps for various procedures could also be used. The book could be used as a reference for surgical instrumentation and procedures and for patient care practices and standards.[5]

CONCLUSION

It is therefore essential that OR nurses, in order to meet the challenges of the future, must be trained to hospitals with an adequate aortic and peripheral vascular workload, so that they will receive good exposure to open aortic and general vascular surgery. In addition, centers performing endovascular aortic aneurysm repairs must also ensure adequate training in basic radiological techniques in conjunction with endovascular aneurysm repair. The training in both is important if the demands of the public are to be met.[22] It is also imperative that both nursing and technical staff are continuously updated and attend education sessions on the developing technology as they progress throughout their career. Life long learning is an integral part of the responsibility of health care delivery professionals.

REFERENCES

1. V. Kozon, N. Fortner, T. He1zenbein, An empirical study of nursing in patients undergoing two different procedures for abdominal aortic aneurysm repair. J Vasc Nurs 1998;16:1-5.
2. Ziegler P, Avgerinos ED, Umscheid T, Perdikides T, Erz K, Stelter WJ. Branched iliac bifurcation: 6 years experience with endovascular preservation of internal iliac artery flow. J Vasc Surg. 2007; 46:204-10.
3. "Standards of perioperative professional performance", in Standards, Recommended Practices. and Guidelines (Denver: Association of Operating Room Nurses, Inc, 1999) 152.
4. Fraulein S. Nelson, Using Adult Learning Principles for Perioperative Orientation Programs. AORN J 1999;70:1046-1058.
5. K. R. Bruni. The role of the vascular nurse in centers of excellence. J Vasc Nurs 2002;20:2-5.
6. Thomas J. Coumey, A Look at a Successful Perioperative Nurse Extern - Intern Program. AORN J 2005;81:564-578.
7. D. Ramage, M. Lovell, G. DeRose, K. A. Harris, S. Kribs, Establishing an endovascular abdominal aortic program-decisions, decisions, decisions: The London Health Sciences Centre experience. J Vasc Nurs 2001;19:10-3.
8. Eric T. Choi, et al. Evolution of vascular fellowship training in the new era of endovascular techniques. J Vasc Surg 2001;33:106-10.
9. Pandey Va, Black Sa, Lazaris Am, Allenberg Jr, Eckstein Hh, Hagmuller Gw et al., European Vascular Workshop, Pontresina. Do workshops improved the technical skill of vascular surgical trainees? Eur J Vasc Endovasc Surg 2005;30:441-447.
10. Sternbergh C, York JW, Conners MS, Money SR. Trends in aortic aneurysm surgical training for general and vascular surgery residents in the era of endovascular abdominal aortic aneurysm repair. J Vasc Surg 2002;36:685-9.
11. Beard JD, Jolly BC, Southgate LJ, Newble DI, Thomas Eg, Rochester J. Developing assessments of surgical skills for the GMC performance procedures. Ann R Coll Surg Engl 2005;87:242-247.
12. Black SA, Pandey VA and Wolfe JHN. Training for Carotid Intervention: Preparing the Next Generation. Eur J Vasc Endovasc Surg 2007;33: 518-524.
13. Martin Ja, Regehr G, Reznick R, Macrae H, Murnaghan J, Hutchison C et al. Objective structured assessment of technical skill (OSATS) for surgical residents. Br J Surg 1997;84: 273-278.
14. Reznick R, Regehr G, Macrae H, Martin J, McCulloch W. Testing technical skill via an innovative "bench station" examination. Am J Surg 1997;173(3):226-230.
15. Datta V, Mackay S, Mandalia M, Darzi A. The use of electromagnetic motion tracking analysis to objectively measure open surgical skill in the laboratory-based model. J Am Coll Surg 2001;193: 479-485.
16. Gallagher Ag, Cates Cu. Virtual reality training for the operating room and cardiac catheterization laboratory. Lancet 2004;364:1538-1540.
17. Aggarwal R, Undre S, Moorthy K, Vincent C, Darzi A. The simulated operating theatre: comprehen-

sive training for surgical teams. Qual Saf Health Care 2004;13:27-32.

18. Schmidt, Fisher, "Effective development and utilization of selflearning modules". The Journal of Continuing Education in Nursing 1992;23:54-59.

19. Brunt, Scott, "Factors to consider in the development of selfinstructional materials". "Effective development and utilization of selflearning modules", The Journal of Continuing Education in Nursing 1992;23:87-93.

20. D. Giachetta-Ryan. Operating Room Internship Program: A collaborative project. Nurs Outlook 2007;55:111.

21. M.M. Rehani. Training of interventional cardiologists in radiation protection-the IAEA's initiatives. International Journal of Cardiology 2007;114:256-60.

22. Y.C. Chan, J.P. Morales, P.R. Taylor. Training in Aortic Surgery Requires Radical Change. Eur J Vasc Endovasc Surg 2007;33:516-517.

33. NURSING TRAINING IN THE NEW ERA OF ADVANCED ENDOVASCULAR TECHNIQUES

When interventional suite meets the operation theater in the modern Era of advanced endovascular procedures

Konstantinos Lagios, Panayiotis Goutzios, Dimitrios Matsarides, Efthimios Avgerinos, Evangelia Shina, Pinelopi Giannopoulou, Dimitrios K. Filippou, Theodossios P. Perdikides

Advances in the interventional management of vascular diseases and endovascular technology have raised the need of a more dedicated operating field for both vascular surgeons and interventional radiologists. More sophisticated imaging technology, full wire-catheter and stent (stent-graft) availability, along with anaesthesia and open surgery-ready facilities are of outmost importance for today's ideal and safe vascular intervention. Traditional distinctions between the operating and interventional imaging rooms are no longer adequate for the contemporary management of vascular diseases.[1-3]

The rapid growth of endovascular surgery has inflicted tremendous challenges to the conventional operating room (OR). The mobile equipment carts that are essential for even the simplest and most basic endovascular procedure inevitably result in an overcrowded and cluttered operating environment with poor ergonomic configuration. The OR turnover time is prolonged and the efficiency reduced. The entangled cables, tubing and wiring also pose significant problems to the safety of both patients and OR staff. These issues can be solved by the emergence of new operating suites with a design that comprehends new technologies on OR construction and functioning,[4] or by incorporating OR facilities in modern interventional suites. The future endovascular suite should improve patient care and operating room efficiencies by improving patient flow and patient comfort, reducing turnover time, improving productivity and enhancing anesthesia efficiency.[5]

One year ago, out of the need to update our workspace, the Department of Interventional Radiology officially inaugurated an Interventional Suite for all kinds of interventional procedures. The suite integrates a dedicated catheterization laboratory imaging system with upgraded surgical facilities. This chapter deals with the planning, construction and equipment of the renovated interventional suite in 251 Hellenic Air Force General Hospital, part of which represents the modern and standards of an endovascular suite.

HISTORICAL BACKGROUND

In August 1992 a Siemens Angiostar D33 was installed for usage by both the Interventional Radiology and the Cardiology Catheterisation Laboratory departments of our hospital. At that time, the Interventional Radiology Department staff consisted of one certified interventional radiologist and later on one more came. These two interventional radiologists performed all kind of interventional procedures. During the same years vascular surgeons had a gradual interventional activity, mainly on aortic aneurysms, which were all performed in the operating theater with a mobile C-arm (Philips, Palsera). Interventional nurses and technicians were also available. Collaboration between the two departments, mainly in aortic aneurysms, irrespective of room (interventional ward or operating theater) performed, was always available.

Since July 2002, a serious effort to replace the old interventional suite, with a modern one, begun. The plan was to expand the list of the interventional procedures that were taking place in our hospital (interventions that require higher quality of imaging and capabilities such as 3D visualization of vessels in CNS procedures, vertebroplasties, percutaneous punctures, biopsies and drainages of solid or cavernous lesions, endoleak embolisations after aortic aneurysm repair and other body interventions) and create surgery and anaesthesia facilities for complex cases (e.g. hybrid interventions in patients with abdominal or thoracoabdominal aortic aneurysms). The medical staff of the department started a training fellowship program abroad in 2003 which was completed in 2007.

In July 2007 the old Siemens-Angiostar angiographic machine was replaced with Siemens biplane unit (Axiom Artis dBA). For the proper installation of the latter unit, all the internal walls of the old Interventional Department had to be demolished and under a new planning it was rebuilt in a more functional and pleasant way, utilizing the experience gained during the last 15 years from Greek and foreign hospitals and their interventional suites. The reconstruction of the Interventional Radiology Department and the installation of the equipment lasted 6 months. The whole project was completed in January 2008 and not until July of the same year all minor problems were solved (Figure 1). These problems had to do with the integrity and functionality of the equipment and the interventional rooms.

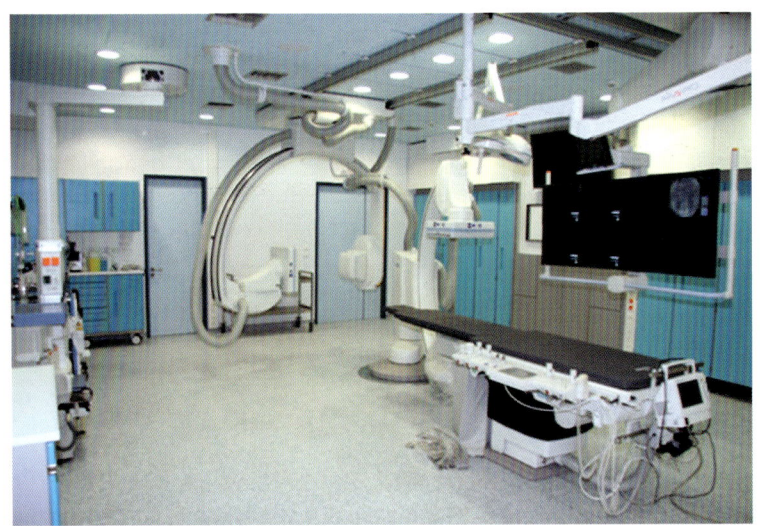

FIGURE 1: The new interventional radiology department.

ROOM CONSTRUCTION

A 200m² surface (7 x 30 m with a North-South direction) had to be utilized in the best possible way (Figure 2). For the angiographic room 60m2 were utilized (Figure 3). Next and in direct communication with it there is the technical room (where all the equipment used for the function of the angiographic suite was placed), the control room, a stockroom and a patient recovery room. More distally, there is the secretary's desk, offices with workstations, examination room, changing rooms, two bathrooms, a housekeeper's room and a recreation room for the staff. The north and south side of the department have no windows. Two side doors for stuff entrance and one in the middle for the patients' entrance are available in the east wall. The west side consists of large windows starting one meter above the floor. They are double glassed with UV protection membranes. Electrically powered moved rolltops, ensure the complete obscuring of light in the rooms, when needed (angiography room, ultrasound examination room). The internal walls were constructed of plasterboard with insulating material in the intermediate leaves (unfortunately bad in terms of soundproofing). Hanging of heavy utilities (lead aprons) was done only after proper

wall enforcement. One of its major advantages is that it allows secondary interventions to be done easier. Also, in conjunction with the furred ceiling, it permits easier passing of power and data cables and wires, even after the completion of masonry.

CENTRAL ANGIOGRAPHY ROOM

In the central main room, where the angiographic unit was installed, the required lead armoring was placed between the plasterboard layers and the surrounding doors. In a total area of 7 x 30 m the central hall was designed to have a length of 8.44 x 7.00 m, in a way to be fully exploited by the biplane system but also to allow sufficient space for the development and the functionality of all the auxiliary equipment available, while for open surgical interventions. The AXIOM Artis dBA unit is located on the longitudinal axis of the hall from north to south. When the second ceiling C-arm is in parking position, the distance from the northern wall is 1.70 m allowing the staff to move unhindered. The minor distance of the top of the angiographic table from the southern wall is 1.15 m. In this way equipment and personnel can move easily around the angiographic unit. Rotating the table by 30°

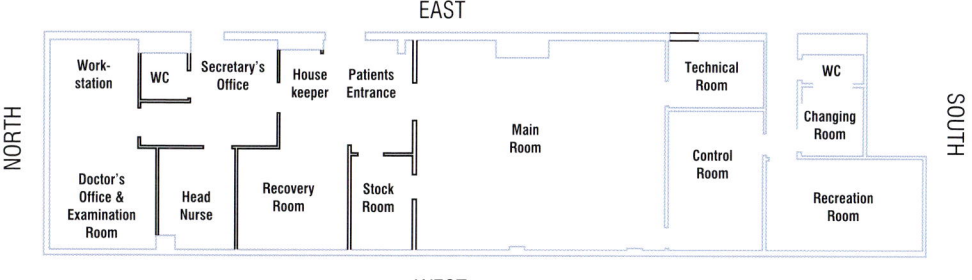

FIGURE 2: The ground plan of the new interventional radiology department.

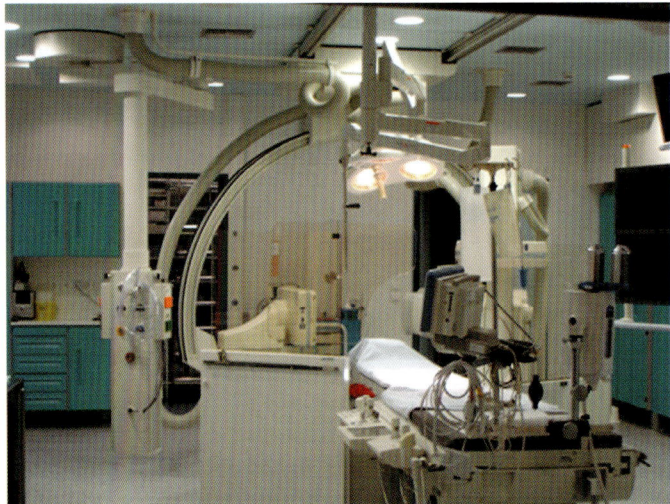

FIGURE 3: A view of the angiography room.

we can have more free space and longer table extensions can be used. Moreover, this rotated configuration allows the anaesthetic machine to be used not only in the main position, but also beside the table foot (south), when required. In the southern wall there is a vertical gas column providing O_2, N_2O, low air pressure, high air pressure, suction, negative pressure and gas removal. In the northern wall there is the entrance of the patients to the main room and a smaller door which brings in communication the main room with the stockroom. West to the smaller door there is a nursing station (45 cm deep and 1.50 m wide). Between the main door and the smaller one there is a free space of 2 m where an emergency unit is positioned (90 cm wide and 53 cm deep). On the same wall there is a vertical column providing auxiliary O_2, N_2O, low air pressure suction, power supply and network connections at its lower part. On the south side of the main room there are the technical and control rooms. The lead covered glass permits the visual contact between the angiography (main) and the control room. Its dimensions are 180 x 100 cm.

Over the eastern wall, where there are no windows, drawers are placed all the way along the 8.44 m creating a total storage space of 6 m in length and 67 cm in depth. This can be used for storing of therapeutic and diagnostic catheters, guide wires, balloons, etc. most of which are hanged from telescopic mechanisms. These are 18 in number and each of them has 7 slots for 10 catheters each. There is an overall ability to store 1260 catheter in a wardrobe 3 m in length. Thus, the storage and retrieval processes of the appropriate catheters or balloons are simple and fast. We covered the wardrobes with opaque doors instead of glass as to be easier to clean. In that way the room becomes uniform and pleasant to both the patient and the staff (Figure 4).

In the middle of the eastern wall a 2.10m free space was left for the placement of a 4″ monitor. This is positioned in an ergonomic height, as to be easy for the interventional radiologist to watch the monitor's screen, while he is standing by the angiographic table. A plain film reading lightscreen is placed 15 cm below the aforementioned monitor. A special cabinet, 20 cm deep, is constructed under-

FIGURE 4: The eastern wall. Plenty of storage, the 46″ TFT screen and the flat light-screen.

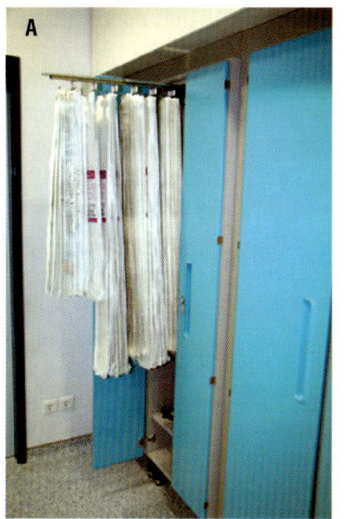
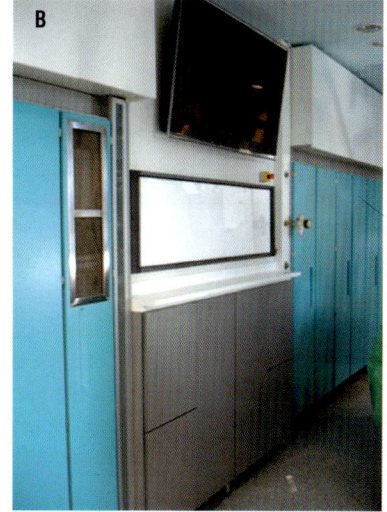

neath and various accessories for supporting the hands and the head of the patient are stored in it. There is also a vertical column providing medical gases similar to that of the southern wall.

On the West wall with windows starting above the 101 cm, there are:
- A wall stand 50 cm long, for the rest of the radioprotection lead when they are not in use.

- An additional air-condition 122 cm long.
- 2 floor cupboards on wheels (94 cm wide, 47 cm deep, 94 cm high) for the storage of the sterile, dressing angiography sets. These 2 cupboards have tops made of corian material.
- The anaesthetic machine with all its parts (85 cm wide, 66 cm deep) (Figure 5B)
- The ceiling anaesthetic column (Figure 5A)

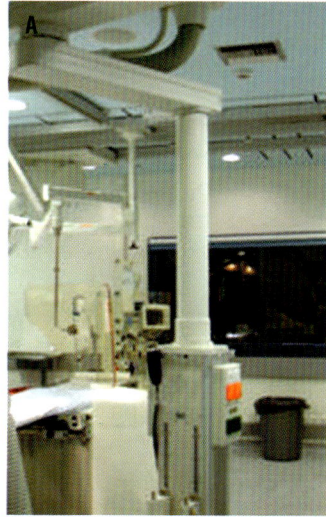
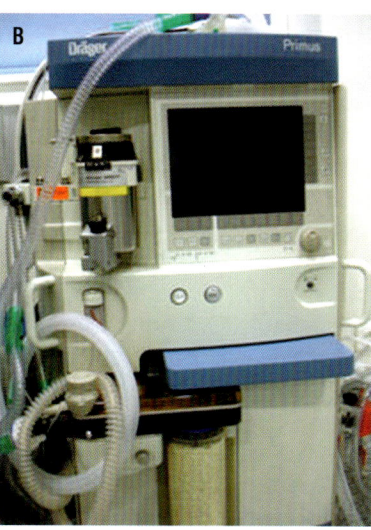

FIGURE 5: The anaesthetic machine and the ceiling anaesthetic column.

- Anaesthetist's cupboard unit (85 cm wide, 66 cm deep)

The furred ceiling is made of plasterboard which ends to the unistrats for holding the Siemens AXIOM Artis dBA. The unistrats' grooves were sealed with special rubber straps that prevented any dust transition from the furred ceiling into the main angiography room. The ceiling was painted in light blue (cerulean) color as to be pleasant for the lying patient and make him/her feel more comfortable.

The ceiling hanging equipment is:
- Ceiling C-arm of Siemens AXIOM Artis Dba
- Monitor's unit (9 monitors in total)
- Surgical lights
- Radioprotection lead-glass

The hanging articulated column for the medical gases and the electric power supply which can lift and move the anaesthetic machine in the most comfortable position for the anaesthetist and the radiologist, depending on the procedure. The middle point of this column is 145 cm away from the west wall. The ceiling dimmer, fluorocent lights are built in the furred ceiling. The intercom and the sound speakers are also built in the ceiling as well as the cables, the medical gases supply and the air circulating tubes. Four ceiling openings allow the access within the hidden roof for inspections or when needed. The main angiographic room floor is covered with a special electric conductible material which is easy to be cleaned and disinfected. Underneath there are electric suppliance and data cables for the connection between the workstations and the main Siemens AXIOM Artis dBA console. So, the floor is free of cables and wires and the staff's move is unblocked. The clear height between the floor and the ceiling is 290 cm. The walls are painted in hepoxidic white color.

The electric power moved supplied

rolltops produce a light free environment and are very practical because they permit the preparation of the patient to be done in a natural light environment with the view of the hospital yard's trees, before darking the room. The main room looks bigger and wider during the preparation and also after the end of the procedure, which acts beneficially in the personnels' and patients' mood. After the room darkness, the environment is suitable for all the angiographic procedures and the ultrasound or intravascular ultrasound diagnostic examinations. The grey scale imaging is very important for both the diagnostic and the interventional procedures and is best achieved when we have a complete darkness room.

In the main as well as in the recovery rooms the air is recycled 12 times per hour and is also filtered and air-conditioned.

Main room's equipment

The heart of the interventional suite is the new, contemporary Siemens AXIOM Artis dBA unit. It has two flat panel detectors with the ability to screen in two planes (biplane system) and a CT (dynaCT) and 3D imaging hardware and software. All the functions can be controlled via a touch screen panel with the control unit attached to the patient's bed.

There are 8 monitors TFT-LCD for the image projection, the road-maps, the reference images and the processed 3D images all in two planes (4 x 2). The ninth monitor shows the parameters of both C-arms and the table's position, during the examination.

The unit's table can rotate left and right for 30°, lean left and right and also move in the trendelenburg and anti-trendelenburg position.

The rest of the equipment consists of:
- 1 contemporary power injector whose

control panel is firmly positioned on the wall and it's injection unit on the patient's table. All the cables and wires are underneath the floor:

- 1 ultrasound unit with 2 linear and 1 convex probes for vessels, superficial and deep organs examinations
- 1 intravascular ultrasound unit.
- 1 monitor for monitoring the patient's vitals.
- 1 defibrilator.
- 1 anaesthetic unit.
- Surgical lighting units.
- ACT (Active Clotting Time) measurement machine.
- Platelets' function counting machine (Verify now).
- Patient's transfer beds, etc.

In the main room a 46″ TFT screen displays CT or MRI images of the patient, during his/her angio examination. The plain film reading lightscreen is a thin (2.5 cm), modern high frequency - high temperature one. There are also two lead covered panels for the personnel protection during the examination. All areas around the main room are self lighted and air-conditioned (Table 1).

AUXILIARY ROOMS

The technical room (2.25 x 3.25 m) is in direct communication with the main room and contains 5 cupboards with all the electronic and electrical circuits for the Siemens AXIOM Artis dBA unit function. It has independent air condition and additional cupboards for the storage of the service and operating books as well as the circumferential parts. All the units, the air-conditioners and the electric power supplies are connected on a UPS for continuous and stable electrical supply.

The control room (4.65 x 3.35 m) (Figure 6) is positioned south of the main room and contains the Siemens AXIOM

Artis dBA main control unit for the processing and storaging of the produced images. It also contains the first workstation (syngo workplace) for the production and process of the 3D and dynaCT images. There are also a dry Laser camera and a Xerox colored laser printer. There is also a pc with a 24″ monitor and a plain film reading lightscreen. In the control room there is an internet connection of the Angiography unit for remote service and ports for connection with HIS-RIS networks.

The stockroom is north to the main room and is connected with it through a small door for quicker transfer of all the expendable equipment during the procedures. It has independent air-condition and contains a drug refrigerator and a thermal chamber.

The scrub area is positioned next to the main room and north to it.

The recovery room (3.81 x 3.35 m) receptions the patients after the procedures in the main room and they are monitored there. There is capacity for 2 patients and can be also used for ultrasound guided procedures (biopsies, drainages, RF ablations, Laser ablations). It can supply O_2, low air pressure and suction to both of the patients simultaneously and is also equipped with a surgical light unit.

In the rest of the rooms, the offices and the secretary's office there are additional cupboards and ergonomically designed top desks for a pleasant work time.

The doctor's office (Figure 7) is a special room with dimensions 7 x 3.5 m and the second workstation syngo X-work place is placed in it. There is also a workstation for other exams such as US, CT, MRI, one pc connected with the internet, two plain film reading lightscreens and a projector for the multidisciplinary meetings. There is also an examination bed for the clinical and US examinations of the patients, primarily or during their follow

TABLE 1

EQUIPMENT AVAILABLE IN OUR INTERVENTIONAL SUITE

Device	Manufacturer
Imaging angio system	Siemens Axiom Artis dBA
Workstations	Leonardo Syngo X Workplace
Contract Injector	Medrad Mark V
Patient Monitor	Drager Infinity Gamma
Patient Monitor	Datex-Ohmeda S/5
Defibrillator/Monitor	Lifepak 20
Ultrasound	Siemens Accuson Antares
Intravascular Ultrasound	Jomed Invision Gold
Active Coagulation Time (ACT) measurement device	Hemochron-Signature+
Device of Platelets' function counting machine	Verify now
Surgical light ceiling mounted	Mavic Portegra 2 (3 lights)
Surgical light ceiling mounted	Drager Sola Ceiling Fixed
Surgical light mobile	Drager Sola 500 mobil
Drug refrigerator	Fiocchetti
Warmer	Rexmed
Anaesthesia machine	Drager Primus
Radiation protection leadglass cart	Mavic Gamma shapped 0,5 mmPb
Radiation protection leadglass cart	Europrotex 0,5 mm Pb
ECG machine	Nihon Kohden-cardiofax
Film Printing Camera	Agfa Drystar 5300
Ceiling mounted column (with ability to carry the anaesthesia machine)	Ondascope 400 single variant
Patient Warming System	Nellcor Warmtouch
Silicone rest pads	EE, Clinicum
Suction unit	Medi-Vac Flex Advantage
Laser colour Printers	Xerox Phazer 8560
Angio Room Exam Projection System	Multirama Pc connected to a 47 inch Sony Monitor
Patient transfer bed	Promotel Midmark
Instrument tray	
Film reading flat lightscreen	Medicanvas
Storage Wardrobes	Favero
Emergency cart	Favero
Examination bed	Quest, Promotel Midmark
Projector	Epson EMPTW200
Computers	

up. There is one recreation room and a small kitchen for the personnel to relax and have some coffee, beverage or lunch, during the working day (Figure 8).

CONCLUSIONS

The presented interventional suite covers the full range of interventional procedures:

FIGURE 6: The control room.

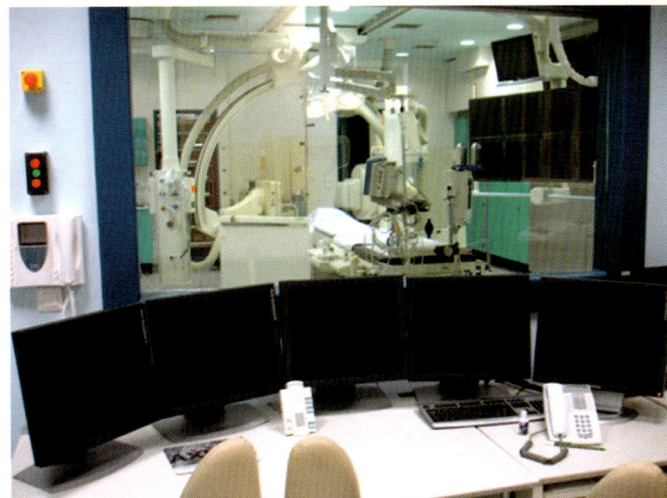

CNS tumor embolizations, embolization of cerebral aneurysms and arteriovenous malformations, percutaneous biliary interventions, brochial artery embolizations, postoperational and traumatic bleeding embolizations and all kinds of endovascular procedures. An endovascular suite can be definitely part of modern interventional suites with upgraded surgical facilities.

Summaring, modern endovascular suites should be large enough in order to accommodate movement of patient and staff and storage of equipment. Installed ceiling with strengthened mounting plates and suspended pendants and floors must be designed for plenty of weight-bearing for new equipment such as Biplane x-ray machines and articulated arms to hold video equipment, monitors, anesthesia ventilators and other devices that are common in new ORs. A top-quality angiographic unit is the cornerstone of a state-of-the-art vascular suite. The ceiling-mounted LCD monitors with easy angle adjustment joints allow comfortable and clear views for the interventionalists, surgeons, assistants and nurses and helps to improve operation efficiency.[1-8]

In our experience, all rooms, areas and the equipment should be validated and

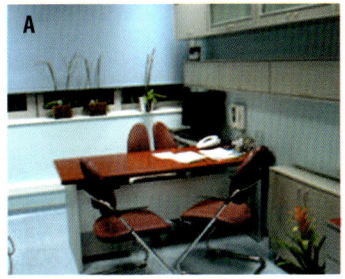 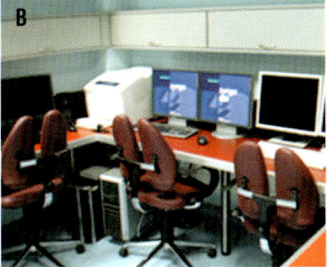 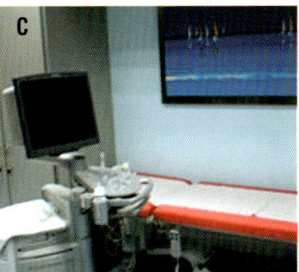

FIGURE 7: Details from the doctors' office.

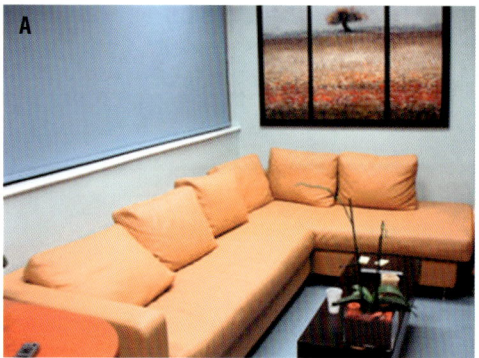
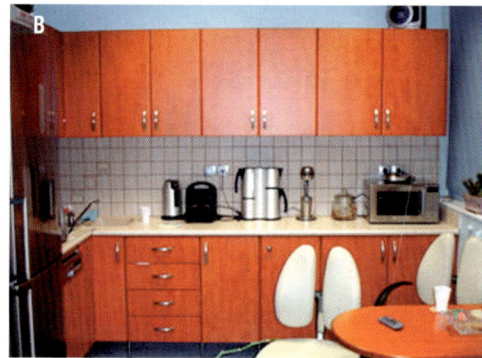

FIGURE 8: Personnel rest area and the kitchen.

tested for 6 months on a regular basis, so that better quality and higher standard services can be provided to our patients.

We hope that this chapter will be very helpful to all our colleagues who are interested in the planning and organization of a contemporary interventional suite.

REFERENCES

1. Greene J. Lines blurring between OR, imaging. OR Manager 2005;3:1-3.
2. Benjamin ME. Building a Modern Endovascular Suite. Endovascular Today March 2008:71-78.
3. Peeters P, Verbist J, Deloose K, Bosiers M. The catheterization lab of the future. Endovascular Today March 2008:94-96.
4. Greene J. Nurses instrumental in design of new outpatient center. OR Manager 2004;9:1-2.
5. Berger J. OR of Future speeds patient throughput. OR Manager 2004;6:1-4.
6. Yau KK, Chung CC, Cheuk-Hoo Wong J, Ka-Wah Li M. Minimally invasive operating suite in the 21st century: Endo-Lap operating room. Surgical Practice 2006;10:87-93.
7. Guidelines for Design and Construction of Health Care Facilities. OR Manager 2006;8:1-2.
8. Mourikis D, Hatziioannou A. Vascular and Interventional Radiology, "Vita" Publications, Athens.

Index